Global Perspectives in Ocular Oncology

Bhavna V. Chawla • Mary E. Aronow
Editors

Global Perspectives in Ocular Oncology

Springer

Editors
Bhavna V. Chawla
Ocular Oncology Service
Rajendra Prasad Centre for Ophthalmic Sciences
All India Institute of Medical Sciences
New Delhi, India

Mary E. Aronow
Retina Service
Massachusetts Eye and Ear
Harvard Medical School
Boston, MA, USA

ISBN 978-3-031-08249-8 ISBN 978-3-031-08250-4 (eBook)
https://doi.org/10.1007/978-3-031-08250-4

This Springer imprint is published by the registered company Springer Nature Switzerland AG
The registered company address is: Gewerbestrasse 11, 6330 Cham, Switzerland

Lovingly dedicated to
our children
Rhea (Bhavna) and Jack (Mary)
for teaching us the most important lessons in life.
You mean the world to us.

Foreword

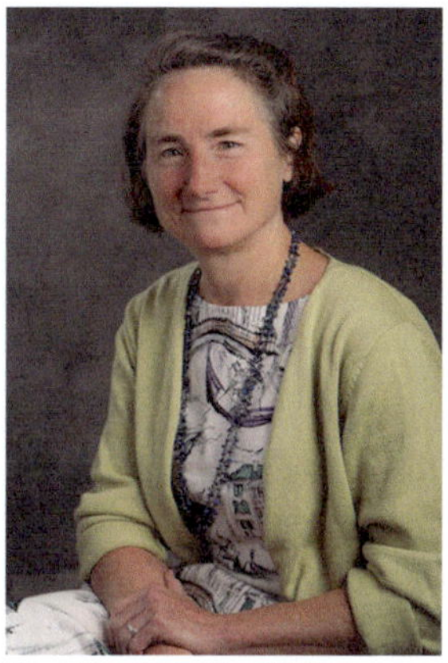
Carol L. Shields, M.D.

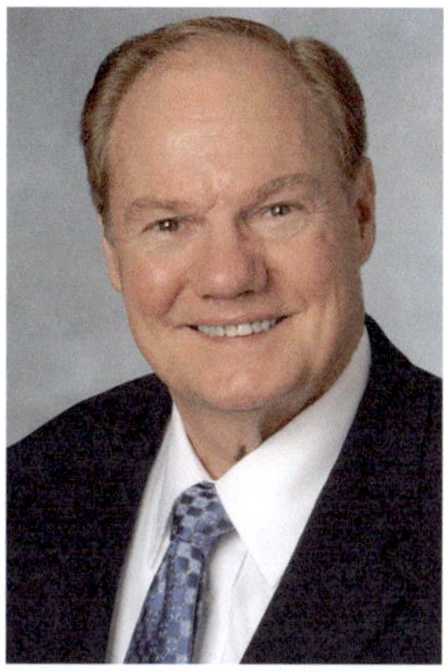
Jerry A. Shields, M.D.

Ocular oncology is an important and challenging subspecialty, involving management of patients with eye tumors and potential eye cancers that can lead to blindness and death. An online survey, sponsored by the Research to Prevent Blindness and conducted by Research!America, a non-profit health research organization, on 2044 persons asked a specific question, "What medical condition is the ***worst*** possible that could happen to you?" [1]. This study found the biggest fear included blindness (20%), cancer (18%), Alzheimer's dementia (18%), AIDS/HIV (8%), loss of limb (4%), heart disease (3%), arthritis (2%), and deafness (2%). The fear of blindness and cancer were profound, as they are related to loss of independence, inability to drive safely, and appearing sick and vulnerable.

This puts it in perspective! In this world, the top two medical concerns include fear of blindness and cancer. And as ocular oncologists, we deal with both, every day.

In this book, *Global Perspectives in Ocular Oncology*, the editors, Drs. Chawla and Aronow, have staged a tremendous journey through the turbulent and tamed pathways of various eye cancers. The book opens with an overview on the topic of *The Power of Collaboration*, setting the stage for the magnitude of this book, especially with somewhat rare tumors.

Specific topics by experts in the field focused on global retinoblastoma numbers and outcomes are described in the chapter entitled *Worldwide Analysis: The Global Presentation of Retinoblastoma* and major clinical trials for retinoblastoma are reviewed in the chapter *Children's Oncology Group Trials in Retinoblastoma*. However, there is still room for new centers and the challenge of development of subspecialty care in other countries is illustrated with chapters *Building a Retinoblastoma Service in China*, *Retinoblastoma, The African Context*, and *The Brazilian Experience: The Retinoblastoma Awareness Campaign*. The topic of retinoblastoma is amply discussed, from genomics, to chemotherapy methods, to local hurdles in establishing and maintaining treatment programs.

Further topics wander into the daunting field of uveal melanoma with the chapter entitled *The MOLES Acronym and Scoring System for Estimating Likelihood of Malignancy in Melanocytic Choroidal Tumors*, a practical method to identify uveal melanoma at an early point, *Application of Deep Learning Models in the Evaluation of Histopathology of Uveal Melanoma,* an elegant look at the future of artificial intelligence in this field, and a new therapy for uveal melanoma in *Novel Therapies for Choroidal Melanoma*. Finally, this book addresses a big topic in the field of ocular oncology and that is the American IRIS® Registry database in the chapter entitled *Big Data: The IRIS® Registry for Ocular Oncology*.

This book covers Ocular Oncology in a comprehensive and fully educational fashion. Additional considerations are presented on diagnosis and management of ocular surface squamous neoplasia, conjunctival melanoma, the serious condition of vitreoretinal lymphoma, and periocular and orbital neoplasms. The final chapters focus on reflections from seasoned members in our field in the topics *Creating a Science Project: Advice from Personal Experience* and *Ocular Oncology Practice during the COVID-19 Pandemic*. And, to complete this book, an enticing chapter, guaranteed to be loaded with good advice, is listed as *Pearls from a Mentor and Legend in Ophthalmic Pathology and Oncology*, likely to share wisdom from one of our senior-most leaders.

The World Health Organization (WHO) has studied many aspects of global eye health, emphasizing the importance of vision beyond 2020 [2]. They underscored that improved eye health can lead to reduction of poverty, improvement in work productivity, and benefits to general health and mental health. Eye health is essential to the overall market of human health care.

In summary, *Global Perspectives in Ocular Oncology* is a bountiful cornucopia of various topics on eye cancers that can affect both eye and systemic health. Orchestrated by leaders in the field of ocular oncology, Drs. Chawla and Aronow have recruited expert authors from around the world to provide a top-notch overview on the landscape of ocular oncology. Together we work to reduce the global impact of ocular cancers and blindness.

References

1. Scott AW, Bressler NM, Ffolkes S, et al. Public Attitudes about eye and vision health. JAMA Ophthalmol. 2016;134:1111–18.
2. Burton MJ, Ramke J, Marques AP, et al. The Lancet Global Health Commission of Global Eye Health: vision beyond 2020. Lancet Glob Health. 2021;9:E489–E551.

Ocular Oncology Service
Wills Eye Hospital, Thomas Jefferson University
Philadelphia, PA, USA

Carol L. Shields, M.D.
Jerry A. Shields, M.D.

Preface

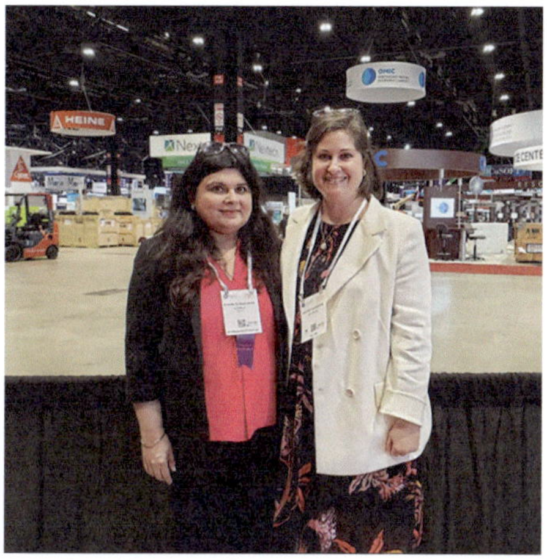

Technology is at the intersection of nearly every aspect of medical practice: from treatment innovation, to genetic discovery, to the creation and exchange of information through the electronic health record. This tide of advances has moved our society into an era of *evidence-based medicine*. The data supporting medical decision-making, and the strength of these associations, drive medical practice towards the goal of delivering high-quality and cost-effective care.

In parallel to the evidence base, and equally instrumental in the art and science of medicine, is the *experience base*. This is the knowledge that lives *within* individuals, that is passed on through generations of mentors, and that is cultivated through the course of our work. This finer knowledge is not subject to statistical rigor. Rather, these are lessons garnered through professional journeys, in the pursuit of excellence in patient care.

A lot can happen over coffee. At a recent Academy meeting, we enjoyed sharing coffee and conversation. With a common passion for ocular oncology, the most natural conversation evolved around the art and science of managing eye cancers. We were struck by the similarities in the practice of ocular oncology between two opposite parts of the world, India and the United States; and yet, there were stark differences. Thus, the idea of creating a "global perspective" was born.

This endeavor comes with the recognition that within our complex and challenging subspecialty, two principles dominate. The first is that the *experience base* is fundamental to our practice. The conditions that we treat are frequently orphan diseases. Taken together, they comprise the rich field of ocular oncology. Large data pools rarely exist, and our current knowledge is the direct result of our own experience, and that of others. The second principle is that the *global nature* of these conditions uniquely informs our *experience base*. The management of retinoblastoma is a prime example. Developed countries have perfected the techniques for local delivery of chemotherapy to the eye, whereas colleagues practising in the developing world have improved survival by pioneering the management of advanced forms of the disease. This book calls on the expertise of luminaries from around the world. Rather than serving as a pure textbook, these chapters present unique *perspectives* that bring the *experience base* from different parts of the globe to readers everywhere.

An important lesson that our subspecialty has taught us is TEAM work: *Together, Everyone Achieves More*. This book is a tribute to the "multidisciplinary" effort that is critical to the practice of ocular oncology. We owe much gratitude to our esteemed colleagues, for it is they who have been our teachers and our inspiration. We hope that readers will enjoy these *perspectives* every bit as much as we have celebrated the collaboration of bringing this book to life.

New Delhi, India Bhavna V. Chawla
Boston, MA, USA Mary E. Aronow

Acknowledgments

This book would not have been possible without the support of many. We are deeply grateful to our spouses, Arunish (Bhavna) and Roger (Mary), for unconditionally supporting our careers and celebrating our achievements. We thank our parents, Naina and Bhushan (Bhavna), and Barbara and Michael (Mary), for raising us with open minds and encouraging us to pursue our dreams. To the entire staff at Springer - Josephine Fabiola, Michelle Tam, Jeffrey Taub, ArulRonika Pathinathan, Asja Rehse - thank you for guiding us on this path and helping us bring the project to life. And finally, we wish to acknowledge our patients who have shared their journeys with us and given us the great honor to continually learn.

With much gratitude,
Bhavna and Mary

Contents

Contributors

Ghada AlBayyat Department of Ophthalmology, Bascom Palmer Eye Institute, University of Miami, Miami, FL, USA

Osmel P. Alvarez Department of Ophthalmology, Bascom Palmer Eye Institute, University of Miami, Miami, FL, USA

Nagham Al-Zubidi Department of Head and Neck Surgery, MD Anderson Cancer, Houston, TX, USA

Mary E. Aronow Retina Service, Massachusetts Eye and Ear, Harvard Medical School, Boston, MA, USA

Matteo Barchitta Department Medicine, Surgery and Neurosciences, Ophthalmology Unit, Siena, Italy

Rubens N. Belfort Department of Ophthalmology, Universidade Federal de São Paulo/Escola Paulista de Medicina (UNIFESP - EPM) and Instituto da Visão (IPEPO), São Paulo, SP, Brazil

Jesse L. Berry USC Roski Eye Institute, Keck School of Medicine of the University of Southern California, Los Angeles, CA, USA

The Vision Center at Children's Hospital Los Angeles, Los Angeles, CA, USA

Norris Comprehensive Cancer Center, Keck School of Medicine, University of Southern California, Los Angeles, CA, USA

The Saban Research Institute, Children's Hospital Los Angeles, Los Angeles, CA, USA

Eugenio Bertelli Department of Molecular and Developmental Medicine, University of Siena, Siena, Italy

Vera M. Beyuo Eye Department, Korle Bu Teaching Hospital, Accra, Greater Accra, Ghana

Sandra Bracco Clinical Department of Neurological and Human Movement Sciences, Interventional Neuroradiology Unit, Hospital S. Maria alle Scotte, Siena, Italy

Rachel C. Brennan Department of Oncology, St. Jude Children's Research Hospital, Memphis, TN, USA

Emily Chang Eye Plastic, Orbital and Facial Cosmetic Surgery, Kellogg Eye Center, University of Michigan, Ann Arbor, MI, USA

Ocular Oncology, Kellogg Eye Center, University of Michigan, Ann Arbor, MI, USA

Bhavna V. Chawla Ocular Oncology Service, Rajendra Prasad Centre for Ophthalmic Sciences, All India Institute of Medical Sciences, New Delhi, India

Yen-Lin E. Chen Department of Radiation Oncology, Massachusetts General Hospital, Harvard Medical School, Boston, MA, USA

Murali M. Chintagumpala Retinoblastoma Center of Houston, Texas Children's Cancer Center, Baylor College of Medicine, Houston, TX, USA

Zelia M. Correa Department of Ophthalmology, Retina Service, Ocular Oncology Program, Bascom Palmer Eye Institute, University of Miami, Miami, FL, USA

Sarah E. Coupland George Holt Chair of Pathology, Liverpool, UK

Department of Molecular and Clinical Cancer Medicine, Institute of Systems, Molecular and Integrative Biology, University of Liverpool, Liverpool, UK

Bertil E. Damato Nuffield Laboratory of Ophthalmology, University of Oxford, Oxford, UK

Ocular Oncology Service, Moorfields Eye Hospital, London, UK

Department of Ocular Oncology, Royal Liverpool University Hospital, Liverpool, UK

Department of Molecular and Clinical Cancer Medicine, Institute of Systems, Molecular and Integrative Biology, University of Liverpool, Liverpool, UK

University of California, San Francisco, CA, USA

Hakan Demirci Eye Plastic, Orbital and Facial Cosmetic Surgery, Kellogg Eye Center, University of Michigan, Ann Arbor, MI, USA

Ocular Oncology, Kellogg Eye Center, University of Michigan, Ann Arbor, MI, USA

Helen Dimaras Ophthalmology & Vision Sciences, The Hospital for Sick Children and University of Toronto, Toronto, ON, Canada

Antonio Eleuteri Department of Medical Physics and Clinical Engineering, Liverpool University Hospitals NHS Foundation Trust, University of Liverpool, Liverpool, UK

Department of Physics, University of Liverpool, Liverpool, UK

Doaa Elfadaly Retinoblastoma Service, Royal London Hospital, London, UK

Department of Ophthalmology, Faculty of Medicine, Minia University, Minia, Egypt

Sidnei Epelman Pediatric Oncology Department, Santa Marcelina Hospital, São Paulo, Brazil

TUCCA - Associação para Crianças e Adolescentes com Câncer, Santa Marcelina Hospital, São Paulo, Brazil

Bita Esmaeli Orbital Oncology & Ophthalmic Plastic Surgery, Department of Plastic Surgery, The University of Texas MD Anderson Cancer Center, Houston, TX, USA

Vera Adobea Essuman Ophthalmology Unit, Department of Surgery, University of Ghana Medical School, College of Health Sciences, University of Ghana, Accra, Greater Accra, Ghana

Ido Didi Fabian The Goldschleger Eye Institute, Sheba Medical Center, Tel Hashomer, Tel Aviv University, Tel Aviv, Israel

International Centre for Eye Health, London School of Hygiene & Tropical Medicine, London, UK

Aluisio Rosa Gameiro Filho Department of Ophthalmology, Universidade Federal de São Paulo/Escola Paulista de Medicina (UNIFESP - EPM) and Instituto da Visão (IPEPO), São Paulo, SP, Brazil

Paul T. Finger The Department of Ocular Tumor, Orbital Disease and Ophthalmic Radiation Therapy, The New York Eye Cancer Center, New York, NY, USA

Shahar Frenkel Ocular Oncology Service, Division of Ophthalmology, Hadassah—Hebrew University Medical Center, Jerusalem, Israel

Brenda L. Gallie Department of Ophthalmology and Vision Sciences, The Hospital for Sick Children, University of Toronto, Toronto, ON, Canada

Paolo Galluzzi Department of Neuroimaging and Neurointervention, Siena University Hospital, Siena, Italy

Anat Galor Department of Ophthalmology, Bascom Palmer Eye Institute, University of Miami, Miami, FL, USA

Department of Ophthalmology, Miami Veterans Administration Medical Center, Miami, FL, USA

Jeremy A. Goldfarb Orbital Oncology & Ophthalmic Plastic Surgery, Department of Plastic Surgery, The University of Texas MD Anderson Cancer Center, Houston, TX, USA

Dan S. Gombos Department of Head and Neck Surgery, MD Anderson Cancer, Houston, TX, USA

Marissa D. Gonzalez World Eye Cancer Hope, California, USA

Pim de Graaf Department of Radiology and Nuclear Medicine, Amsterdam UMC, Vrije Universiteit Amsterdam, Cancer Center Amsterdam, Amsterdam, The Netherlands

Evangelos S. Gragoudas Retina Service, Massachusetts Eye and Ear, Harvard Medical School, Boston, MA, USA

Theodora Hadjistilianou Department of Medicine, Surgery and Neurosciences, Ophthalmology Unit, Oncology Service, Siena, Italy

Umiya Harley Sheffield Ocular Oncology Service, Royal Hallamshire Hospital, Sheffield, UK

Steffen Heegaard Department of Pathology, Eye Pathology Section, Rigshospitalet, University of Copenhagen, Copenhagen, Denmark

Heinrich Heimann Department of Ocular Oncology, Royal Liverpool University Hospital, Liverpool, UK

Michael O. Hughes Artificial Eye Clinic, Vienna, VA, USA

Neill Hughes Artificial Eye Clinic, Vienna, VA, USA

Fabio M. Iwamoto Department of Neurology, Neuro-Oncology Division, New York Presbyterian Hospital, Columbia University, New York, NY, USA

Martine J. Jager Department of Ophthalmology, Leiden University Medical Center (LUMC), Leiden, The Netherlands

Puneet Jain Oculoplasty and Ocular Oncology Department, Eye-Q Super-Specialty Eye Hospitals, Gurgaon, India

Robin W. Jansen Department of Radiology and Nuclear Medicine, Amsterdam UMC, Vrije Universiteit Amsterdam, Cancer Center Amsterdam, Amsterdam, The Netherlands

Hayley Jones Institute of Risk Management/Institute of Systems, Molecular and Integrative Biology, University of Liverpool, Liverpool, UK

Marcus C. de Jong Department of Radiology and Nuclear Medicine, Amsterdam UMC, Vrije Universiteit Amsterdam, Cancer Center Amsterdam, Amsterdam, The Netherlands

Carol L. Karp Department of Ophthalmology, Bascom Palmer Eye Institute, University of Miami, Miami, FL, USA

Florence K. Keane Department of Radiation Oncology, Massachusetts General Hospital, Harvard Medical School, Boston, MA, USA

Ivana K. Kim Retina Service, Massachusetts Eye and Ear, Harvard Medical School, Boston, MA, USA

Jane S. Kim Eye Plastic, Orbital and Facial Cosmetic Surgery, Kellogg Eye Center, University of Michigan, Ann Arbor, MI, USA

Jonathan W. Kim Department of Ophthalmology, Kaiser Permanente, Orange County, CA, USA

Mary E. Kim USC Roski Eye Institute, Keck School of Medicine of the University of Southern California, Los Angeles, CA, USA

The Vision Center at Children's Hospital Los Angeles, Los Angeles, CA, USA

Hayyam Kiratli Ocular Oncology Service, Department of Ophthalmology, Hacettepe University School of Medicine, Ankara, Turkey

Marina K. Kirkegaard Department of Pathology, Eye Pathology Section, Rigshospitalet, University of Copenhagen, Copenhagen, Denmark

Stephanie N. Kletke Department of Ophthalmology and Vision Sciences, The Hospital for Sick Children, University of Toronto, Toronto, ON, Canada

İrem Koç Ocular Oncology Service, Department of Ophthalmology, Hacettepe University School of Medicine, Ankara, Turkey

Ilyse S. Kornblau Department of Surgical Services, Division of Ophthalmology, Veteran's Health Administration, Memphis, TN, USA

Anne Marie Lane Retina Service, Massachusetts Eye and Ear, Harvard Medical School, Boston, MA, USA

Ann M. Leahey Perelman School of Medicine at the University of Pennsylvania and the Children's Hospital of Philadelphia, Philadelphia, PA, USA

T. Y. Alvin Liu Department of Ophthalmology, Retina Service, Wilmer Eye Institute, Johns Hopkins Medicine, Baltimore, MD, USA

Shannon M. MacDonald Department of Radiation Oncology, Massachusetts General Hospital, Harvard Medical School, Boston, MA, USA

Arman Mashayekhi Ophthalmology Department, Mayo Clinic Florida, Jacksonville, FL, USA

Anam Mazharuddin Department of Ophthalmology, University of Texas Medical Branch, Galveston, TX, USA

Abdul Wajid Moothedath Division of Pediatric Oncology, Department of Pediatrics, All India Institute of Medical Sciences, New Delhi, India

Alexander Melendez Moreno Department of Ophthalmic Oncology, Cole Eye Institute, Cleveland Clinic, Cleveland, OH, USA

Timothy G. Murray Miami Ocular Oncology and Retina (MOOR), Miami, FL, USA

Lakshmi Nayak Center for Central Nervous System Lymphoma, Dana-Farber Cancer Institute, Harvard Medical School, Boston, MA, USA

Jacob Pe'er Ocular Oncology Service, Division of Ophthalmology, Hadassah—Hebrew University Medical Center, Jerusalem, Israel

Daphna Landau Prat The Goldschleger Eye Institute, Sheba Medical Center, Tel Hashomer, Tel Aviv University, Tel Aviv, Israel

M. Ashwin Reddy Retinoblastoma Service, Royal London Hospital, London, UK

Queen Mary University of London, London, UK

Duangnate Rojanaporn Department of Ophthalmology, Faculty of Medicine, Ramathibodi Hospital, Mahidol University, Bangkok, Thailand

Mandeep S. Sagoo Retinoblastoma Service, Royal London Hospital, London, UK

National Institute for Health Research Biomedical Research Centre at Moorfields Eye Hospital NHS Foundation Trust and UCL Institute of Opthalmology, London, UK

Sachin M. Salvi Sheffield Ocular Oncology Service, Royal Hallamshire Hospital, Sheffield, UK

Amy C. Schefler Retina Consultants of Texas, Retina Consultants of America, Houston, TX, USA

Blanton Eye Institute, Houston Methodist Hospital, Houston, TX, USA

Rachna Seth Division of Pediatric Oncology, Department of Pediatrics, All India Institute of Medical Sciences, New Delhi, India

Amish Shah Perelman School of Medicine at the University of Pennsylvania and the Children's Hospital of Philadelphia, Philadelphia, PA, USA

Helen A. Shih Department of Radiation Oncology, Massachusetts General Hospital, Harvard Medical School, Boston, MA, USA

Janani Singaravelu Department of Ophthalmic Oncology, Cole Eye Institute, Cleveland Clinic, Cleveland, OH, USA

Arun D. Singh Department of Ophthalmic Oncology, Cole Eye Institute, Cleveland Clinic, Cleveland, OH, USA

Nakul Singh Department of Ophthalmology, Massachusetts Eye and Ear, Boston, MA, USA

Alison H. Skalet Departments of Ophthalmology, Radiation Medicine, and Dermatology, Casey Eye Institute and Knight Cancer Institute, Oregon Health & Science University, Portland, OR, USA

Sandra E. Staffieri Department of Ophthalmology, Royal Children's Hospital, Parkville, VIC, Australia

Centre for Eye Research Australia, Royal Victorian Eye and Ear Hospital, East Melbourne, VIC, Australia

Ophthalmology, University of Melbourne Department of Surgery, Parkville, VIC, Australia

Anna M. Stagner Department of Ophthalmology, Massachusetts Eye and Ear; Department of Pathology, Massachusetts General Hospital, Boston, MA, USA

Gangadhara Sundar Orbit and Oculofacial Surgery, Ophthalmic Oncology, Department of Ophthalmology, National University Hospital, National University of Singapore, Singapore, Singapore

Azzam F. G. Taktak Department of Medical Physics and Clinical Engineering, Liverpool University Hospitals NHS Foundation Trust, University of Liverpool, Liverpool, UK

Department of Physics, University of Liverpool, Liverpool, UK

Alexei V. Trofimov Department of Radiation Oncology, Massachusetts General Hospital, Harvard Medical School, Boston, MA, USA

Ogul E. Uner Department of Ophthalmology, Casey Eye Institute, Oregon Health & Science University, OR, USA

Victor M. Villegas Department of Ophthalmology, University of Puerto Rico, San Juan, PR, USA

Bascom Palmer Eye Institute, University of Miami Miller School of Medicine, Miami, FL, USA

Department of Surgery, Ponce Health Sciences University, Ponce, PR, USA

Abby White World Eye Cancer Hope, Oxfordshire, England

Matthew W. Wilson Department of Ophthalmology, Hamilton Eye Institute, University of Tennessee Health Science Center, Memphis, TN, USA

Jacquelyn M. Wrenn Department of Ophthalmic Oncology, Cole Eye Institute, Cleveland Clinic, Cleveland, OH, USA

Honggai Yan Department of Ophthalmology, Beijing Children's Hospital, Capital Medical University, National Center for Children's Health, Beijing, China

Hannah J. Yu Retina Consultants of Texas, Retina Consultants of America, Houston, TX, USA

Carlen A. Yuen Department of Neurology, Neuro-Oncology Division, New York Presbyterian Hospital, Columbia University, New York, NY, USA

Hongrun Zhang Institute of Life Course and Medical Sciences/Institute of Systems, Molecular and Integrative Biology, University of Liverpool, Liverpool, UK

Junyang Zhao Department of Pediatric Oncology Center, Beijing Children's Hospital, Capital Medical University, National Center for Children's Health, Beijing, China

Yalin Zheng Healthcare Eye and Vision Science, Institute of Life Course and Medical Sciences, University of Liverpool, Liverpool, UK

Marcia Zondervan International Centre for Eye Health, London School of Hygiene & Tropical Medicine, London, UK

Part I

The Power of Collaboration

Working Together: Specialty Interest Groups with Global Presence

Mary E. Kim, Abby White, Marissa D. Gonzalez, and Jesse L. Berry

1 Introduction

As a small subspecialty within ophthalmology responsible for treating some of the rarest cancers, ocular oncology is a unique field. A highly specialized career choice with relatively few colleagues worldwide means that ocular oncologists must prioritize collaboration and companionship—for both our professional and personal selves, as well as for our patients. This facilitates the sharing of research discoveries, continuing education, networking, mentorship, friendship, and opportunities for improving patient care and seeking patient-guided solutions to critical problems. Fortunately, there are a plethora of conferences and societies to encourage these relationships. Herein, we highlight specialty interest groups that work with young physicians in training or shortly thereafter, empower women ocular oncologists, and unite patients, parents, and survivors, focusing on their histories, distinct goals, and global presence. We hope reading about these networks inspires your participation and reminds you that your voice as an ocular oncologist and as a patient survivor can have worldwide influence.

M. E. Kim
USC Roski Eye Institute, Keck School of Medicine of the University of Southern California, Los Angeles, CA, USA

The Vision Center at Children's Hospital Los Angeles, Los Angeles, CA, USA
e-mail: maryekim@usc.edu

A. White
World Eye Cancer Hope, Oxfordshire, England
e-mail: abby@wechope.org

M. D. Gonzalez
World Eye Cancer Hope, California, USA
e-mail: marissa@wechope.org

J. L. Berry (✉)
USC Roski Eye Institute, Keck School of Medicine of the University of Southern California, Los Angeles, CA, USA

The Vision Center at Children's Hospital Los Angeles, Los Angeles, CA, USA

Norris Comprehensive Cancer Center, Keck School of Medicine, University of Southern California, Los Angeles, CA, USA

The Saban Research Institute, Children's Hospital Los Angeles, Los Angeles, CA, USA
e-mail: jesse.berry@med.usc.edu

2 Young Physicians in Training or Early Years in Ocular Oncology

In 2019, during the biennial International Society of Ocular Oncology (ISOO) meeting, the Young Ocular Oncologists (YOOs) were founded under the leadership of Victoria Cohen, MB BChir, FRCOphth. The inaugural meeting focused on the pros and pitfalls of an ocular oncology fellowship and transitioning from training to practice with advice from senior leaders; it was met with much excitement by the YOOs (Fig. 1).

In the same year, the Young Ophthalmic Oncologists and Pathologists (YOOPers), part of the American Association of Ophthalmic Oncologists and Pathologists, were founded by the executive board with the leadership of Claudia Prospero Ponce, MD, and Jesse Berry, MD. Inspired by the Young Ophthalmologists of the American Academy of Ophthalmology, YOOPers aim to connect aspiring ophthalmic oncologists and pathologists across the globe.

Through educational programs, forums for case discussion, and professional development resources catered to young professionals' needs, YOOs and YOOPers help physicians from training and into early practice years establish their careers. Most important are the networking opportunities that encourage mentorship, clinical case review, and research collaboration. Both groups meet as part of their parent organization meetings.

If you are interested in becoming involved in either organization, please visit their websites:

YOOs: www.isoo.org

YOOPers: www.aaoop.org

B. V. Chawla, M. E. Aronow (eds.), *Global Perspectives in Ocular Oncology*, https://doi.org/10.1007/978-3-031-08250-4_1

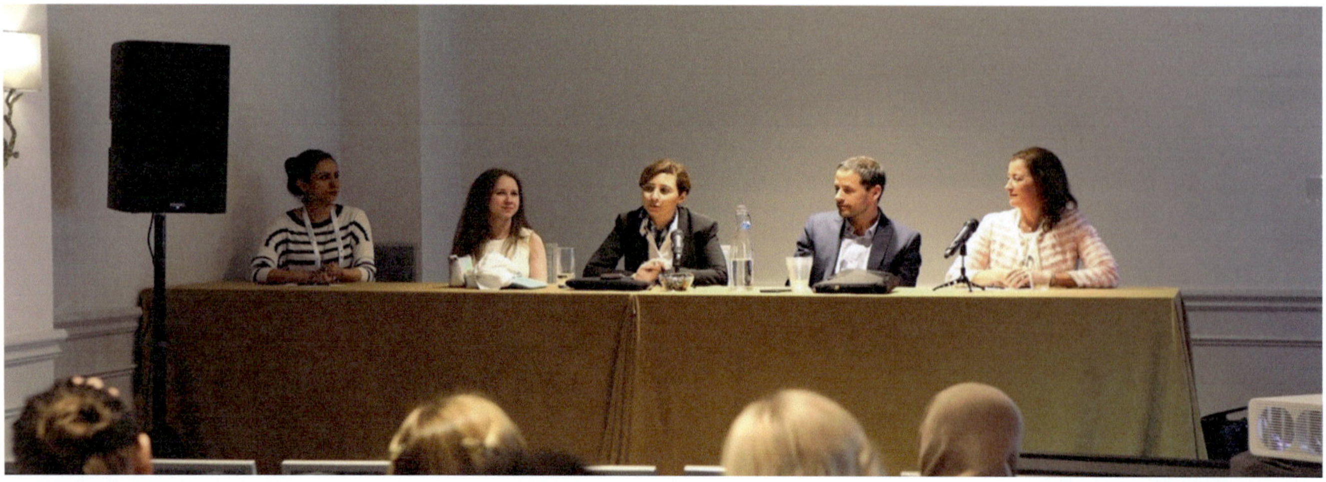

Fig. 1 The Inaugural session of the YOOs at ISOO 2019, led by Victoria Cohen. Pictured on this panel: Melina C. Morales, MD, Lauren A. Dalvin, MD, Lamis Al Harbi, MD, Ido Didi Fabian, MD, Victoria Cohen, MB BChir, FRCOphth, Chair of YOO

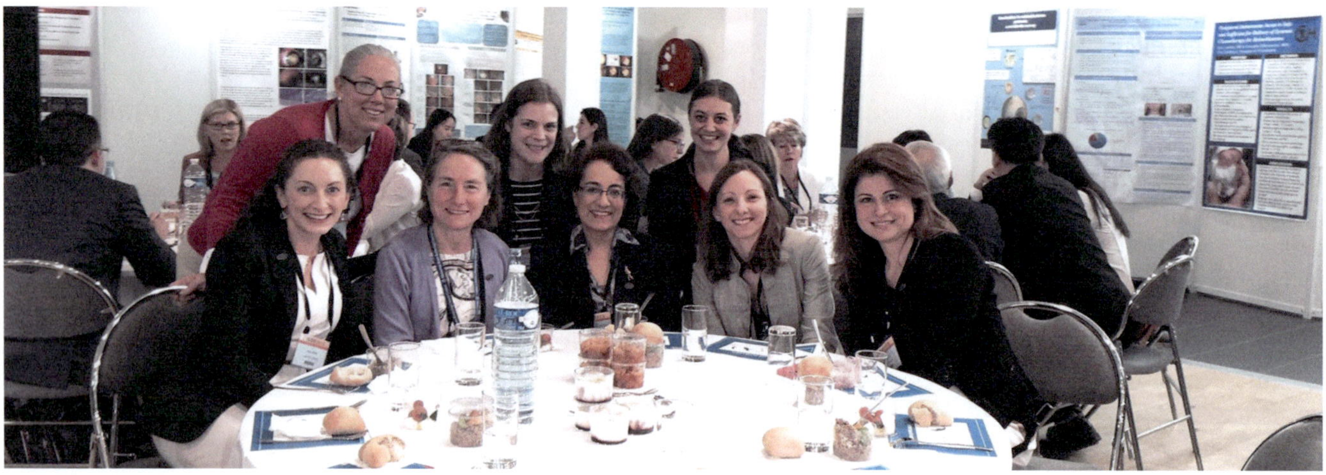

Fig. 2 The first meeting of WOO at the 2015 ISOO meeting in Paris, France

3 Women in Ocular Oncology

At the International Society of Ocular Oncology (ISOO) conference in 2013, Jesse Berry, MD, was inspired by the number of young female ocular oncologists she saw present. She thought that bringing these women together to discuss their lives in medicine and issues pertinent to women in ocular oncology might inspire mentorship and a supportive community. Joined by Zelia Correa, MD, PhD, Isabella Phan, MD, Jasmine Francis, MD, and Nahyoung Grace Lee, MD, Women in Ocular Oncology (WOO) was founded. By the 2015 ISOO meeting, WOO had a logo, Facebook page, pin, and a mission statement: "The mission of WOO is to support and promote opportunities for mentorship and growth of women in the field of ocular oncology through academic collaboration, networking and fellowship among members. Furthermore, our mission is to foster a friendly environment for women in the subspecialty while seeking opportunities for participation and representation." [1] WOO had lunch in 2015 for the first time with eight members present (Fig. 2).

At the 2017 ISOO meeting, the membership list grew to nearly 60 members, and a small symposium focused on mentorship and opportunities was held (Fig. 3).

WOO grew further in 2019, expanding beyond just women to include supporters of WOO regardless of their gender identity. Multiple events were hosted at the ISOO meeting in Los Angeles, California, including the WOO symposium entitled "Challenges in Ocular Oncology—how to spend more time doing what you love and growing your career," WOO morning yoga, and a WOO cocktail reception. A record of 141 ISOO members registered as WOO (Fig. 4).

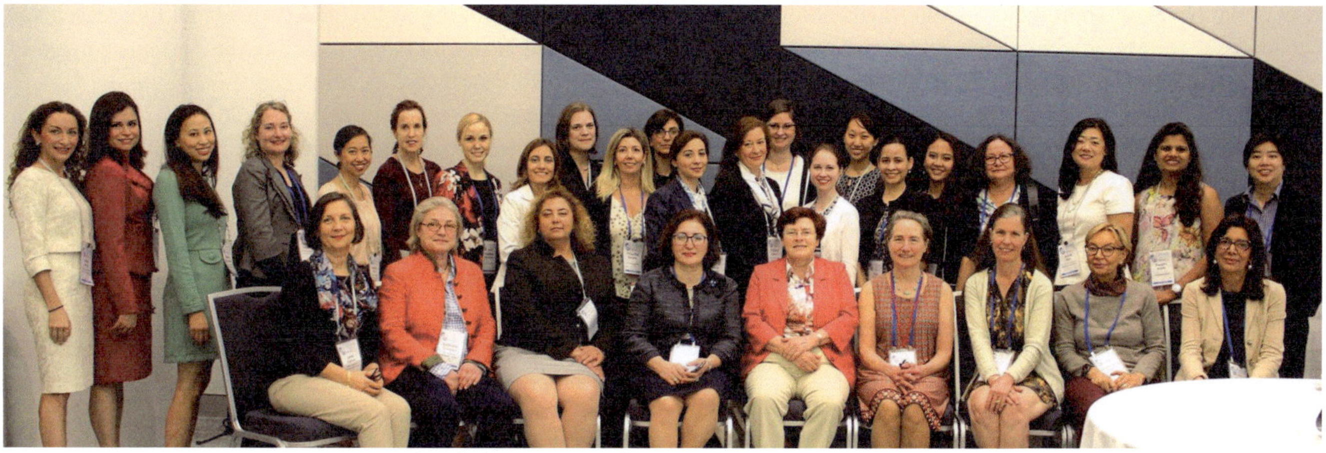

Fig. 3 The second meeting of WOO at the 2017 ISOO meeting in Sydney, Australia

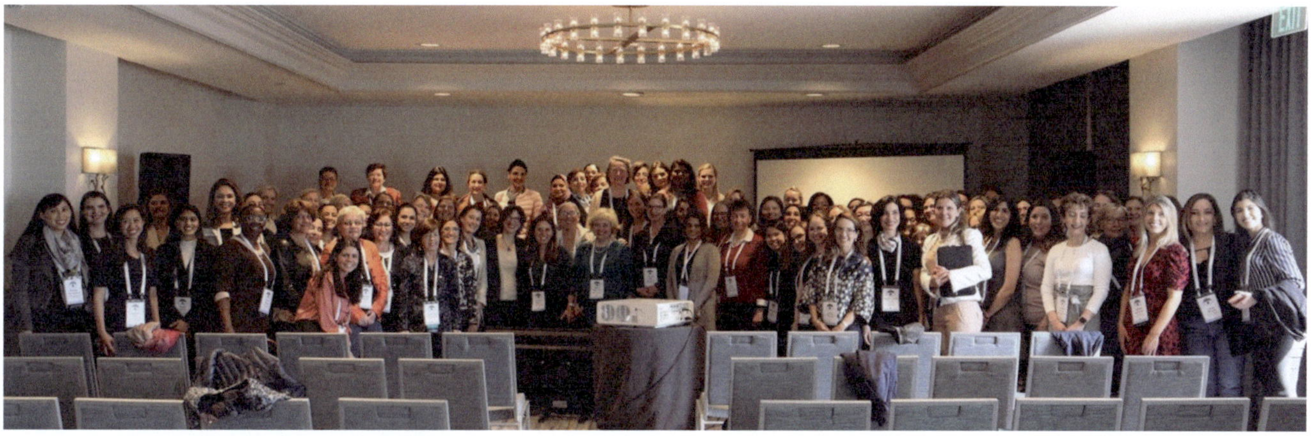

Fig. 4 The 2019 meeting of WOO: standing room only

The current leadership includes Drs. Jesse Berry (chair) and board members: Martina Angi, Bhavna Chawla, Zelia Correa, Helen Dimaras, Brenda Gallie, Doris Hadjistilianou, Martine Jager, Maria Manquez Hatta, Katherine Paton and Carol Shields. The organization looks forward to opportunities for further growth and female representation at the 2022 ISOO meeting in the Netherlands.

A particularly unique manifestation of WOO was a research study published in 2019 entitled "Trends in Radiation Practices for Female Ocular Oncologists in North America: A Collaborative Study of the International Society of Ocular Oncology." [2] Nineteen female ocular oncologists from ISOO completed a radiation exposure survey, which was created with the goal of further understanding the attitudes and consequent risk modifications of women who routinely perform radioactive plaque brachytherapy surgeries. Thankfully, similar to previously published work, results suggested that surgeons' radiation exposure during plaque brachytherapy is minimal. However, the publication highlighted concerns that female ocular oncologists have due to the potential effects of radiation on fertility and fetal health. Dedicated to WOO, the study suggests continued conversation about pregnancy guidelines and increased education to empower female ocular oncologists to best care for themselves and their patients.

If you are interested in becoming involved in WOO, as a member of ISOO, please contact woncology@gmail.com or join our Facebook group (https://www.facebook.com/groups/1431530637089637/).

4 Patient-Centered Clinical and Research Collaborations: One Retinoblastoma World—World Eye Cancer Hope

While the previous specialty interest groups are focused on ocular oncologists' personal and professional development, One Retinoblastoma World (One RB World) was inspired by our patients. One RB World is a global network with the bold idea that all children with retinoblastoma as well as survivors can have equal opportunity to access optimal care. When diagnosed early and treated effectively, childhood eye cancer is curable. No child should die or suffer avoidable blindness because of it. Many challenges prevent development of evidence-based care, particularly in developing countries, but One RB World is tearing down these obstacles.

The One RB World Conference gathers together ocular oncologists, parents, and survivors from around the world. The founding idea is that collaborative research, clinical care, and family support can only be developed through inclusive meetings that embrace a real-world focus and patient-centered experience. Empowering clinicians in developing countries, parents, and survivor advocates to take a leading role in the evolution of effective patient care will ultimately lead to improved quality of life and increased survival for all children, while reducing the burdens carried by families and health care systems.

This inclusive conference was first held in London in 2012 (Fig. 5), followed by Toronto in 2014, Dublin in 2016, Washington D.C. in 2017 (Fig. 6), and virtually in Ottawa in 2020. Each event has seen a growth in participation from medical professionals, retinoblastoma families, and survivors, growing from 62 attendees from 24 countries in 2012 to 250 attendees from 40 countries on 6 continents in 2020. This notable expansion is a testament to the importance of allowing patient advocates and survivors to exist on the same

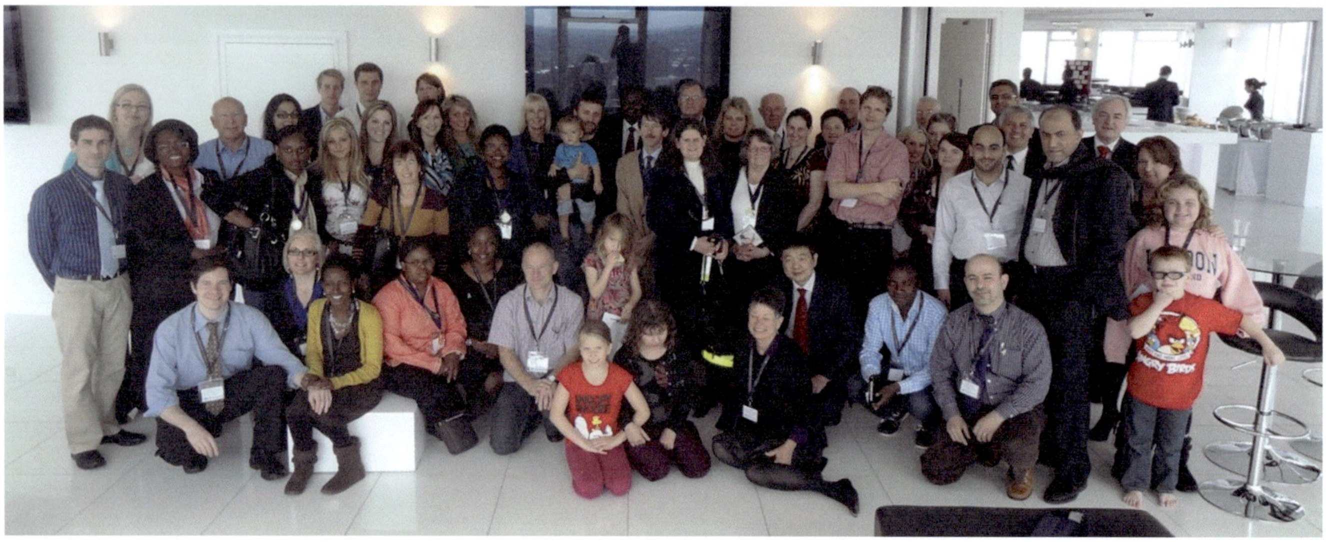

Fig. 5 The first One RB World conference was held in London in 2012

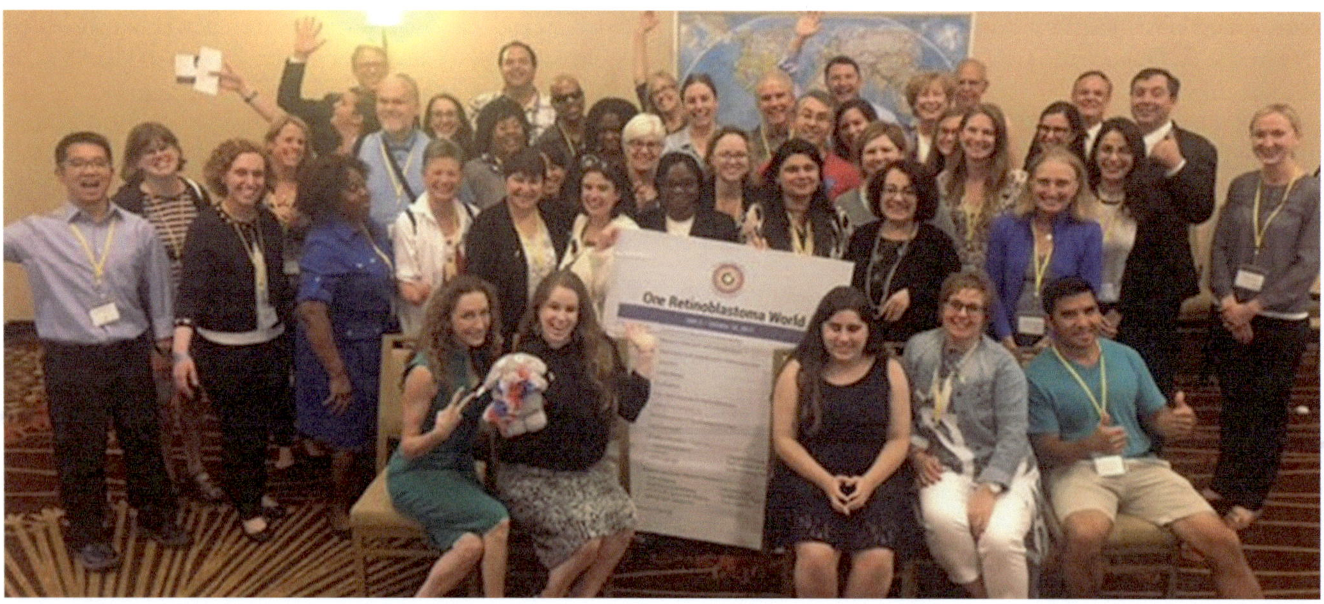

Fig. 6 The most recent in-person One RB World conference held in Washington D.C. in 2017

playing field as medical professionals. By referring to physicians by their first name and fostering a more relaxed environment, parents and survivors feel more confident and comfortable interacting with some of the top worldwide retinoblastoma specialists. Everyone is equal at One RB World, and over the years, this has proven extremely effective.

The inspiration for One RB World and World Eye Cancer Hope came from a British child with retinoblastoma treated in Toronto named Daisy. In 2004, Abby White, a bilateral retinoblastoma survivor, received an email from a mother in Botswana. Her 2-year-old daughter, Rati, had a relapse of retinoblastoma 19 months after enucleation. Doctors gave no hope of survival, and the mother asked Abby for information, advice, and prayer. Abby began advocating for Rati, and with an initial donation from Daisy's family to kick-start fundraising, she soon started treatment at the Hospital for Sick Children in Toronto. Within 1 month, Rati had no evidence of disease, and moved forward to bone marrow transplant in March 2005. Intrathecal chemotherapy continued, but the cancer relapsed in January 2006 with extensive meningeal metastasis. Rati died on August 21, 2006.

During treatment in Canada, Abby began to talk with Rati's ocular oncologist, Dr. Brenda Gallie, about the many missed opportunities to save her life in Africa: an appointment at 5 months of age during which doctors queried retinoblastoma but concluded Rati was too young to develop cancer, resulting in delays in diagnosis and enucleation; lack of adequate pathology and postoperative care; and discharge from follow-up after just one eye exam. Rati did not die due to lack of a cure, but due to lack of knowledge and health care structure to support a cure.

In November 2006, Abby and Dr. Gallie traveled to Kenya for 1 week to find out what might be possible to address some of these challenges. Abby's father was born and raised in Kenya, diagnosed with bilateral retinoblastoma in Nairobi in 1946. Abby had also worked in Kisumu on Lake Victoria between her undergraduate and postgraduate studies, including at the pediatric ward of the city's provincial hospital. Kenya seemed a good place to begin. Dr. Gallie and Abby visited a family to learn about their challenges of diagnosis, completing their child's treatment, accessing care, and receiving support from their impoverished rural community. At Nyanza Provincial Hospital in Kisumu, Dr. Gallie and Abby addressed a large community gathering—attended by medical professionals, students, surrounding district hospitals, the American Centre for Disease Control, the Aga Khan private hospital, and Siaya Eye Hospital—sharing information about early signs of retinoblastoma.

Inspired by the importance of combining the parent and professional voice, Abby began attending international meetings that included a retinoblastoma focus. They presented an opportunity to share latest treatment innovations and research developments. However, as a survivor and patient advocate and following her experience in Kenya, Abby was concerned about the accessibility of the conferences, both financially and topically, for individuals from developing countries who were therefore significantly underrepresented. Most retinoblastoma research takes place in high-income countries where the priority is saving eyes and sight. The priority for children in lower-income countries—life-saving therapy for advanced cancer—remains unaddressed. Additionally, there was a consistently low focus on psychosocial impacts and long-term survivorship aspects of retinoblastoma. Abby was dismayed to note that when these topics were included, they were frequently scheduled for the final day, when medical professionals had begun to leave, reducing engagement.

Reflecting on these concerns, Abby founded One RB World, and its first meeting took place in London in 2012. It was funded by a mix of registration fees, donations, small grants, and one significant sponsorship. A reduced registration rate was offered to all parents and survivors, and to researchers and professionals providing retinoblastoma care in low or lower-middle income countries. Sessions during this meeting explored retinoblastoma awareness, medical care, and family support with the goal of advancing effective comprehensive care for all children. Each subject was presented by one key speaker. Open floor discussion followed to foster innovative thinking and generate collaborative research solutions to advance evidence-based care. One RB World has since held four conferences, recently adding a family and child life program for patients as well as survivors. Both programs were led by World Eye Cancer Hope Child Life Director, Morgan Livingstone, and created an opportunity to see first-hand the benefits of simple child life interventions.

Due to the Coronavirus Disease-2019 (COVID-19) pandemic, the 2020 conference was held virtually and was the most widely attended yet. Attendance grew with each event, nearly doubling the countries that registered for the conference originally. With one-fifth of the world's countries represented in 2020, the international reach of One RB World and its impact has been groundbreaking for a relatively rare pediatric eye cancer.

Dr. Vera Essuman, pediatric ophthalmologist from Korle-Blu Teaching Hospital in Ghana, began attending One RB World conferences in 2017 hoping to develop a national strategy for treating retinoblastoma in Ghana. In a highly attended talk during the 2020 conference, Dr. Essuman outlined the tremendous progress she has made and attributed her success to the physicians she met through One RB World. Dr. Essuman hopes to have her national strategy in place within the next 3 years; this will be a testament to the collaboration and global impact of One RB World.

Current leadership of World Eye Cancer Hope includes Abby White (CEO), Marissa Gonzalez (Board President),

Dr. Brenda Gallie (Medical Director), Dr. Helen Dimaras (Scientific Advisor), and Morgan Livingstone (Child Life Director). The sixth One RB World conference is scheduled for October 2021 in Honolulu, Hawaii. World Eye Cancer Hope looks forward to a successful event, whether in-person, hybrid, or virtual. If you would like to attend, donate to support our mission, or contact us at: https://wechope.org/onerbworld/.

Herein, we have discussed four specialty interest groups in ocular oncology. While they have slightly varied goals, overall they aim to unite ocular oncologists, researchers, and, uniquely, patients to facilitate the care for these rare diseases. These societies inspire research, collaboration, mentorship, and education while promoting women and those early in their career. By both celebrating fellowship and encouraging continued scientific discovery, these specialty interest groups allow ocular oncologists to expand their influence beyond the clinic and operating room.

Acknowledgments The authors would like to thank everyone - patients, families, doctors - for their support and engagement in these groups. You help make the world a better place. Dr. Berry has research support not directly applicable to this work: The Berle & Lucy Adams Chair in Cancer Research National Cancer Institute of the National Institute of Health Award K08CA232344 Wright Foundation Hyundai Hope on Wheels American Cancer Society IRG-16-181-57 Knights Templar Eye Foundation Institute for Families, Inc., Children's Hospital Los Angeles Larry and Celia Moh Foundation Childhood Eye Cancer Trust Children's Cancer Research Fund Nautica Foundation Research to Prevent Blindness, an unrestricted departmental grant

References

1. Oncology, W.i.O., Women in ocular oncology newsletter, International Society of Ocular Oncology; 2019.
2. Shah SN, et al. Trends in radiation practices for female ocular oncologists in North America: a collaborative study of the international society of ocular oncology. Ocular Oncol Pathol. 2019;5(1):54–9.

Children's Oncology Group Trials in Retinoblastoma

Murali M. Chintagumpala

1 Introduction

The Retinoblastoma Committee was formed within the Children's Oncology Group (COG) in 2001. One of the main goals of this committee was to identify and study issues related to the management of retinoblastoma in a prospective manner. Many of the previous reported studies were retrospective and from single institutions and therefore not readily applicable as accepted standard of care. With only 300 new patients with retinoblastoma diagnosed every year within the United States, the formation of the Retinoblastoma Committee within the COG was considered essential to perform prospective multi-institutional studies. There were five initial protocols that were opened through COG. These protocols addressed the issues of defining histopathologic risk factors following enucleation (COG ARET 0332), using reduced therapy for group B retinoblastoma, intensified systemic chemotherapy with periocular therapy for group C and D disease, multidisciplinary therapy for metastatic retinoblastoma, and epidemiologic studies. These studies are discussed below.

2 ARET 0332

This was a study to determine the prevalence of high-risk histopathologic features (HRFs) in patients with unilateral retinoblastoma who undergo enucleation and to evaluate the role of chemotherapy in preventing recurrences [1]. Previous reports describing the histopathologic risk factors were retrospective and precise definitions were not used to define the risk factors. For example, many of the previous reports suggested that choroid invasion by retinoblastoma was either minor or major, which was a subjective measure and which could not be applied as a standard in daily practice. At the same time, there were reports that choroid invasion, whether minor or major, did not require prophylactic therapy [2–13]. A standard definition for choroid involvement was used for the first time in a prospective study (ARET 0332) within the COG. Any choroid involvement less than 3 mm did not meet the criteria for prophylactic chemotherapy whereas patients with choroid involvement equal to or larger than 3 mm in any direction were required to receive chemotherapy on the study.

Any post-laminar optic nerve involvement also required prophylactic chemotherapy on this study. However, if the tumor extended to the surgical margin of the optic nerve, the patient was not considered eligible for the study. Similarly, if the tumor involved the subarachnoid space of the optic nerve, the patient was considered ineligible. In this study, patients with a combination of any degree of optic nerve and choroid involvement were also considered eligible for the study for prophylactic chemotherapy based on previous reports [8].

Of the 331 enrolled patients in the study, 321 eligible patients had central histopathologic review. This study represents the largest prospective trial of children with unilateral retinoblastoma whose affected eyes were enucleated [1]. Central review of histopathology was required for eligibility, and timelines was observed for submission of pathology material and return of results of central review to individual institutions. Guidelines for the processing of pathology specimens and interpretation were also established. Central review prevented 22% of patients from receiving chemotherapy by changing the institutional high-risk interpretation, and in 12% of patients, central review classified them as having high-risk features and therefore were to receive chemotherapy. This study is the first to provide evidence that lack of universal guidelines for handling and interpreting retinoblastoma specimens contributes to the controversy surrounding recognition and categorizations of high-risk features and outcomes [14]. Using the criteria in this study, outcomes can be improved for children whose tumors have high-risk histopathologic features while avoiding chemotherapy for those who do not require prophylaxis. A particular subset of

M. M. Chintagumpala (✉)
Retinoblastoma Center of Houston, Texas Children's Cancer Center, Baylor College of Medicine, Houston, TX, USA
e-mail: mxchinta@texaschildrens.org

B. V. Chawla, M. E. Aronow (eds.), *Global Perspectives in Ocular Oncology*, https://doi.org/10.1007/978-3-031-08250-4_2

patients with concomitant peripapillary choroidal invasion greater than 3 mm along with post-laminar optic nerve invasion of 1.5 mm or greater emerged in the analyses of this study. This subset had the poorest outcome with the prescribed six courses of chemotherapy, suggesting that the subset of patients with these concomitant high-risk features requires more intensified therapy [1].

A previous report suggested that fewer courses of chemotherapy are sufficient for those with high-risk choroid invasion [15]. Whether chemotherapy courses can be reduced for isolated choroid invasion can be addressed in future prospective studies.

3 ARET 0331

One of the early studies within COG addressed the role of systemic chemotherapy in group B disease and to what extent two drugs carboplatin and vincristine along with local ophthalmic therapies can prevent enucleation or external beam radiation, which were considered as events [16]. The 2-year event-free survival (EFS) was 65% with 25 eligible eyes analyzed on this study. This result is inferior to reports using three drugs vincristine, etoposide, and carboplatin (VEC), but compares favorably to a similar study using carboplatin and vincristine [17]. In this study, local therapies were allowed with the second cycle of chemotherapy. The addition of etoposide with local ophthalmic therapies with every course of systemic chemotherapy can achieve the optimum results. However, this should be weighed against the low but definite risk of second malignancy with the use of etoposide, especially in a patient with heritable form of retinoblastoma. Increasingly, intra-arterial chemotherapy is being used in the management of group B retinoblastoma. Systemic chemotherapy still plays a role in children less than 3 months of age and in places where resources for intra-arterial chemotherapy are lacking.

4 ARET 0231

This a protocol that enrolled patients from 2007 to 2011. This was a single-arm prospective study to determine the proportion of failures at 12 months for eyes with group D retinoblastoma. The treatment regimen consisted of systemic chemotherapy with VEC (vincristine, etoposide, and carboplatin). Sub-Tenon carboplatin was part of the treatment regimen [18]. A total of six courses were prescribed and each course was given every 28 days and was supported by growth factor to hasten neutrophil recovery between courses. Carboplatin 20 mg was the sub-Tenon therapy and was given on day 0 or 1 of systemic courses 2–4 only. The dose of carboplatin for each of the courses was at 14 mg/kg/day for 2 days at the beginning of each course. The results of this study were based on 25 group D eyes from 20 patients. The one-year treatment failure rate was 0.52. Thirteen eyes experienced failure within 1 year and enucleation was performed in five of these patients and eight eyes received external beam radiation therapy (RT). The overall one-year eye preservation of group D eyes was 80%. All three doses of sub-Tenon carboplatin were given to 19/25 patients. Periorbital fat atrophy developed in 45% of the eyes that received sub-Tenon carboplatin. Contemporary reports during the course of this study also described periorbital toxicities and this method of increasing intraocular concentration of chemotherapy is largely abandoned [19, 20]. Increasing the systemic dose of carboplatin with concomitant sub-Tenon carboplatin resulted in a one-year failure rate of 52% for group D eyes, which was lower than the planned historical rate of 70% at the time of the study. With the advent of intra-arterial chemotherapy, the ability to increase the concentration of chemotherapy has increased substantially with lesser systemic toxicity.

One of the novel inclusions in the above two studies was a central review by a panel of ocular oncologists to confirm the stage of the disease for study enrollment. This should be a model for all future studies so that completed studies can be compared for outcomes stage by stage.

5 ARET 0321

Retinoblastoma is usually diagnosed as an intraocular tumor in high-income countries while extraocular involvement is common in low-income countries and is uniformly fatal. The staging of extraocular involvement has been described before [21]. Local and regional diseases can involve the orbit and regional lymph nodes and can still be cured. Widespread hematogenous spread and spread directly to the central nervous system indicate advanced stages and lead to a poor prognosis. Many of the reports describing the treatment and outcome of patients with extraocular disease are retrospective [22–28]. COG initiated a prospective multicenter international study and patients were enrolled between 2008 and 2014 [29]. Treatment for loco-regional disease consisted of four cycles of chemotherapy consisting of cisplatin, cyclophosphamide, etoposide, and vincristine, followed by radiation therapy to the affected areas. Patients with stages 4a and 4b disease received high-dose chemotherapy with autologous stem cell rescue after four cycles of induction therapy. In those patients who had marrow disease at study entry, bone marrow examinations were performed after every induction cycle and cells were harvested after bone marrow was rendered free of disease. The regimen for high-dose chemotherapy consisted of carboplatin, thiotepa, and etoposide. Stage 4a patients were not irradiated after complete response to induction chemotherapy or to sites measuring <5 mm after high-dose chemotherapy. RT was omitted for stage 4b patients who achieved a complete response to induction chemotherapy.

Of the 60 patients enrolled, 57 were eligible for analysis [29]. The event-free survival at 36 months was 87.7% for those with stages 2 and 3, 79.3% for patients with stage 4a disease, and 8% for those with 4b/trilateral disease. Children with disease spread to the central nervous system need more effective therapy. Subsequent studies within COG will focus on optimal delivery of radiation therapy to the central nervous system and the use of effective intrathecal agents.

6 ARET 12P1

A subsequent study within the COG was a feasibility study of intra-arterial therapy with a single agent melphalan. The purpose of this study was to study the feasibility of delivering intra-arterial therapy in a multi-institutional study given the requirement of an interventional radiologist who is experienced in delivering intra-arterial therapy in children and technique of delivering chemotherapy through the ophthalmic artery of the affected eye. This study was completed and the results are not published yet.

7 Epidemiological Studies

COG also conducted an epidemiology study AEPI05N1, which explored the relationship between carcinogen metabolism, deoxyribonucleic acid (DNA) repair, parental exposures, and retinoblastoma. This study suggested that parental hazardous occupational exposures can play a role in the development of childhood retinoblastoma. There also appeared to be preliminary evidence that mothers who consume diets higher in fruit and lower in fried foods and cured meats during pregnancy may reduce the risk of unilateral retinoblastoma in their children [30–32].

7.1 Future Studies

One of the impediments to preserving the globe of an eye with advanced disease with systemic chemotherapy alone is the presence of diffuse vitreous seeds and the barriers to achieving high intraocular concentrations of an effective anti-neoplastic agent. Increasingly, intravitreal injections have become an essential concomitant therapeutic intervention in a significant number of patients receiving intra-arterial chemotherapy [33, 34]. This has become a safe and easily administered method of significantly increasing intraocular concentrations of a chemotherapy agent. A concept for a trial within the COG to evaluate the globe salvage rate with systemic therapy and intravitreal chemotherapy was recently approved.

Prospective clinical trials in retinoblastoma are limited by the rarity of the disease and a general inability to arrive at a consensus among the multidisciplinary participants who are essential for delivery of care. There are several questions that can be answered through prospective clinical trials but may require international collaborations: What combination of drugs are most effective for intra-arterial chemotherapy? What are the indications for two drugs versus three drugs for Intra-arterial infusions? When to assess response after initiation of an intra-arterial combination of drugs? How responses and progressions are defined with intra-arterial and intravitreal chemotherapies? The toxicities associated with intra-arterial and intravitreal therapies have not been systematically studied in a prospective manner. For many of these questions, a central review panel must be established within the context of a clinical trial.

Future trials should also incorporate studies of cell-free DNA (cfDNA) from aqueous humor. Preliminary studies seem to suggest that 6p gain identified in cfDNA (cell-free DNA) obtained from aqueous humor can predict poor prognosis for globe salvage [35, 36]. A recent report also suggests that cfDNA from the blood can help in monitoring patients with retinoblastoma [37].

References

1. Chevez-Barrios P, Eagle RC Jr, Krailo M, et al. Study of unilateral retinoblastoma with and without histopathologic high-risk features and the role of adjuvant chemotherapy: a Children's oncology group study. J Clin Oncol. 2019;37:2883–91.
2. Khelfaoui F, Validire P, Auperin A, et al. Histopathologic risk factors in retinoblastoma: a retrospective study of 172 patients treated in a single institution. Cancer. 1996;77:1206–13.
3. Kopelman JE, McLean IW, Rosenberg SH. Multivariate analysis of risk factors for metastasis in retinoblastoma treated by enucleation. Ophthalmology. 1987;94:371–7.
4. Magramm I, Abramson DH, Ellsworth RM. Optic nerve involvement in retinoblastoma. Ophthalmology. 1989;96:217–22.
5. Messmer EP, Heinrich T, Hopping W, de SE, Havers W, Sauerwein W. Risk factors for metastases in patients with retinoblastoma. Ophthalmology. 1991;98:136–41.
6. Kaliki S, Shields CL, Shah SU, Eagle RC Jr, Shields JA, Leahey A. Postenucleation adjuvant chemotherapy with vincristine, etoposide, and carboplatin for the treatment of high-risk retinoblastoma. Arch Ophthalmol. 2011;129:1422–7.
7. Honavar SG, Singh AD, Shields CL, et al. Postenucleation adjuvant therapy in high-risk retinoblastoma. Arch Ophthalmol. 2002;120:923–31.
8. Shields CL, Shields JA, Baez KA, Cater J, De Potter PV. Choroidal invasion of retinoblastoma: metastatic potential and clinical risk factors. Br J Ophthalmol. 1993;77:544–8.
9. Shields CL, Shields JA, Baez K, Cater JR, De PP. Optic nerve invasion of retinoblastoma. Metastatic potential and clinical risk factors. Cancer. 1994;73:692–8.
10. Uusitalo MS, Van Quill KR, Scott IU, Matthay KK, Murray TG, O'Brien JM. Evaluation of chemoprophylaxis in patients with unilateral retinoblastoma with high-risk features on histopathologic examination. Arch Ophthalmol. 2001;119:41–8.

11. Chantada GL, Dunkel IJ, de Davila MT, Abramson DH. Retinoblastoma patients with high risk ocular pathological features: who needs adjuvant therapy? Br J Ophthalmol. 2004;88:1069–73.
12. Chantada GL, Casco F, Fandino AC, et al. Outcome of patients with retinoblastoma and postlaminar optic nerve invasion. Ophthalmology. 2007;114:2083–9.
13. Chantada GL, Fandino AC, Guitter MR, et al. Results of a prospective study for the treatment of unilateral retinoblastoma. Pediatr Blood Cancer. 2010;55:60–6.
14. Sastre X, Chantada GL, Doz F, et al. Proceedings of the consensus meetings from the international retinoblastoma staging working group on the pathology guidelines for the examination of enucleated eyes and evaluation of prognostic risk factors in retinoblastoma. Arch Pathol Lab Med. 2009;133:1199–202.
15. Aerts I, Sastre-Garau X, Savignoni A, et al. Results of a multicenter prospective study on the postoperative treatment of unilateral retinoblastoma after primary enucleation. J Clin Oncol. 2013;31:1458–63.
16. Friedman DL, Krailo M, Villaluna D, et al. Systemic neoadjuvant chemotherapy for group B intraocular retinoblastoma (ARET0331): a report from the Children's Oncology Group. Pediatr Blood Cancer. 2017;64
17. Rodriguez-Galindo C, Wilson MW, Haik BG, et al. Treatment of intraocular retinoblastoma with vincristine and carboplatin. J Clin Oncol. 2003;21:2019–25.
18. Jubran RF, Villablanca JG, Krailo M, et al. A single-arm study of systemic and sub-Tenon chemotherapy for Groups C and D intraocular retinoblastoma: a Children's Oncology Group study (ARET 0231). Pediatr Blood Cancer. 2020;67:e28502.
19. Mulvihill A, Budning A, Jay V, et al. Ocular motility changes after subtenon carboplatin chemotherapy for retinoblastoma. Arch Ophthalmol. 2003;121:1120–4.
20. Marr BP, Dunkel IJ, Linker A, Abramson DH. Periocular carboplatin for retinoblastoma: long-term report (12 years) on efficacy and toxicity. Br J Ophthalmol. 2012;96:881–3.
21. Chantada G, Doz F, Antoneli CB, et al. A proposal for an international retinoblastoma staging system. Pediatr Blood Cancer. 2006;47:801–5.
22. Matsubara H, Makimoto A, Higa T, et al. A multidisciplinary treatment strategy that includes high-dose chemotherapy for metastatic retinoblastoma without CNS involvement. Bone Marrow Transplant. 2005;35:763–6.
23. Namouni F, Doz F, Tanguy ML, et al. High-dose chemotherapy with carboplatin, etoposide and cyclophosphamide followed by a haematopoietic stem cell rescue in patients with high-risk retinoblastoma: a SFOP and SFGM study. Eur J Cancer. 1997;33:2368–75.
24. Kremens B, Wieland R, Reinhard H, et al. High-dose chemotherapy with autologous stem cell rescue in children with retinoblastoma. Bone Marrow Transplant. 2003;31:281–4.
25. Dunkel IJ, Chan HS, Jubran R, et al. High-dose chemotherapy with autologous hematopoietic stem cell rescue for stage 4B retinoblastoma. Pediatr Blood Cancer. 2010;55:149–52.
26. Dunkel IJ, Khakoo Y, Kernan NA, et al. Intensive multimodality therapy for patients with stage 4a metastatic retinoblastoma. Pediatr Blood Cancer. 2010;55:55–9.
27. Rodriguez-Galindo C, Wilson MW, Haik BG, et al. Treatment of metastatic retinoblastoma. Ophthalmology. 2003;110:1237–40.
28. Doz F, Khelfaoui F, Mosseri V, et al. The role of chemotherapy in orbital involvement of retinoblastoma. The experience of a single institution with 33 patients. Cancer. 1994;74:722–32.
29. Dunkel IJ, Krailo M, Chantada G et al. Intensive multi-modality therapy for extra-ocular retinoblastoma (RB): A Children's Oncology Group (COG) trial (ARET0321). [abstract]. American Society of Clinical Oncology Annual Meeting; 2017.
30. Omidakhsh N, Bunin GR, Ganguly A, et al. Parental occupational exposures and the risk of childhood sporadic retinoblastoma: a report from the Children's Oncology Group. Occup Environ Med. 2018;75:205–11.
31. Omidakhsh N, Ganguly A, Bunin GR, von Ehrenstein OS, Ritz B, Heck JE. Residential pesticide exposures in pregnancy and the risk of sporadic retinoblastoma: a report from the Children's Oncology Group. Am J Ophthalmol. 2017;176:166–73.
32. Lombardi C, Ganguly A, Bunin GR, et al. Maternal diet during pregnancy and unilateral retinoblastoma. Cancer Causes Control. 2015;26:387–97.
33. Abramson DH, Daniels AB, Marr BP, et al. Intra-arterial chemotherapy (ophthalmic artery chemosurgery) for group D retinoblastoma. PLoS One. 2016;11:e0146582.
34. Berry JL, Shah S, Bechtold M, Zolfaghari E, Jubran R, Kim JW. Long-term outcomes of Group D retinoblastoma eyes during the intravitreal melphalan era. Pediatr Blood Cancer. 2017;64
35. Berry JL, Xu L, Kooi I, et al. Genomic cfDNA analysis of aqueous humor in retinoblastoma predicts eye salvage: the surrogate tumor biopsy for retinoblastoma. Mol Cancer Res. 2018;16:1701–12.
36. Berry JL, Xu L, Murphree AL, et al. Potential of aqueous humor as a surrogate tumor biopsy for retinoblastoma. JAMA Ophthalmol. 2017;135:1221–30.
37. Abramson DH, Mandelker D, Francis JH, et al. Retrospective evaluation of somatic alterations in cell-free DNA from blood in retinoblastoma [abstract]. Am J Ophthalmol. 2021;

Worldwide Analysis: The Global Presentation of Retinoblastoma

Daphna Landau Prat, Marcia Zondervan, and Ido Didi Fabian

1 Introduction

Retinoblastoma is the most common intraocular malignancy of childhood, with an average incidence ranging from 1:15,000 to 1:20,000 livebirths [1] and, overall, approximately 8000 new cases globally per annum [2]. Retinoblastoma is initiated by either a germline or somatic mutation in the *RB1* tumor suppressor gene, located on the long arm of chromosome 13 (13q14). The malignancy can be inherited by an affected family member or develop sporadically, and may involve one or both eyes. Rarely, an intracranial midline primitive neuroectodermal tumor develops in conjunction with ocular retinoblastoma, termed trilateral retinoblastoma [3].

At an early stage, the tumor is confined to the retina, appearing as a small, translucent, gray to white mass [4]. As the tumor grows, it extends away from the vitreous cavity (i.e., exophytic growth pattern) or toward it (i.e., endophytic growth pattern). Retinoblastoma may also consist of a combination of these two forms. Exophytic tumors arise from the outer retinal layers, grow beneath the retina, may have an associated serous retinal detachment, and can shed tumor seeds into the subretinal space [5]. Endophytic tumors arise from the inner retinal layers and grow on the retinal surface into the vitreous cavity. This variant is more likely to give rise to vitreous seeds, which are cells shed from retinal tumors that remain viable in the relatively hypoxic vitreous cavity.

Left untreated, retinoblastoma will grow within the eye, but eventually will breach the eye wall to spread locally to the orbit and adjacent lymphatics, via the optic nerve to reach the brain, or hematogenously to distant sites. Extraocular spread is associated with a worse prognosis for survival as compared to intraocular disease [6]. Early detection of retinoblastoma and urgent referral to a specialized treatment center is of utmost importance in order to save life, salvage the eye, and, in selected cases, retain vision [7].

Progress in patient care is usually measured in terms of the advances made in well-developed countries, where higher education, excellent health care, and scientific research converge [8]. A large disparity exists in the presentation patterns of retinoblastoma, and consequently the prognosis, between countries from different income levels [2, 9]. Overall, only about 20–30% of retinoblastoma cases worldwide are thought to be adequately diagnosed and treated, the vast majority of these being from high-income countries (HICs) [10].

The Global Retinoblastoma Study Group consists of retinoblastoma specialists, ophthalmologists, and pediatric oncologists from over 100 countries. The group published their first paper on retinoblastoma presentation patterns analyzed by national income levels in 2020 [2]. Over half of the estimated annual incidence of new cases, globally, from over 150 countries, were included in the study, making it the most comprehensive analysis in the field. In the study, the authors investigated epidemiological and clinical variables related to presentation of retinoblastoma on a global level. Additional investigations performed by this collaboration included travel distance from home to a treatment center as a potential

Supplementary Information The online version contains supplementary material available at [https://doi.org/10.1007/978-3-031-08250-4_3].

D. L. Prat
The Goldschleger Eye Institute, Sheba Medical Center, Tel Hashomer, Tel Aviv University, Tel Aviv, Israel

M. Zondervan
International Centre for Eye Health, London School of Hygiene & Tropical Medicine, London, UK
e-mail: Marcia.Zondervan@lshtm.ac.uk

I. D. Fabian (✉)
The Goldschleger Eye Institute, Sheba Medical Center, Tel Hashomer, Tel Aviv University, Tel Aviv, Israel

International Centre for Eye Health, London School of Hygiene & Tropical Medicine, London, UK
e-mail: didi@didifabian.com

B. V. Chawla, M. E. Aronow (eds.), *Global Perspectives in Ocular Oncology*, https://doi.org/10.1007/978-3-031-08250-4_3

risk factor for late disease presentation [11], and the issue of traveling across borders to obtain medical treatment for retinoblastoma [12]. Recently, the American Joint Committee on Cancer Ophthalmic Oncology Task Force published the presentation and outcome data from 18 centers in 13 countries across 6 continents, over a period of 13 years [9]. This work compared metastasis-related mortality, local treatment failure, and globe salvage following the diagnosis of retinoblastoma in countries at various national income levels.

This chapter focuses on the presentation patterns of retinoblastoma analyzed by national income level and is mainly based on the recent work done by both the Global Retinoblastoma Study Group and the American Joint Committee on Cancer Ophthalmic Oncology Task Force [2, 9].

2 A Global Perspective of Disease Burden

Although there is no validated evidence of racial or geographical variations in retinoblastoma incidence, disease burden is greatest in large populations with high birth rates, such as in Asia and Africa, where most countries are of low- to medium-income levels [1, 13–15]. Accordingly, the prevalence of this disorder is significantly higher in low- and middle-income countries (LMICs), which have approximately 80% of global cases, compared with HICs (Fig. 1) [13]. For example, in 2017 the number of new cases of retinoblastoma in France was 49 out of a population of 66.77 million, compared with 84 new cases out of 41.16 million population in Uganda—demonstrating a 1:2.8 ratio of new

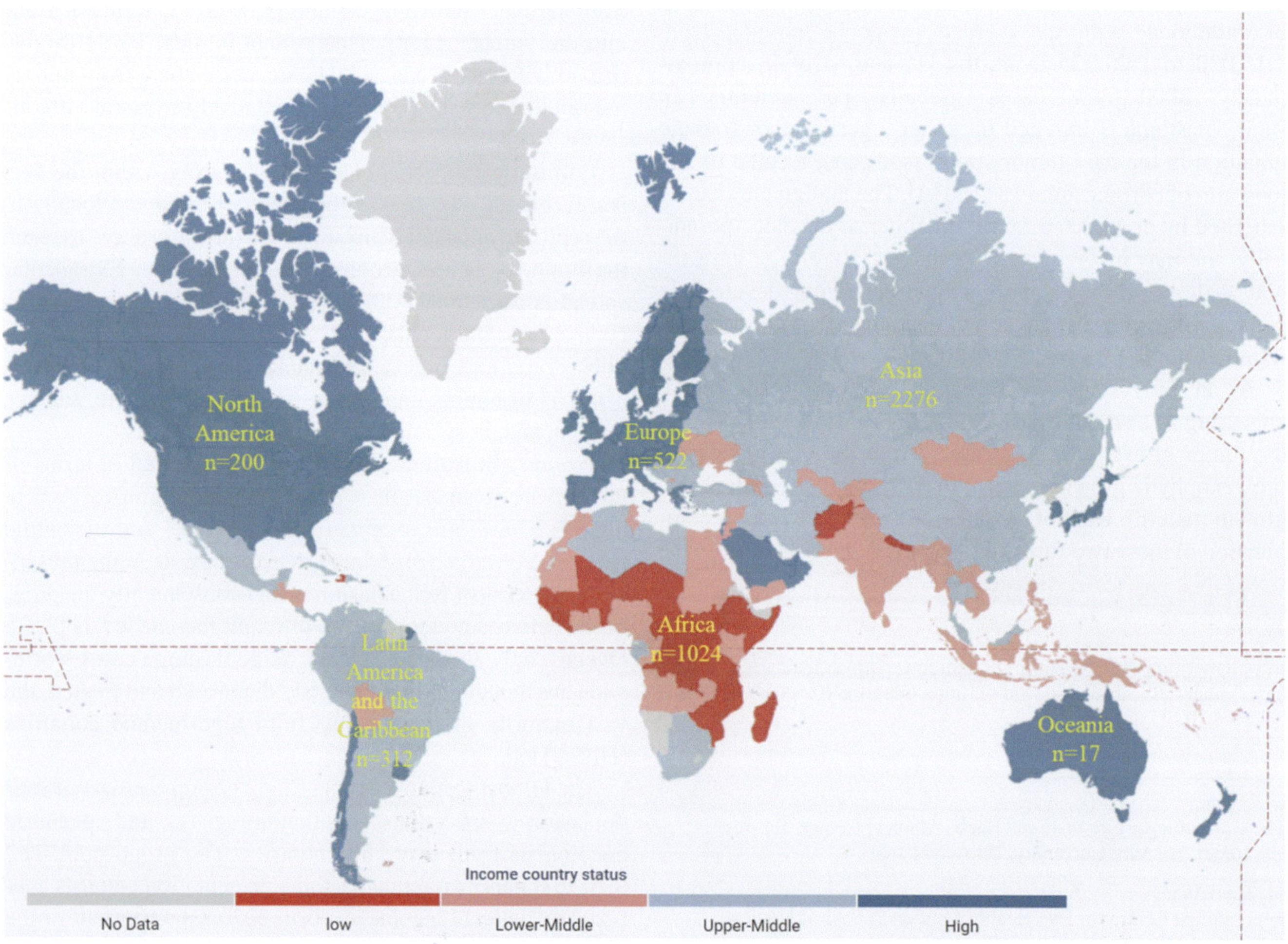

Fig. 1 Number of treatment-naïve retinoblastoma patients who presented to local retinoblastoma centers worldwide during 2017. The numbers represent new cases per continent. The different national income level is represented by different colors as demonstrated in the color legend. The highest disease burden was observed in LMICs. *The data were retrieved from Fabian et al, Global Retinoblastoma Presentation and Analysis by National Income Level, JAMA Oncol 2020, with permission*

cases per population [2]. The number of predicted retinoblastoma cases in Afghanistan in 2012 was roughly 60, compared with 3 in Singapore; nonetheless, both rates were similar (~0.00005) when dividing number of cases by number of live births per country [13].

3 Symptoms Leading to Referral

Worldwide, the most common first symptom of disease is leukocoria, reported in over 60% of cases, followed by strabismus in 10%, or a combination of leukocoria and strabismus in 4%. Proptosis is reported in 7% of patients; generally, symptoms of advanced disease (i.e., proptosis, swollen eyelids, red eye) are reported in 12% of patients. A higher income level was found to be associated with a lower proportion of patients with such symptoms of advanced disease [2].

4 Symptoms at Time of Diagnosis at Retinoblastoma Centers

Globally, the most common signs at presentation to a retinoblastoma treatment center are leukocoria, strabismus, or a combination of both. In low-income countries (LICs), symptoms of advanced disease (proptosis, red eye, orbital cellulitis, and/or extraocular retinoblastoma) are present in nearly half of patients. Analysis by economic grouping [2] shows that significantly more patients from LICs as compared with patients from higher-income-level countries shift from early symptoms (i.e., leukocoria and/or strabismus) as noted by parents, to advanced-disease signs that are diagnosed in specialized treatment centers. Underlying reasons include poor awareness, barriers to access, and underserved areas [11]. In addition, parents of children with retinoblastoma who present late at a tertiary center in LICs often report several interactions with different health professionals, sometimes over many months or years, prior to reaching a specialized treatment center in which diagnosis is made and treatment given. [16]

5 Sex, Gender, and Retinoblastoma

Sex has long been recognized as a significant factor influencing cancer risk and response to treatment and outcome, including in the pediatric population [17, 18]. In retinoblastoma, it is unclear whether there are differences between sexes. This is mainly because retinoblastoma is a rare disease; hence, studies are comprised of relatively small cohorts, making it difficult to demonstrate any real difference between the sexes.

In a recent cross-sectional analysis that included more than half of the estimated global annual incidence of retinoblastoma [2], no differences were found between the sexes (unpublished data). There was suggestive evidence of gender discrimination in parts of Asia. This finding adds to the growing literature on gender inequity that has been reported across the spectrum of child health, with girls having poorer nutritional status, lower rates of immunization, and lower uptake of surgery for serious conditions such as bilateral cataract and congenital heart disease [19–23].

6 Age at Time of Diagnosis

There is a significant association between age of presentation and national income level, with children from LMICs presenting at an older age than those from HICs. Overall, the median age at diagnosis of retinoblastoma worldwide is 24 months; 31 months in LICs, and 14 months in HICs. Differences between the various economic groups remain when subdividing into unilateral and bilateral disease at presentation.

The observation that national income level and, independently, older age at presentation are associated with advanced disease, suggests that other factors besides age may affect disease progression. Infection by the human papilloma virus, which is more prevalent in LMICs, has been suggested to be associated with nonhereditary retinoblastoma, and possibly a more aggressive disease [24]. Another association might relate to the genetic landscape of retinoblastoma, especially in cases with a high level of amplification of the oncogene *MYCN* rather than the *RB1* mutation [25]. These cases develop at early age, and demonstrate aggressive features. They are much less common than the *RB1* mutation and were found only in 1.4% of unilateral retinoblastoma cases, although all of these findings were evaluated in cohorts from HICs. [25]

7 Tumor Staging

Higher economic grouping is associated with higher proportions of intraocular disease and earlier stages at diagnosis. Orbital retinoblastoma is an advanced form of the disease that is seen mostly in LMICs in Asia and Africa [5]. Globally, according to the report by the Global Retinoblastoma Study Group, the most common clinical Tumor, Node, and Metastasis (cTNM) stages were cT3 (47%), N0 (77%), and M0 (93%). Extraocular retinoblastoma at time of diagnosis was observed in 21% of the cases, with nearly 50% of the patients from LICs vs <2% from HICs. Distant metastases at presentation were reported in 19%, 8%, 5%, and less than

1% of patients from low, lower-middle, upper-middle, and high income-level countries, respectively. It is likely that the real gap in the pattern of retinoblastoma presentation is even wider owing to unreported patients in LICs who never arrived at a retinoblastoma treatment center and for whom death from metastatic disease is inevitable.

A recent multicenter, retrospective study analyzed the management and outcome of 2085 retinoblastoma cases from 13 countries in 6 continents over a period of 13 years [9]. Forty percent of patients came from HICs, 44% from upper middle-income countries, and 16% from lower-middle income countries. None from low-income countries were included in this analysis. Tumor staging at presentation were: cT1a in 3%, cT1b in 8%, cT2a in 9%, cT2b in 39%, cT3 in 40%, and cT4 in 1%. As expected, more advanced disease was inversely related to national income level. Lymph node involvement at presentation was seen in 0.2% in HIC, 0.4% in upper middle-income countries, and 2.7% in lower-middle income countries. Synchronous metastatic disease at presentation was seen in 0.6% of cases in HIC, 0.8% in upper middle-income countries, and 3.9% in lower-middle income countries. Overall, lower national income level and older age at presentation were found to be both significant and independent predictive factors for advanced disease (cT3 and cT4).

8 Familial History and Bilateral Retinoblastoma

Significantly higher rates of bilateral cases and, independently, familial cases are observed in HICs compared with LMICs [2, 9]. Familial history of retinoblastoma is in direct proportion to income level: reported in 3%, 4%, 4.5%, and 8% of patients from low, lower-middle, upper-middle, and high income-level countries, respectively, with an overall 5% rate worldwide. Similarly, bilateral disease at time of diagnosis was more common in HICs, with an overall incidence of 31%, including 23% in LICs vs 35% in HICs.

A possible explanation to the lower rates of familial history in lower-income countries could be inadequate medical record keeping or underreporting in resource-constrained settings. However, a more plausible explanation would be that in LMICs, where diagnosis and treatment are late, patients do not reach a childbearing age. In addition, as there is a high incidence of non-ocular subsequent primary tumors in survivors of heritable retinoblastoma, some of the deaths, particularly those occurring more than 5 years from the diagnosis of retinoblastoma, can be attributed to such tumors [26].

9 Travel Burden

A recent study investigated the travel burden and its impact on clinical presentation in a large sample of patients with retinoblastoma from Africa and Europe [11]. This cross-sectional analysis included 1542 treatment-naïve patients with retinoblastoma residing in 40 European and 43 African countries. Overall, while the distribution of retinoblastoma centers in Europe was found to cover the entire continent, large parts of Africa were underserved. Findings of the Global Retinoblastoma Study Group suggest that in European countries, travel distance from home to retinoblastoma center is not a barrier to early disease diagnosis. In Africa, other factors besides geographic distance to a retinoblastoma treatment center also play a role in late diagnosis. They include poor awareness by caregivers and health workers, lack of knowledge about clinical presentation by health workers, cost to reach a specialized retinoblastoma treatment center, and probably the absence of retinoblastoma centers in some parts of Africa.

10 Bridging the Gap

Several factors underlie the differences in retinoblastoma presentation globally, including difficulties in accessing medical facilities resulting in diagnostic delays. Once arrived at a specialized treatment center, however, nearly all essential diagnostic modalities are available in most treatment centers, including imaging (computed tomography and/or magnetic resonance imaging) and histopathology services [2]. The need for a well-coordinated specialized multidisciplinary team (MDT) including an ophthalmologist, pediatric oncologist, imaging specialist, and pathologist to manage retinoblastoma, which is lacking in many LMICs, is yet another contributing factor [8]. In general, disparities in awareness and socioeconomic and cultural factors, coupled with inefficient or suboptimal health care, result in immense differences in the timing of presentation and extent of disease [27].

The data presented in this chapter point to an urgent need to improve retinoblastoma detection and access to treatment in LMICs. Several initiatives are addressing this challenge by implementing twinning programs that link centers from higher- and lower-resource countries [10, 16, 28–32]. Screening for ocular conditions by nurses and health workers examining children in the community during routine visits (e.g., immunization appointments) may reveal otherwise undetected cases of retinoblastoma [16]. Community nurses in Tanzania have been trained to look for the red reflex using an affordable, solar-powered, and easy to use ophthalmoscope [16]. Twinning programs between retinoblastoma treatment centers from high- and lower-income settings have shown improved outcomes over the years [33]. The Retinoblastoma-Network (Rb-NET) has generated a resource manual focusing on the management of retinoblastoma in LMICs (Supplemental Material, with permission from the authors at International Centre for eye Health/The London School of Hygiene & Tropical Medicine (ICEH/LSHTM)), and created specific management protocols tailored for each country, focusing on Sub-Saharan East Africa [16]. Recently, the Rb-NET has initiated national online retinoblastoma MDT meetings, including treatment centers from LMICs together with international experts, to discuss challenging cases of retinoblastoma (https://www.rb-net-mdt.org/). One of the lead participants from an African country wrote: "The Rb-NET MDT program has held several online meetings during the COVID-19 crisis in which we presented retinoblastoma children under our care who have complex problems. The opportunity for discussion and input from colleagues around the world has been of great value. The interaction with worldwide experts has been an important boost to the team's confidence. The parents also are very appreciative of this international support in the care of their children. We are keen that the program must continue even when normality returns."

There is an urgent need for joint action on a global level, to make this rare yet curable cancer a zero-death disease [13]. The World Health Organization Global Initiative for Childhood Cancer intends to increase survival rate to 60% for retinoblastoma as well as other key childhood cancers by the year 2030. This is planned to be addressed by helping LMIC health systems to improve their ability to diagnose and provide curative treatment, and integrate childhood cancer into their national strategies [34]. Improving the outcomes for patients with retinoblastoma is feasible by establishing strong global partnerships.

11 Conclusion

Significant differences exist in the clinical presentation of retinoblastoma between patients from different countries, depending on their economic grouping. Patients with retinoblastoma from HICs present with early disease associated with high survival rates, while patients from lower-income settings present with advanced disease, thus with a guarded prognosis. A positive family history of retinoblastoma is less common in lower-income countries, probably because of death due to late presentation happening prior to childbearing years. Improving health education about retinoblastoma and coordinated action at both national and international levels are needed to enhance access to early diagnosis and treatment in retinoblastoma treatment centers in LMICs worldwide.

References

1. Kivelä T. The epidemiological challenge of the most frequent eye cancer: retinoblastoma, an issue of birth and death. Br J Ophthalmol. 2009;93:1129–31.
2. Global Retinoblastoma Study Group, Fabian ID, Abdallah E, et al. Global retinoblastoma presentation and analysis by National Income Level. JAMA Oncologia. 2020;
3. de Jong MC, Kors WA, de Graaf P, et al. The incidence of trilateral retinoblastoma: a systematic review and meta-analysis. Am J Ophthalmol. 2015;160:1116–1126.e5.
4. Ophthalmology AA of 2018–2019 BCSC (Basic and Clinical Science Course), Section 04: ophthalmic pathology and intraocular tumors. (Jr RHR, MD, editors.).
5. Rao R, Honavar SG. Retinoblastoma. Indian J Pediatr. 2017;84:937–44.
6. Chawla B, Hasan F, Azad R, et al. Clinical presentation and survival of retinoblastoma in Indian children. Br J Ophthalmol. 2016;100:172–8.
7. Fabian ID, Johnson KP, Stacey AW, et al. Focal laser treatment in addition to chemotherapy for retinoblastoma. Cochrane Database Syst Rev. 2017;6:CD012366.
8. Rodriguez-Galindo C, Wilson MW, Chantada G, et al. Retinoblastoma: one world, one vision. Pediatrics. 2008;122:e763–70.
9. Tomar AS, Finger PT, Gallie B, et al. Global retinoblastoma treatment outcomes: association with National Income Level. Ophthalmology. 2020;
10. Ribeiro RC, Steliarova-Foucher E, Magrath I, et al. Baseline status of paediatric oncology care in ten low-income or mid-income countries receiving my child matters support: a descriptive study. Lancet Oncol. 2008;9:721–9.
11. Fabian ID, Stacey AW, Foster A, et al. Travel burden and clinical presentation of retinoblastoma: analysis of 1024 patients from 43 African countries and 518 patients from 40 European countries. Br J Ophthalmol. 2020;
12. Bowman RJC, Foster A, Stacey A, et al. International travel to obtain medical treatment for primary retinoblastoma: a global cohort study. Int J Cancer. 2020;
13. Dimaras H, Corson TW, Cobrinik D, et al. Retinoblastoma. Nat Rev Dis Primers. 2015;1:15021.
14. Broaddus E, Topham A, Singh AD. Incidence of retinoblastoma in the USA: 1975-2004. Br J Ophthalmol. 2009;93:21–3.
15. Krishna SM, Yu G-P, Finger PT. The effect of race on the incidence of retinoblastoma. J Pediatr Ophthalmol Strabismus. 2009;46:288–93.
16. Bowman R. Retinoblastoma: a curable, rare and deadly blinding disease. Community Eye Health. 2018;31:1–4.

17. Pui CH, Boyett JM, Relling MV, et al. Sex differences in prognosis for children with acute lymphoblastic leukemia. J Clin Oncol. 1999;17:818–24.
18. Pala L, Nezi L, De Pas T, et al. Sex differences in efficacy and toxicity of systemic cancer treatments: role of the microbiome. J Clin Oncol. 2019;37:439.
19. Pokhrel S, Snow R, Dong H, et al. Gender role and child health care utilization in Nepal. Health Policy (Amsterdam, Netherlands). 2005;74:100–9.
20. Dancer D, Rammohan A, Smith MD. Infant mortality and child nutrition in Bangladesh. Health Econ. 2008;17:1015–35.
21. Mitra AK, Rahman MM, Fuchs GJ. Risk factors and gender differentials for death among children hospitalized with diarrhoea in Bangladesh. J Health Popul Nutr. 2000;18:151–6.
22. Gilbert CE, Lepvrier-Chomette N. Gender inequalities in surgery for bilateral cataract among children in low-income countries: a systematic review. Ophthalmology. 2016;123:1245–51.
23. Ramakrishnan S, Khera R, Jain S, et al. Gender differences in the utilisation of surgery for congenital heart disease in India. Heart. 2011;97:1920–5.
24. Shetty OA, Naresh KN, Banavali SD, et al. Evidence for the presence of high risk human papillomavirus in retinoblastoma tissue from nonfamilial retinoblastoma in developing countries. Pediatr Blood Cancer. 2012;58:185–90.
25. Rushlow DE, Mol BM, Kennett JY, et al. Characterisation of retinoblastomas without RB1 mutations: genomic, gene expression, and clinical studies. Lancet Oncol. 2013;14:327–34.
26. Fletcher O, Easton D, Anderson K, et al. Lifetime risks of common cancers among retinoblastoma survivors. J Natl Cancer Inst. 2004;96:357–63.
27. Chawla B, Kumar K, Singh AD. Influence of socioeconomic and cultural factors on retinoblastoma. Asia Pac J Oncol Nurs. 2017;4:187–90.
28. Traoré F, Sylla F, Togo B, et al. Treatment of retinoblastoma in sub-Saharan Africa: experience of the paediatric oncology unit at Gabriel Toure teaching hospital and the Institute of African Tropical Ophthalmology, Bamako. Mali Pediatr Blood Cancer. 2018;65:e27101.
29. Hill JA, Kimani K, White A, et al. Achieving optimal cancer outcomes in East Africa through multidisciplinary partnership: a case study of the Kenyan National Retinoblastoma Strategy group. Glob Health. 2016;12:23.
30. Wilimas JA, Wilson MW, Haik BG, et al. Development of retinoblastoma programs in Central America. Pediatr Blood Cancer. 2009;53:42–6.
31. Qaddoumi I, Nawaiseh I, Mehyar M, et al. Team management, twinning, and telemedicine in retinoblastoma: a 3-tier approach implemented in the first eye salvage program in Jordan. Pediatr Blood Cancer. 2008;51:241–4.
32. Antillon F, Baez FL, Barr R, et al. AMOR: a proposed cooperative effort to improve outcomes of childhood cancer in Central America. Pediatr Blood Cancer. 2005;45:107–10.
33. Yousef YA, Al-Nawaiseh I, Mehyar M, et al. How telemedicine and centralized care changed the natural history of retinoblastoma in a developing country: analysis of 478 patients. Ophthalmology. 2021;128:130–7.
34. Anon. WHO | Global Initiative for Childhood Cancer. WHO. Available at: http://www.who.int/cancer/childhood-cancer/en/. Accessed 30 Aug 2020.

International Collaborations for Characterizing Ocular Adnexal Lymphoma

Marina K. Kirkegaard and Steffen Heegaard

1 Introduction

Throughout history, scientific reporting has progressed through three ages of research: the individual, the institutional, and the national. Today, we are standing at the forefront of the fourth age of research, driven by international collaborations. Whether it is to develop new ideas, acquire specialized equipment, or gain access to new sources of funding, researchers are increasingly reaching out to their colleagues around the world. International multicenter collaboration is particularly advantageous when needed to accumulate large numbers of patients for statistical analysis to acquire medical evidence. This improves the quality of the research and the impact of the publications. Although scientific research increasingly requires international collaboration, less is known about the barriers that impede such collaboration [1–3]. In the following, we describe the advantages and the challenges of international multicenter registry-based research, exemplified by our collaboration on ocular adnexal lymphoma with six other international eye cancer centers.

2 Why International Multicenter Registry-Based Studies?

2.1 Investigating Rare Diseases

Rare diseases are often difficult to diagnose, prognosticate, and treat, which makes research in this field particularly urgent. Conducting research on a rare disease, however, is challenging, as it is frequently difficult to recruit enough patients to generate statistically meaningful results. In these cases, international multicenter retrospective study design is particularly beneficial, as it has the unique advantage of garnering much data quickly [4].

Lymphoma of the ocular adnexa is an example of a rare disease, accounting for approximately 3% of all primary extranodal non-Hodgkin lymphomas (Fig. 1) [5]. The clinical characteristics, outcome, and prognostic factors of ocular adnexal lymphoma have long been poorly understood, as the previous studies have not been able to recruit sufficiently large patient populations [6]. This has prompted our research group in Copenhagen to investigate the subject by creating an international registry database from the registries of seven international eye cancer centers. The participating eye cancer centers included: Liverpool, England; Hyderabad, India; New York, New York; Houston, Texas; Atlanta, Georgia; Melbourne, Australia; and Copenhagen, Denmark (Fig. 2). Each of these eye cancer centers has been collecting clinical information on patients with ocular adnexal lymphoma for 20–40 years and has treated 25–392 patients during that period. Collectively, however, the eye cancer centers were able to provide 1188 patients for the analysis. These were unprecedented numbers of ocular adnexal lymphoma patients from which we could discover statistically meaningful evidence on this rare disease.

The international collaboration yielded eight publications on the clinical features of lymphoma at the various ocular adnexal locations during a 6-year period. Together, the studies characterized ocular adnexal lymphoma as a disease of the elderly that mainly consists of four histological subtypes: extranodal marginal zone lymphoma, follicular lymphoma, diffuse large B-cell lymphoma, and mantle cell lymphoma. The histological subtype was identified as the main outcome predictor for the patients, with the last two subtypes carrying markedly poorer prognoses [7–14]. With this prognostic information available, physicians are better equipped to make clinical decisions, including the choice of treatment, which ultimately may lead to improved outcomes for our patients. Thereby, the international collaboration has provided a sufficiently large patient population, in a short period of time, enabling us to answer previously unanswerable clinical questions regarding a rare disease.

M. K. Kirkegaard · S. Heegaard (✉)
Department of Pathology, Eye Pathology Section, Rigshospitalet, University of Copenhagen, Copenhagen, Denmark
e-mail: marina.hoey.knudsen@regionh.dk; sthe@sund.ku.dk

B. V. Chawla, M. E. Aronow (eds.), *Global Perspectives in Ocular Oncology*, https://doi.org/10.1007/978-3-031-08250-4_4

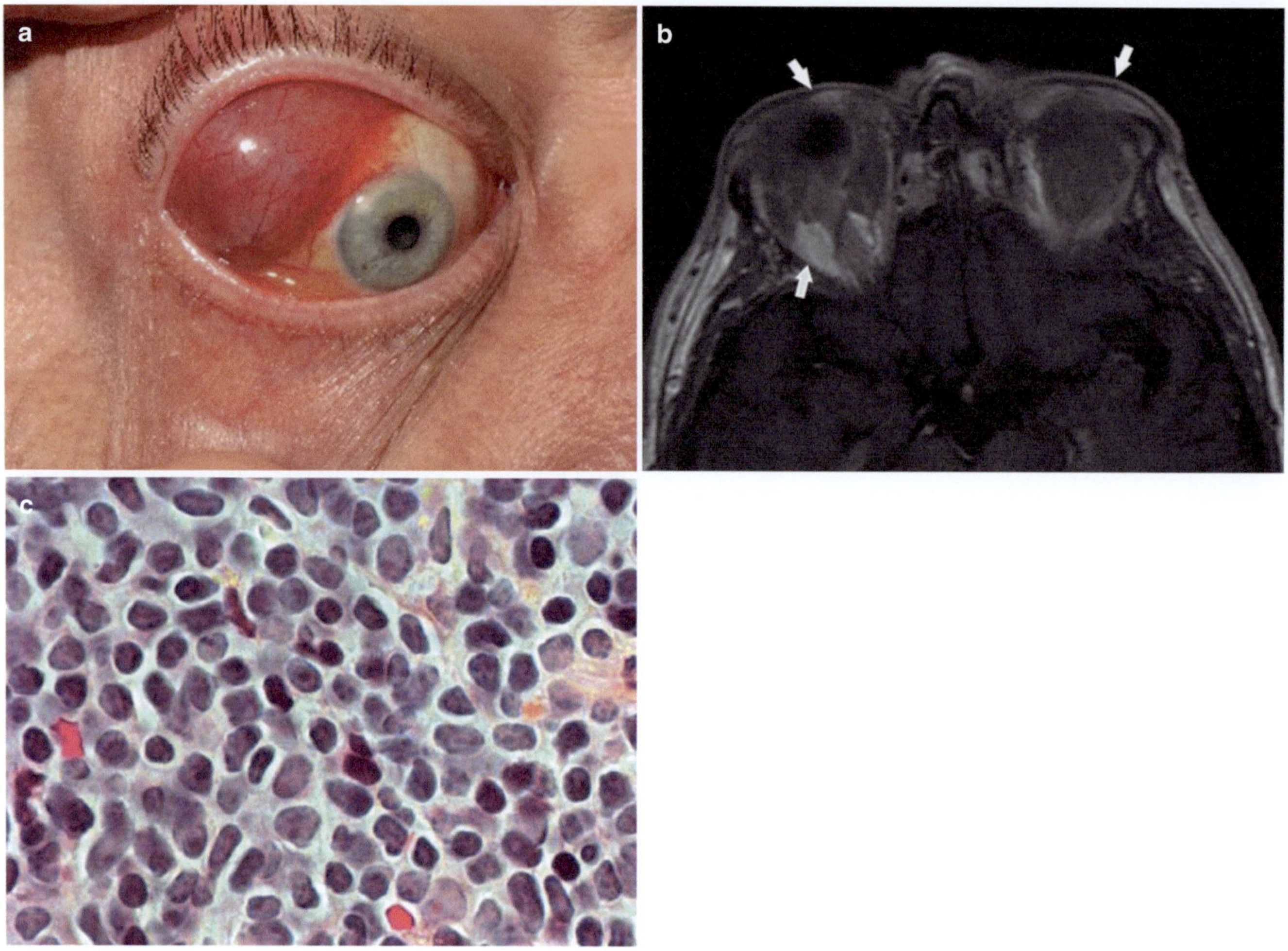

Fig. 1 Presentation of an ocular adnexal mantle cell lymphoma. **(a)** Clinical presentation with a salmon-pink mass of the conjunctiva in a 64-year-old male patient. **(b)** Magnetic resonance imaging scan shows conjunctival and orbital tumor masses (arrows). **(c)** Histological presentation with a monotonous pattern of small cells containing irregular nuclei with inconspicuous nucleoli and scant cytoplasm consistent with a mantle cell lymphoma (hematoxylin-eosin; bar = 50 μm)

2.2 Investigating Diseases with Rarity of Adverse Outcomes

The ability of international multicenter registry-based studies to provide a larger sample size is advantageous when examining not only rare diseases but also diseases with rarity of adverse outcomes. An example of such a disease is ocular adnexal extranodal marginal zone lymphoma, which we investigated in our international collaboration. Although it is the most common lymphoma subtype in this anatomical region, cases with adverse outcomes are sparse due to the indolence of the disease (20 years after diagnosis, 90% of patients are alive or have died of other causes) [12]. Despite having one of the largest registries, Copenhagen eye cancer center only had 16 cases with lymphoma death among these patients. The 7 centers together, however, were able to contribute 71 of such cases, providing a reasonable sample size for survival analysis. Similarly, studies of rare therapeutic side effects can benefit greatly from a multicenter setting because of its ability to provide the necessary statistical power.

2.3 Validating Staging Systems

Staging systems have long been used in ocular oncology. Eye cancer specialists, oncologists, and researchers have incorporated staging into their daily practice and peer review journals have made staging part of their standards. However, few staging systems have been tested with "real-world" data from international cancer centers. Validation is of great importance because it leads to world acceptance, in turn leading to improvements in clinical care and research communication. The American Joint Committee on Cancer

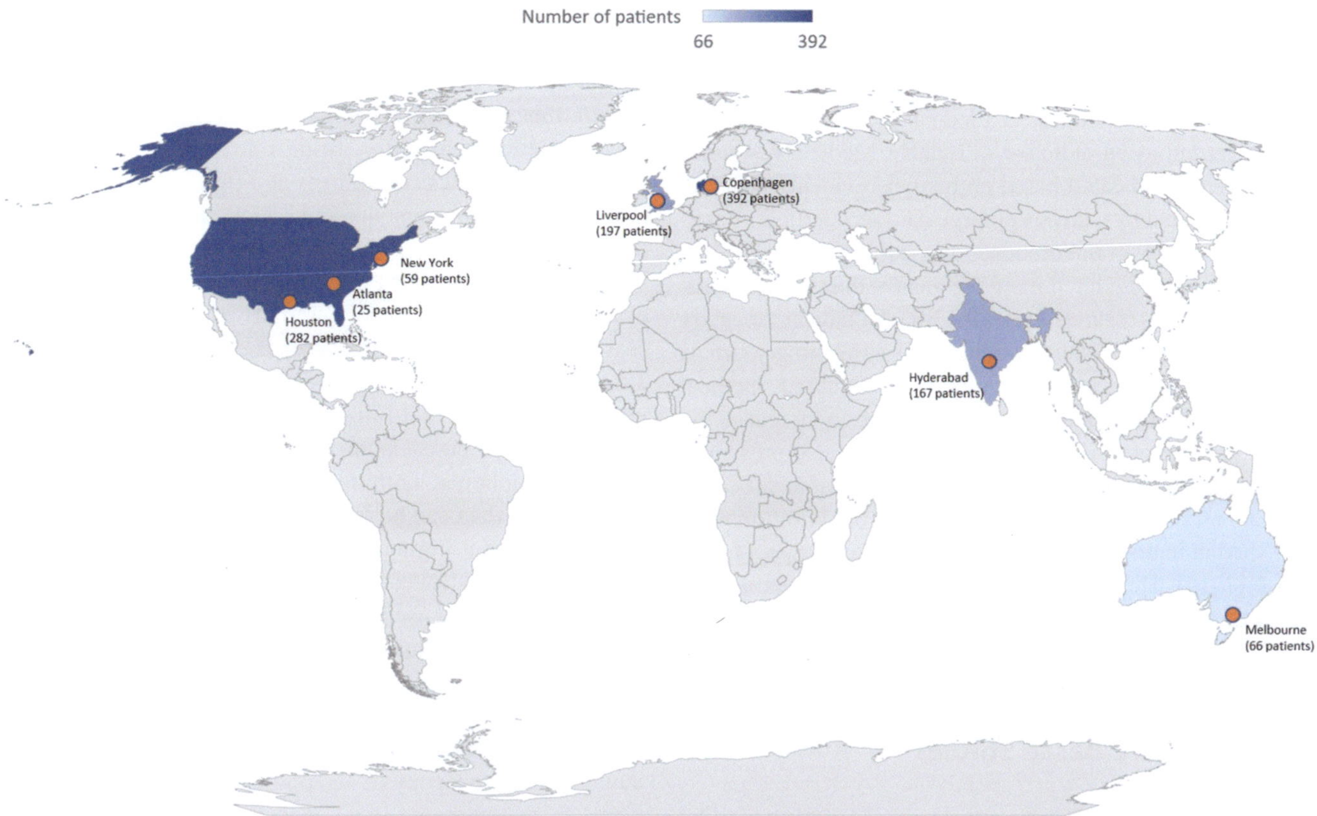

Center, number of patients included

North America		**Europe**		**Asia**		**Australia**	
New York, USA	59	Liverpool, England	197	Hyderabad, India	167	Melbourne	66
Atlanta, USA	25	Copenhagen, Denmark	392				
Houston, USA	282						

Fig. 2 Geographic location and number of included patients for the eye cancer centers participating in the collaboration on ocular adnexal lymphoma

(AJCC) tumor, node, metastasis (TNM) staging system for eye cancers is currently being tested within the framework of multicenter retrospective studies. This anatomically based staging system was found to predict both mortality and globe salvage in several eye cancers by these studies [15, 16]. One of the aims of our project was to investigate the validity of this staging system for ocular adnexal lymphoma in a large cohort, attained through international collaboration. We found that the histopathologic subtype of lymphoma was more important than the location of the tumor for outcome prediction, suggesting that the AJCC TNM staging system is of limited utility for ocular adnexal lymphomas [7–14].

2.4 Comparing Patient Populations

International multicenter studies increase the geographical, social, and cultural diversity of the cohort. This renders the results more transferable and provides abundant opportunities to compare patient populations. Comparison of patient populations can help discover geographical differences in epidemiology, clinical features, treatment, and outcomes of ophthalmic cancers. Detected geographical disparities in cancer incidence may be used to identify possible carcinogens as well as help ensure appropriate distribution of resources and stimulate new research and clinical care initiatives in high-incidence areas [17, 18]. In our multicenter collaboration on ocular adnexal lymphoma, the cohort consisted of patients from five countries on four different continents. However, only one center, Hyderabad, India, was non-Western and the detected geographical differences were limited to this center. Patients from Hyderabad were younger and overrepresented by women, which may reflect a differing demographic pattern in this region or be attributed to a referral bias [7, 9].

2.5 Improving the Dissemination of Research

International collaboration in medical research is increasingly regarded as an indicator of quality. Medical resources are frequently allocated based on medical evidence that can only be obtained by analysis of large data sets. Articles based on international collaborations are published in higher-impact journals and cited more frequently than those resulting from local research [15, 19, 20]. A Taiwanese study compared median impact factors of the publishing journals between locally and internationally co-authored medical papers, finding that international collaboration increased the impact factor by 0.8 [21]. This tendency was also present in our international collaboration on ocular adnexal lymphoma—all the papers resulting from the collaboration were published in high-impact journals, with a mean impact factor of 5.2 [7–14]. Hence, international collaboration is a great means of enhancing the impact of your scientific work.

3 Conducting International Multicenter Registry-Based Studies

An international multicenter registry-based project can be divided into four phases: (1) *planning phase*, for defining the research question, reviewing the literature, and identifying the outcome measures; (2) *project development phase*, where the lead research site identifies international collaborators, grant applications are prepared, and ethical approvals are obtained; (3) *study execution phase*, involving creation of an international registry database and analysis of the data; and (4) *dissemination phase*, when the project team shares their results through publications, conference presentations, and social and traditional media as well as implements strategies to translate the results into clinical practice [22]. During each of these phases, the scientific and logistic complexity of the international multicenter retrospective study design poses distinct obstacles for the investigator. In the following, we address some of the main challenges and provide our perspective on how to overcome them.

3.1 Obtaining Ethical Approvals

Data security, privacy, and integrity are of particular concern in international multicenter studies because of the large-scale data collection. The principal investigator from each participating center is responsible for their local ethical approvals. Acquiring consensus among the research ethics boards is not always easy and is always time consuming. It is not uncommon for the different ethics committees to have different perceptions of what is ethical. Sometimes this is due to the lack of knowledge regarding the particular disease entity. In other cases, as an ethics committee is supposed to represent the ethical opinion of the community in which the study is conducted, this variation represents a difference in deeply held ethical views that differ from one culture to another. Therefore, the ethics committees at different sites frequently have different requirements and review levels ranging from exempt to review by a full board [23–26].

Common across many ethics committees is that the level of identifiable patient information drives the regulation process for collection, storage, use, and sharing of the data. There are typically three classifications of data sets: de-identified, limited, and fully identified. If the data set is de-identified, as in case of our multicenter research on ocular adnexal lymphoma, nothing further usually needs to take place and the data can be freely transferred between the centers. In case of a limited data set, the recipient of the data typically needs a data use agreement that establishes how the information may be used and how it will be protected by the recipient. If the information is fully identified, it is governed by the regulations of the human subject research [27].

To reduce the workload and streamline the process of obtaining the ethical approvals, principal investigators should distribute a copy of an approved submission with relevant documentation (e.g., consents and demographic forms), which can be used as a template for other site researchers. A presentation by the principal investigator discussing the content of the ethical approval submission will help engage investigators who are working on their own submissions. Additionally, acquiring assistance of an ethics committee staff member is of great help when navigating international ethical approvals [22].

3.2 Funding the Project

Funding support from grants is frequently necessary to conduct an international multicenter retrospective research study. The research team begins the process of obtaining funding by identifying candidate grants, which differ depending on the focus of the research and the country of origin. Applying for multiple grants (if allowed by the grant agencies) is recommended to increase the chances of securing funding. The applications should include any preliminary data and be written with emphasis on the strengths of the project team and any previous collaborative accomplishments. When preparing a budget, the principal investigator at the lead research site should collect institutional budgets from each participating center to form the overall project budget. Management of the overall project budget and its distribution is usually also the responsibility of the principal investigator at the lead research center. The funding allocation should match the responsibilities of each institution with a transparent process of sharing the funding across the sites. Ultimately, a study may be left underfunded. In this case, the project team needs to evaluate whether it is possible to conduct the study within the existing infrastructure. From our experience and the experience of other research teams, a multicenter registry-based research project can be conducted with a fairly modest budget if the researchers are passionate about the project and have the time to fully commit to it [22].

3.3 Forming an International Registry Database

When forming an international registry database, the first step is identifying which centers to include. This choice should be based on careful consideration of which centers would best help elucidate the studied subject. In case of lymphoma, its epidemiology is complicated by a great number of subtypes and their association with infection, genetic predisposition, and immunological abnormality, which entails ethnic idiosyncrasy among many lymphoma subtypes. For instance, Asian populations have higher proportions of extranodal marginal zone lymphoma and mature T/NK cell lymphomas than Western populations, due to a high prevalence of *Helicobacter pylori* and human T-lymphotropic virus 1, respectively. Similarly, African populations are characterized by a high prevalence of Acquired Immune Deficiency Syndrome (AIDS)-related lymphomas, such as Burkitt lymphoma and B-cell immunoblastic lymphoma [28]. In our studies, six of seven included eye cancer centers were from Western countries. The detected subtype distributions were, therefore, reflective of those in Western populations. This allowed a comprehensive clinical characterization of these lymphoma subtypes, in line with our objective, while the clinical features of such lymphomas as AIDS-related lymphomas in the ocular adnexa remain to be determined.

3.4 Choosing a Database Platform

Choosing a platform for your registry database is an important step in an international multicenter project. To select the most appropriate software, one needs to ask the following questions: How much storage is needed for the information? How many users need to access the database? Is the data de-identified?

The first decision one needs to make is between a desktop and a server database platform. Desktop database solutions are licensed for single users and include such options as Microsoft Excel and Microsoft Access. Server database management systems typically include designs that are accessible by multiple users and include vendors such as REDCap and IBM Clinical Development [29].

When starting up our international registry database, we decided to collect the data in Microsoft Excel. The practicality of this tool depends greatly on the scale of one's database. Excel is a convenient and simple-to-use tool for relatively small tasks but is not appropriate for handling very large *amounts of data*. Excel has a limited capacity per sheet, so as the volume of the data grows, it must be separated between multiple sheets, making it difficult to work with. There is also a limit to the amount of data Excel can handle before it suffers performance issues, potentially leading to data loss. Another drawback of Excel is its lack of support for *collaboration*, as it is not designed to be accessible by multiple users. Emailing an Excel file is tedious and the file quickly becomes difficult to keep track of—collaborators will have several versions at one time and not know which is the latest. Further, an important issue with Excel as a database is its lack of *security*. Although Excel allows you to protect the information with a password, there are tools available on the Internet that can unlock a file without entering the password. Thus, one's data must be fully de-identified for Excel to be an appropriate tool for a database [30–32].

In our collaboration, we have worked with a medium amount of data that was de-identified, making Excel an appropriate, easy-to-use software for our database. If one's data do not meet these criteria, a server database may be a more suitable solution. These options usually meet the regulatory requirements on hosting, access, and transfer of data to ensure its security and confidentiality. In REDCap, for example, fields can be indicated as identifiable and users have the option of de-identifying the data when exporting it. Additionally, this software can be accessed from any device with an Internet connection and offers daily backups and basic support [33, 34].

3.5 Collecting Data

Identifying the right data to collect is an essential step of a quality database setup. At the lead research site in Copenhagen, we synthesized an Excel document, where we defined the data to be registered and sent the document to the participating centers for completion. Only the most relevant data were requested, as collaborators might find it tedious to fill out large amounts of information, which could threaten the quality of the data needed to reach the aims of the study. To collect the most relevant data, one needs to make sure that each piece of information has a clear role in each part of the research: data for quality and safety purposes, data to characterize the patient sample, data to address the aims of the study, etc. [35]. The information we collected in our database included age and sex of the patient, symptoms, clinical findings, laterality, extent of ocular adnexal involvement according to the AJCC TNM staging system and systemic involvement according to the Ann Arbor staging system, treatment modalities and response to therapy, survival duration, and cause of death.

Heterogeneity of data is a critical scientific limitation, potentially yielding results with poor statistical power. It is particularly relevant for international multicenter retrospective studies because reporting regulations and perceptions of adverse events are likely to vary widely among the participating centers, as are diagnostic and treatment methods throughout the data collection period. The lead research site should, therefore, strive to standardize the reporting when collecting data from the collaborators. This will, additionally, relieve the local investigator of decisions such as whether the outcome is serious and/or related to the research objective. In the data collection document, synthesize the name and the definition of the information, accompanied by its unit of measure (preferably using the international system of units) and the rounding value. Some data may be collected using free-form text, e.g., in a category "other" for specifications and additional information. This prevents loss of information without making an excessively long list of categories but requires specific processing to homogenize the data and should, therefore, be used sparingly. Provide instructions for filling out missing values to clearly report any missed visit, examination, biological test, etc. Additionally, instructions for recording adverse events should be provided, for instance, to record the diagnosis instead of symptoms [25, 35, 36].

3.6 Analyzing Data

To optimize the analysis of multicenter data, we recommend collaborating with a statistician. A statistician will help select appropriate statistical methods and assist in the interpretation of results and drawing conclusions. Additionally, a statistician can provide valuable information on key design questions, such as whether the design is valid and whether the data will be analyzable. Therefore, it is beneficial to involve a statistician as early as possible. Specifying statistical methods in advance will also help minimize the risk of bias and maintain the integrity of the analysis as well as maximize one's chances of obtaining funding. If the investigators do not have the funding to support a statistician, an option is to include the statistician as a co-investigator in the grant application to cover the salary and the supplies needed to implement the statistical methods described in the application [37].

Statistics is a large and diverse field; hence statisticians have specific areas of expertise. It is, therefore, very important to collaborate with a statistician who is an expert within your study design. For some of the studies in our international collaboration, we have acquired advice from an epidemiologic statistician, specializing in disease etiology and risk factors. This collaboration has been of great value, particularly in identifying the outcome variables related to the research questions and addressing the issues of bias and stratification. Additionally, just as a statistician who can understand the clinical aspect of the study is very advantageous, the clinical investigator should endeavor to understand the rationale of the proposed statistical methodology. This will make the collaboration more dynamic and lead to more efficient execution of the research [37].

Several statistical issues are particularly prominent when analyzing a multicenter data set. Due to the magnitude of the data, small differences may be statistically significant. Reporting the effect size may be far more meaningful for a clinician in this case [25]. Another issue is the fact that multicenter retrospective studies are particularly prone to missing data. Missing data should be analyzed to detect any systematic biases [22]. Furthermore, referral bias is a concern in the interpretation of multicenter data, particularly when investigating the characteristics or outcomes of patients with rare diseases. Referral bias is a type of selection bias occurring as a result of systematic selection of patients from tertiary-care centers. For instance, some of our collaborating eye cancer centers specialize in chemotherapy, which explains why treatment data for patients referred to these centers do not include other treatments, such as external beam radiation therapy. Referral bias may, thereby, affect the generalizability of the results. Adjustment for referral bias is not routinely done in research but it is possible, for example, using Bayesian methods [38, 39].

3.7 Publication of the Results

When the results of the multicenter international collaboration are ready, the dissemination phase begins in the form of conference presentations and publications. Presentation abstracts can be submitted to multiple conferences (if permitted by the conference guidelines) for greater dissemination. International multicenter collaborations provide multiple publication opportunities, such as narrative or systematic reviews that define the research question, the main study, related sub-studies, as well as educational content. The main study should be published before the related substudies. The sub-studies should be planned in advance to make sure that they address new objectives and report endpoints that do not entirely overlap with those in the main study [22].

3.8 General Challenges

Despite meticulous planning of each of the described steps, unanticipated events occur frequently in international multicenter research. These are often due to upheavals in the local health care systems, such as changes in staff, institutional mergers, changes in computer systems, or new policies for accessing medical data. Researchers should be prepared to devote resources to finding alternatives and solutions to these problems [17]. Clear communication between the principal investigator and the collaborators at each site will help minimize unforeseen complications as well as keep the project on the proposed timeline. To maintain effective communication, investigators from each site as well as any administrative support should meet regularly by conference call to discuss the progress and make key decisions [22]. Even though it is easier than ever to connect with overseas colleagues, there are distinct barriers that impede communication in international research. It is, for instance, frequently difficult to arrange meetings when dealing with multiple time zones and investigators have to be in conference calls at inconvenient times of the day. Most importantly, researchers have to be cognizant of cultural differences, mannerisms, and sensitivities, when communicating with international colleagues [2, 40].

4 What Is Next for International Research Collaboration?

In this chapter, we have seen how international multicenter retrospective studies can be used to obtain much information on a subject in a short time, which is particularly advantageous for studying rare diseases, such as ocular adnexal lymphoma. The international collaboration has improved our understanding of the clinical features of this disease and its prognostic markers, making physicians better equipped to make clinical decisions. This progress was made in 6 years with the participation of seven eye cancer centers, while it would have taken an entire academic career to study for one single center. Clearly, international multicenter research speeds up the wheels of progress. So, what is next for international collaboration in ophthalmic cancer research? The next logical step is prospective multicenter data sharing by real-time reporting of patient data. Prospective multicenter data sharing will provide even larger numbers of patients for analysis and thereby the greatest potential for discovery. It will, for example, be particularly useful in time sensitive outcome analysis and for limiting damage from poor diagnostic and treatment methods. Additionally, electronic medical record-based data sharing will facilitate the development of artificial intelligence and machine learning. These advances will in turn improve the quality of care for the benefit of our ocular oncology patients [15].

References

1. Adams J. Collaborations: the fourth age of research. Nature. 2013;497(7451):557–60.
2. Owens B. The benefits and challenges of international research collaboration [internet]. Ottawa, Canada: University Affairs; 2018. [cited 2021 Apr 19]. Available from: https://www.universityaffairs.ca/features/feature-article/the-benefits-and-challenges-of-international-research-collaboration/.
3. Matthews KRW, Yang E, Lewis SW, Vaidyanathan BR, Gorman M. International scientific collaborative activities and barriers to them in eight societies. Account Res. 2020;27(8):477–95.
4. Alfonso Farnos I, Alcalde BG. Clinical research in rare diseases: new challenges, opportunities and ethical issues. An Pediatr (Engl Ed). 2020;93(4):219–21.
5. Otter R, Gerrits WBJ, Sandt MMVD, Hermans J, Willemze R. Primary extranodal and nodal non-Hodgkin's lymphoma. A survey of a population-based registry. Eur J Cancer Clin Oncol. 1989;25(8):1203–1210.
6. Sjo LD. Ophthalmic lymphoma: epidemiology and pathogenesis. Acta Ophthalmol 2009;87:1–20. Thesis 1.
7. Kirkegaard MM, Rasmussen PK, Coupland SE, Esmaeli B, Finger PT, Graue GF, et al. Conjunctival lymphoma—an international multicenter retrospective study. JAMA Ophthalmol. 2016;134(4):406–14.
8. Knudsen MKH, Rasmussen PK, Coupland SE, Esmaeli B, Finger PT, Graue GF, et al. Clinicopathological features of ocular adnexal mantle-cell lymphoma in an international multicenter cohort. JAMA Ophthalmol. 2017;135(12):1367–74.
9. Munch-Petersen HD, Rasmussen PK, Coupland SE, Esmaeli B, Finger PT, Graue GF, et al. Ocular adnexal diffuse large B-cell lymphoma: a multicenter international study. JAMA Ophthalmol. 2015;133(2):165–73.
10. Rasmussen PK, Coupland SE, Finger PT, Graue GF, Grossniklaus HE, Honavar SG, et al. Ocular adnexal follicular lymphoma: a multicenter international study. JAMA Ophthalmol. 2014;132(7):851–8.
11. Svendsen FH, Rasmussen PK, Coupland SE, Esmaeli B, Finger PT, Graue GF, et al. Lymphoma of the eyelid—an international multicenter retrospective study. Am J Ophthalmol. 2017;177:58–68.
12. Hindso TG, Esmaeli B, Holm F, Mikkelsen LH, Rasmussen PK, Coupland SE, et al. International multicentre retrospective cohort study of ocular adnexal marginal zone B-cell lymphoma. Br J Ophthalmol. 2020;104(3):357–62.
13. Vest SD, Mikkelsen LH, Holm F, Rasmussen PK, Hindso TG, Knudsen MKH, et al. Lymphoma of the lacrimal gland—an international multicenter retrospective study. Am J Ophthalmol. 2020;219:107–20.
14. Olsen TG, Holm F, Mikkelsen LH, Rasmussen PK, Coupland SE, Esmaeli B, et al. Orbital lymphoma-an international multicenter retrospective study. Am J Ophthalmol. 2019;199:44–57.
15. Finger P. International eye cancer registries: the need for world cooperation in ophthalmic oncology [Video]; 2021. Available from https://www.youtube.com/watch?v=UXizUboGEYw
16. Finger P. Cancer staging. In: Singh AD, Damato B, editors. Clinical ophthalmic oncology: basic principles and diagnostic techniques. 2nd ed. New York: Springer; 2014. p. 69–75.

17. Hawkins JW, Haggerty LA. Diversity in health care research strategies for multisite, multidisciplinary, and multicultural projects. New York: Springer; 2003.
18. Pakilit AT, Kahn BA, Petersen L, Abraham LS, Greendale GA, Ganz PA. Making effective use of tumor registries for cancer survivorship research. Cancer. 2001;92(5):1305–14.
19. Freshwater D. International research collaboration: issues, benefits and challenges of the global network. J Res Nurs. 2006;11(4):295–303.
20. Butrous G. International cooperation to promote advances in medicine. Ann Thorac Med. 2008;3(3):79–81.
21. Chen TJ, Chen YC, Hwang SJ, Chou LF. International collaboration of clinical medicine research in Taiwan, 1990-2004: a bibliometric analysis. J Chin Med Assoc. 2007;70(3):110–6.
22. Cheng A, Kessler D, Mackinnon R, Chang TP, Nadkarni VM, Hunt EA, et al. Conducting multicenter research in healthcare simulation: lessons learned from the INSPIRE network. Adv Simul (Lond). 2017;2:6.
23. Wachtell K. What is not to like about large national or international registries and databases? Int J Cardiol. 2018;262:117–8.
24. Belle GV, Kerr KF. Design and analysis of experiments in the health sciences. Hoboken: Wiley; 2013.
25. Robertson D, Williams GH. Clinical and translational science: principles of human research Cambridge. Massachusetts: Academic Press; 2017.
26. Marsolo K. Approaches to facilitate institutional review board approval of multicenter research studies. Med Care. 2012;50(Suppl):S77–81.
27. Lane-Fall M, Fleisher LA. Quality improvement and implementation science, an issue of anesthesiology clinics. Amsterdam: Elsevier - Health Science; 2018.
28. Huh J. Epidemiologic overview of malignant lymphoma. Korean J Hematol. 2012;47(2):92–104.
29. Kozlowicz J. Lunavi blog [Internet]. Cheyenne, Wyoming. Which database management platform is right for you? 2016 Jun 9 [cited 2021 Apr 19]. Available from: https://www.lunavi.com/blog/which-database-management-platform-is-right-for-you.
30. Cacace M. BoundState software blog [Internet]. Vancouver, Canada. Reasons to Beware of Using Excel as a Database; 2014 May 19 [cited 2021 Apr 19]. Available from: https://boundstatesoftware.com/blog/7-reasons-to-beware-of-using-excel-as-a-database.
31. Leitch D. Gridlines blog [Internet]. London, United Kingdom. Is excel the right tool for the job? 2021 Feb [cited 2021 Apr 19]. Available from: https://www.gridlines.com/is-excel-the-right-tool-for-the-job/.
32. Jones M. TechHQ blog [Internet]. Bristol, England. Should you use excel as a database? 2020 Oct 5 [cited 2021 Apr 19]. Available from: https://techhq.com/2020/10/should-you-use-microsoft-excel-as-a-database/.
33. Ganu G. Advance concepts of clinical research guidance for industry. Bilaspur, India: Sankalp Publishers; 2020.
34. Patridge E. Research electronic data capture (REDCap). J Med Libr Assoc. 2018;106(1):142–4.
35. Brembilla A, Martin B, Parmentier AL, Desmarets M, Falcoz PE, Puyraveau M, et al. How to set up a database?—a five-step process. J Thorac Dis. 2018;10(Suppl 29):S3533–S8.
36. Pezoulas VC, Exarchos TP, Fotiadis DI. Medical data sharing, harmonization and analytics. Cambridge, Massachusetts: Academic Press; 2020.
37. Adams-Huet B, Ahn C. Bridging clinical investigators and statisticians: writing the statistical methodology for a research proposal. J Investig Med. 2009;57(8):818–24.
38. Al-Hasan MN, Eckel-Passow JE, Baddour LM. Influence of referral bias on the clinical characteristics of patients with gram-negative bloodstream infection. Epidemiol Infect. 2011;139(11):1750–6.
39. Glen S. Referral Bias [Available from: https://www.statisticshowto.com/referral-bias/].
40. Sloan SS, Alper J, National Research C, Planning Committee for the Workshop on Culture Matters: An Approach to International Research A, Government-University-Industry Research R. Culture matters: international research collaboration in a changing world. Washington, D.C.: National Academies Press; 2014.

Big Data: The IRIS® Registry for Ocular Oncology

Ogul E. Uner and Alison H. Skalet

1 Introduction

Big data analyses provide important insights into presentation, demographics, treatment patterns, and outcomes and have particular importance in the study of rare disease. The Intelligent Research In Sight (IRIS®) Registry is a large electronic health record (EHR)-based disease registry in the United States designed for ophthalmology [1]. It collects ophthalmic data of interest, demographic information, and diagnosis and procedure codes in an automated fashion. It has been successfully queried to answer broad questions regarding incidence and prevalence of ophthalmic disease, treatment patterns, and outcomes in other eye conditions, but has not yet been evaluated for use in ocular oncology. This chapter will introduce the IRIS® Registry, discuss current challenges related to its use for study of ophthalmic tumors, and outline a strategy for future collaboration using this unique tool—the largest national clinical specialty data registry in the United States [2].

2 Large Data Sets in Ocular Oncology

The power of working with large clinical data sets is well recognized in ocular oncology. Over the past decades, several large data sets on patients with ocular cancers have been established. Studies using this data have led to important insights into the rare diseases we treat.

O. E. Uner
Department of Ophthalmology, Casey Eye Institute, Oregon Health & Science University, OR, USA
e-mail: uner@ohsu.edu

A. H. Skalet (✉)
Departments of Ophthalmology, Radiation Medicine, and Dermatology, Casey Eye Institute and Knight Cancer Institute, Oregon Health & Science University, Portland, OR, USA
e-mail: skalet@ohsu.edu

The American Joint Committee on Cancer (AJCC) Ophthalmic Oncology Task Force has one of the most well-known international registries for ocular oncology. The data are collected using patient-specific data fields selected by the committee of ophthalmic oncologists and pathologists and recorded by ophthalmic oncology centers worldwide [3]. Subsequently, the information is uploaded onto a secure Internet-based platform. These collaborations have led to many impactful studies. These include validation of AJCC classifications for uveal and conjunctival melanoma, assessing staging and treatment outcomes in retinoblastoma, and evaluating systemic findings in patients with stage IV metastatic uveal melanoma [4–7]. Most recently, the Task Force has been working to create the first international vitreoretinal lymphoma tumor registry, a significant undertaking to improve our understanding of the disease.

In Europe, there is a strong tradition of registry-based epidemiologic research. These regional registries provide comprehensive information owing to robust data collection practices. The European Cancer Registry includes data from 22 countries, 67 cancer registries, and over 100 million patients. Studies have evaluated incidence and survival of ocular cancers using this large data set [8, 9]. In individual countries, ocular tumors are generally included in national cancer databases. Dedicated registries have also been developed, including an eye tumor registry begun in Denmark in 2011, and, remarkably, a retinoblastoma registry that has been collecting patient information since 1862 in the Netherlands [10].

Registries for specific ocular cancers are on the horizon. For example, a Canada-based retinoblastoma-specific database called Disease-specific electronic Patient Illustrated Clinical Timeline^{RetinoBlastoma} (DePICT^{RB}) has been in development for decades and is now beginning to roll out in Canada, as well as internationally [11]. This registry involves an interactive computer-based data collection platform that is accessible to patients and families and contains a high level of detail. It was designed to facilitate communication among

B. V. Chawla, M. E. Aronow (eds.), *Global Perspectives in Ocular Oncology*, https://doi.org/10.1007/978-3-031-08250-4_5

colleagues and with patient families, as well as for research purposes. Data entry is complex on the front-end, but this detailed approach and intent for global involvement promise to position the DePICT[RB] platform as a strong contributor in retinoblastoma research worldwide.

In the United States, the Surveillance, Epidemiology, and End Results (SEER) Program has proven to be a useful tool in the study of ophthalmic cancers. SEER is a national cancer-related statistics platform from the U.S. National Cancer Institute that collects cancer incidence data. Since its inception in 1973, the program has evolved into multiple population-based cancer registries that cover 34.6% of the US population [12]. Records are updated annually. With over 10 million cases of cancer in the registry, the SEER Program has been used to report longitudinal incidence and prevalence, as well as 5-year survival rates of ocular cancers [13].

Administrative claim records provide access to both government and private insurance data for research purposes. These databases are not focused on ophthalmology or cancer specifically, and do not contain the level of detail present in ocular tumor registries, but have the significant advantage that they do not require dedicated data entry. In the United States, Medicare is one of the largest national health databases and includes up-to-date eye cancer information on approximately 53 million beneficiaries [14]. This group makes up approximately 98% of the US population older than 65 years of age [14]. Medicaid's Analytic eXtract (MAX) can provide de-identified data regarding both benign and malignant eye neoplasms [15]. The MarketScan Commercial Claims and Encounters Data produced by IBM Watson Health is another large database in the United States. It contains employer-sponsored insurance claim data totaling 43.6-million-person years in 2016 [16]. However, vision insurance is not included in these claims. As the largest managed vision care provider in the United States, the Vision Service Plan (VSP) provides claims data representing over a quarter of the US population. These data are represented in some states more than others [17]. The Centers for Disease Control and Prevention has formed the Vision and Eye Health Surveillance System (VEHSS) to compile and monitor these data [18]. This national system represents a growing data set that may have utility for claims-based research in ocular oncology.

3 The Intelligence Research in Sight (IRIS®) Registry

The IRIS® Registry is an ophthalmology-specific national database in the United States developed by the American Academy of Ophthalmology that has been active since 2014. The aims of the Registry are to improve vision care delivery and outcomes, help practices meet the Physician Quality Reporting System requirements, promote population health, and cultivate scientific knowledge [2]. As of July 1, 2017, a total of 37.3 million unique patient visits were connected to the Registry, representing 13,199 ophthalmologists [2]. Ophthalmologist registration is on a voluntary basis and the patient electronic health records (EHRs) are the primary source of data. Participating clinics and hospitals have data acquisition software installed on the server that houses the user's EHR database. Most client–server EHRs are compatible with the software, which periodically extracts information using an automated data-pull method. This method provides swift upload of information, significantly reducing physician effort in this process. A cloud-based site (AWS Gov Cloud; Amazon Web Services, Seattle, WA) houses the information uploaded and can send or store files in various servers. Here, the EHR data are separated into two components: protected health information and de-identified information. Only de-identified data are sent and stored in the IRIS® Registry database. As such, patient consent is not required according to the Health Insurance Portability and Accountability Act that protects the privacy of individually identifiable health information [1]. The Registry provides each patient with a unique identifier and collects patient information in defined data elements. These include patient demographics, vision care payers, pertinent clinical findings, diagnostic test results, and billing information in the form of Current Procedural Terminology or International Classification of Diseases codes [1].

The IRIS® Registry has been used to study epidemiology, practice patterns, and outcomes. As of July 2021, a total of 26 publications have utilized the IRIS® Registry. Most studies have investigated operative complication rates, such as endophthalmitis after cataract surgery, returns to the operating room after vitrectomy and cataract surgery for various reasons, and strabismus surgery reoperations [19–23]. In the area of oncology, the IRIS® Registry has been used to identify ophthalmic immune-related adverse events after immune checkpoint therapy [24]. The Registry has further been used to establish relationships between smoking and high intraocular pressure (IOP), intravitreal anti-vascular endothelial growth factor (VEGF) agents and high IOP, and intravitreal anti-VEGF and visual recovery in age-related macular degeneration [25–27]. Clinical outcome studies using the Registry include investigating factors associated with a less favorable laser trabeculoplasty response, refractive outcomes of sequential bilateral cataract surgery, and results of rhegmatogenous retinal detachment treated with pneumatic retinopexy [28–30]. More recently, it has been used to shed light on health and insurance disparities for anti-VEGF injections in the treatment of diabetic macular edema [31]. In addition, the Registry has been used for economic analyses, investigating cost savings with increased intravitreal bevacizumab reimbursements using both IRIS® and Medicare claims data

[32]. The quality and breadth of these studies are testaments to the IRIS® Registry's power in ophthalmology research.

There are several advantages to researchers interested in utilization of the IRIS® Registry. First and foremost, the Registry allows researchers to study diseases that would be expensive and difficult to study with randomized clinical trials. The software is easy to implement, predetermined data elements are pulled in an automated fashion without need for manual data entry, and the database is updated more frequently than many large data sets. In addition, its large size and inclusion of both administrative and clinical information make IRIS® the most comprehensive national eye registry in the United States, capable of improving performance rates in cataract surgery, retina, and glaucoma [33]. The Registry may have the potential to influence preferred practice patterns in ophthalmology in the future.

The IRIS® Registry has shortcomings as well. The software extracts data using completed patient records that are part of the patient's medical chart. As these cannot be altered, the Registry cannot request any changes or additions to the data acquired. Most ophthalmology EHRs do not include hospital-based visits or details of outpatient surgeries. Hence, information regarding preoperative care, anesthesia, and intraoperative care may not be present in the database. Furthermore, there may be inherent limitations in the captured data set depending on the pre-existing fields of the EHR studied [1]. As more EHRs are linked into the Registry database, increased communication between EHR vendors and Registry users will likely address these limitations.

4 The IRIS® Registry and Ocular Oncology

Large data sets have great potential in ocular oncology. Though prospective clinical studies including clinical trials remain essential for evidence-based cancer care, the power of studying rare diseases using automated data collection has potential for significant impact in our field. Many areas of ophthalmology were swift in starting to use the IRIS® Registry from its inception. Ocular oncology was not among these early adopters. This was due, in part, to the lack of inclusion of important data elements in the IRIS® Registry related to care and outcomes for ocular malignancies. For example, a patient with uveal melanoma might have a chief complaint, visual acuity, examination findings, and local treatment compiled as de-identified information. However, the Registry would not include biopsy results, information regarding metastatic progression, mortality data, or systemic imaging and treatment information. Another current challenge is that while many academic ophthalmology centers are now included in the Registry, care for ocular oncology patients is often multidisciplinary, takes places in both hospital and outpatient settings including some private practices, and data from these practice settings are not yet incorporated.

Nonetheless, the IRIS® Registry provides opportunities for research to ocular oncologists in its current form and there is potential for future adaptation to expand its utility. For example, as patients have unique identifiers, patients diagnosed with ophthalmic tumors could be tracked geographically from time of diagnosis to determine how frequently these patients are referred to a tertiary eye care center versus receiving local care. In addition, encounters for post-treatment care can be collected and analyzed for outcomes such as visual acuity—a data element not present in other US-based registries such as insurance databases and SEER. Similarly, treatment for radiation retinopathy can be studied, as intravitreal injections and vision outcomes are well documented in the Registry.

5 Strategies for Growth

To study the outcomes of greatest interest in our field, expansion of the data elements being extracted in the IRIS® Registry will be necessary. There are several strategies being investigated to better harness the power of the IRIS® Registry for the study of ophthalmic cancers. The first strategy is development and implementation of minimum data sets for specific cancers. Minimum data sets developed by disease experts constitute a standardized group of data elements deemed to be of importance for the study of a specific disease. A proposed minimum data set for uveal melanoma, for example, might include the anatomic location, tumor dimensions, primary treatment, molecular prognostic information, and outcomes related to local and distant recurrence. The American Association of Ophthalmic Oncologists and Pathologists is actively engaged in the development of minimum data sets for intraocular cancers, with plans to expand to conjunctival tumors next. In parallel, minimum data sets for ophthalmic pathology are being developed.

Once a minimum data set is developed, there are various strategies for inclusion of data elements not currently being collected by the automated data-pull method of the IRIS® Registry. One involves use of standardized discrete data entry forms within the EHR, which then can be mapped for automated retrieval by the IRIS® Registry. Many physicians in the United States are already working within their EHRs to develop similar clinic- or institution-based data-pull systems for data collection. Ultimately, direct partnership with the IRIS® Registry to develop systems for extracting elements of interest would promote future ocular oncology studies using the Registry. In addition, centers are continually being added to the Registry, expanding its footprint. There is potential for future cooperative data sharing and inclusion of non-ophthalmic records.

The IRIS® Registry has the power to provide valuable information regarding ophthalmic disease presentation and outcomes, identify areas for improvement in care, and influence practice patterns in all areas of ophthalmology practice, including ocular oncology. While there are existing hurdles for implementation of the IRIS® Registry for study of ophthalmic cancers, there is also significant promise. Leveraging the IRIS® Registry to perform big data analyses for ophthalmic cancers has significant potential to improve our understanding of the rare diseases we treat and ultimately lead to improved care for our patients.

References

1. Chiang MF, et al. The 2016 American Academy of Ophthalmology IRIS® registry (intelligent research in sight) database. Ophthalmology. 2018;125(8):1143–8.
2. Parke DW 2nd, et al. The American Academy of Ophthalmology's IRIS(®) registry (intelligent research in sight clinical data): a look Back and a look to the future. Ophthalmology. 2017;124(11):1572–4.
3. Tomar AS, et al. A multicenter, international collaborative study for American joint committee on cancer staging of retinoblastoma. Ophthalmology. 2020;127(12):1719–32.
4. Garg G, et al. Patients presenting with metastases: stage IV uveal melanoma, an international study. Br J Ophthalmol. 2021;
5. Jain P, et al. Multicenter, international assessment of the eighth edition of the American Joint Committee on Cancer Staging Manual for Conjunctival Melanoma. JAMA Ophthalmology. 2019;137(8)
6. Jain P, et al. Conjunctival melanoma treatment outcomes in 288 patients: a multicentre international data-sharing study. Br J Ophthalmol. 2020;
7. Force AOOT. International validation of the American Joint Committee on Cancer's 7th edition classification of uveal melanoma. JAMA Ophthalmol. 2015;133(4):376–83.
8. Virgili G, et al. Survival in patients with uveal melanoma in Europe. Arch Ophthalmol. 2008;126(10):1413–8.
9. Sjö LD, et al. Primary lymphoma of the lacrimal sac: an EORTC ophthalmic oncology task force study. Br J Ophthalmol. 2006;90(8):1004–9.
10. Nilbert M, et al. The power of empirical data; lessons from the clinical registry initiatives in Scandinavian cancer care. Acta Oncol. 2020;59(11):1343–56.
11. wechope, DePICT the Cancer Care Journey, Overcome Rarity Through Collaborative Research—WE C Hope; 2018.
12. Statistics, N.C.I. Surveillance, epidemiology, and end results program; 2021 [cited 2021 July 4]. Available from: https://seer.cancer.gov/index.html.
13. Aronow ME, Topham AK, Singh AD. Uveal melanoma: 5-year update on incidence, treatment, and survival (SEER 1973-2013). Ocular Oncol Pathol. 2018;4(3):145–51.
14. 2019 Medicare Enrollment Section | CMS. 2021 July 4, 2021]. Available from: https://www.cms.gov/research-statistics-data-systems/cms-program-statistics/2019-medicare-enrollment-section#Fee-For-Service%20Medicare%20Enrollment.
15. Initiative, T.C.f.D.C. and H. Prevention Vision. Medicaid administrative claims records; 2021 2021-06-09T10:16:21Z [cited 2021 July 4]. Available from: https://www.cdc.gov/visionhealth/vehss/data/claims/medicaid.html.
16. Corporation, I.B.M. MarketScan research databases; 2021 2021-03-23 [cited 2021 July 4]. Available from: https://www.ibm.com/products/marketscan-research-databases.
17. Initiative, T.C.f.D.C. and H. Prevention Vision. *VSP Global Administrative Claims Records*. 2021 2021-06-15T03:15:43Z [cited 2021 July 4]. Available from: https://www.cdc.gov/visionhealth/vehss/data/claims/vsp.html.
18. Initiative, T.C.f.D.C. and H. Prevention Vision. *Vision and Eye Health Surveillance System*. 2021 2021-06-17T02:07:08Z [cited 2021 July 4]. Available from: https://www.cdc.gov/visionhealth/vehss/index.html.
19. Pershing S, et al. Endophthalmitis after cataract surgery in the United States: a report from the intelligent research in sight registry, 2013-2017. Ophthalmology. 2020;127(2):151–8.
20. Mahr MA, et al. Return to the operating room for removal of retained lens fragments after cataract surgery: IRIS® registry (intelligent research in sight) analysis. Ophthalmology. 2020;127(5):698–9.
21. Repka MX, Lum F, Burugapalli B. Strabismus, strabismus surgery, and reoperation rate in the United States: analysis from the IRIS registry. Ophthalmology. 2018;125(10):1646–53.
22. Rubino SM, Parke DW 3rd, Lum F. Return to the operating room after vitrectomy for vitreous opacities: intelligent research in sight registry analysis. Ophthalmol Retina. 2021;5(1):4–8.
23. Parke DW 3rd, Lum F. Return to the operating room after macular surgery: IRIS registry analysis. Ophthalmology. 2018;125(8):1273–8.
24. Sun MM, et al. Ophthalmic immune-related adverse events after anti-CTLA-4 or PD-1 therapy recorded in the American Academy of Ophthalmology Intelligent Research in Sight Registry. Ophthalmology. 2021;128(6):910–9.
25. Lee CS, et al. Smoking is associated with higher intraocular pressure regardless of glaucoma: a retrospective study of 12.5 million patients using the intelligent research in sight (IRIS®) registry. Ophthalmol Glaucoma. 2020;3(4):253–61.
26. Atchison EA, et al. The real-world effect of Intravitreous anti-vascular endothelial growth factor drugs on intraocular pressure: an analysis using the IRIS registry. Ophthalmology. 2018;125(5):676–82.
27. Rao P, et al. Real-world vision in age-related macular degeneration patients treated with single anti-VEGF drug type for 1 year in the IRIS registry. Ophthalmology. 2018;125(4):522–8.
28. Chang TC, et al. Factors associated with favorable laser trabeculoplasty response: IRIS registry analysis. Am J Ophthalmol. 2021;223:149–58.
29. Yannuzzi NA, et al. Clinical outcomes of rhegmatogenous retinal detachment treated with pneumatic retinopexy. JAMA Ophthalmol. 2021;
30. Owen JP, et al. Refractive outcomes after immediate sequential vs delayed sequential bilateral cataract surgery. JAMA Ophthalmol. 2021;
31. Malhotra NA, et al. Racial, ethnic, and insurance-based disparities upon initiation of anti-vascular endothelial growth factor therapy for diabetic macular edema in the US. Ophthalmology. 2021;
32. Glasser DB, et al. Intravitreal anti-vascular endothelial growth factor cost savings achievable with increased bevacizumab reimbursement and use. Ophthalmology. 2020;127(12):1688–92.
33. Rich WL 3rd, et al. Performance rates measured in the American Academy of Ophthalmology IRIS(©) registry (intelligent research in sight). Ophthalmology. 2018;125(5):782–4.

Part II

Multidisciplinary Perspectives

Intravenous Chemotherapy for Retinoblastoma: A Pediatric Oncologist's Perspective

Amish Shah and Ann M. Leahey

1 Introduction

The primary goal in treating a child with retinoblastoma (RB) is to save the patient's life. Intravenous (IV) chemotherapy is the most frequently used RB treatment worldwide and, unlike newer focal chemotherapy delivery routes, is available in 98% of centers surveyed in a recent global analysis [1]. In high-income countries, where RB is overwhelmingly contained within the globe at the time of diagnosis, multiple authors have proposed that intraocular RB should be a zero death cancer [2, 3] and that conservative treatment of RB should never compromise "the state of metastatic grace" [4].

However, the Global Retinoblastoma Study Group gathered data on greater than 4000 patients from 153 countries and found that 85% of patients with RB live in low- and middle-income countries. Sadly, 25% of patients from middle-income countries will have extraocular disease at the time of presentation and almost 50% of patients with RB in low-income countries will have extraocular spread at diagnosis [1].

Although intravenous chemotherapy (also referred to as systemic chemotherapy) was employed to treat RB outside the globe for more than 50 years, it was not until the 1990s that a regimen effective for intraocular RB was found. The regimen of carboplatin, etoposide, and vincristine (CEV) had shown success in treating childhood brain tumors, successfully crossing the blood brain barrier. American, Canadian, and European investigators trialed variations of the CEV regimen and the use of intravenous chemotherapy for intraocular RB was born [5–8]. CEV has also recently been shown in rigorous prospective studies to be highly effective in the adjuvant setting (following frontline enucleation) and in the setting of stage III RB [8, 9]. Higher doses of CEV are required for the latter indication. As systemic chemotherapy is active against intraocular and extraocular disease, understanding how and when to administer it is critical to saving the life and preserving as much vision as possible in children with RB worldwide.

A. Shah · A. M. Leahey (✉)
Perelman School of Medicine at the University of Pennsylvania and the Children's Hospital of Philadelphia, Philadelphia, PA, USA
e-mail: shahac@chop.edu; Leahey@chop.edu

2 General Principles of Cancer Chemotherapy

The strategy for curing cancer is based upon exploiting differences between cancer cells and the normal host cells. The rationale for the use of combination chemotherapy regimens is to overcome resistance to individual agents. This bedrock principle is based on the seminal observation in childhood acute lymphoblastic leukemia (ALL) that approximately 60% of patients achieved remission with a single drug while three- and four-drug regimens including the same single agent induced remission in greater than 95% of patients [10].

Two main factors are critical to a particular regimen's success. Firstly, successful regimens contain agents that are non-cross-resistant and preferably have synergistic or additive mechanisms of action against the tumor. Additionally, regimens should have non-overlapping toxicity profiles. This factor is critical as dose reductions or delays can compromise cure. To ensure timely and safe administration of intravenous chemotherapy, it is important to understand individual drug mechanisms of action and the spectrum of toxicities.

3 General Mechanisms of Action

Conventional drugs used in the treatment of childhood cancers are cytotoxic agents that non-selectively damage deoxyribonucleic acid (DNA), ribonucleic acid (RNA), or vital pathways critical to normal cells. For example, topoisomer-

B. V. Chawla, M. E. Aronow (eds.), *Global Perspectives in Ocular Oncology*, https://doi.org/10.1007/978-3-031-08250-4_6

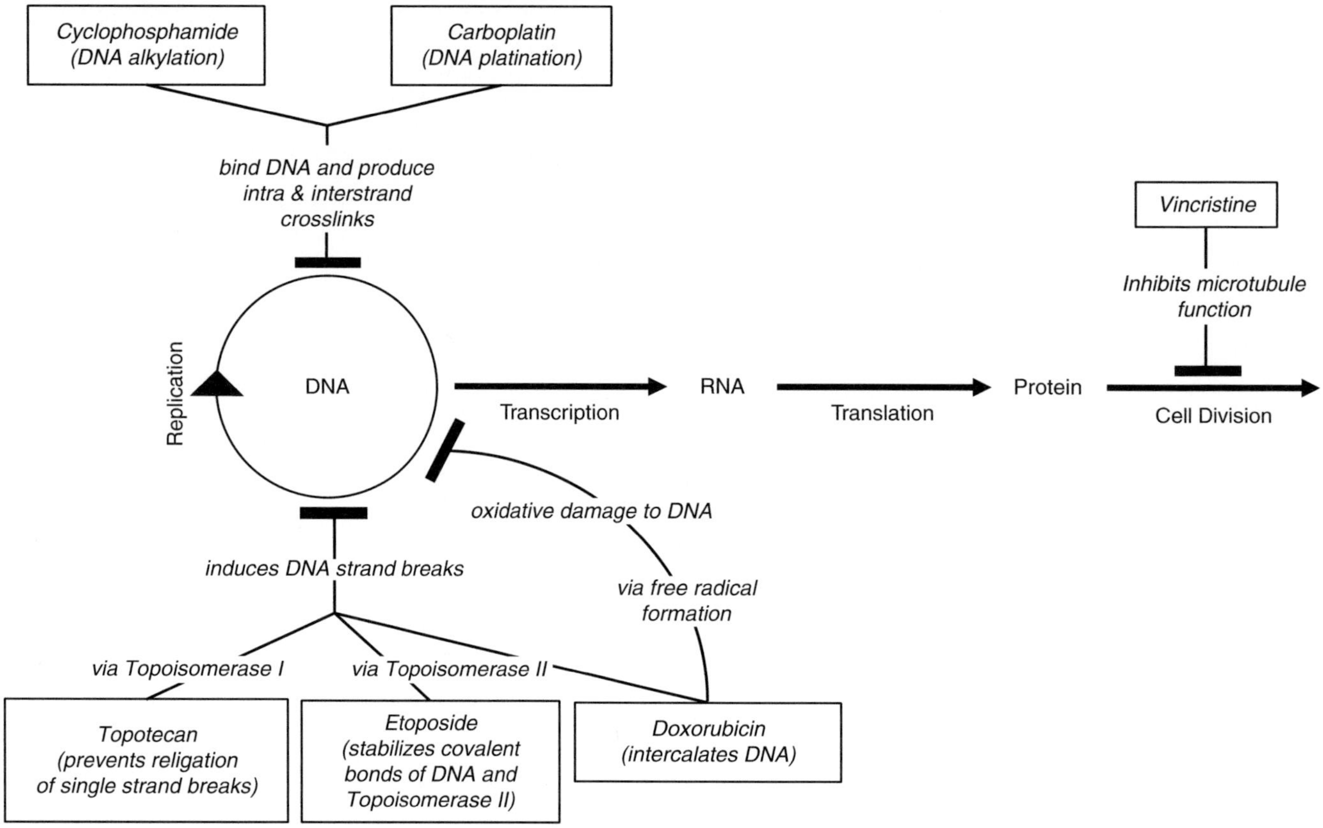

Fig. 1 Mechanisms of action of commonly used chemotherapeutic agents

ase inhibitors such as epipodophyllotoxins interfere with DNA religation, resulting in DNA strand breaks. Figure 1 depicts the mechanisms of activity of chemotherapy agents commonly used in the treatment of RB.

The term pharmacokinetics refers to quantitative aspects of drug delivery in the body including absorption, distribution, metabolism, and excretion (abbreviated ADME). Substantial interpatient variability in drug disposition and systemic exposure occurs with most anticancer drugs. For instance, administering a standard dose of etoposide leads to a two- to ten-fold range in systemic drug exposure [11]. Particularly important in the chemotherapeutic management of children with RB are the age-related developmental changes in body composition and organ function such as variation in the kidney function affecting excretion of chemotherapy agents. Kearns and colleagues warned that failure to account the ontogeny of organ failure can result in exposure to potentially toxic serum levels of drugs [12]. For example, renal blood flow, glomerular filtration, and tubular secretion are all decreased in children under the age of one. Notably, most children with bilateral RB present in the first year of life.

4 Individual Mechanisms of Action and Unique Toxicities in Agents Commonly Used to Treat Retinoblastoma

4.1 Carboplatin

Carboplatin and its related compound cisplatin are referred to as non-classical alkylating agents. They exert their effects by platination of DNA, a mechanism analogous to alkylation. In the case of carboplatin, reactive intermediates covalently bind to DNA and form intrastrand and interstrand DNA crosslinks [13]. The primary route of elimination of carboplatin is renal. In children less than 1 year of age the clearance is reduced, likely related to age-related differences in glomerular filtration rate. The clearance of carboplatin has been shown to be highly correlated with creatinine clearance. This association has led to formulas for individualized carboplatin doses. However, caution must be employed when using these formulas as a dose normalized to body surface area (such as the Calvert formula) can place children under the age of one at risk for excessive toxicity [14].

One toxicity of particular concern in children with RB treated with carboplatin is ototoxicity. Reports from the Dutch, French, and Philadelphia groups place this risk at approximately 1%, while reports from St. Jude and Canadian teams found substantially higher rates [15–19]. The teams finding low rates of ototoxicity employed six cycles of standard dose CEV. St Jude utilized eight cycles with a body surface area dosing strategy, which leads to increased drug exposure in infants. Additionally, almost half of their patients received external beam radiotherapy (EBRT), which can also be a risk factor for ototoxicity. The recent report from the Canadian team utilized cyclosporine in addition to CEV in an attempt to modulate drug resistance. Cyclosporine is known to cause nephrotoxicity and subclinical changes in renal function could have altered drug exposure and potentially led to increased ototoxicity.

4.2 Etoposide

Etoposide exerts its antitumor effect through stabilization of normally transient covalent intermediates formed between DNA and topoisomerase II. This results in single- and double-strand DNA breaks [20]. Renal clearance accounts for only one-third of the total systemic clearance. Pharmacokinetic parameters do not vary substantially in children and thus no specialized dosing guidelines are needed for infants [21].

The most feared toxicity of etoposide is the development of secondary leukemia that occurs due to a chromosomal translocation of the KMT2A gene at chromosome band 11q23 resulting in monocytic or myelomonocytic leukemia [22]. These leukemias are characterized by a short latency period with a median time to presentation of 30 months. The risk is dose and schedule dependent. In children with ALL treated with high cumulative doses of epipodophyllotoxins on a weekly or twice weekly (not on consecutive days) schedule, this risk can be as high as 12% [23]. In contrast, the incidence of this secondary leukemia in germ cell tumor survivors treated with lower doses is less than 1% [24]. It is important to note that a frequently referenced report of 15 patients with RB treated with intravenous chemotherapy who developed myelodysplastic syndrome or acute myelogenous leukemia did not include any patients who received standard dose CEV [25]. The majority had received external beam radiation and/or alkylating agents. German physicians who previously treated patients with cyclophosphamide concurrently with CEV have now eliminated cyclophosphamide from their treatment regimens to avoid this complication [26].

A report from the Surveillance Epidemiology and End Result (SEER) registry found no cases of secondary acute myelogenous leukemia (sAML) in 158 survivors of RB treated with chemotherapy [27]. Lastly, of the first 245 consecutive Philadelphia patients treated with CEV there were no cases of sAML in patients treated with chemotherapy alone. There was one case of acute promyelocytic leukemia that developed 7 years after a combination of EBRT and CEV [28]. The combination of EBRT and chemotherapy is known to be synergistic in causing secondary cancers in patients with RB [29].

4.3 Vincristine

Vincristine is a vinca alkaloid that binds to tubulin, a dimeric protein that polymerizes to form microtubules. Thus, vincristine inhibits mitotic spindle formation, causing metaphase arrest during mitosis. Neurotoxicity is the dose-limiting toxicity of vincristine and occurs more commonly on a weekly schedule not regularly employed in the treatment of RB. Practically, neuropathic pain in young children can manifest as oral pain that can interfere with feeding. This usually responds well to acetaminophen. If acetaminophen is insufficient, a 25% dose reduction for subsequent cycles can be used. Additionally, autonomic nerve involvement can lead to constipation. The risk of vincristine neurotoxicity is substantially elevated in children with Charcot-Marie-Tooth syndrome [30]. Lastly, vincristine can rarely cause seizures due to hyponatremia related to the syndrome of inappropriate antidiuretic hormone (SIADH).

In developed nations, central venous lines (often implanted ports) are usually placed prior to administration of the first cycle of chemotherapy. This is in part due to concern that vincristine extravasation from peripheral intravenous lines can cause chemical burns. Central venous lines increase the risk of blood stream infections and also the financial costs of care. They also may be associated with blood clots leading to the need for systemic anticoagulation. Both of these complications are potentially fatal compared to the morbidity (but not mortality) of peripheral intravenous lines. A report from a center with a large RB practice found no episodes of extravasation in 270 doses of vincristine administered by peripheral intravenous lines [31]. It is important that peripheral intravenous lines not be placed over a joint as extravasation could result in a joint contracture. In sum, peripheral intravenous lines are a low cost and safe alternative that can be utilized worldwide.

4.4 Doxorubicin

Doxorubicin is an anthracycline that is red in color. It can intercalate into DNA and induce topoisomerase-II-mediated single- and double-stranded breaks. Although this is experimentally the most important mechanism of action, anthracyclines can also block helicase catalyzed dissociation of duplex DNA and oxidize DNA bases. Additionally, anthracyclines can undergo chemical reduction yielding free radical intermediates. The main acute toxicity of doxorubicin is mucositis. This is in contradistinction to CEV, which does not cause mucosal toxicity. Extravasation of anthracyclines can result in severe local tissue damage with deep ulcerations that are slow to heal and difficult to skin graft. Thus, unlike vincristine, the risk–benefit ratio favors central line administration of doxorubicin.

Anthracyclines can cause acute and chronic cardiac toxicities. Acutely, arrhythmias can be seen as well as drops in left ventricular function with variable recovery. Chronic anthracycline toxicity is dose related. However, there is no safe dose as cumulative doses as low as 101 mg/m^2 have been associated with cardiomyopathy [32]. At greatest risk are those patients under the age of five. Girls have a significantly higher risk than boys. An approach to the prevention of anthracycline toxicity is the co-administration of the chelating agent dexrazoxane. This agent undergoes intracellular hydrolysis to a compound similar to ethylenediamine tetraacetic acid (EDTA), which tightly binds iron, a cofactor in anthracycline free radical reactions. The dexrazoxane dose in milligrams is ten times the dose of the anthracycline administered [33]. In trials of patients with acute lymphoblastic leukemia, dexrazoxane did not diminish the antileukemia effect of doxorubicin. In diseases other than Hodgkin's Disease in childhood (which carries an elevated risk of second malignant neoplasms), no increased risk of secondary acute myelogenous leukemia has accompanied the use of dexrazoxane [34, 35]. Lastly, it should be noted that doxorubicin can cause a radiation recall phenomenon if used after EBRT [36].

4.5 Cyclophosphamide

Cyclophosphamide is a nitrogen mustard derivative and an oxazaphosphorine. This type of agent exists as an inactive prodrug that requires biotransformation by the liver to express its alkylating activity. A unique toxicity of cyclophosphamide is hemorrhagic cystitis, which can range from mild dysuria to severe bladder hemorrhage. To lessen the incidence and severity of this complication, patients should be aggressively hydrated. Additionally, after those patients receiving a dose greater than 1 g/m^2, concurrent 2-mercaptoethane sulfonate (MESNA) should be administered either intravenously or orally [37].

4.6 Topotecan

Topotecan is a semisynthetic camptothecin analog that induces DNA strand breaks by complexing with topoisomerase I. In the treatment of intraocular RB, topotecan can be used intravenously in combination with vincristine. A recent study from the St. Jude team used pharmacokinetically guided dosing of topotecan with vincristine alternating with cycles of vincristine and carboplatin. Unlike standard CEV, grade 4 neutropenia was seen in the majority of patients with two-thirds of patients experiencing fever and neutropenia and/or requiring platelet transfusion. Bacteremia occurred in 13% of patients [38]. Thus, this strategy is challenging in developing countries. Topotecan can also be administered intrathecally or intraventricularly. Although safe and well tolerated, objective antitumor activity was not observed in a Phase I study of brain tumors [39].

5 General Toxicities of Cytotoxic Chemotherapy Regimens

As discussed, each individual chemotherapy agent can have distinct toxicities but there are also toxicities that are common across agents. Assessment of the exact incidence and severity of toxicity has been difficult due to the retrospective nature of many studies of chemotherapy for RB. However, the Children's Oncology Group recently reported a study of 102 RB patients who received 6 cycles of standard dose CEV. Toxicity data from this prospective trial were collected by certified clinical research associates and graded according to the gold standard Common Terminology Criteria of Adverse Events (CTCAE). As is customary, grade 3/4 toxicities were catalogued.

In this study, 76% of patients did not experience grade 3 or greater toxicity. The most common grade 3/4 toxicity was neutropenia occurring in 14% of patients with febrile neutropenia in 11% [8]. Allergic reactions to carboplatin and thrombocytopenia were each seen in 5% of patients. Grade 3/4 vomiting and dehydration were seen in 4% and 2% of patients, respectively, despite the use of pre-emptive antiemetics. Two patients had grade 3/4 anemia. Another two had elevation in aminotransferase levels. Grade 3/4 anorexia, constipation, headaches, and rash were seen in <1% of patients. It should be noted that grade 3 alopecia does not exist as a category and that almost all patients will experience this side effect. It is standard that patients treated with six cycles of CEV receive prophylactic oral Bactrim to prevent pneumocystis pneumonia.

6 Intravenous Chemotherapy Regimens for Intraocular Retinoblastoma

It is important to state explicitly the three goals of therapy from the perspective of the pediatric oncologist. It is critical to understand that these goals are not co-equal: that is, a child's life should never be put at risk in pursuit of goals 2 and 3.

1. Save the child's life.
2. Save as much vision as possible.
3. Avoid the use of external beam radiotherapy in patients with heritable RB because its use can triple the risk of a second cancer.

Appropriate use of systemic chemotherapy is predicated upon correct assessment of the amount of intraocular and extraocular disease. Until recently, intraocular disease was stratified by the International Classification System for Intraocular Retinoblastoma (ICRB) [40]. This classification system assigned Groups A through E based on the size of tumors, amount of seeding, and the presence or absence of poor prognostic factors (Table 1). However, variations of the ICRB existed and thus publications were sometimes difficult to compare. More recently, the American Joint Committee on Cancer (AJCC) proposed a new classification schema to describe more explicitly the clinical and pathological status as well as the hereditary status of the patient (Table 2). The AJCC classification has now been validated in a data set of 2097 patients [41]. The AJCC system also included a schema to stratify extraocular disease. In this chapter, planning based on the ICRB and prior International Staging System of stages 0–4 (Table 3) [42] will be discussed as these were utilized in the reports cited in this chapter.

Table 1 International Classification of Retinoblastoma (ICRB)

Group	Quick reference	Specific features
A	Small tumor	Retinoblastoma (RB) <3 mm in size
B	Larger tumor • Macula. • Juxtapapillary. • Subretinal fluid.	RB >3 mm in size, or • Macular RB location (<3 mm to foveola). • Juxtapapillary RB location (<1.5 mm to disk). • Clear subretinal fluid <3 mm from margin.
C	Focal seeds	RB with • Subretinal seeds <3 mm from RB. • Vitreous seeds <3 mm from RB. • Both subretinal and vitreous seeds <3 mm from RB.
D	Diffuse seeds	RB with • Subretinal seeds >3 mm from RB. • Vitreous seeds >3 mm from RB. • Both subretinal and vitreous seeds >3 mm from RB.
E	Extensive RB	Extensive RB • Neovascular glaucoma. • Opaque media from hemorrhage in anterior chamber, vitreous, or subretinal space. • Invasion of post-laminar optic nerve, choroid (>3 mm), sclera, orbit, and anterior chamber.

7 Chemoreduction

The term chemoreduction refers to the use of intravenous chemotherapy to reduce the size of tumors such that focal modalities such as laser, plaque brachytherapy, or cryotherapy can control residual disease. It should be stressed that this is a combined modality approach and that chemoreduction without consolidative focal therapies will fail to control intraocular disease in over 90% of eyes [43]. Ideally, sys-

Table 2 American Joint Committee on Cancer (AJCC) eighth edition Tumor, Node, Metastasis, Heredity (TNMH) clinical staging compared to International Intraocular Retinoblastoma Classification (IIRC) group classification of intraocular retinoblastoma

AJCC	IIRC
cTX: Unknown evidence of intraocular tumor	
cT0: No evidence of intraocular tumor	
cT1: Intraretinal tumor(s) with subretinal fluid <5 mm from tumor base; no seeding	
cT1a: Tumors ≤3 mm in size and >1.5 mm away from the optic disk and fovea	A
cT1b: Tumors >3 mm in size and <1.5 mm away from the optic disk and fovea	B
cT2: Tumors with retinal detachment/subretinal seeding/vitreal seeding	
cT2a: Subretinal fluid >5 mm from tumor base	C/D
cT2b: Tumors with subretinal seeding/vitreal seeding	C/D/E
cT3: Advanced intraocular tumor(s)	
cT3a: Phthisis or prephthisis bulbi	E
cT3b: Tumor invasion of choroid, pars plana, ciliary body, lens, zonules, iris, or anterior chamber	E
cT3c: Raised intraocular pressure with neovascularization or buphthalmos	E
cT3d: Hyphema and/or massive vitreal hemorrhage	E
cT3e: Aseptic orbital cellulitis	E
cT4: Extraocular tumor involving orbit, including optic nerve	

Table 3 International Retinoblastoma Staging System (IRSS)

Stage	
0	Intraocular disease, conservative treatment
1	Eye enucleated, tumor completely resected
2	Eye enucleated, microscopic residual tumor
3	Regional extension, overt orbital disease ± preauricular or cervical lymph node extension
4a	Hematogenous metastases
4b	Central nervous system disease

Table 4 Standard dose CEV (for 6 cycles every 28 days)

		Age <36 months	Age ≥36 months	
Carboplatin	IV	18.6 mg/kg	560 mg/m^2	Day 1
Etoposide	IV	5 mg/kg	150 mg/m^2	Days 1 and 2
Vincristine	IV	0.05 mg/kg	1.5 mg/m^2	Day 1

Abbreviations: CEV Carboplatin, etoposide, and vincristine, *IV* Intravenous
Note: Maximum vincristine dose <2 mg

temic chemotherapy is given within 24 h of focal ophthalmic therapies. Focal cryorupture allows improved chemotherapy penetration into the vitreous and/or subretinal fluid.

The most commonly employed chemotherapy regimen is CEV. Standard dosing typically refers to carboplatin 18.6 mg/kg IV daily × 1, etoposide 5 mg/kg daily IV × 2, and vincristine 0.05 mg/kg IV daily × 1. Patients aged three or greater are dosed based on a per meter squared basis by the Children's Oncology Group (Table 4) [35]. This regimen is given on every 28 day schedule for a planned 6 cycles. Nearly 100% of Group A tumors can be controlled with focal ophthalmic therapies alone and systemic chemotherapy is not needed. A report published in 2006 detailed ocular salvage rate of 93% and 90% for Group B and C eyes, respectively. However, with standard dose CEV, only 47% of Group D eyes were effectively salvaged [44].

A more recent report from this institution detailed the outcomes of 964 eyes in 554 patients treated with frontline chemoreduction [45]. With a median follow-up of 57 months, ocular salvage without the need for external beam radiotherapy was 96% for Group A eyes, 91% for Group B eyes, 91% for Group C eyes, and 71% for Group D eyes. In this subsequent report, the majority of patients with Group D or E disease in their more affected eye received 50% higher dosing of carboplatin—14 mg/kg daily × 2 days for patients less than 36 months of age (420 mg/m^2 daily × 2 days for greater than 3 years of age)—and 20% higher dosing of etoposide—6 mg/kg × 2 days for patients less than 36 months (180 mg/m^2/daily × 2 days for patients greater than 3 years of age)—given with standard dose vincristine. This intensified regimen was given in conjunction with granulocyte colony stimulating factor beginning in 1998, which changed to pegfilgrastim in 2002. The dose of pegfilgastim is 100 ug/kg given subcutaneously 24 h after the completion of a chemotherapy cycle. After frontline therapy, 4% of these patients received intra-arterial chemotherapy and 3% received intravitreal chemotherapy. Only 32% of a selected group of E eyes managed with frontline chemotherapy—usually in patients with bilateral advanced disease—were salvaged. Notably, only 2% of Group E eyes so salvaged had a final visual acuity greater than 20/40. This is in comparison to the majority of Group A eyes, one-third of Group B and C eyes, and one-tenth of Group D eyes. There were few events after 2 years of follow-up, with the range of follow-up extending to 25 years. Critically, less than 0.4% of patients so treated died of metastatic disease.

Demirci and colleagues in a smaller subset of patients had found that two-thirds of eyes salvaged with intravenous chemotherapy alone have 20/200 vision or better at a mean follow-up of 68 months [46]. French investigators recently reported their experience with chemoreduction for bilateral macular RB (or unilateral macular RB if the patient was monocular). Treatment with CEV and macular sparing transpupillary thermotherapy saved 24 of 26 eyes with a median visual acuity of 20/50. One-quarter of the eyes salvaged had visual acuity worse than 20/200. A strength of this paper was that the median follow-up was 77 months [47].

The major cause of intraocular treatment failure is resistant seeding. This is usually intravitreal but can be subretinal, in the aqueous, or retrohyaloid. As these spaces should be avascular, systemic chemotherapy must enter by diffusion. Conceptually, these are sanctuary sites akin to the central nervous system in the treatment of acute leukemia. As most anticancer drugs penetrate into the cerebrospinal fluid poorly, strategies to circumvent the blood brain barrier have been in use for the treatment of acute leukemia for 50 years. In fact, the greatest advance in the treatment of acute lymphoblastic leukemia (ALL) was the introduction of pre-emptive (prior to the onset of clinical disease) intrathecal chemotherapy. The overall survival in ALL was approximately 20% prior to the advent of intrathecal chemotherapy and tripled to 60% with the introduction of intrathecal therapy [48].

A similar breakthrough occurred in RB in 2012 when Munier directly injected melphalan into the vitreous humor [49]. Compared to systemic and intra-arterial delivery routes of chemotherapy where milligram doses are needed, the doses of intravitreal chemotherapy (typically melphalan ± topotecan) are measured in micrograms. Ocular survival of patients with Group D and selected Group E eyes was found to be 77% at 5 years by the team from Lausanne. However, Berry and colleagues have warned that combining systemic chemotherapy and concurrent intravitreal chemotherapy may risk increase in ocular toxicity [50]. The Children's Oncology Group is presently planning to study this in a prospective trial of CEV in combination with intravitreal chemotherapy.

8 Adjuvant Chemotherapy

For over 200 years, enucleation has been used for the treatment of RB and is still performed in every RB center in the world. It is the least costly and most expeditious treatment. There has been a substantial decrease in the use of enucleation over the last three decades. In the 1970s, Shields and colleagues used enucleation for treatment of unilateral RB in

96% of cases (before the discovery of effective chemotherapy for intraocular RB) [51]. Abramson and coworkers utilized enucleation in only 8% of patients with bilateral RB in the years between 2012 and 2017 [52].

Importantly, strategies to avoid enucleation employed by highly experienced teams in nations with unlimited resources [53] are often not available and potentially dangerous in treatment of patients in developing nations. Socioeconomic and cultural factors must be considered. Poor outcomes have been correlated with decreased national income [54]. Increased paternal education was shown in Brazil to correlate with better survival [55]. In Uganda, the costs are unaffordable to most families and thus donors subsidize care [56]. If compliance with follow-up after conservative management cannot be assured, there is a risk of disease progression and death. Additionally, even mild chemotherapy regimens can lead to death in resource-poor communities. The primary goal without exception must be to save the life of the child.

Adjuvant chemotherapy refers to systemic chemotherapy administration employed after enucleation to decrease the risk of developing overt metastatic disease. Appropriate use of adjuvant chemotherapy is critical to its success. Knowledge of the routes of egress of RB out of the globe is fundamental (Fig. 2). RB typically grows under the retina and toward the vitreous with invasion of the ocular coats and optic nerve as the tumor progresses. After invasion of the choroid, the tumor may gain access to the systemic circulation causing bone and marrow disease with later involvement of the visceral organs. Additionally, progression can lead to invasion of the sclera and then the orbit. Tumor invading the anterior chamber can spread to the systemic circulation through the canal of Schlemm or progress into the conjunctiva. Conjunctival disease can then spread via lymphatic channels to the preauricular lymph nodes and subsequently to the submandibular or cervical lymph nodes.

The most lethal site of spread is the central nervous system, which occurs when RB spreads contiguously down the optic nerve or through invasion of the subarachnoid space. Infiltration of the pia into the subarachnoid space allows RB to seed the craniospinal fluid. Thus, central nervous system involvement can and does occur without presence of RB at the surgical margin of the cut nerve.

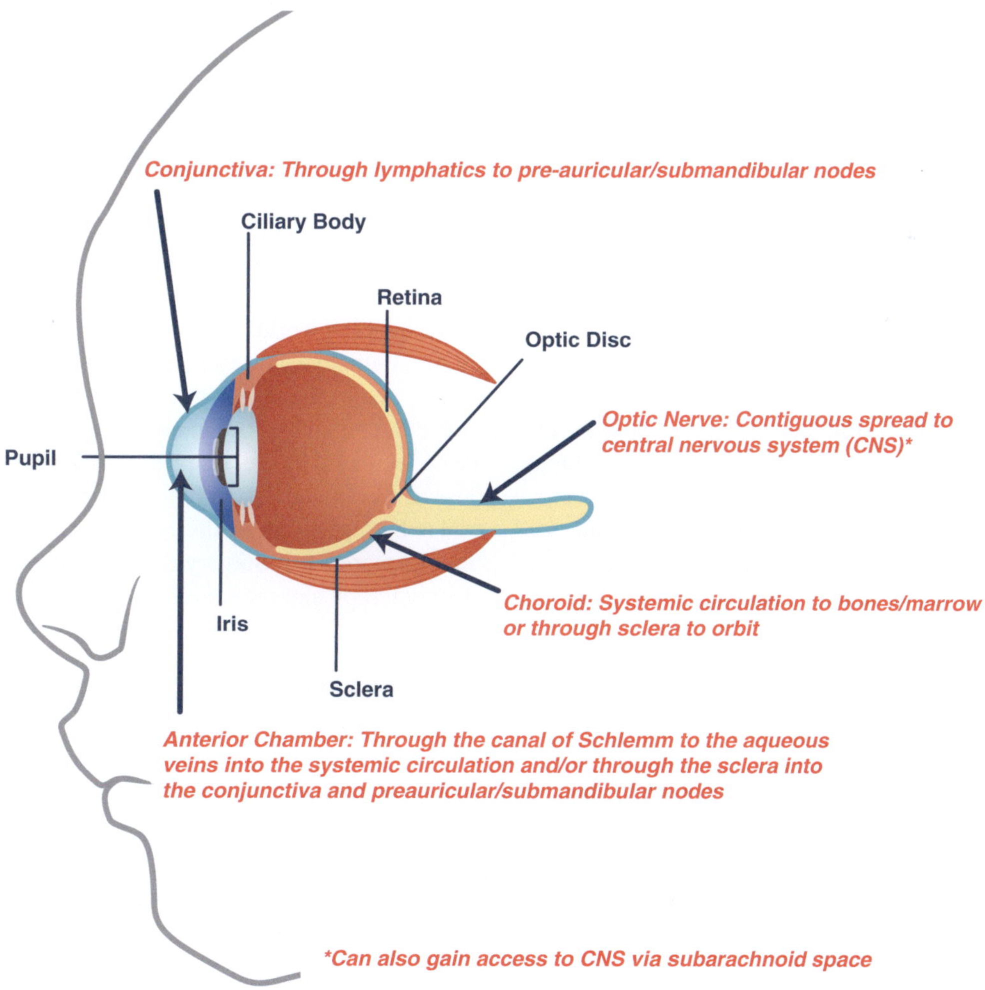

Fig. 2 Anatomy of the eye with routes of extraocular spread indicated in red (courtesy of Angela Knott and Alexis Arvanitides)

A prospective trial of frontline enucleation ± adjuvant chemotherapy in 321 children from the United States and India found a 2-year overall survival rate of 99% [8]. Six cycles of standard dose CEV were prescribed for patients with high-risk pathological features including massive choroidal involvement (largest diameter greater than 3 mm) and retrolaminar optic nerve invasion. A last indication for adjuvant chemotherapy was non-massive choroidal involvement with concomitant optic nerve involvement. The authors suggested this final indication (which occurred in less than 5% of the patients enrolled) might be observed without adjuvant chemotherapy in future clinical trials. There were two critical findings: first, 15% of local institution pathology findings were overturned on central review. These occurred in both directions of ascertainment. That is, 12% of patients were originally felt not to require adjuvant chemotherapy when in fact they did evidence high-risk features (HRF) on consensus review. Conversely, 22% of patients felt to have HRF locally were reassigned to no HRF.

As patients without HRF have died from toxicity while receiving adjuvant chemotherapy, it is essential that enucleated eyes be processed in a standard fashion [57]. Additionally, there were no survivors of patients with 3 mm or greater choroidal invasion around the head of the optic nerve (peripapillary posterior choroidal invasion) in combination with greater than or equal to 1.5 mm of retrolaminar optic nerve invasion. The authors hypothesized that these patients had microinvasion into the meningeal spaces. They suggested that these patients should undergo a spinal tap for cytology. Even if negative, consideration should be given to combined modality therapy with more intensive chemotherapy and orbital radiation as this is used in the treatment of patients with tumor extending to the cut edge of the optic nerve.

The most commonly used adjuvant regimen is six cycles of standard dose CEV. However, in patients with life-threatening allergy to carboplatin or etoposide, the combination of vincristine, doxorubicin, and cyclophosphamide (Table 5), which is active in other small round blue cell tumors of childhood such as Ewing's sarcoma and neuroblastoma, can be utilized. As previously mentioned, this regimen should be given with dexrazoxane cardioprotection. Another indication for this regimen is in the adjuvant setting for patients previously treated with CEV for chemoreduction.

A small number of teams do not utilize adjuvant chemotherapy, reserving therapy for patients who develop overt metastatic disease [58]. While as many as 70% of patients with bone and/or marrow metastases can be cured with highly intensive chemotherapy followed by stem cell transplantation, fewer than 5% can be cured of RB metastatic to the central nervous system [59]. Notably, survivors of this approach bear substantial burdens of therapy including sterility.

9 Treatment of Extraocular Retinoblastoma

Orbital RB occurs as a result of progression of the tumor through the sclera and emissary vessels. This is why transscleral disease is considered extraocular and is treated as such. There are two main approaches to stage 2 and 3 RB. When treated in countries with substantial resources, a four-drug regimen of vincristine, cisplatin, etoposide, and cyclophosphamide, in doses also used for stage 4a (bone/marrow metastases) and stage 4b (central nervous system disease), is utilized. In the case of stage 2 or 3 disease, orbital radiotherapy is used to consolidate patients while stage 4 patients are consolidated with hematopoietic stem cell transplantation. This expensive, toxic regimen does cure greater than 70% of stage 2 and 3 patients, but is not a realistic strategy for the majority of RB patients worldwide who live in the developing world.

An alternative approach to orbital RB is dose intensification of two of the drugs in the CEV regimen. This regimen (Table 6) contains a 50% increased dose of carboplatin and a 100% increased dose of etoposide used with a 50% decreased dose of vincristine. It was found in a prospective randomized trial to be superior to an alternate regimen used principally in South America [9]. Surgery follows or three to six cycles of chemotherapy and orbital radiation follow the surgery. With

Table 5 Alternative adjuvant regimen: vincristine, doxorubicin, and cyclophosphamide (VDC)

		Age <36 months	Age ≥36 months	
Vincristine	IV	0.05 mg/kg	1.5 mg/m^2	Day 1
Doxorubicin	IV	1.25 mg/kg	37.5 mg/m^2	Days 1 and 2
Cyclophosphamide	IV	40 mg/kg	1200 mg/m^2	Day 1
Mesna	IV	8 mg/kg	240 mg/m^2	Day 1
Dexrazoxane	IV	12.5 mg/kg	375 mg/m^2	Days 1 and 2
Pegfilgastrim	SQ	100 mcg/kg	100 mcg/kg	24–48 h after chemotherapy

Abbreviations: IV intravenous; *SQ* subcutaneous
Note: Maximum vincristine dose <2 mg

Table 6 High-dose CEV used for orbital retinoblastoma

		Age <36 months	Age ≥36 months	
Carboplatin	IV	28 mg/kg	420 mg/m^2	Days 1
Etoposide	IV	12 mg/kg	180 mg/m^2	Days 1 and 2
Vincristine	IV	0.025 mg/kg	0.75 mg/m^2	Day 1

Abbreviations: CEV Carboplatin, etoposide, and vincristine, *IV* Intravenous

this approach, approximately two-thirds of patients with stage 3 disease were event-free survivors at a median follow-up of 55 months.

10 Metastatic Disease

In high-income countries, less than 3% of patients with RB have extraocular disease at the time of presentation. Patients who develop metastatic disease usually do so after frontline attempts at globe salvage. In low-income countries, metastatic disease is often observed at diagnosis in older children presenting with extensive orbital disease or after declined enucleation in patients who previously presented with intraocular disease [60].

Despite the intrinsic chemosensitivity of RB, metastatic disease is not curable with conventional dose chemotherapy and thus efforts to improve survival in patients with RB should focus on increased screening of familial RB and decreased treatment abandonment. In a South American report, less than one-quarter of patients with a family history were diagnosed via screening [61]. In Indonesia, 45% of patients with intraocular RB will opt out of recommended treatment, leading to a death rate of 80% [62]. If the parents of these children did not opt out of treatment, the impact would be equivalent to a 50% reduction in the number of cases of metastatic disease at diagnosis.

Refusal of enucleation is not just a concern in the developing world. In Taiwan, a relatively affluent country with subsidization of care, 60% of families will opt out of an enucleation of the second affected eye after attempts at globe preservation in the setting of bilateral disease. This leads to a survival rate of less than 60% in Taiwanese patients with bilateral RB [63].

11 Pineoblastoma (Trilateral RB)

It is estimated that approximately 4% of patients with heritable RB will develop trilateral (tumor in the pineal gland) or quadrilateral (suprasellar or parasellar tumor) disease. Five-year survival rates were less than 10% in the 1990s, but are now approximately 40% for patients with pineal tumors [64]. Ranges of survival for patients with quadrilateral RB are wider (0–57%) as these tumors are less common, which precludes statistical precision. Nevertheless, the majority of patients with trilateral or quadrilateral RB will not survive.

Intracranial tumors found concurrently at the time of diagnosis of intraocular RB are usually smaller in size and appear to have a better prognosis. Additionally, patients with tumors less than 15 mm in size have a better survival [65]. Many centers screen with a brain magnetic resonance imaging (MRI) twice a year until the age of five, a recommendation espoused by the American Association of Cancer Research's Workshop on Childhood Cancer Predisposition [66]. Some authors question whether this is a cost-effective strategy. A controversial subject is whether systemic chemotherapy can prevent the development of these intracranial tumors. With the advent of intravenous chemotherapy in 1993, investigators in Philadelphia noted a statistically significant decreased observed-to-expected ratio when comparing the incidence of pineoblastoma in patients with heritable RB who did or did not receive chemotherapy [67]. A recent meta-analysis did not find systemic chemotherapy to be protective [68].

12 Summary

The World Health Organization Global Initiative for childhood cancer aims to raise the survival for 21 key childhood cancers including RB to 60% in the next 10 years [69]. Intravenous chemotherapy, usually CEV, is a treatment available in almost all centers caring for children with RB worldwide. It is an effective treatment in multiple situations. In conjunction with focal ophthalmic therapies, it is used for globe and vision salvage (chemoreduction) as well as following enucleation (as adjuvant therapy) to prevent the development of overt metastatic disease. When used in higher doses, it can cure two-thirds of patients with stage 2 and 3 disease if combined with surgery and radiation. Focal delivery routes of chemotherapy such as intra-arterial and intravitreal can be used sequentially or paired with systemic chemotherapy [50, 70]. The strength of intravenous chemotherapy is that it intentionally delivers chemotherapy into the systemic circulation to treat any micrometastatic disease that might exist. This is a protection that focal routes of chemotherapy cannot provide.

Concerns about the use of CEV have included effects on fertility, hearing, and secondary leukemia. It should be unequivocally stated that standard dose CEV does not cause infertility. Ototoxicity is seen in approximately 2% of patients dosed on a per kilogram basis if under 10 kg and who did not have abnormal hearing prior to the onset of their treatment. Lastly, although secondary leukemia is a feared complication of systemic chemotherapy, the largest report to date of 523 RB patients treated with etoposide-containing regimens saw no secondary leukemia in patients treated with chemotherapy alone [71]. There was a single case of secondary leukemia in a patient treated with a combination of chemotherapy and radiation. The median follow-up was 57 months, a time by which topoisomerase-induced leukemias would be expected to have appeared.

In sum, it would be a disservice to patients worldwide to abandon intravenous chemotherapy in favor of higher technology delivery routes as a result of concerns about late effects that are either rare or do not exist. This is especially true when one considers that the majority of children diagnosed with RB worldwide live in less economically developed countries where salvage treatments such as external beam radiotherapy and stem cell transplantation are not readily available. Simply put, frontline intravenous chemotherapy is a safe, effective way to save lives of children afflicted with RB.

References

1. Global Retinoblastoma Study Group. Global retinoblastoma presentation and analysis by national income level. JAMA Oncol. 2020;1:685–95.
2. Dimaras H, Corson TW, Cobrinik D, et al. Retinoblastoma. Nat Rev Dis Primers. 2015;1:15021.
3. Leahey AM. Let's make retinoblastoma a zero-death cancer. Ophthalmol Retina. 2020;4:640–1.
4. Munier FL, Beck-Popovic M, Chantada GL, et al. Conservative management of retinoblastoma: challenging orthodoxy without compromising the state of metastatic grace. "alive, with good vision and no comorbidity". Prog Retin Eye Res. 2019;73:100764.
5. Shields CL, De Potter P, Himelstein BP, Shields JA, Meadows AT, Maris JM. Chemoreduction in the initial management of intraocular retinoblastoma. Arch Ophthalmol. 1996;114:1330–8.
6. Murphree AL, Villablanca JG, Deegan WF 3rd, et al. Chemotherapy plus local treatment in the management of intraocular retinoblastoma. Arch Ophthalmol. 1996;114:1348–56.
7. Gallie BL, Budning A, DeBoer G, et al. Chemotherapy with focal therapy can cure intraocular retinoblastoma without radiotherapy. Arch Ophthalmol. 1996;114:1321–8.
8. Chavez-Barrios P, Eagle RC Jr, Krailo M, et al. Study of unilateral retinoblastoma with and without histopathologic high-risk features and the role of adjuvant chemotherapy. J Clin Oncol. 2019;37:2883–91.
9. Chawla B, Hasan F, Seth R, et al. Multimodal therapy for stage III retinoblastoma (international retinoblastoma staging system): a prospective comparative study. Ophthalmology. 2016;123:1933–9.
10. Fox E, Blaney SM, Moreno L, et al. General principles of chemotherapy chapter 10. In: Blaney SM, Adamson PC, Helman LJ, editors. Pizzo and Poplack's pediatric oncology. 8th ed. Philadelphia: Wolters Kluwer Health; 2021. p. 239–302.
11. Crom W, Glynn-Barnhart AM, Rodman JH, et al. Pharmacokinetics of anti-cancer drugs in children. Clin Pharmacokin. 1987;12:168–213.
12. Kearns GL, Abdel-Rahman SM, Alander SW, Blowey DL, Leeder JS, Kauffman RE. Developmental pharmacology—drug disposition, action, and therapy in infants and children. N Engl J Med. 2003;349:1157–67.
13. Go RS, Adjei AA. Review of the comparative pharmacology and clinical activity of cisplatin and carboplatin. J Clin Oncol. 1999;17:409–22.
14. Leahey A. A cautionary tale: dosing chemotherapy in infants with retinoblastoma. J Clin Oncol. 2012;30:1023–4.
15. Lambert MP, Shields C, Meadows AT. A retrospective review of hearing in children with retinoblastoma treated with carboplatin-based chemotherapy. Pediatr Blood Cancer. 2008;50:223–6.
16. Jehanne M, Lumbroso-Le Rouic L, Savignoni A, et al. Analysis of ototoxicity in young children receiving carboplatin in the context of conservative management of unilateral or bilateral retinoblastoma. Pediatr Blood Cancer. 2009;52:637–43.
17. Smits C, Swen SJ, Theo Goverts S, et al. Assessment of hearing in very young children receiving carboplatin for retinoblastoma. Eur J Cancer. 2006;42:492–500.
18. Qaddoumi I, Bass JK, Wu J, et al. Carboplatin-associated ototoxicity in children with retinoblastoma. J Clin Oncol. 2012;30:1034–41.
19. Soliman SE, D'Silva CN, Dimaras H, Dzneladze I, Chan H, Gallie BL. Clinical and genetic associations for carboplatin-related ototoxicity in children treated for retinoblastoma: a retrospective noncomparative single-institute experience. Pediatr Blood Cancer. 2018;65(5):e26931.
20. Long BH. Mechanisms of action of teniposide (VM-26) and etoposide (VP-16). Sem Oncol. 1992;19(Suppl 6):3–19.
21. Boos J, Krumpelmann S, Schulze-Westhoff P, et al. Steady-state levels and bone marrow toxicity of etoposide in children and infants: does etoposide require age-dependent dose calculations. J Clin Oncol. 1995;13:2954–60.
22. Meyer C, Burmeister T, Groger D, et al. The MLL recombinome of acute leukemias in 2017. Leukemia. 2018;32:273–84.
23. Winick NJ, McKenna RW, Schuster JJ, et al. Secondary acute leukemia in children with acute lymphoblastic leukemia treated with etoposide. J Clin Oncol. 1993;11:209–17.
24. Smith MA, Rubenstein L, Ungerleider RS. Therapy-related acute myeloid leukemia following treatment with epipodophyllotoxins: estimating the risk. Med Pediatr Oncol. 1994;23:86–98.
25. Gombos DS, Hungerford J, Abramson DH, et al. Secondary acute myelogenous leukemia in patients with retinoblastoma: is chemotherapy a factor. Ophthalmology. 2007;114:1378–83.
26. Temming P, Arendt M, Viehmann A, et al. Incidence of second cancers after radiotherapy and systemic chemotherapy in heritable retinoblastoma survivors: a report from the German reference center. Pediatr Blood Cancer. 2017;64:71–80.
27. Rihani R, Bazzeh F, Faqih N, et al. Secondary hematopoietic malignancies in survivors of childhood cancer: an analysis of 111 cases from the surveillance, epidemiology, and end Result-9 registry. Cancer. 2010;116:4385–94.
28. Turaka K, Shields CL, Meadows AT, et al. Second malignant neoplasms following chemoreduction with carboplatin, etoposide, and vincristine in 245 patients woith intraocular retinoblastoma. Pediatr Blood Cancer. 2012;59:121–5.
29. Wong JR, Morton LM, Tucker MA, et al. Risk of subsequent malignant neoplasms in long-term hereditary retinoblastoma survivors after chemotherapy and radiotherapy. J Clin Oncol. 2014;32:3284–90.
30. Neumann Y, Toren A, Reghavi G, et al. Vincristine treatment triggering the expression of Charcot-Marie-tooth disease. Med Pediatr Oncol. 1996;26:280–3.
31. DiDomenico C, Clerico D, Leahey A. Lack of vincristine infiltrates in patients with retinoblastoma receiving chemotherapy by peripheral intravenous lines. Pediatr Blood Cancer. 2015;62:1859–61.
32. Singhal PK, Iliskovic N. Doxorubicin-induced cardiomyopathy. N Engl J Med. 1998;339:900–5.
33. Liesse K, Harris J, Chan M, et al. Dexrazoxane significantly reduces anthracycline-induced cardiotoxicity in pediatric solid

tumor patients: a systemimatic review. J Pediatr Hematol Oncol. 2018;40:417–25.
34. Tebbi CK, London WB, Friedman D, et al. Dexrazoxane-associated risk for acute myeloid leukemia/myelodysplastic syndrome and other secondary malignancies in pediatric Hodgkin's disease. J Clin Oncol. 2007;25:493–500.
35. Kim H, Kang HJ, Park KD, et al. Risk factor analysis of secondary malignancy in dexrazoxane-treated pediatric cancer patients. Cancer Res Treat. 2019;51:357–67.
36. Wong KY, Lampkin BC. Anthracycline toxicity. Am J Pediatr Hematol Oncol. 1983;5:93–7.
37. Burket H. Clinical overview of mesna. Cancer Treat Rev. 1983;10(Suppl):175–81.
38. Brennan RC, Qaddoumi I, Mao S, et al. Ocular salvage and vision preservation using a topotecan-based regimen for advanced intraocular retinoblastoma. J Clin Oncol. 2017;35:72–7.
39. Blaney SM, Tagen M, Onar-Thomas A, et al. A phase I pharmacokinetic optimal dosing study of intravenous topotecan for children with neoplastic meningitis: a pediatric brain tumor consortium study. Pediatr Blood Cancer. 2013;60:627–32.
40. Murphree AL. Intraocular retinoblastoma: the case for a new group classification. Ophthalmol Clin N Am. 2005;18:41–53.
41. Tomar AS, Finger PT, Gallie B, et al. A multicenter, international collaborative study for American joint committee on cancer staging of retinoblastoma: part II: treatment success and globe salvage. Ophthalmology. 2020;127:1733–46.
42. Chantada G, Doz F, Antoneli CB, Grundy R, et al. A proposal for an international retinoblastoma staging system. Pediatr Blood Cancer. 2006;47:801–5.
43. Wilson TW, Chan HS, Moselhy GM, Heydt DD Jr, Frey CM, Gallie BL. Penetration of chemotherapy into vitreous is increased by cryotherapy and cyclosporine in rabbits. Arch Ophthalmol. 1996;114:1390–5.
44. Shields CL, Mashayekhi A, Au AK, et al. The international classification of retinoblastoma predicts chemoreduction success. Ophthalmology. 2006;113:2276–80.
45. Shields CL, Bas Z, Tadepalli S, et al. Long-term (20 year) real-world outcomes of intravenous chemotherapy (chemoreduction) for retinoblastoma in 964 eyes of 554 patients at a single Centre. Br J Ophthamol. 2020;104:1548–55.
46. Demirci H, Shields CL, Meadows AT, Shields JA. Long-term visual outcome following chemoreduction for retinoblastoma. Arch Ophthamol. 2005:1525–30.
47. Russo I, Levy-Gabriel C, Dupont A, et al. Prospective phase II study of children affected by bilateral intraocular retinoblastoma with macular involvement of both eyes or in the only preserved eye. Macular tumor control, eye preservation rate, and visual outcome. Pediatr Blood Cancer. 2021;68:e28721.
48. Hunger SP, Mullighan CG. Acute lymphoblastic leukemia in children. N Engl J Med. 2015;373:1541–52.
49. Munier FL, Gaillard MC, Balmer A, et al. Intravitreal chemotherapy for vitreous disease in retinoblastoma revisited: from prohibition to conditional indications. Br J Ophthalmol. 2012;96:1078–83.
50. Berry JL, Shah S, Kim F, et al. Integrated treatment during the intravitreal melphalan era: concurrent intravitreal melphalan and systemic chemoreduction. Oncol Pathol. 2018;4:335–40.
51. Shields JA, Shields CL, Sivalingam V. Decreasing frequency of enucleation in patients with retinoblastoma. Am J Ophthamol. 1989;108:185–8.
52. Lu JE, Francis JH, Dunkel IJ, et al. Metastases and death rates after primary enucleation of unilateral retinoblastoma in the USA 2007-2017. Br J Ophthalmol. 2019;103:1272–7.
53. Francis JH, Roosipu N, Levin AM, et al. Current treatment of bilateral retirnoblastoma: the impact of intraarterial and intravitreous chemotherapy. Neoplasia. 2018;20:757–63.
54. Tomar AS, Finger PT, Gallie B, et al. Global retinoblastoma treatment outcomes: association with national income level. Ophthalmology. 2021;128:740–53.
55. Mattosinho C, Moura AT, Grigorovski N, Araújo LH, Ferman S, Ribeiro K. Socioeconomic status and retinoblastoma survival: experience of a tertiary cancer center in Brazil. Pediatr Blood Cancer. 2021;68:e28757.
56. Waddell K, Matua M, Bidwell C, et al. A ten-year study of retinoblastoma in Uganda: an approach to improving outcome with limited resources. Cancer Epidemiol. 2020;10:101,777.
57. Sastre X, Chantada GL, Doz F, et al. Proceedings of the consensus meetings from the international retinoblastoma staging working group on the pathology guidelines for the examination of enucleated eyes and evaluation of prognostic risk factors in retinoblastoma. Arch Pathol Lab Med. 2009;133:1199–202.
58. Abramson DH, Shields CL, Munier FL, Chantada GL. Treatment of retinoblastoma in 2015: agreement and disagreement. JAMA Ophthalmol. 2015;133:1341–7.
59. Clarissa A, Sutandi N, Fath AA. Stem-cell therapy following high-dose chemotherapy in advanced retinoblastoma: a systematic review. Asia Pac J Ophthalmol (Phila). 2021;10:397–407. Online ahead of print.
60. Canturk S, Qaddoumi I, Khetan V, et al. Survival of retinoblastoma in less-developed countries impact of socioeconomic and health-related indicators. Br J Ophthalmol. 2010;94:1432–6.
61. Chantada GL, Dunkel IJ, Qaddoumi I, et al. Familial retinoblastoma in developing countries. Pediatr Blood Cancer. 2009;53:338–42.
62. Sitorus RS, Moll AC, Suhardjono S, et al. The effect of therapy refusal against medical advice in retinoblastoma patients in a setting where treatment delays are common. Ophthalmic Genet. 2009;30:31–6.
63. Su WW, Kao LY. Retinoblastoma in Taiwan: the effect of a government-sponsored national health insurance program on the treatment and survival of patients with retinoblastoma. J Pediatr Ophthalmol Strabismus. 2006;43:358–62.
64. de Jong MC, Kors WA, de Graaf P, Castelijns JA, Moll AC, Kivelä T. The incidence of trilateral retinoblastoma: a systematic review and meta-analysis. Am J Ophthalmol. 2015;160:1116–26.
65. Kivela T. Trilateral retinoblastoma: a meta-analysis of hereditary retinoblastoma associated with primary ectopic intracranial retinoblastoma. J Clin Oncol. 1999;17:1829–37.
66. Kamihara J, Bourdeaut F, Foulkes WD, et al. Retinoblastoma and neuroblastoma predisposition and surveillance. Clin Cancer Res. 2017;23:e98–e106.
67. Ramasubramanian A, Meadows AT, Shields JA, Leahey A, Shields CL. Reply to Am J Ophthalmol 2013;156:1320–1.
68. de Jong MC, Kors WA, Moll AC, et al. Screening for pineal trilateral retinoblastoma revisited: a meta-analysis. Ophthalmology. 2020;127:601–7.
69. World Health Organization. Global initiative for childhood cancer; 2018 Accessed 3 March 2020.
70. Shields CL, Kaliki S, Al-Dahmash S, et al. Management of advanced retinoblastoma with intravenous chemotherapy then intra-arterial chemotherapy as alternative to enucleation. Retina. 2013;33:2103–9.
71. Turaka K, Shields CL, Meadows AT, et al. Second malignant neoplasms following chemoreduction with carboplatin, etoposide, and vincristine in 245 patients with intraocular retinoblastoma. Pediatr Blood Cancer. 2012;59:121–5.

Intra-arterial Chemotherapy for Retinoblastoma: A Team Effort

Theodora Hadjistilianou, Sandra Bracco, Matteo Barchitta, and Eugenio Bertelli

1 Introduction

Intra-arterial chemotherapy (IAC) was first performed in 1954 by Algernon B. Reese with direct internal carotid artery injection of the alkylating agent triethylene melamine (TEM) [1]. Unfortunately, as systemic toxicity associated with this procedure was too high, it was discontinued.

Melphalan has been demonstrated to be one of the most effective drugs against retinoblastoma (RB), and hence chosen as the agent for carotid injection [2].

A technique has been then developed to deliver chemotherapy to the orbit by temporarily occluding the carotid artery distal to the ophthalmic artery and injecting the drug in the cervical internal carotid artery [3]. Furthermore, intravitreal injection of melphalan has been associated to treat vitreous seeding [4].

In 2004, Yamane and Kaneko proposed the technique of "selective ophthalmic artery infusion" (SOAI) using a microballoon catheter positioned distal to the ostium of the ophthalmic artery and injecting chemotherapy with the flow directed into the ophthalmic artery enabling the delivery of the drug even closer to the RB (local delivery) [5].

Two years later, in 2006, Abramson and Gobin revisited the SOAI technique giving birth to the "direct intra-arterial ophthalmic artery infusion." Via a transfemoral approach, a microcatheter is directed under fluoroscopic and roadmap guidance to superselectively catheterize the ophthalmic artery origin [6].

The evolution of intra-arterial chemotherapy contributed to increased safety and efficacy of this treatment method. Nowadays, IAC is used in more than 45 countries worldwide, and it has been shown to be more effective in saving the globe in group D and E retinoblastomas compared to systemic chemotherapy. It has also minimal systemic toxicity and allows for shorter treatment duration and hospitalization [7].

2 IAC Objective

The main goal of IAC is to deliver a high dose of drugs to the tumor while avoiding the side effects and risks of systemic chemotherapy. It generally consists of one, two, or three drugs, respectively, melphalan, melphalan + topotecan, or melphalan + topotecan + carboplatin, typically delivered once a month for a median of three sessions. IAC also avoids the risks of external beam radiotherapy, which include midfacial contracture, cataract, radiation retinopathy, and, in patients with germinal mutations, the development of second malignant neoplasms [8].

Interestingly, the tumor response to IAC, in most cases, is dramatic, with an immediate tumor shrinkage after the first infusion (Fig. 1). Additional treatment, usually consisting of laser therapy and/or cryotherapy, may usefully increase the permeability of the blood–retina barrier prior to IAC if no retinal detachment is present.

3 Indications

IAC is generally avoided in neonates and infants younger than 6 months (and weight less than 7 kg) due to difficulties in femoral artery cannulation, so the first-line treatment for

T. Hadjistilianou (✉)
Department of Medicine, Surgery and Neurosciences, Ophthalmology Unit, Oncology Service, Siena, Italy
e-mail: dorisocularoncology@libero.it

S. Bracco
Clinical Department of Neurological and Human Movement Sciences, Interventional Neuroradiology Unit, Hospital S. Maria alle Scotte, Siena, Italy

M. Barchitta
Department Medicine, Surgery and Neurosciences, Ophthalmology Unit, Siena, Italy

E. Bertelli
Department of Molecular and Developmental Medicine, University of Siena, Siena, Italy
e-mail: eugenio.bertelli@unisi.it

B. V. Chawla, M. E. Aronow (eds.), *Global Perspectives in Ocular Oncology*, https://doi.org/10.1007/978-3-031-08250-4_7

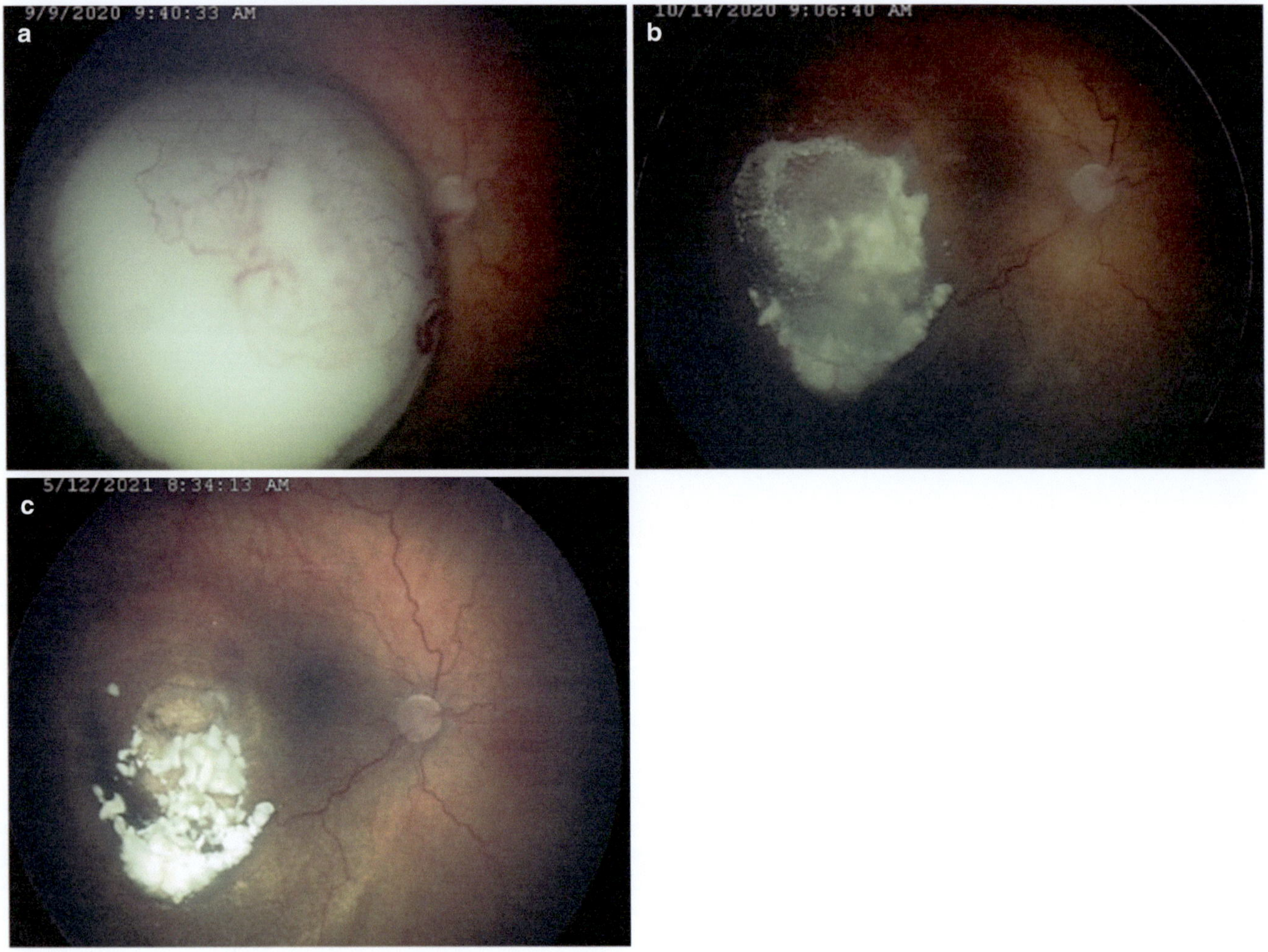

Fig. 1 Ten-month-old female. (**a**) Unilateral group C RB at diagnosis. (**b**) Almost complete regression following the first IAC infusion. (**c**) Five months of follow-up; regression type I

retinoblastoma in patients from zero to six months of age remains systemic chemotherapy [9].

IAC is indicated:

- *As first choice therapy* in unilateral retinoblastoma (stages B, C, D, and selected E eyes) that cannot be treated by laser therapy or cryotherapy alone (stage A) in infants older than 6 months and with a weight greater than 7 kg.
- *As second choice therapy* after failure of systemic chemotherapy and/or focal treatments where there is an incomplete response or recurrent tumor in unilateral cases or in bilateral cases (where one eye is enucleated or treated with focal treatments and IAC is performed in the fellow eye) [10].
- *In combination with intravitreal chemotherapy (IViC)* in unilateral and bilateral cases where there are subretinal and/or vitreous seeds (Fig. 2).

In 2012, the introduction of IViC dramatically changed the approach for eyes with previously intractable vitreous seeds, improving globe salvage rate [11].

Three further treatment scenarios that deserve a mention are bridge, tandem, and rescue therapies.

3.1 Bridge Chemotherapy

Patients less than 3 months old are treated with intravenous chemotherapy with carboplatin alone (single-agent chemotherapy) every 3–4 weeks to be followed by intra-arterial chemotherapy once the patient reaches 7 kg. This strategy allows immediate treatment while postponing IAC, further avoiding potential toxicity of multiagent chemotherapy in very young patients [12].

3.2 Tandem Therapy

It consists of simultaneous bilateral IAC treatment in naive eyes or after failure of systemic chemotherapy (bilateral simultaneous relapses). Melphalan is infused in one eye and carboplatin is injected in fellow eye due to systemic toxicity

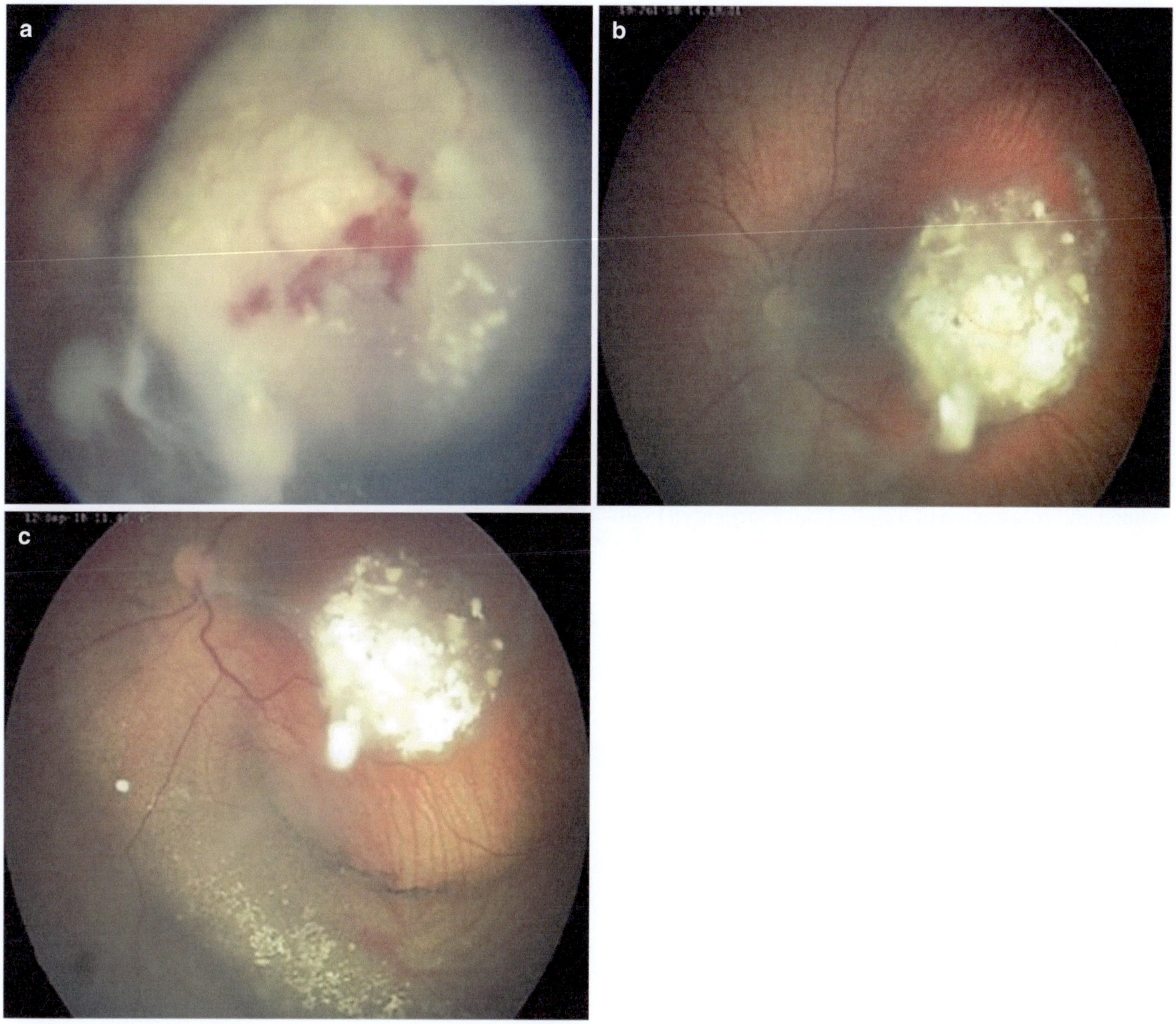

Fig. 2 Twelve-month-old male. (**a**) Unilateral group D RB, type 3 clouds seeding. (**b**) Complete regression (type I) following six IAC infusions and three IViC injections. (**c**) Three years of follow-up

of melphalan, to avoid bone marrow suppression. Melphalan is often given to the eye with more advanced disease, but commonly the drugs are switched in the second or third session so that the melphalan eye then receives carboplatin-based therapy [13]. Topotecan can also be added. The decision about changing drug combinations on subsequent sessions is discussed within the multidisciplinary oncology group (MOG) on a clinical basis and does not follow a rigid protocol.

In our experience, the drug combination for tandem therapy is based on the previous treatments, age of the child, and extension and type of the relapse (vitreous seeding and/or subretinal seeding, diffuse and/or focal) [14].

3.3 Rescue Therapy

Rescue therapy is the re-use of IAC for recurrent tumor or subretinal seeds or vitreous seeds following previous IAC.

4 Contraindications

- Aseptic preseptal or orbital cellulitis, and phthisis
- Optic nerve or scleral extension
- Extraocular or orbital extension
- Trilateral retinoblastoma or systemic metastasis

- Tumors treatable with focal therapies
- Neovascular glaucoma, hyphema, and vitreous hemorrhage
- Anterior chamber invasion
- Secondary glaucoma [7–9]

5 Protocol Treatment

5.1 Customized Treatment

Every treatment is built around the patient and is based on age and weight of the child, on the severity of disease, and its response to previous therapies. Nowadays, there is lack of a standardized protocol or universal consensus regarding drugs and dosage for IAC, so every case is discussed by a specialized team.

The decision-making process regarding IAC for RB requires the cooperation of a skilled and experienced multidisciplinary team in order to perform such subtle procedure with success. These appropriately trained specialists include ocular oncologists, pediatric oncologists, pediatric anesthesiologists, neuroradiologists, interventional neuroradiologists, geneticists, pharmacists, and specialized nurses. Therefore, the crucial points that need to be discussed in the decision-making process regarding the IAC are the ophthalmoscopic evaluation and staging of intraocular disease under anesthesia, the neuroimaging evaluation and assessment of the possible risk factors for conservative therapy, and the pediatric evaluation and genetic consultation.

A final case discussion is then programmed by the MOG (multidisciplinary oncology group). The stage of retinoblastoma has to be assessed through the ophthalmological examination performed under general anesthesia using a fundus photography (Ret-Cam), ocular ultrasonography (A and B scan), ultrasound biomicroscopy (UBM), and optic coherence tomography (OCT) (when necessary). We now use the International Classification System for Intraocular Retinoblastoma (ICRB) (Table 1) and the 8th Edition American Joint Committee on Cancer (AJCC) TNMH (tumor, node, metastasis, heritable trait) staging system [15].

Magnetic resonance imaging and pediatric evaluation should be performed to exclude extraocular disease and for systemic assessment, respectively. Before each treatment, clinical examination and blood test should be performed to evaluate the feasibility of a safe general anesthesia and chemotherapy. During the follow-up, in order to monitor treatment efficacy and retinal toxicity, a complete ophthalmic examination should be performed every 3–4 weeks with Ret-Cam digital photography, B-Scan ultrasonography, and electroretinogram (ERG).

Furthermore, a pediatric evaluation is recommended 8–10 days after the procedure, together with a full blood count to monitor for myelosuppression (particularly neutropenia). If necessary, supportive therapy with fluid and electrolyte infusion, heparin, antiemetics, and painkiller agents is indicated. After the treatment, during the follow-up, it is important to evaluate the short- and long-term side effects. Usually, the tumor response to IAC is dramatic and reduction can be observed since the first infusion (Fig. 1). Treatment efficacy is judged on tumor shrinkage and regression, disappearance or calcifications or inactivation of vitreous and subretinal seeds, and absence of new tumor growth. Retinal toxicity is estimated from electroretinogram (ERG) results.

Summarizing, the aim of IAC is to salvage the eye avoiding the side effects and risks of systemic chemotherapy with the delivery of a high dose of chemotherapeutic agents directly to the tumor [16].

Table 1 International Classification System for Intraocular Retinoblastoma (ICRB)

Group A	Very low risk	Small intraretinal tumors away from foveola and disk	• Less than 3 mm in size • More than 1.5 mm from the disk • More than 3 mm from the fovea
Group B	Low risk	Eyes with no vitreous seeds or subretinal seeding and discrete retinal tumor of any size or location	• Tumors not in group A • No vitreous or subretinal seeding
Group C	Moderate risk	Eyes with only focal vitreous or subretinal seeding and discrete retinal tumors of any size or location	• Seeding local, fine, and limited • Up to one-quadrant of subretinal fluid
Group D	High risk	Eyes with diffuse vitreous or subretinal seeding and/or massive, non-discrete endophytic or exophytic disease; eyes with more extensive seeding than group C	• Massive intraocular disseminated disease • More than one-quadrant of retinal detachment • Fine vitreous seeding • Subretinal seeding
Group E	Very high risk	Eyes that have been destroyed anatomically or functionally by the tumor; eyes with one or more than the following	• Neovascular glaucoma. • Massive intraocular hemorrhage • Aseptic orbital cellulitis • Tumor touching the lens • Diffuse infiltrating retinoblastoma • Phthisis

5.2 IAC Technique

The setting of IAC is a neuroangiographic suite where the child is under general anesthesia. The procedure should be performed by an experienced interventional neuroradiologist. For each procedure, the femoral artery is catheterized by the insertion of a 4 Fr short femoral sheath.

After systemic heparinization according to a dedicated pediatric protocol, the catheter is advanced under fluoroscopy guidance into the internal carotid artery ipsilateral to the affected eye in order to verify the presence of the ophthalmic artery by a lateral angiogram (Fig. 3). After detecting the ophthalmic artery under roadmap, a superselective microcatheterization (1.2 Fr microcatheter) of the artery is performed. Once the microcatheter is stably placed at the ophthalmic artery ostium, an angiogram is performed to confirm the right posterior eyeball enhancement, which represents the capillary phase of choroid and retinal blood flow (Fig. 3). The retina receives blood from the central retinal artery or from the cilioretinal arteries that detach from the posterior ciliary arteries. In both cases, the blood supply ultimately derives from the ophthalmic artery [17]. The choroidal–retinal enhancement (the so-called choroidal blush), obtained with the injection of contrast medium through the microcatheter into the ophthalmic artery, is the sign that the chemotherapeutic agent delivered by the same route will reach the target. Once this check has been positively achieved, the prescribed drugs can be administrated, generally over a 30-min time of infusion. At the end of the procedure, a final control angiogram of the intracranial vascular integrity is carried out and when the activated clotting time (ACT) test is back to normal, the femoral sheath is removed and a manual compression is performed to ensure hemostasis before awakening of the child.

The technique of intraophthalmic arterial drug delivery may seem easy for a skilled interventional neuroradiologist but two challenging scenarios can occur with a certain frequency.

The first scenario is a troublesome and unstable catheterization of the ophthalmic artery, in spite of its visualization by selective angiography of the internal carotid artery. This situation is usually the result of a too much angulated origin of the ophthalmic artery and may require the manual customization of the tip of the catheter to properly fit the vascular anatomy [18].

The second unfavorable situation occurs when the ophthalmic artery does not appear in the carotid angiogram (Fig. 4) or when the choroidal blush cannot be visualized even when ophthalmic artery catheterization is properly achieved (Fig. 4).

In the latter circumstance the contrast medium, instead of diffusing along the ophthalmic artery, usually flows back into the internal carotid artery. In both cases, an anastomosis between the ophthalmic artery and the external carotid is probably in place producing a flow reversal in the ophthalmic artery [18]. Taking into account also cases of aberrant origin of the ophthalmic artery from the middle meningeal artery, in 3.4–6.6% of individuals the territory supplied by the ophthalmic artery falls entirely or in large part into the area of distribution of the external carotid artery [17] with

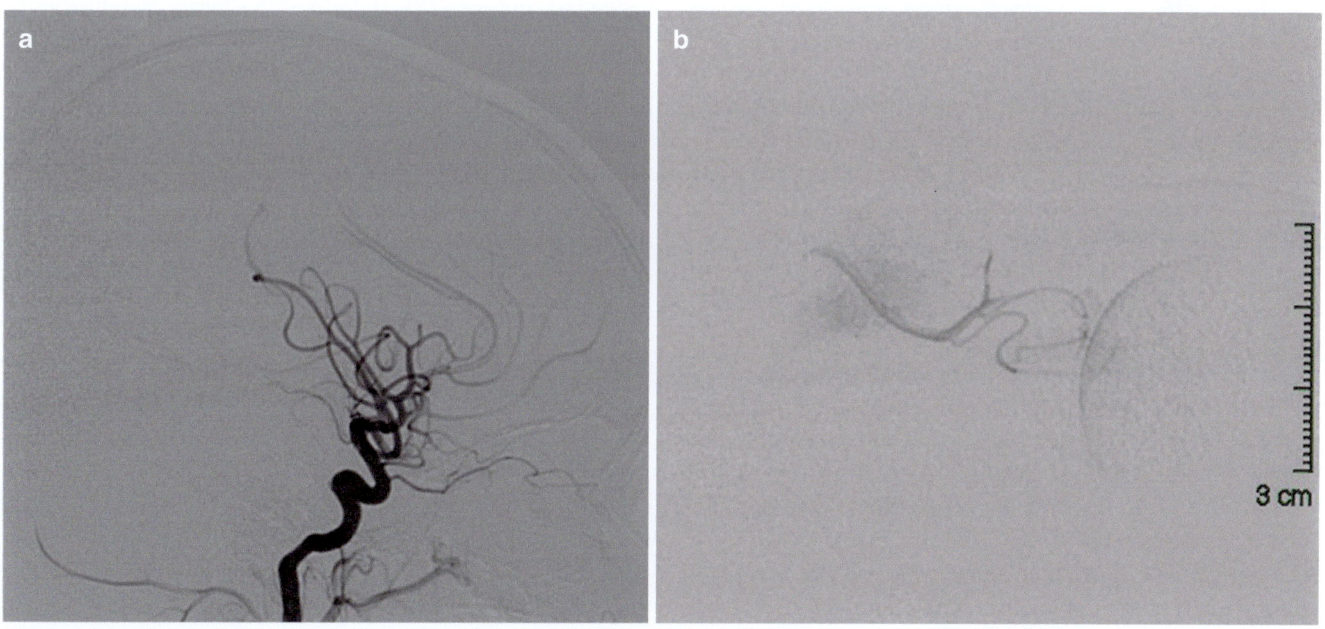

Fig. 3 (**a**) Lateral angiogram of the internal carotid artery. The ophthalmic artery is well visible. (**b**) Superselective lateral angiogram of the ophthalmic artery. The posterior globe enhancement is evident

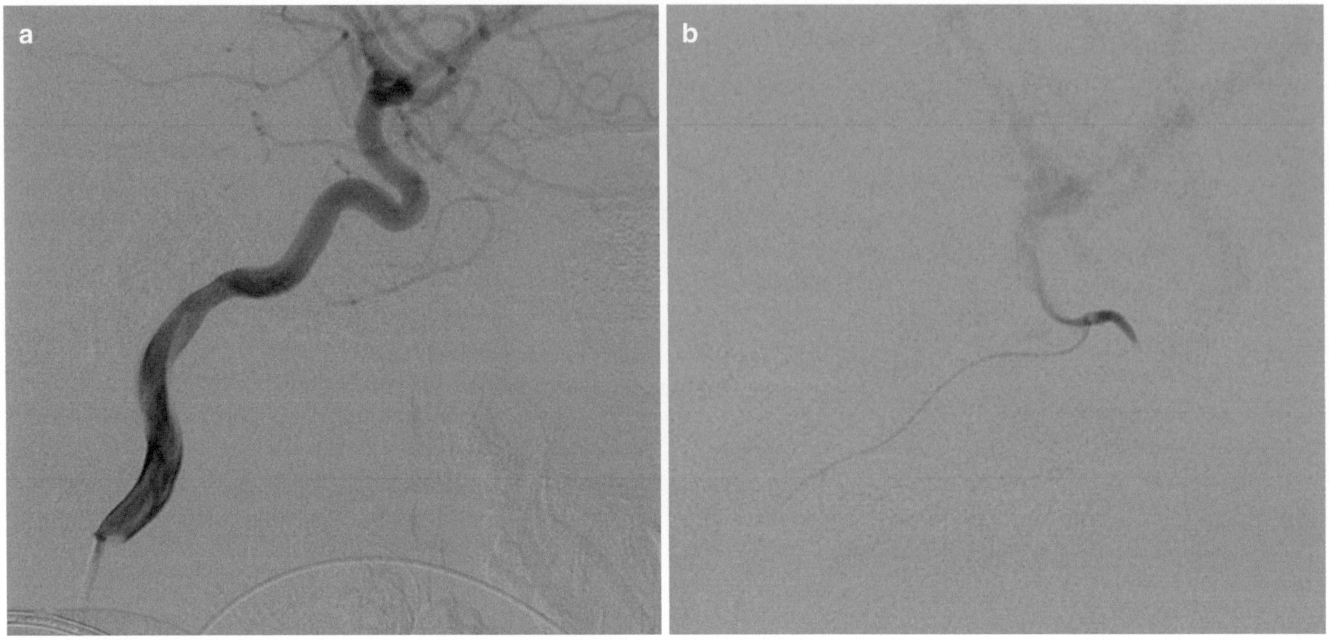

Fig. 4 (**a**) Internal carotid lateral view angiogram. The ophthalmic artery is not visualized. (**b**) Superselective lateral angiogram of the ophthalmic artery. The posterior globe enhancement is not visible because the contrast medium injected through the microcatheter flows back into the internal carotid artery

several anastomoses that may provide alternative pathways for the orbital blood supply [19] and drug administration. In this respect, a series of publications [20–25] have testified that the intra-arterial release of chemotherapy can be achieved by the micronavigation of alternative routes from the external carotid artery instead of the direct cannulation of the ophthalmic artery. Some retrospective studies have reported that up to 16% of the procedures have been carried out via branches of the external carotid artery [18]. Though the anastomoses most frequently employed to deliver chemotherapeutic agents to the eye involve the middle meningeal artery, many other interarterial connections have successfully served the same scope (Figs. 5, 6, and 7).

In addition, the hemodynamic balance between the external and the internal carotid systems connected by permanent anastomoses is susceptible to temporary changes. This may lead to choose different pathways of drug delivery for each session of intra-arterial chemotherapy in the same patient (interprocedural variability) or, exceptionally, even within the same procedure (intraprocedural variability) [18].

Some authors suggest to perform the transient occlusion of the external carotid artery with a balloon catheter to redirect the ophthalmic flow from the external to the internal carotid in order to perform the regular procedure from the internal carotid artery (Fig. 8) [26].

This approach has some drawbacks (puncture of both femoral arteries, two catheters in the same small vessel), and its safety/efficacy vs catheterization of the external carotid artery (ECA) branches still requires validation [18].

Intra-arterial chemotherapy is performed using X-rays. Young patients are exposed to radiation during fluoroscopic observation and images acquisition [27]. Some concerns about the risk of cumulative toxicity from repeated exposure to ionizing radiations have been raised, especially in children with germline mutation and potential susceptibility for secondary tumors [28]. Bertelli et al. reported significantly higher levels of radiation exposure in the procedures performed through branches of the external carotid compared to the direct access to the ophthalmic artery [18]. Nevertheless, it is believed that the exposure is minimal and the dose received by the brain, thorax, abdomen, and pelvis should be considered safe. Guasti et al. recently published a method to estimate dose of radiation absorbed by internal organs [29].

5.3 Principal Chemotherapeutic Agents

IAC sessions are usually repeated every 3–4 weeks although the number of sessions is not standardized and mainly depends on the stage of the disease (naïve cases), on previous treatments (if residual or relapsed disease), and on the fundus features observed during the treatment and follow-up under anesthesia.

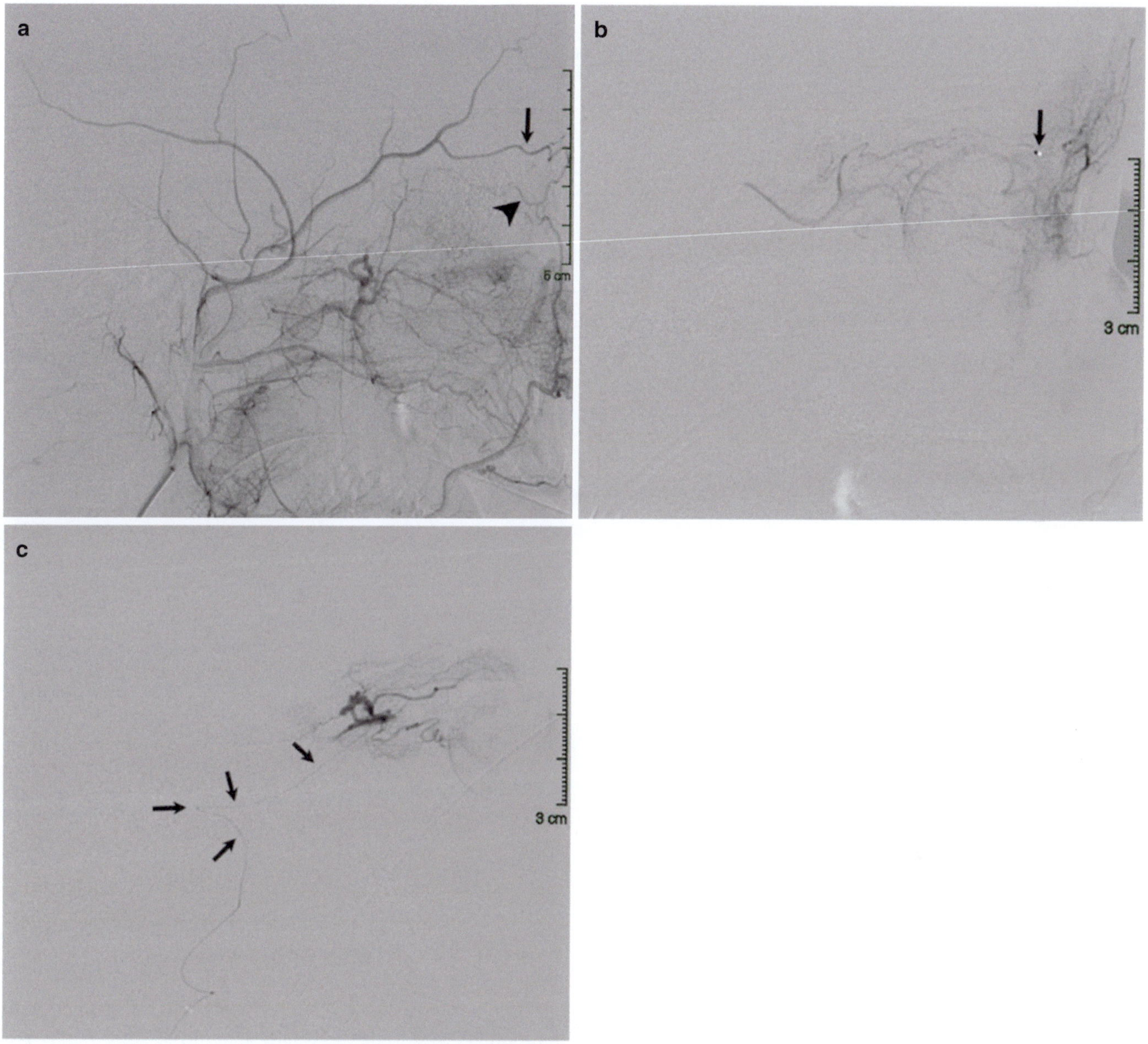

Fig. 5 (**a**, **b**) Alternative route of drug delivery through the external carotid artery via the microcatheterization of the superficial temporal artery. (**a**) The superficial temporal artery is visible (arrow) as well as the anastomosis with the ophthalmic artery (arrowhead). (**b**) The choroidal blush is achieved by contrast medium injection through the microcatheter (arrow points to the tip of the catheter). (**c**) Alternative route of drug delivery through the external carotid artery via the microcatheterization of the middle meningeal artery. A meningolacrimal anastomosis is in place and functional to produce the choroidal blush. Arrows = microcatheter within the middle meningeal artery

The intra-arterial drug dosage reported in literature (melphalan 2.5–5 mg or topotecan 0.3–0.4 mg or carboplatin 30 mg; Table 2) is adjusted according to the patient's age and weight, besides the severity or extent of the disease and its response to the treatment [30].

Melphalan is the most extensively used alkylating agent, topotecan is used in IAC for aggressive cases not responsive to melphalan alone, and carboplatin is used in cases in which the tumor failed to respond to melphalan and/or topotecan and, more commonly, in a simultaneous triple therapy in eyes that have failed single- or double-agent IAC or systemic intravenous chemotherapy.

IAC is administered every 3–4 weeks for three sessions, which can be extended in selective cases to improve response. In rescue IAC, higher doses of melphalan and topotecan are needed for tumor control, while the carboplatin dose is maintained at 30 mg [31].

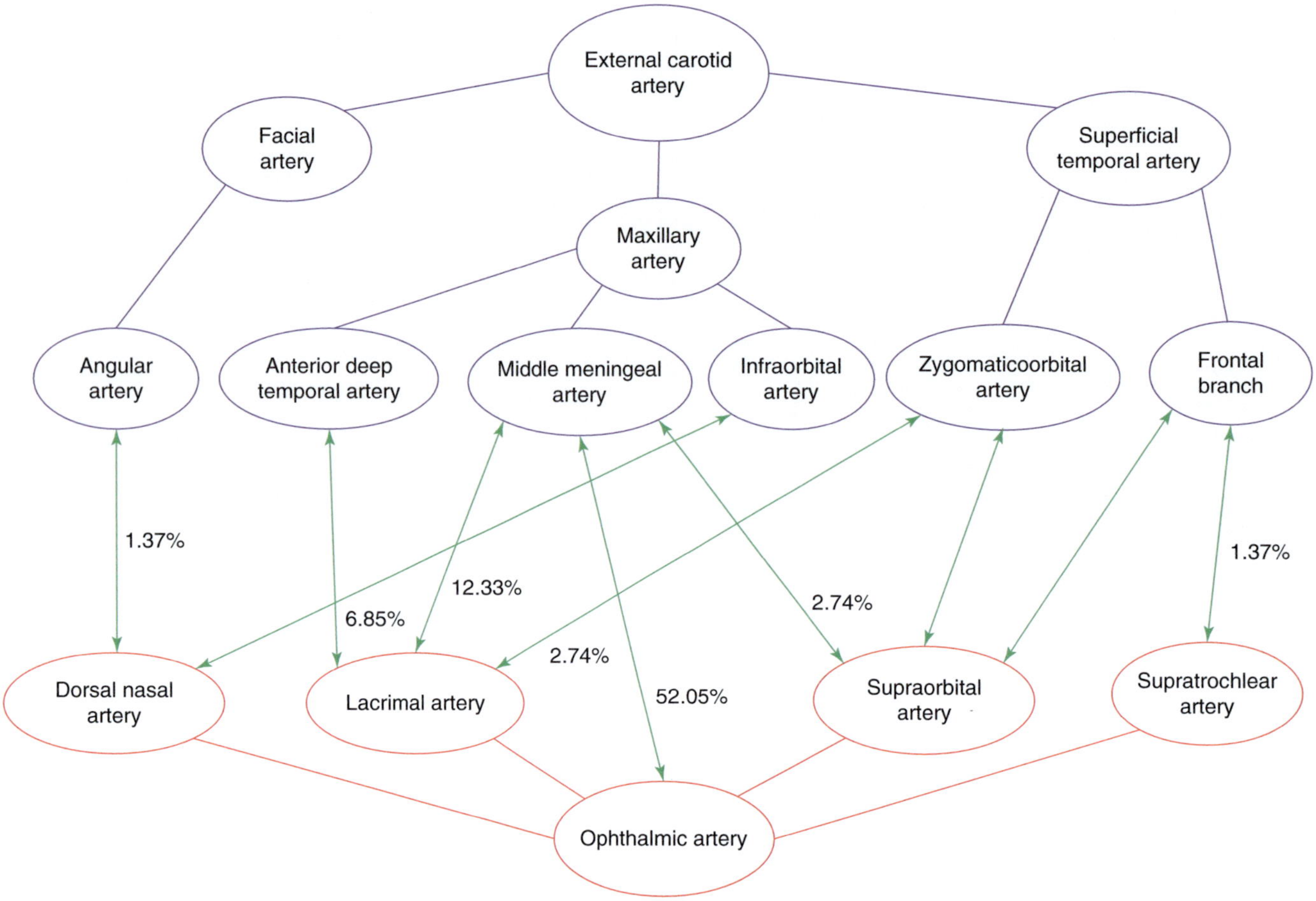

Fig. 6 Schematic diagram of the anastomoses between the ophthalmic artery and the external carotid artery systems. The alternative pathways of drug delivery used by Bertelli et al. [18] are indicated with the frequency of their employment

6 Retinoblastoma Regression Pattern

The ophthalmoscopic appearance of successfully treated tumors (disappearance of tumor activity) has been classified into four regression patterns (Table 3) [32].

7 Complications

Intra-arterial chemotherapy has potential complications due to its invasive nature and due to the delivery of high doses of chemotherapeutic agents directly to the orbit, doses up to ten times higher than in systemic chemotherapy [33]. We can divide complications into ocular and periocular vs systemic, transient vs permanent, and drug-related vs endovascular procedure-related complications [34].

7.1 Ocular and Periocular Side Effects

Ocular complications are an important indicator of local toxicity. Most side effects are transient, more evident at the first infusion, and less pronounced in the following cycles.

Chemosis, eyelid edema, and erythema (Fig. 9) are the most commonly reported ocular complications. Nevertheless, they are transient and usually resolve within few days.

Blepharoptosis and orbital congestion, sometimes with temporary dysmotility, frontal hair loss, and madarosis (Fig. 9), typically recover within a few months.

Forehead hyperemia, erythema, dyschromia, and skin necrosis (Fig. 10) are transient periocular side effects typically related to the territories of distribution of the terminal branches of the ophthalmic artery (i.e., supratrochlear and dorsal nasal arteries; Fig. 10). A retrospective unpublished evaluation of the initial ophthalmic angiogram of the group of children affected by these complications revealed that the supratrochlear artery could be visualized (Fig. 10) in a statistically significant higher number of cases compared to a group of children who did not show any side effect. Thus, when observing such angiographic findings, simple and effective measures like manual compression of the superomedial orbital angle or application of topical phenylephrine on the forehead may be useful to prevent skin frontal side effects by reducing the drug diffusion [35].

The effect on tumor response and on possible side effects of anatomical and/or hemodynamic variations of orbital ves-

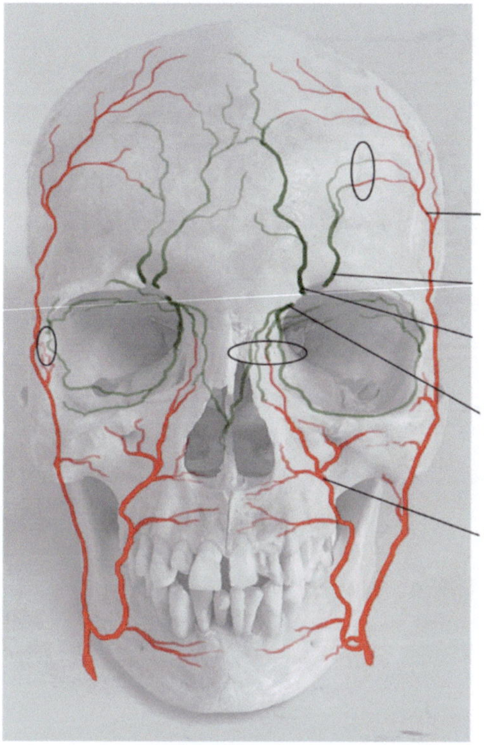

Fig. 7 Schematic diagram of the periorbital arterial circulation. Vessels in green are branches of the ophthalmic artery; vessels in red are branches of the external carotid artery. The two arterial trees meet together at the anterior border of the orbit. The sites of some periorbital anastomoses are encircled

sels and flow pattern is still to be determined. However, the presence of a small territory of distribution of the ophthalmic artery beyond the origin of the central retinal artery would reasonably seem to be the prerequisite for obtaining a greater therapeutic effect and fewer periocular side effects (Fig. 3b).

Serious ophthalmic vascular events with various degrees of permanent damage include vitreous or macular hemorrhage (Fig. 11), occlusion of the central retinal artery or of one of its branches, ophthalmic artery occlusion, and choroidal occlusive vasculopathy (Fig. 12) [36].

In contrast to the abrupt findings of ophthalmic or retinal obstruction, the choroidal ischemic process manifests more slowly with focal areas of retinal pigment epithelium (RPE) alterations (mottling) that gradually evolve over several months into RPE atrophy. The features of choroidal atrophy are mild in most cases and probably due to chemotherapy-related toxic effects on the endothelium more than acute embolic or traumatic events. The incidence of permanent ocular side effects should be considered in the decision-making process regarding IAC for RB in children with residual vision.

An impaired global growth may occur as a consequence of choroidal occlusive vasculopathy or due to the direct action of antitumoral drugs on the cells replicating within the eye (Fig. 13).

Retinal detachment, possibly secondary, due to accelerated regression of endophytic tumors, has been reported in 8–16% of naïve retinoblastoma [33].

7.2 Systemic Side Effects

Despite localized delivery of drugs, systemic toxicity has been observed following IAC, mostly mild and transient. Nausea and vomiting is the most common systemic adverse event. The second one is transient neutropenia observed in 12% of patients [33] and/or anemia, especially with higher doses of chemotherapy [37]. True anaphylaxis or anaphylactoid reactions are rare. Fever associated with neutropenia or myelosuppression or cytopenias requiring hospitalization is very rare [7].

7.3 Procedure-Related Complications

IAC has a learning curve and is safe when performed by a neuroendovascular interventional team in a high-volume institution. Possible complications related to the vascular access are bleeding and hematoma at the groin puncture site. Femoral artery occlusion and other severe complications related to supra-aortic catheterization, like carotid artery dissection, embolism, stroke, and death, are seldom reported but can occur [33].

Other complications, strictly associated with the catheterization procedure, include autonomic episodes due to vagal reflex induced by the navigation of the cavernous internal carotid artery or cannulation of the ophthalmic artery [27]. The patients may present increase in airway pressure with reduction in oxygen saturation up to 30% due to bronchospasm. In some cases, various degrees of bradycardia and hypotension can occur [27].

8 IAC: Advantages and Disadvantages

8.1 Advantages

Intra-arterial chemotherapy delivering chemotherapeutic drugs selectively into the ophthalmic artery:

- Minimizes systemic absorption and drug-related toxicity, such as neutropenia, infection, and secondary neoplasms.
- Decreases the need for hospitalization.

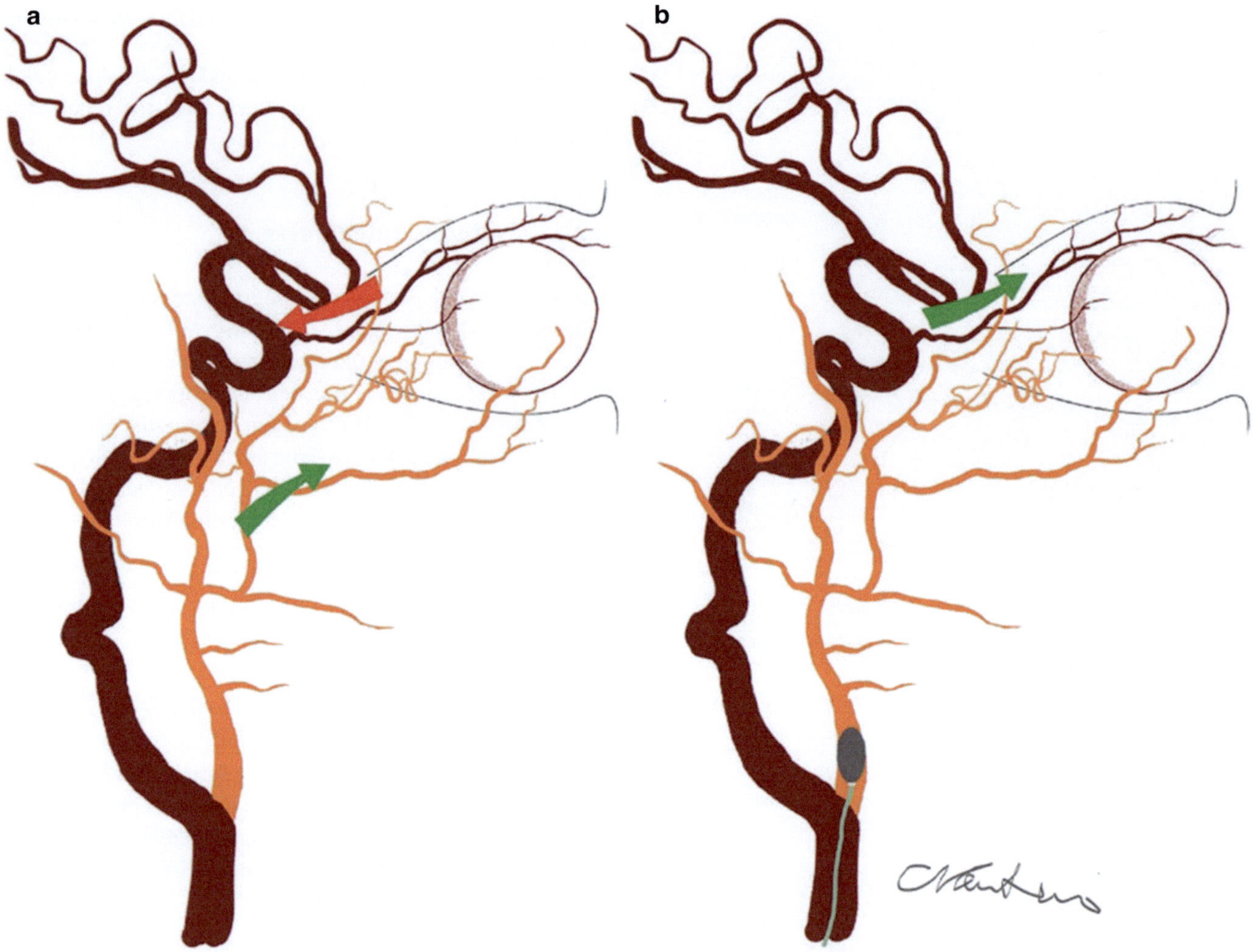

Fig. 8 Schematic diagrams of the technique employed by Abruzzo et al. [26]. (**a**) Ophthalmic flow coming from the external carotid arterial circulation. (**b**) According to Abruzzo et al. [26], a balloon catheter temporarily inflated in the external carotid trunk is capable of reverting the flow within the ophthalmic artery

Table 2 Drugs dosage in IAC according to Gobin et al. [30]

Drug	3–6 months	6–12 months	1–3 years	Over 3 years
Melphalan	2.5 mg	3 mg	4 mg	5 mg
Topotecan	0.3 mg	0.3 mg	0.3 mg	0.4 mg
Carboplatin	Not tested	30 mg	30 mg	30 mg

Table 3 Retinoblastoma regression patterns

Type 0	Complete disappearance of tumor (a very rare event in retinoblastoma)
Type I	The tumor assumes a glistening white appearance resembling cottage cheese
Type II	The regressed tumor has a homogeneous, gray, translucent aspect, which has been likened to fish flesh and which is difficult to distinguish from viable tumor
Type III	It is a combination of types I and II
Type IV	Flat chorioretinal scar

- In case of recurrent retinoblastoma after systemic chemotherapy, the risk of resistance is minimal as melphalan is not employed in the intravenous therapy.
- Administers significantly higher doses of chemotherapy directly to the tumor and to any seeds, thereby increasing the biological effect, enhancing tumor control, and reducing the rate of recurrence.

All the above contribute to a dramatic reduction in enucleation in advanced and treatment-resistant retinoblastomas (Figs. 14, 15, 16, 17, and 18) [27, 38, 39].

8.2 Disadvantages

- IAC alone is not effective against vitreous seeds. Since the introduction of IViC in combination with IAC, a clear decrease in enucleation rate has been reported.
- Lack of control of potential metastatic diseases.
- Most adverse side effects are transient. However, choroidal vasculopathy is permanent and, in some cases, progressive [40].

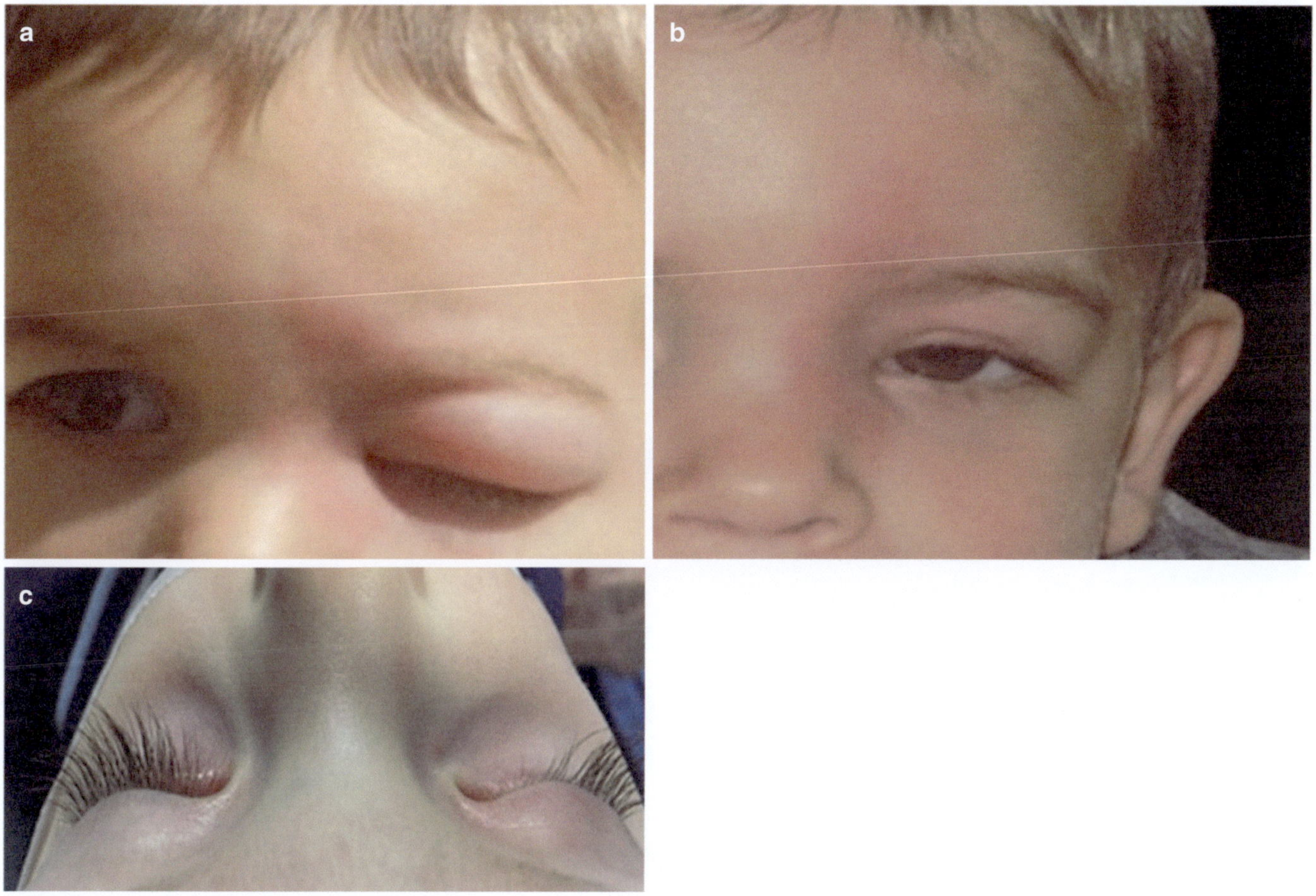

Fig. 9 Typical local side effects of IAC. (**a**) Upper eyelid edema. (**b**) Frontal rash. (**c**) Madarosis in the medial third of the upper eyelid

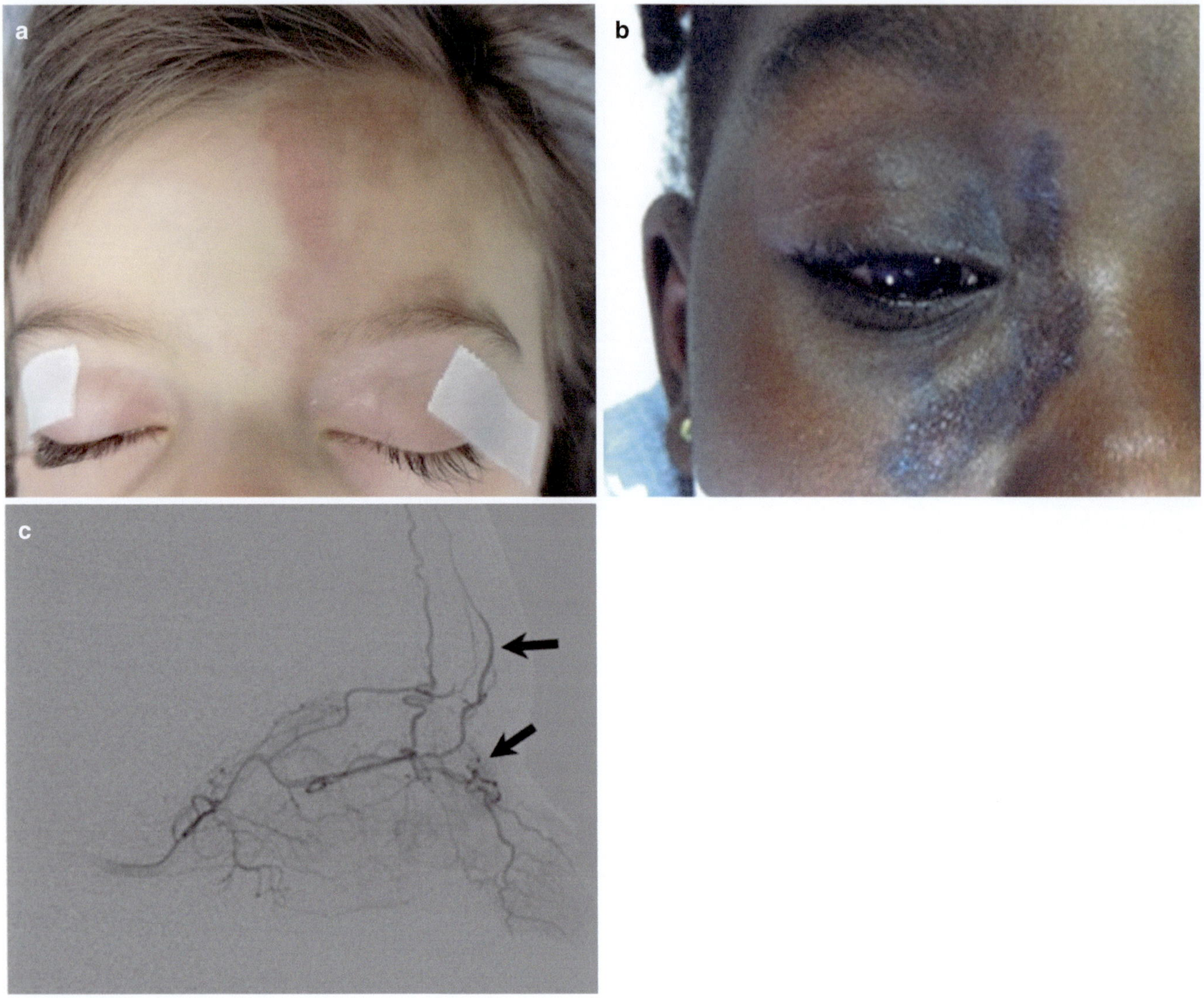

Fig. 10 Typical local side effects of IAC. (**a**) Forehead hyperemia, erythema, and dyschromia in the territory of distribution of the supratrochlear and supraorbital arteries. (**b**) Skin necrosis in the territory of distribution of the dorsal nasal/facial artery. (**c**) Side effects shown in (**a**) and (**b**) are frequently related with a dominant ophthalmic artery blood supply of the upper face. This hemodynamic pattern can be demonstrated when the selective angiography of the ophthalmic artery allows a good visualization of one or both terminal branches

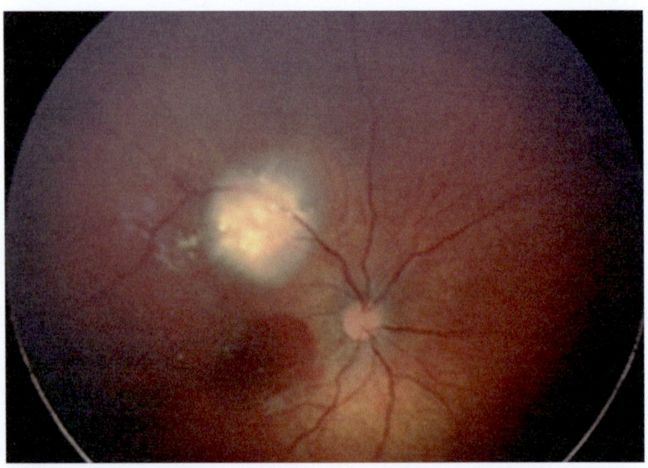

Fig. 11 Macular hemorrhage

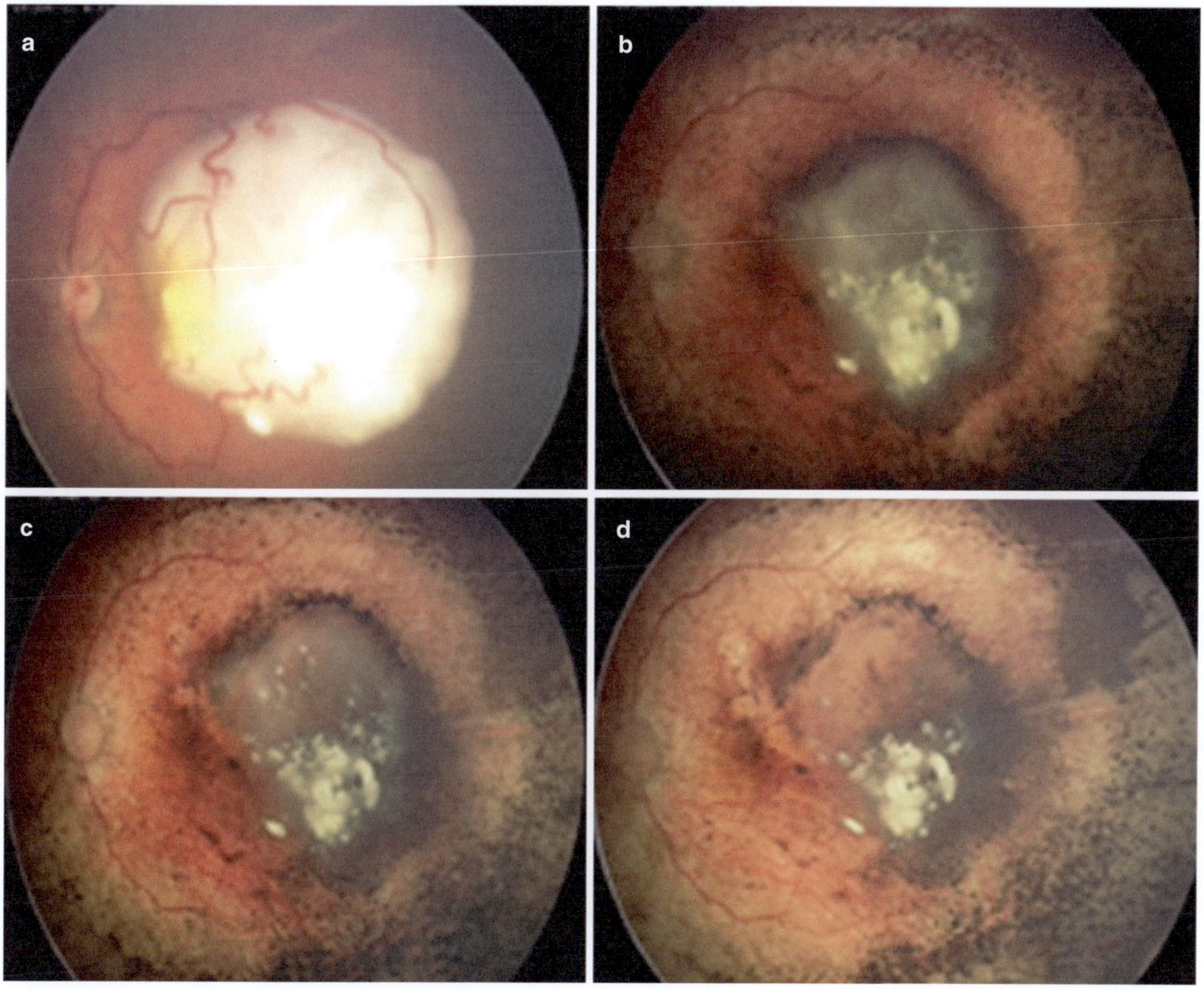

Fig. 12 Progression of choroidal occlusive vasculopathy **a** (top left), **b** (top right), **c** (lower left), and **d** (lower right)

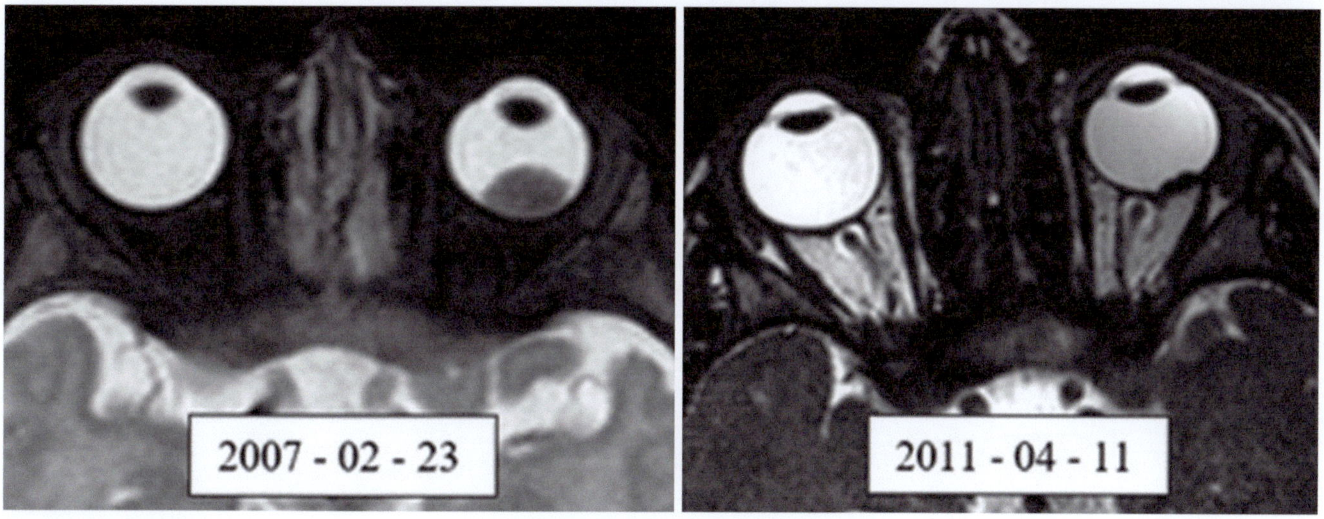

Fig. 13 Magnetic resonance imaging (MRI) at diagnosis and after complete remission: impaired globe growth of the treated eye

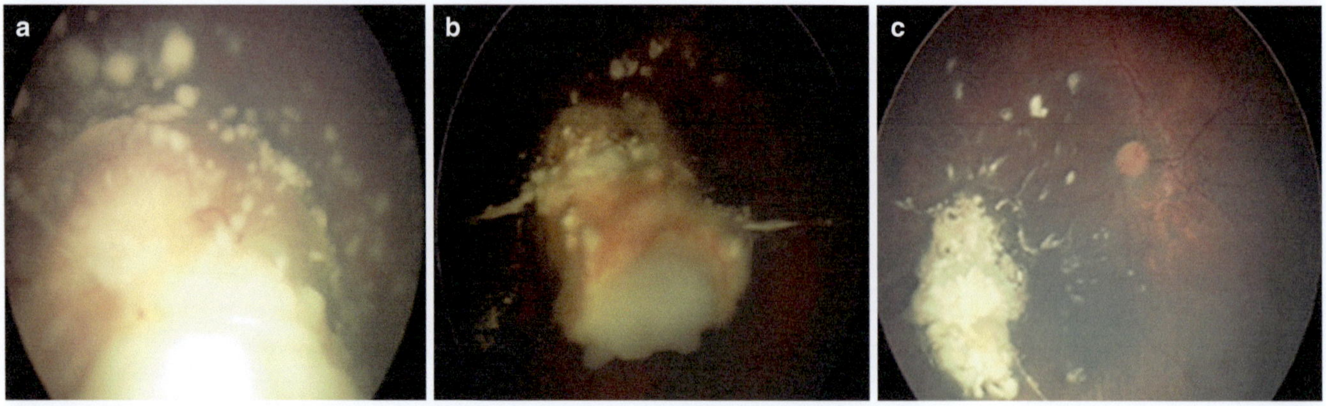

Fig. 14 (**a**) Three-year-five-month-old male, unilateral RB, large endophytic tumor, group D with type 2 vitreous seeding. (**b**) Complete regression (type I) following six IAC infusions and four IViC injections with no complications. (**c**) Seven years of follow-up

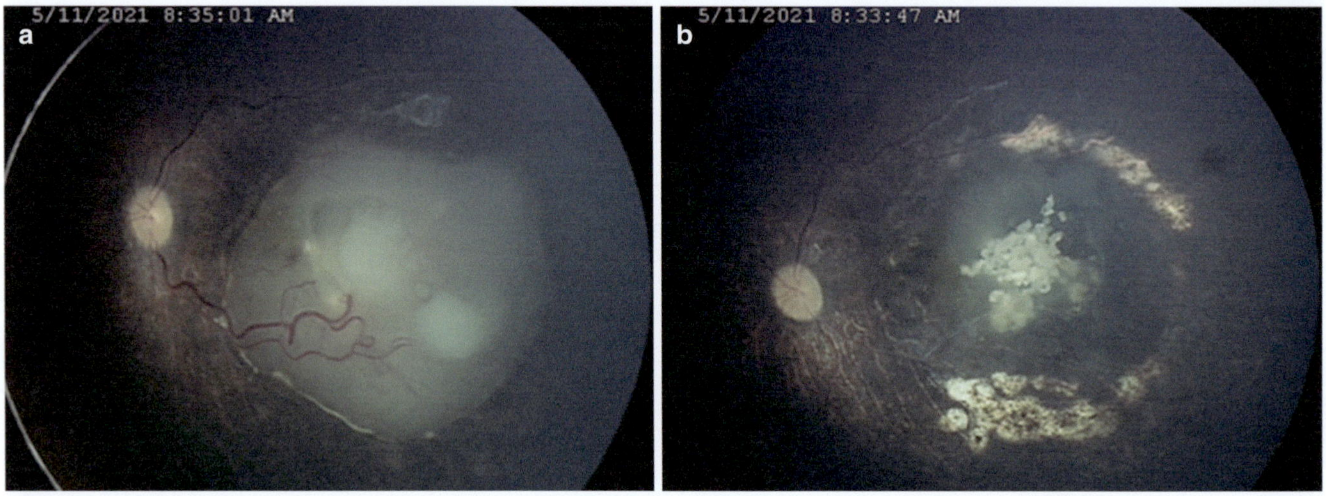

Fig. 15 One-year-four-month-old male. (**a**) Unilateral macular RB, Group B. (**b**) Complete regression type I following IAC infusions

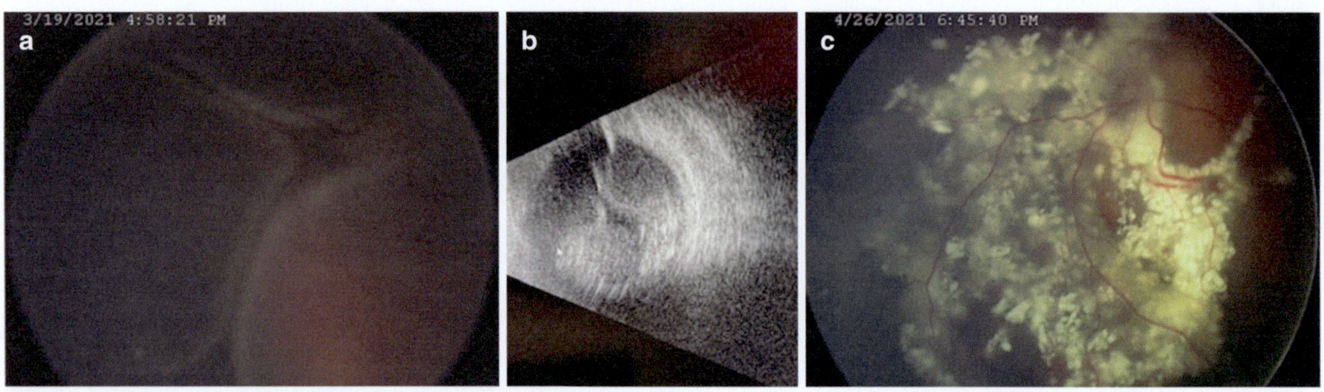

Fig. 16 One-year-two-month-old female, unilateral RB group E, exophytic. (**a**) Complete retinal detachment. (**b**) Ultrasound (US) documenting a bilobed tumor. (**c**) Complete regression type III following four IAC

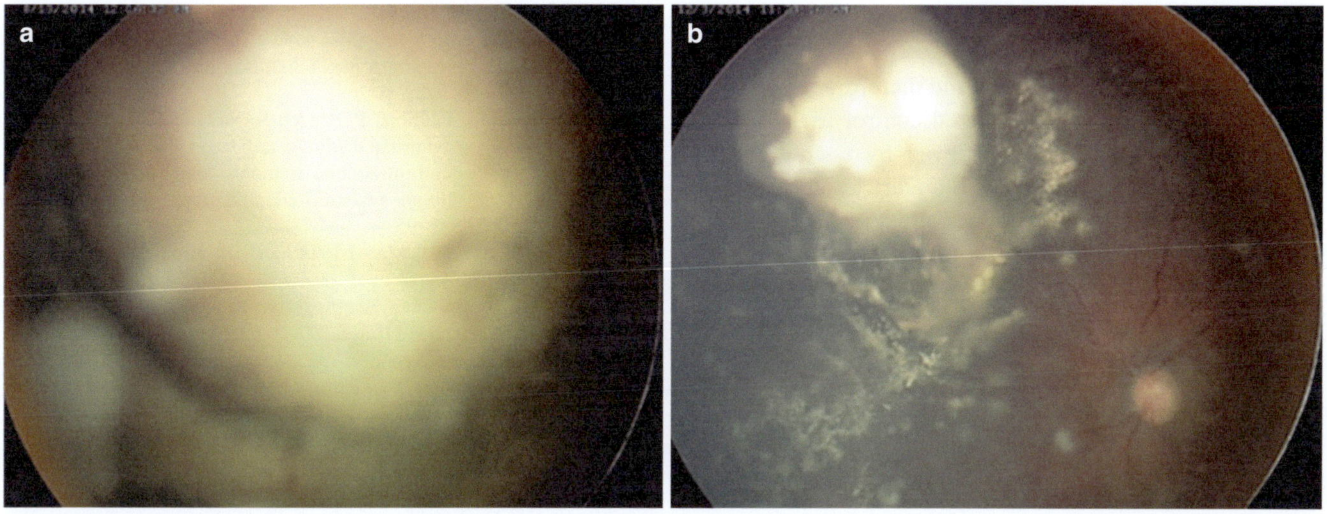

Fig. 17 One-year-one-month old male. (**a**) Unilateral RB group D, type vitreous seeding. (**b**) Complete remission type III following six IAC infusions and five IViC

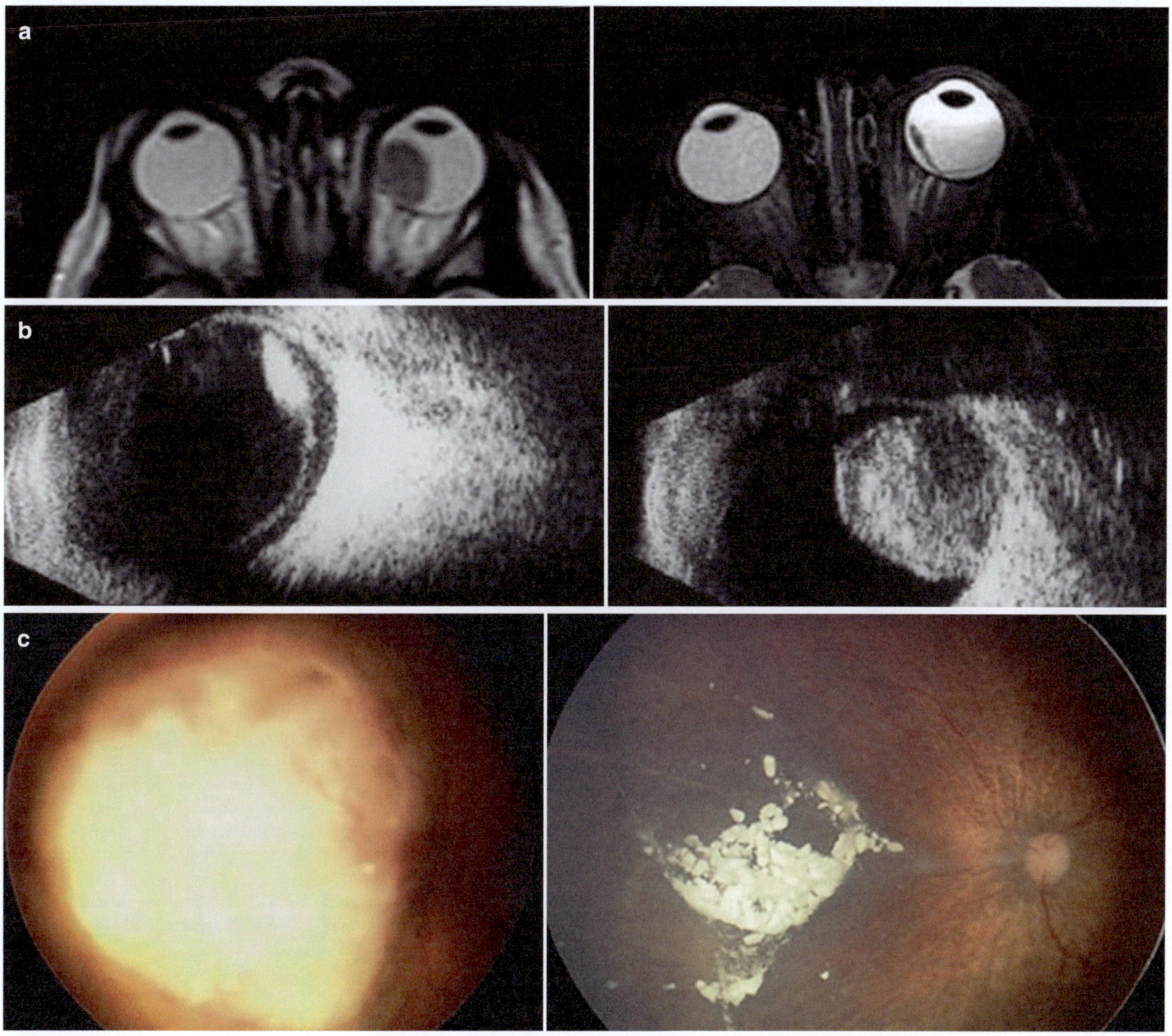

Fig. 18 Two-year-old male, unilateral RB group B. (**a**) MRI at diagnosis and regression. (**b**) US at diagnosis and regression. (**c**) Ophthalmoscopic appearance at diagnosis and complete regression type I

9 Conclusions

Retinoblastoma is a rare cancer, and therefore it is difficult to perform prospective randomized control trials to compare the diverse outcomes achieved by each treatment modality [41]. The international literature has a large number of case series on the IAC in patients with retinoblastoma, the majority of them being retrospective. The most common limitations of these studies are small sample size, short follow-up, use of concurrent adjuvant therapies, different types and doses of chemotherapeutic agents, diverse number of IAC sessions, and variation in the interval between them [30].

Currently, IAC has been implemented in more than 45 countries and is used as primary and secondary treatment for intraocular retinoblastoma. Since its introduction, the evolution of IAC has contributed to increased efficacy and safety, especially for group D retinoblastoma. Risks and benefits in less advanced tumors are yet to be established [7].

Eyes with advanced tumors constitute the major therapeutic challenge because they are often associated with high-risk histopathological features predictive of dissemination, so IAC should be used with caution in group E.

The implementation of IAC worldwide has made it possible to reduce the rate of enucleation without increasing deaths from metastases [42].

References

1. Reese AB, Hyman G, Tapley N, Forrest AW. The treatment of retinoblastoma by X-ray and triethilene melamine. AMA Arch Ophthalmol. 1958 Nov;60(5):897–906.
2. Inomata M, Kaneko A. Chemosensitivity profiles of primary and cultured human retinoblastoma cells in a human tumor clonogenic assay. Jpn J Cancer Res. 1987 Aug;78(8):858–68.
3. Suzuki S, Kaneko A. Management of intraocular retinoblastoma and ocular prognosis. Int J Clin Oncol. 2004 Feb;9(1):1–6.
4. Kaneko A, Suzuki S. Eye-preservation treatment of retinoblastoma with vitreous seeding. Jpn J Clin Oncol. 2003 Dec;33(12):601–7.
5. Yamane T, Kaneko A, Mohri M. The technique of ophthalmic arterial infusion therapy for patients with intraocular retinoblastoma. Int J Clin Oncol. 2004 Apr;9(2):69–73.
6. Abramson DH, Dunkel IJ, Brodie SE, Kim JW, Gobin YP. A phase I/II study of direct intraarterial (ophthalmic artery) chemotherapy with melphalan for intraocular retinoblastoma initial results. Ophthalmology. 2008 Aug;115(8):1398–404.
7. Pekacka A. The role of intraarterial chemotherapy in the management of retinoblastoma. J Ophthalmol. 2020 Jan;24:3638410. https://doi.org/10.1155/2020/3638410.
8. Abramson DH. Super selective ophthalmic artery delivery of chemotherapy for intraocular retinoblastoma: 'chemosurgery' the first Stallard lecture. Br J Ophthalmol. 2010 Apr;94(4):396–9.
9. Hadjistilianou T, Coriolani G, Bracco S, Gennari P, Caini M, Cerase A, et al. Successful treatment of macular retinoblastoma with superselective ophthalmic artery infusion of melphalan. J Pediatric Ophthalmol Strabismus. 2014 Jan-Feb;51(1):32–8.
10. Abramson DH, Dunkel IJ, Brodie SE, Marr B, Gobin YP. Superselective ophthalmic artery chemotherapy as primary treatment for retinoblastoma (chemosurgery). Ophthalmology. 2010 Aug;117(8):1623–9.
11. De Francesco S, Galluzzi P, Bracco S, Menicacci F, Motolese E, Hadjistilianou T. Alternated intra-arterial and intravitreal chemotherapy for advanced intraocular retinoblastoma: preliminary successful results without systemic chemotherapy. Int Ophthalmol. 2015 Dec;35(6):887–95.
12. Gobin PY, Dunkel IJ, Marr BP, Francis JH, Brodie SE, Abramson DH. Combined, Sequential intravenous and intra-arterial chemotherapy (bridge chemotherapy) for young infants with retinoblastoma. PLoS One [Internet]. 2012;7(9):e44322. https://doi.org/10.1371/journal.pone.0044322.
13. Abramson DH, Marr BP, Francis JH, Dunkel IJ, Fabius AWM, Brodie SE, et al. Simultaneous bilateral ophthalmic artery chemosurgery for bilateral retinoblastoma (tandem therapy). PLoS One [Internet]. 2016;11(6):e0156806. https://doi.org/10.1371/journal.pone.0156806.
14. Stacey AW, De Francesco S, Borri M, Hadjistilianou T. The addition of Topotecan to Melphalan in the treatment of retinoblastoma with intra-arterial chemotherapy. Ophthalmol Retina. 2020 Nov;19 https://doi.org/10.1016/j.oret.2020.11.007.
15. De Francesco S, Pichi F, Lembo A, Mastrangelo D, Paradiso A, De Luca M, et al. Massive anterior chamber involvement after intra-arterial chemotherapy for retinoblastoma: ultrasound biomicroscopy and histopathology. Int Ophthalmol. 2014 Aug;34(4):967–70.
16. Zanaty M, Barros G, Chalouhi N, Starke RM, Manasseh P, Tjoumakaris SI, et al. Update on intra-arterial chemotherapy for retinoblastoma. ScientificWorldJournal. 2014;2014:869604.
17. Bertelli E. Anatomy of the eye and human visual system. Piccin Nuova Libraria: Padova, Italy; 2019. 423 p.
18. Bertelli E, Leonini S, Galimberti D, Moretti S, Tinturini R, Hadjistilianou T, et al. Hemodynamic and anatomic variations require an adaptable approach during intra-arterial chemotherapy for intraocular retinoblastoma: alternative routes, strategies, and follow-up. AJNR Am J Neuroradiol. 2016 Jul;37(7):1289–95.
19. Bracco S, Venturi C, Leonini S, Romano DG, Cioni S, Vallone IM, et al. Transorbital anastomotic pathways between the external and internal carotid systems in children affected by intraocular retinoblastoma. Surg Radiol Anat. 2016 Jan;38(1):79–87.
20. Klufas MA, Gobin YP, Marr B, Brodie SE, Dunkel IJ, Abramson DH. Intra-arterial chemotherapy as a treatment for intraocular retinoblastoma: alternatives to direct ophthalmic artery catheterization. AJNR Am J Neuroradiol. 2012 Sep;33(8):1608–14.
21. Cooke D, Farid H, Kim W, Dowd W, Higashida R, Halbach V. Zygomatico-orbital intra-arterial melphalan infusion for intraocular retinoblastoma. J Neurointerv Surg. 2012 Jul;4(4):e16. https://doi.org/10.1136/neurintsurg-2011-010019.
22. Pham C-T, Blanc R, Lumbroso-Le Rouic L, Pistocchi S, Bartolini B, Piotin M. Access to the ophthalmic artery by retrograde approach through the posterior communicating artery for intra-arterial chemotherapy of retinoblastoma. Neuroradiology. 2012 Aug;54(8):845–8. https://doi.org/10.1007/s00234-011-0978-4.
23. Saglam M, Sarici A, Anagnostaku V, Yildiz B, Kocer N, Islak C, et al. An alternative technique of the superselective catheterization of the ophthalmic artery for intra-arterial chemotherapy of the retinoblastoma: retrograde approach through the posterior communicating artery to the ophthalmic artery. Neuroradiology. 2014 Sep;56(9):751–4.
24. Amans MR, Narvid J, Van Halbach V. Intra-arterial chemotherapy for bilateral retinoblastoma via left ophthalmic artery and right anterior deep temporal artery. BMJ Case Rep. 2014;2014:bcr2014204549. https://doi.org/10.1136/bcr-2014-204549.

25. Bartolini B, Puccinelli F, Hajdu SD, Stathopoulos C, Beck-Popovic M, Munier FL, et al. Middle meningeal artery occlusion for intra-arterial chemotherapy of retinoblastoma. Interv Neuroradiol. 2019 Jun;25(3):335–7.
26. Abruzzo TA, Geller JI, Kimbrough DA, Geller JI, Kinbrough DA, Michaels S, Correa ZM, Cornell K, et al. Adjunctive techniques for optimization of ocular hemodynamics in children undergoing ophthalmic artery infusion chemotherapy. J Neurointerv Surg. 2015;7(10):770–6.
27. Venturi C, Bracco S, Cerase A, Cioni S, Galluzzi S, Gennari P, et al. Superselective ophthalmic artery infusion of melphalan for intraocular retinoblastoma: preliminary results from 140 treatments. Acta Ophthalmol. 2013;91(4):335–42.
28. Buddu S, Abramson DH, Marr BP, Francis JH, Gobin YP. Selective ophthalmic artery chemosurgery (SOAC) for retinoblastoma: fluoroscopic time and radiation dose parameters. A baseline study. J Neurointerv Radiol. 2017 Nov;9(11):1107–12.
29. Guasti A, Leonini S, Bertelli E, Baldi R, Gennari P, Cioni S, Vallone IM, Romano DG, Casseri T, Guerrini L, La Rocca AE, Scala PGD, De Francesco S, Hadjistilianou T, Bracco S. Intra-arterial chemotherapy for retinoblastoma: the dosimetric impact. Neuroradiology. 2019 Sep;61(9):1083–91.
30. Gobin YP, Dunkel IJ, Marr BP, Brodie SE, Abramson DH. Intra-arterial chemotherapy for the Management of Retinoblastoma: four year experience. Arch Ophthalmol. 2011;129(6):732–7.
31. Marr BP, Brodie SE, Dunkel IJ, Gobin YP, Abramson DH. Three-drug intra-arterial chemotherapy using simultaneous carboplatin, topotecan and melphalan for intraocular retinoblastoma: preliminary results. Br J Ophthalmol. 2012 Oct;96(10):1300–3. https://doi.org/10.1136/bjophthalmol-2012-301925.
32. Abramson, Gerardi CM, Ellsworth RM, McCormick B, Sussman D, Turner L. Radiation regression patterns in treated retinoblastoma: 7 to 21 years later. J Pediatr Ophthalmol Strabismus. 1991 Mar-Apr;28(2):108–12.
33. Ancona-Lezama D, Dalvin LA, Shields CL. Modern treatement of retinoblastoma: a 2020 review. Indian J Ophthalmol. 2020;68(11):2356–65.
34. Shields CL, Bianciotto CG, Jabbour P, Griffin GC, Ramasubramanian A, Rosenwasser R, Shields JA. Intra-arterial chemotherapy for retinoblastoma: report no. 2, treatment complications. Arch Ophthalmol. 2011;129(11):1407–15.
35. Abramson DH, Daniels AB, Marr BP, Francis JH, Brodie SE, Dunkel IJ, et al. Intra-arterial chemotherapy (ophthalmic artery chemosurgery) for group D retinoblastoma. PLoS One. 2016 Jan;11(1):e0146582. https://doi.org/10.1371/journal.pone.0146582.
36. Munier FL, Beck-Popovic M, Balmer A, Gaillard MC, Bovey E, Binaghi S. Occurrence of sectoral choroidal occlusive vasculopathy and retinal arteriolar embolization after superselective ophthalmic artery chemotherapy for advanced intraocular retinoblastoma. Retina. 2011;31(3):566–73.
37. Muen WJ, Kingston JE, Robertson F, Brew S, Sagoo MS, Reddy MA. Efficacy and complications of super-selective intra-ophthalmic artery melphalan for the treatment of refractory retinoblastoma. Ophthalmology. 2011;118(10):2081–7.
38. Stathopoulos C, Gaillard MC, Puccinelli F, Maeder P, Hadjistilianou D, Beck-Popovic M, Munier FL. Successful conservative treatment of massive choroidal relapse in 2 retinoblastoma patients monitored by ultrasound biomicroscopy and/or spectral domain optic coherence tomography. Ophthalmic Genet. 2018 Apr;39(2):242–6.
39. Jabbour P, Chalouhi N, Tjoumakaris S, Gonzalez LF, Dumont AS, Chitale R, Rosenwasser R, Bianciotto CG, Shields C. Pearls and pitfalls of intraarterial chemotherapy for retinoblastoma. J Neurosurg Pediatr. 2012 Sep;10(3):175–81.
40. Hadjistilianou T, De Francesco S, De Luca M, Borri M, Micheli L, Bracco S, et al. Superselective intraarterial chemotherapy complications in advanced retinoblastoma. Acta Ophthalmologica. 2011;89(supplement):S248.
41. Kaewkhaw R, Rojanaporn D. Retinoblastoma: etiology, modeling, and treatment. Cancers. 2020 Aug;12(8):2304. https://doi.org/10.3390/cancers12082304.
42. Abramson DH, Shields CL, Jabbour P, Teixeira LF, Fonseca JRF, Marques MCP, et al. Metastatic deaths in retinoblastoma patients treated with intraarterial chemotherapy (ophthalmic artery chemosurgery) worldwide. Int J Retin Vitr. 2017 Oct 23;3:40. https://doi.org/10.1186/s40942-017-0093-8.

Treatment Algorithms for Intraocular Retinoblastoma: An Ocular Oncologist's Perspective

Jonathan W. Kim

1 Introduction

An ocular oncologist faces critical decisions when making recommendations for both primary and secondary therapies for retinoblastoma (RB). The decision-making process is complicated because the clinician must weigh the realistic chances for globe salvage, spectrum of complications from potential harmful therapies, and the remote but serious risk of extraocular spread. Treatment decisions are also based on the clinical experiences of the treating physician, availability of treatment modalities at the facility, and the preferences of the parents. Over the past 10 years, I was the director of one of the busiest retinoblastoma centers in the country at Children's Hospital Los Angeles (CHLA). I also had the opportunity of examining the first patient ever treated with intra-arterial chemotherapy (IAC) in 2006 at Memorial Sloan-Kettering Cancer Center (MSKCC). In 2012, I had the privilege of working with Dr. A. Linn Murphree at CHLA, who treated all children with systemic chemotherapy (carboplatin, etoposide, and vincristine [CEV]) and focal consolidation. Therefore, I can offer a balanced perspective when it comes to comparing the two techniques (IAC vs CEV) for treating intraocular retinoblastoma. In addition, I have had the opportunity to review charts of retinoblastoma patients sent to me by hospitals from across the country, and I recognize that the empiric evidence available in the published literature is incomplete. I have been involved in the development of national protocols for the Children's Oncology Group (COG) and served as lead moderator of retinoblastoma panels at the American Academy of Ophthalmology (AAO) annual meetings. My recommendations are based on this experience and my personal belief that the retinoblastoma treatment team should take a decisive course of action, based on all of the available evidence to date.

J. W. Kim (✉)
Department of Ophthalmology, Kaiser Permanente, Orange County, CA, USA
e-mail: jonathan.w.kim@kp.org

2 Primary Therapy

I will not discuss primary enucleation in detail in this chapter but will remind the reader that this option should be offered to all unilateral retinoblastoma cases with an advanced tumor and dismal visual potential. Both group D and E eyes can harbor high-risk histopathologic features, and primary enucleation is the *best* option for reducing the chances for metastatic disease. Even though success rates for globe salvage after IAC can be as high as 90% for group D eyes, exposing a young child or infant to potentially harmful therapies to save a blind eye is not the right approach in all cases. A major issue in having these discussions with parents is that there is a great deal of discrepancy between the classification of group D and E eyes, and therefore inconsistency in how these very advanced eyes are managed at various centers [1]. To me, a group E eye has evidence of high intraocular pressure (or buphthalmia), significant intraocular hemorrhage, or anterior segment infiltration (on clinical exam or ultrasound). Next, there are group D/E eyes that harbor very large tumors with no visible normal retina on fundoscopy. The rest of the eyes that have distant tumor seeding at diagnosis I consider to be "typical" group D eyes. I believe that any unilateral group E eye should be enucleated, because an eye with buphthalmia or massive intraocular hemorrhage has a low risk of globe salvage and is likely to develop phthisis or severe strabismus, even with successful treatment. During attempted globe salvage of these group E eyes, the clinician will not have an adequate view of the fundus and the child is going to be at an increased risk for metastatic disease. For those group D/E eyes with no visible normal retina and the majority of the globe filled with tumor, the parents should be advised that the salvage rate is going to be approximately 50%, and that a long course of treatment with more than 20 anesthesia sessions lies ahead.

In 2006, I co-wrote the original manuscript on IAC with David Abramson at MSKCC [2]. At that time, we did not know that IAC would become the dominant primary modality

B. V. Chawla, M. E. Aronow (eds.), *Global Perspectives in Ocular Oncology*, https://doi.org/10.1007/978-3-031-08250-4_8

to treat intraocular retinoblastoma in 2021, but that is exactly what has happened over the past decade [3–7]. I regret that we were not more specific in our recommendations for how IAC should be used, including which patients should receive IAC or when IAC should be abandoned in a particular case. We also should have recommended that all patients have a preoperative magnetic resonance imaging (MRI) scan to identify the relevant intracerebral vasculature. I have summarized below my opinion on how IAC should be used to treat intraocular retinoblastoma as primary therapy, depending on the clinical setting that faces the treating physician.

2.1 Unilateral Retinoblastoma

For unilateral group D disease, there is currently a consensus among retinoblastoma experts that IAC is the preferred primary modality for globe salvage. I have already explained my bias in not treating unilateral group E disease, and the realistic chances of salvaging group D/E disease. Clinical series from MSKCC and Will's Eye Hospital demonstrate >90% success in salvaging group D disease with IAC, with or without intravitreal melphalan (IVM) [5, 7]. Clinicians I have consulted outside of these two centers expect a salvage rate between 75 and 85% after IAC for group D disease. However, the rate of globe salvage of group D eyes using systemic chemotherapy (CEV) and IVM as salvage for vitreous seeding is 70–80% [8]. Therefore, the reported success rate with IAC (in the community) is probably slightly but not dramatically higher than CEV (plus IVM). A meta-analysis comparing the two techniques showed an advantage for IAC when evaluating the outcomes for group D eyes but not B or C disease [9, 10]. Regarding the side effect profiles of both treatment options, my belief is that for children older than 6 months of age, the overall side effect profile for IAC should be more favorable than with CEV (see below).

2.2 Bilateral Retinoblastoma

Bilateral patients can present with various combinations of tumors between the two eyes and it is not unusual for a child to have group E in one eye and group A or B in the second eye. Any child with a group E tumor and a contralateral eye that can be treated with focal modalities should undergo primary enucleation of the group E eye and laser or cryotherapy in the less advanced eye. If both eyes are group C or higher, then the general recommendation is for systemic chemotherapy, with IAC being reserved as secondary therapy. MSKCC currently utilizes bilateral IAC and more centers are starting to adopt this approach [11, 12]. However, I would caution against bilateral IAC in routine use for several reasons. Bilateral patients obviously have germinal disease, and therefore radiation exposure during fluoroscopy is a concern, although it is difficult to quantify this risk [13, 14]. Secondly, the treatment team must use a different agent for the second eye because of the systemic dose limits of melphalan, which is typically about 0.5 mg/kg per child per treatment [15]. At MSKCC, Dr. Abramson uses various combinations of melphalan, carboplatin, and topotecan between the two eyes to avoid this toxicity level, but there is absence of a well-defined regimen that his team follows when performing bilateral IAC [11, 12, 16]. For these reasons, most centers currently recommend using systemic CEV for bilateral, advanced disease.

2.3 Intravitreal Melphalan (IVM) During Primary Therapy

The original IVM paper by Munier did not describe how and when intravitreal melphalan should be used by retinoblastoma specialists [17]. But the reader should recognize that IVM is used for secondary treatment of vitreous seeding not responding to primary therapy (either IAC or CEV). The majority of eyes with vitreous seeding respond to primary therapy (either IAC or CEV) and therefore IVM is not needed at diagnosis. Also, inserting a needle into an eye without an initial control of vitreous seeding (with primary therapy) may pose a significant risk of extraocular spread. Whether IAC or CEV is better for vitreous seeding as primary therapy is difficult to determine since a comparative trial has not been performed, but most clinicians believe that IAC is more effective. One caveat is that for patients with a calcified tumor and vitreous seeding arising from a tumor recurrence not in contact with the retina, IAC does not tend to get into the vitreous very well in that setting because the blood–retinal barrier has sealed after primary therapy.

I was recently involved with the planning of a national protocol that was designed to use IVM at diagnosis, and I had ethical objections to performing injections on patients who may not need it since both IAC and CEV eliminate vitreous seeding in at least 50% of patients. The potential risks of vision loss (see below) and extraocular relapse should always be a concern when performing IVM. Our center has given IVM with the last three cycles of a six-cycle CEV regimen when it was clear that the vitreous seeding was progressing. Theoretically, IVM could also be used during the three to four courses of IAC but this may not be practical since it takes at least several months to determine if the vitreous seeding is responding to primary therapy.

2.4 Infants

For children younger than 3 months of age (or 6 kg), I do not recommend IAC because of the unknown long-term effects of melphalan in infants and the very small size of the ophthalmic artery. Primary enucleation of advanced, unilateral disease is the preferred option in infants, rather than giving chemotherapy to a one- to two-month-old baby to save a blind eye. In my opinion, concerns about the health of the anophthalmic socket in infants have been greatly exaggerated. If a silicone implant is used at the time of primary enucleation in an infant, an implant exchange can be performed later in life with excellent cosmetic and functional results. For bilateral cases, CEV can be used in very young infants at a reduced dose, with IAC being used after 6 months of age if needed for salvage (i.e., bridge therapy) [18]. However, I do not recommend stopping CEV during primary therapy for IAC if there is a good response.

3 Secondary Therapy

There are no established guidelines for when and how an ocular oncologist should attempt to rescue an eye that has failed primary therapy. The following recommendations are based on my clinical experience and management principles taught to me by Dr. Abramson and Dr. Murphree.

3.1 Vitreous Seeding

For persistent or recurrent vitreous seeding after primary therapy, there are very few eyes that cannot be rescued with multiple sessions of IVM. A total of 10 IVM injections can be given, 1–3 weeks apart. However, any recurrence of vitreous seeding after the initial series of 3–4 injections probably indicates a persistent active retinal source of seeding. In the modern era of IVM, the only other situation that IVM therapy can fail is if a vitreous seed lands on the optic nerve and starts to grow in the prelaminar area. Theoretically, vitreous seeding could also grow in an uncontrolled fashion with the appearance of hundreds of new pre-retinal foci, but we have not observed this scenario with frequent, serial melphalan injections and concurrent treatment of any active retinal tumors.

3.2 Retinal Recurrence in a Unilateral Patient

Whenever a unilateral RB patient has a retinal recurrence, I recommend laser or cryotherapy (for anterior tumors) as focal modalities have the best side effect profiles. However, if the tumor is not responding or is larger than 3 mm, another modality will be needed. There are unique clinical situations where focal therapies are not effective, such as a tumor recurrence arising on top of a calcified mass. There is one report from MSKCC of IVM being used successfully for retinal foci in this scenario (using multiple agents) [19], but this strategy is far from reliable. For a large retinal recurrence (>3 mm) in a unilateral patient, a decision must be made whether to enucleate or use chemotherapy (IAC or CEV) as secondary therapy. Our team has used CEV successfully when IAC had to be stopped for various technical reasons but would not consider CEV as secondary therapy if a full cycle of IAC (minimum of three to four cycles) has been used. If a tumor has not responded to IAC for three to four cycles, it is extremely unlikely that CEV will be effective. When trying to decide whether to use IAC again in a salvage situation for a large retinal recurrence in a unilateral case, the parents should be warned that the chance of salvage is approximately 50%. Despite the high rate of globe salvage that has been reported for secondary IAC [20], this type of success has not been my experience. For patients with poor visual potential, secondary enucleation is always a good option. For unilateral cases with retinal, vitreous, and subretinal recurrence, secondary enucleation should also be strongly considered. If the patient has recently failed IAC with multiple drugs (within 2 months), then secondary enucleation is recommended. If the child has received recent IAC with one drug, then multiple drug secondary IAC can be attempted. If the child has not had IAC for at least 3 months, multiple agent IAC can be restarted for secondary salvage. Restarting IAC is a commitment for three more cycles unless technical difficulties are encountered or significant side effects occur.

What is the maximum number of IAC cycles for a unilateral case? As lead moderator, I posed this question to Dr. Abramson at the AAO meeting in 2017, but a definite answer was not provided. As mentioned, centers typically give three to four cycles for group D disease, but there are some specialists who have given over ten cycles of IAC for unilateral retinoblastoma. In my opinion, if the tumor has not completely regressed after seven cycles of IAC (four for primary and three for salvage), then it is very unlikely that the eye will ultimately be salvaged. Therefore, the practical limit for the number of cycles for unilateral disease is seven total cycles. Also, if at any time the fundus view becomes suboptimal and there is suspicion for recurrent disease, the eye must be enucleated.

3.3 Retinal Recurrence in a Bilateral Patient

For bilateral patients, if the contralateral eye without the recurrence is stable and has excellent vision, the above recommendations for unilateral patients can be followed. If the retinal recurrence is in the eye with better vision, then all attempts must be made for globe salvage (even with recurrent disease in multiple locations). Just a reminder that when you are treating the only remaining eye with useful vision, the treating physician must be even more cognizant of the possibility of treatment-related vision loss. When the better seeing eye has received multiple treatments and you are now adding additional courses of multiple drug IAC, there is the possibility of retinal or optic nerve toxicity. I am aware of a case of severe vision loss from retrobulbar optic neuropathy that occurred after multidrug IAC in this exact scenario. It has also been my impression that the threshold for radiation retinopathy is significantly lower if the child has recently received any form of chemotherapy. Obviously, the tumor recurrence poses a greater risk for loss of the eye than the threat of treatment-related visual decline, so this scenario is the most difficult situation for a pediatric ocular oncologist. Although a potential limit for IAC was discussed in the section for recurrent unilateral disease, when you are trying to save the only seeing eye, there are no such limits. However, secondary enucleation of the only seeing eye and definitely active (growing) tumor must be considered if there are no viable treatment options remaining. Fortunately, this is a very rare scenario in the current era of modern retinoblastoma treatment, and the episcleral chemotherapy implant may be available as a salvage option in the very near future. The episcleral implant is a silicone reservoir that holds topotecan in a fibrin sealant vehicle. At the time of the writing of this chapter, the implant has been used only in a salvage situation for monocular patients in a small series of patients at several centers. I am aware of the initial results, which are encouraging as the majority of the eyes are currently showing tumor response. However, I have been informed of several cases of retinal toxicity in eyes that have received multimodal therapy (e.g., brachytherapy). The efficacy of the episcleral implant in achieving long-term tumor control is also unknown. The clinical indications for the episcleral implant for primary or secondary therapy will be determined over time, although I caution clinicians against being too optimistic about its potential from these early clinical results. I am quite certain there will be both complications and limitations of this device identified with increasing clinical use, similar to other modalities that have been introduced for intraocular retinoblastoma over the past 50 years (though it is not the focus of this chapter, a paragraph on the episcleral chemo implant would be nice to add).

If both eyes have active retinal disease after IAC, then the choices would be bilateral, multiple drug IAC, systemic chemotherapy (CEV vs topotecan), or bilateral radiation (intensity-modulated radiation therapy [IMRT]). If the patient has already had CEV, then bilateral IAC can be considered or enucleation of the worse seeing eye and IAC in the better seeing eye. We have used systemic topotecan successfully after a full six cycles of CEV to allow for some regression of retinal recurrences, allowing laser consolidation to be performed. If the patient has bilateral small active recurrences in the posterior pole and all chemotherapy options have been exhausted, then IMRT can be considered as a last resort (using a maximum of 42 Gy). My impression of IMRT in these salvage situations is that the globe salvage rate for small posterior active retinal recurrences is 50% or lower. Parents and the treatment team must weigh the odds for globe salvage with the possible long-term risk of second cancers when considering IMRT.

4 Treatment Complications

There are both ocular and non-ocular (regional/systemic) complications to consider when recommending IAC, CEV, or IVM. For ocular complications, IVM has the highest risk, IAC intermediate risk, and CEV has essentially no risk (except after radiation therapy). When considering regional complications, IAC has the potential for serious neurologic and vascular sequelae. The risk of systemic complications is the highest with CEV and may be lifelong for the patient. Treatment complications are always underreported in the literature and therefore clinicians should not take an aggressive approach when adopting a novel technique. For a newer modality, it takes literally a decade for clinicians to get a full picture of the type of complications that can occur in various clinical settings.

4.1 IAC Complications

IAC was introduced in 2007 and is no longer considered experimental. Despite its technical complexity, I advise parents that the procedure is generally safe. However, there is a small risk of serious complications that the parents should be aware of when considering IAC as a treatment option. Neutropenia was recognized in the initial series of patients and is mainly a risk when the treatment dose exceeds 0.5 mg/kg [15]. For this reason, all children have a complete blood count (CBC) several weeks after a course of IAC. One of my patients received up to 8 mg of melphalan with IAC and in that case there was no demonstrable benefit to giving the higher dose. In my experience, the efficacy of IAC is determined by giving the recommended doses of melphalan (3–4 mg) at regular intervals (every 3–4 weeks) until the tumor is completely regressed, rather than the peak or absolute doses.

The potential ocular effects of IAC are a serious concern. There have been numerous reports of retinal and choroidal vascular occlusion with IAC [21–24], although this complication is not common in my experience. There have also been observations of choroidal atrophy after IAC at multiple centers [25, 26]. Patients commonly develop enophthalmos after IAC, and this is likely due to fat atrophy in the orbit. My colleagues at MSKCC have informed me that they have observed diffuse changes in the retinal pigment epithelium (RPE) with repeated treatments. There have been several studies documenting changes on electroretinogram (ERG) after IAC with a total dose >14 mg of melphalan but no documented effects on vision [27, 28]. During my time at MSKCC, we treated several adult patients with uveal melanoma with IAC (unsuccessfully) and there were no documented effects on vision post-treatment. All of this evidence poses the question: is there a risk of vision loss with IAC? In my opinion there is the potential risk of vision loss with repeated IAC although it is certainly less than with IVM. As previously mentioned, I am aware of one case of optic neuropathy that led to severe vision loss but that case had received extensive multimodal treatments.

When considering regional complications after IAC, there was early recognition that moderate but transient soft tissue swelling, madarosis, and skin erythema can be observed [29]. I am aware of a case of "skin necrosis" after IAC, although further details were not available. I was also referred a patient with an anomalous Circle of Willis who had developed a frontal lobe stroke after IAC was performed at another center [30]. There are also anecdotal cases of transient hemiparesis and cranial nerve palsies after IAC, which are very concerning. If these serious regional or neurologic side effects are noted after IAC, it is recommended that IAC be discontinued. These serious complications may be a sign that your patient has anomalous vasculature or perhaps a blood dyscrasia.

The national Children's Oncology Group (COG) protocol evaluating IAC was suspended because of cardiopulmonary side effects, which I believe to be greatly underreported. Because of autonomic reflexes, both bradycardia and a drop in oxygen saturation can be observed when the catheter is manipulated in the region of the cavernous sinus, and the IAC team must be ready to provide cardiopulmonary support during IAC. If these side effects can be reversed and the patient stabilized, IAC can be continued. I am not aware of any permanent cardiopulmonary side effects from IAC but the treatment team must be ready to counteract them during treatment.

4.2 Intravitreal Melphalan Injections for Vitreous Seeding (IVM)

Intravitreal melphalan injections have revolutionized the treatment of vitreous seeding over the past decade, and initially there were no reports of any serious ocular complications [31]. Our service began using IVM in 2012 and the initial results were very encouraging, with numerous eyes avoiding radiation or enucleation. However, over the next few years we observed several cases of severe retinal toxicity after IVM leading to complete vision loss. As I began to speak to other retinoblastoma specialists regarding this concerning side effect of IVM, I learned of other anecdotal cases with similar complications. We published our first case report of retinal toxicity after IVM in 2014 [32], which described a fundus appearance that was a combination of an arterial occlusion (widespread ischemia) and a vein occlusion (widespread hemorrhages and retinal edema). We had two cases of grade V retinal toxicity in the first 5 years of using IVM at our center but none thereafter. In attempting to determine the risk factors for this devastating complication, we could not correlate post-injection vision loss to any preoperative factor including the number of injections, variation in technique, or the presence of a posterior vitreous detachment. However, my clinical impression was that the risk of this devastating complication is related to dose, combined with an individual sensitivity to the drug (melphalan). Although many eyes will tolerate up to 30 μg of melphalan, it is much safer to use 20 μg as the standard dose, particularly in patients less than 2 years of age. Interestingly, we have not observed any eye with grade 3–5 retinal toxicity develop any tumor recurrence during long-term follow-up. There was recently a theory presented at an international meeting that perhaps the needle was injecting the drug into Cloquet's canal and by fluid passage into the sub-hyaloid space over the macula. Currently, we inject into the center of the vitreous cavity with the needle visible through the microscope (parallel with the lens) and inject slowly. Anterior segment toxicity is actually quite common, and there are theories that darker irides may be more prone to the development of iris atrophy, iritis, posterior synechiae, and cataract formation. In monocular patients, intravitreal topotecan may be a better choice with melphalan being used for failures, since topotecan does not have any significant ocular toxicity. One final clinical issue to mention is that it is very difficult to know when to stop IVM once a course has been initiated. At our center, we typically give three to four IVM total injections every 1–3 weeks and then observe for clinical documentation of progression. If a clinician injects until the vitreous seeds have completely disappeared, you may end up overtreating. My experience is that there is usually some lag time between the performance of IVM and the clinical response, which is detectable on fundoscopy, and not all cases demonstrate complete clearance of the vitreous debris.

4.3 Systemic Chemotherapy (CEV)

Over the past decade, our center (CHLA) has used more systemic chemotherapy than IAC to treat intraocular retinoblastoma. Because there was a tradition of using CEV at our center and our treatment team had a comfort level with using systemic chemotherapy, that was our primary modality for both unilateral and bilateral patients when I arrived at CHLA in 2012. Adopting IAC at our center involved overcoming some political resistance, as the oncologists were reluctant to give up control of their patients. Also, there was some faculty turnover in our neuro-interventional department and it was a reminder that the success of IAC is completely reliant on the experience of the interventionalist performing the treatment. Whenever a service adopts IAC, there is going to be a learning curve and I highly recommend that any new interventionalist spend time at MSKCC to learn the technique from Pierre Gobin's team. In my opinion, it takes at least 5 years for a center to develop expertise with IAC and it is not advisable to treat younger kids and use multiple drugs while the service is getting comfortable with the technique.

Given our center's expertise with systemic chemotherapy, I can confirm that complications with CEV are more common than is reported in the literature. Almost all patients receiving six cycles of CEV will require a transfusion or neutropenia support at some point in their course. Temporary hair loss occurs in all patients after several months of starting CEV. However, even young children tolerate systemic therapy surprisingly well, and weight loss or significant fevers are unusual. One complication that patients should be aware of is permanent hearing loss, particularly in younger infants less than 6 months of age. I believe hearing loss is more common than we understand because hospitals do not perform routine hearing tests on the majority of children who receive CEV. Over the past 10 years, we have diagnosed several cases of secondary leukemia at my center; these children had received six additional cycles of adjuvant chemotherapy after a full six cycles of CEV for intraocular retinoblastoma. There are some centers that routinely give ten cycles of CEV for group D retinoblastoma and I do not have information on the rates of complications associated with such a long course, but the eyes that I examined from these centers showed completely atrophic retinal scars with almost no calcium or type 2 regression patterns.

5 Metastatic Risk After IAC and CEV

With increasing use of IAC over the past decade, questions have arisen regarding the possible risk of extraocular spread and/or metastatic disease when patients are treated with IAC rather than CEV. This concern has been raised because CEV provides systemic coverage of micro-metastasis, which is of theoretical benefit since a significant percentage of group D eyes harbor high-risk histopathologic features. If a clinician believes in the effectiveness of adjuvant therapy post-enucleation, then this must be considered a benefit of CEV as well. Another concern is that more advanced eyes are being treated with IAC than in the previous era with CEV. The original IAC protocol at MSKCC enrolled patients who were "destined for enucleation." Not all of these very advanced eyes are going to respond to IAC and therefore some patients will have persistent and reactivated disease. Accordingly, there will be cases of tumor recurrence and possibly extraocular spread after IAC, whereas some of these eyes in the past would have been primarily enucleated. The risk of metastatic disease in the IAC era must not be dramatically higher compared to the era of CEV because no study has demonstrated a difference in rates of extraocular disease between the two modalities. However, the reader should recognize that there are cases of metastatic death that go unreported in the literature. Therefore, these theoretical concerns remain when using IAC for advanced intraocular retinoblastoma.

I am aware of three cases where children have died from metastatic disease after IAC, and the clinical situation was similar in all cases. The patient presented with advanced unilateral retinoblastoma, initially responded to IAC, but then developed recurrent disease that was treated with more cycles of IAC. Eventually, the clinician lost the fundus view or the mass itself obscured the location of the optic disk, and the patient developed an intraocular recurrence that eventually extended down the optic nerve and into the brain before the clinician could detect this horrible complication on MRI scan. As a clinician who treats intraocular retinoblastoma, under no circumstances can you allow an intraocular tumor to extend into the optic nerve during primary or secondary therapy and clinical protocols must be designed accordingly [33].

References

1. Kim JW, Shah SN, Green S, O'Fee J, Tamrazi B, Berry JL. Tumour size critera for group D and E eyes in the international classification system for retinoblastoma: effects on rates of globe salvage and high-risk histopathologic features. Acta Ophthalmol. 2019; Aug 17 (Epub ahead of print).
2. Abramson DH, et al. A phase I/II study of direct intraarterial (ophthalmic artery) chemotherapy with melphalan for intraocular retinoblastoma initial results. Ophthalmology. 2008;115(8):1398–404, 1404 e1.
3. Gobin YP, et al. Intra-arterial chemotherapy for the management of retinoblastoma: four-year experience. Arch Ophthalmol. 2011;129(6):732–7.
4. Peterson EC, et al. Selective ophthalmic artery infusion of chemotherapy for advanced intraocular retinoblastoma: initial experience with 17 tumors. J Neurosurg. 2011;114(6):1603–8.
5. Shields CL, et al. Intra-arterial chemotherapy for retinoblastoma in 70 eyes: outcomes based on the international classification of retinoblastoma. Ophthalmology. 2014;121(7):1453–60.
6. Abramson DH. Super selective ophthalmic artery delivery of chemotherapy for intraocular retinoblastoma: 'chemosurgery' the first Stallard lecture. Br J Ophthalmol. 2010;94(4):396–9.
7. Abramson DH, Francis JH, Gobin YP. What's new in intra-arterial chemotherapy for retinoblastoma? Int Ophthalmol Clin. 2019;59(2):87–94.

8. Berry JL, Shah S, Bechtold M, Zolfaghari E, Jubran R, Kim JW. Long-term outcomes of Group D retinoblastoma eyes during the intravitreal melphalan era. Pediatr Blood Cancer. 2017; https://doi.org/10.1002/pbc.26696.
9. Ravindran K, et al. Intra-arterial chemotherapy for retinoblastoma: an updated systematic review and meta-analysis. J Neurointerv Surg. 2019;11(12):1266–72.
10. Chen Q, et al. Comparison between intravenous chemotherapy and intra-arterial chemotherapy for retinoblastoma: a meta-analysis. BMC Cancer. 2018;18(1):486.
11. Abramson DH, et al. Bilateral superselective ophthalmic artery chemotherapy for bilateral retinoblastoma: tandem therapy. Arch Ophthalmol. 2010;128(3):370–2.
12. Francis JH, et al. Carboplatin +/– topotecan ophthalmic artery chemosurgery for intraocular retinoblastoma. PLoS One. 2013;8(8):e72441.
13. Gobin YP, et al. Radiation exposure during intra-arterial chemotherapy for retinoblastoma. Arch Ophthalmol. 2012;130(3):403–4; author reply 404-5.
14. Vijayakrishnan R, et al. Irradiation toxic effects during intra-arterial chemotherapy for retinoblastoma: should we be concerned? Arch Ophthalmol. 2010;128(11):1427–31.
15. Dunkel IJ, et al. Risk factors for severe neutropenia following intra-arterial chemotherapy for intra-ocular retinoblastoma. PLoS One. 2014;9(10):e108692.
16. Marr BP, et al. Three-drug intra-arterial chemotherapy using simultaneous carboplatin, topotecan and melphalan for intraocular retinoblastoma: preliminary results. Br J Ophthalmol. 2012;96(10):1300–3.
17. Munier FL, Soliman S, Moulin AP, et al. Profiling safety of intravitreal injection for retinoblastoma using an anti-reflex procedure and sterilization of the needle track. Br J Ophthlmolo. 2012;96(8):1084–7.
18. Gobin YP, et al. Combined, sequential intravenous and intra-arterial chemotherapy (bridge chemotherapy) for young infants with retinoblastoma. PLoS One. 2012;7(9):e44322.
19. Francis JH, Marr BP, Brodie SE, Gobin P, Dunkel IJ, Abramson DH. Intravitreal melphalan as salvage therapy for refractory retinal and subretinal retinoblastoma. Retin Cases Brief Rep. 2016;10(4):357–60.
20. Francis JH, et al. Efficacy and toxicity of second-course ophthalmic artery chemosurgery for retinoblastoma. Ophthalmology. 2015;122(5):1016–22.
21. Munier FL, et al. Occurrence of sectoral choroidal occlusive vasculopathy and retinal arteriolar embolization after superselective ophthalmic artery chemotherapy for advanced intraocular retinoblastoma. Retina. 2011;31(3):566–73.
22. Monroy JE, Orbach DB, VanderVeen D. Complications of intra-arterial chemotherapy for retinoblastoma. Semin Ophthalmol. 2014;29(5–6):429–33.
23. Shields CL, et al. Intra-arterial chemotherapy for retinoblastoma: report no. 2, treatment complications. Arch Ophthalmol. 2011;129(11):1407–15.
24. Sweid A, et al. Incidence and predictors of ophthalmic artery occlusion in intra-arterial chemotherapy for retinoblastoma. J Neurointerv Surg. 2021;13(7):652–6.
25. Tse BC, et al. Enophthalmos and choroidal atrophy after intraophthalmic artery chemotherapy for retinoblastoma. Ophthalmology. 2015;122(2):435–7.
26. Maidana DE, et al. Choroidal thickness after intraarterial chemotherapy for retinoblastoma. Retina. 2014;34(10):2103–9.
27. Brodie SE, et al. Persistence of retinal function after intravitreal melphalan injection for retinoblastoma. Doc Ophthalmol. 2013;126(1):79–84.
28. Brodie SE, et al. ERG monitoring of retinal function during systemic chemotherapy for retinoblastoma. Br J Ophthalmol. 2012;96(6):877–80.
29. Marr B, et al. Spontaneously resolving periocular erythema and ciliary madarosis following intra-arterial chemotherapy for retinoblastoma. Middle East Afr J Ophthalmol. 2010;17(3):207–9.
30. De la Huerta I, et al. Delayed cerebral infarction following intra-arterial chemotherapy for retinoblastoma. JAMA Ophthalmol. 2016;134(6):712–4.
31. Nguyen SM, Sison J, Jones M, Berry JL, Kim JW, Murphree AL, Salinas V, Olch AJ, Chang EL, Wong KK. Lens dose-response prediction modeling and cataract incidence in retinoblastoma patients after lens-sparing or whole-eye radiotherapy. Int J Radiat Oncol Biol Phys. 2018;8(18):34,083–34, 085.
32. Aziz HA, Kim JW, Munier FL, Berry JL. Acute hemorrhagic retinopathy following intravitreal melphalan injection for retinoblastoma: a report of two cases and technical modifications to enhance the prevention of retinal toxicity. Ocul Oncol Pathol. 2017;3(1):34–40.
33. Berry JL, Zolfaghari E, Chen A, Murphree AL, Jubran R, Kim JW. Optic nerve obscuration in retinoblastoma: a risk factor for optic nerve invasion? Ocul Oncol Pathol. 2017;3(4):283–91.

Treatment for Primary Vitreoretinal Lymphoma: The Neuro-Oncologist's View

Carlen A. Yuen, Fabio M. Iwamoto, and Lakshmi Nayak

1 Introduction and Nomenclature

Primary vitreoretinal lymphoma (PVRL) is a subgroup of primary intraocular lymphoma (PIOL) and a subtype of primary central nervous system lymphoma (PCNSL) [1, 2]. PVRL can arise in different eye compartments, including the vitreous and retina. The eye is considered a sanctuary site for neoplastic cells. Like PCNSL, the majority of PVRL (>90%) are non-Hodgkin diffuse large B-cell lymphoma (DLBCL). The remainder are T-cell and natural killer (NK)-cell lymphomas.

First recognized in 1951 by Cooper and Riker, "ocular reticulum cell sarcoma" was named in a patient with disease occurring in the retina and uvea [3]. Ocular reticulum cell sarcoma was then renamed to "primary intraocular lymphoma" (PIOL) after the discovery that the tumor cells originate from only ocular tissues [4, 5].

PIOL can be further subdivided [6, 7]. PVRL, the most common form of intraocular lymphoma (IOL), is a high-grade B-cell malignancy that originates from the posterior eye segments (vitreous and retina). In contrast, primary uveal lymphoma involves the choroid, iris, ciliary body, or a combination of these structures. Choroidal lymphomas are usually low-grade B-cell lymphomas (BCLs), not associated with central nervous system (CNS) disease, and are most frequently extranodal marginal zone lymphomas (EMZLs). Primary iridal lymphomas are exceedingly rare and tend to be B-cell or T-cell lymphomas. Secondary intraocular lymphoma occurs in patients with advanced systemic disease. The terms IOL and vitreoretinal lymphoma (VRL) are sometimes used interchangeably in various studies, which adds to confusion with nomenclature. For the purpose of this chapter, we are consistently using the term VRL.

C. A. Yuen · F. M. Iwamoto
Department of Neurology, Neuro-Oncology Division, New York Presbyterian Hospital, Columbia University, New York, NY, USA
e-mail: cay2115@cumc.columbia.edu; fi2146@cumc.columbia.edu

L. Nayak (✉)
Center for Central Nervous System Lymphoma, Dana-Farber Cancer Institute, Harvard Medical School, Boston, MA, USA
e-mail: Lakshmi_Nayak@dfci.harvard.edu

2 Epidemiology

PVRL is approximately 1% of non-Hodgkin's lymphomas, 1% of intracranial tumors, and <1% of intraocular tumors [8]. Given its rarity, the true incidence of PVRL is unknown, but 300–380 new cases of PVRL are reported annually [7]. PVRL typically presents in patients of median age in the 60s.

More epidemiologic data exist for PCNSL. The rising incidence of PCNSL, which peaked in 1995, was partially driven by the acquired immune deficiency syndrome (AIDS) epidemic and susceptibility in the elderly population [9, 10]. Since the 2000s, the incidence has decreased in younger adults with the decreased incidence of AIDS, whereas the incidence in the elderly population is increasing as the overall population ages [11]. The incidence of PCNSL is slightly higher in men. There is an association between PCNSL and iatrogenic immunosuppression and autoimmune diseases such as rheumatoid arthritis, Sjögren syndrome, systemic lupus erythematosus, and sarcoidosis.

3 Prognostic Factors

There are no identifiable prognostic factors for PVRL, but age and performance status have been proposed based on data from PCNSL studies [12, 13]. Significantly improved outcomes occur in newly diagnosed PCNSL patients that are younger and with a Karnofsky performance score (KPS) of >70. Due to the high incidence of CNS progression, the prognosis of PVRL is poor. It is not clear whether isolated PVRL at presentation carries a better prognosis than VRL with CNS involvement as most patients eventually develop

B. V. Chawla, M. E. Aronow (eds.), *Global Perspectives in Ocular Oncology*, https://doi.org/10.1007/978-3-031-08250-4_9

brain or leptomeningeal disease. In a series of 22 patients with PVRL with or without CNS involvement, there was a trend toward longer survival in patients with isolated PVRL compared to those with concurrent central nervous system lymphoma (CNSL), 43.4 vs. 30.3 months, respectively [14]. A 20-year retrospective review of 19 PVRL patients, 7 of whom had concurrent CNS lymphoma, reported a median progression-free survival (PFS) of 11 months, and median survival of 33 months [15]. In a large multicenter retrospective study of patients with isolated PVRL, 29% (23/78) died; of these, 30% of patients died from CNSL, 13% died from indirect complications of CNSL (including treatment complications), and 13% died from unrelated causes [16]. The five-year cumulative survival rate was also lower in patients with CNSL compared to patients without CNSL (35% and 68%, respectively; $p = 0.003$) [16]. Local relapse typically occurs within 2 years of initial diagnosis and CNS dissemination is the most common cause of fatality [17–19].

4 Clinical Presentation

PVRL patients can initially present with unilateral disease, but approximately 80–90% develop bilateral disease [7, 20–24]. Ocular involvement does not necessitate ocular symptoms and patients can present with a broad range of visual acuities, ranging from normal vision to blindness [25, 26]. Other presenting symptoms are blurry vision, floaters, and less commonly photophobia and ocular pain [2, 22, 27–30]. These non-specific symptoms often lead to diagnostic delay [31] of over 1 year on average from symptom onset to diagnosis [7, 25, 31].

5 Diagnosis and Pathophysiology

PVRL can be a diagnostic challenge and is known as a masquerade syndrome, mimicking other diseases, such as chronic uveitis and other inflammatory processes, including endophthalmitis, sarcoidosis, multiple sclerosis, rheumatoid arthritis, Behcet's and Vogt-Koyanagi-Harada disease, and other inflammatory processes [4, 6, 20, 27, 30, 32–34]. Other neoplastic processes can also imitate PVRL, including amelanotic choroidal melanoma, multiple myeloma, and metastatic systemic non-Hodgkin lymphoma [34–36].

Patients with suspected PVRL should be referred for thorough ophthalmic examination and for consideration of diagnostic vitrectomy, or retinal biopsy in appropriate cases. Further diagnostic evaluation for CNS involvement with magnetic resonance imaging (MRI) brain and spine, cerebrospinal fluid (CSF) analysis, and staging evaluation for systemic lymphoma with computed tomography or positron emission tomography (PET) of the chest, abdomen, and pelvis should also be performed.

Slit lamp and dilated fundus examination can reveal cells in the anterior chamber, which are non-specific as they can also be seen in the setting of non-neoplastic inflammatory disease [4, 7]. Infiltrating lymphomatous cells are classically observed in the vitreous cavity and are characterized by hallmark sheets or clumps of cells; retinal and subretinal pigment epithelium (RPE) infiltrates can also be visualized in some cases [2, 4, 6, 7, 30, 36–39].

Non-invasive ancillary imaging including optical coherence tomography (OCT), and ultrasonography in some cases, can be helpful. OCT may show hyper-reflective infiltrates containing discrete nodules or confluent bands with a predilection for the sub-RPE space [40, 41]. Fluorescein angiography can demonstrate punctate hyper-fluorescent foci corresponding to lymphoma infiltrates; however, findings of inflammation (petaloid leakage consistent with cystoid macular edema and perivascular staining with or without leakage) are frequently suggestive of a diagnosis other than PVRL [39, 42].

Definitive diagnosis requires vitreal or retinal biopsy as the gold standard [43]. If the initial biopsy is non-diagnostic, repeat biopsy should be considered when diagnostic suspicion is high. Since malignant cells are typically found within the vitreous, it is the preferred sampling site. The retina and subretinal space are alternative sites for biopsy. Vitrectomy is associated with fewer complications compared to chorioretinal biopsy and may provide added therapeutic benefits of decreasing cell load or inducing remission [44, 45].

The numerous reactive lymphocytes that are admixed with the malignant PVRL cells can compromise the diagnosis [4, 7, 39, 46]. Additionally, scant cellularity resulting from the fragility of the lymphoma cells and the cytotoxic effects of corticosteroids on lymphoma cells can necessitate multiple biopsies [4, 7, 29, 47]. Prompt processing of the samples minimizes cytolysis and optimizes cytologic analysis.

Cytologic analysis shows large pleomorphic atypical lymphoid cells with irregular nuclei and prominent nucleoli with rare mitoses. Monoclonal B-cells stain positive for Cluster of Differentiation 19 (CD19), CD20, and CD22. Detection of CD79B^{Y196} and expression of transcriptional factors B-cell lymphoma (BCL)-6 and Multiple Myeloma Oncogene (MUM)-1 in vitreous DNA may support the diagnosis of PVRL [48, 49]. Flow cytometry assesses for monoclonality for both exclusively kappa-bearing or lambda-bearing B- and T-lymphocytes [39, 50, 51].

Molecular analysis and polymerase chain reaction (PCR) are beneficial adjuncts in diagnosing PVRL [4, 52]. Next-generation sequencing of vitrectomy fluid can detect mutations of Myeloid Differentiation Factor 88 (MYD88)^{L265P}

gain, and CDKN2A and PTEN losses [53]. MYD88 mutations are common in PVRL and can increase the diagnostic yield for PVRL [53–56]. A retrospective review found that 69% (20/29) of 75 vitrectomy samples in 69 PVRL patients harbor MYD88 mutations [56]. Hotspot somatic mutation L265P is the most frequently observed mutation, while 103 and 143 position mutations are less frequent [56, 57]. Similar findings were reported in a proof-of-concept study of 23 VRL patients, with 74% of patients harboring the $MYD88^{L265P}$ mutation [58]. Similar to interleukin (IL)-10 levels, MYD88 mutations are detectable in both the vitreous fluid and aqueous humor (sensitivity 75% and 67%, respectively). When clinical presentation is highly suggestive of PVRL, a positive MYD88-allele-specific PCR in combination with CD20+ vitreous cells could potentially be adequate for diagnosis in absence of definitive diagnosis on cytopathologic analysis. The aqueous humor is more easily accessible than vitreous fluid and MYD88 mutations in the aqueous humor can also be informative. MYD88 mutations may have higher concordance rates than IL-10 in the vitreous compared to aqueous fluid. One study reported a concordance rate of 89% in 12-paired samples. Patients with PVRL have IgH rearrangements similarly found in systemic non-Hodgkin lymphoma, but can be falsely negative [43]. T-cell receptor gene rearrangements have been reported in T-cell lymphoma [4].

Finally, intraocular cytokine analysis of interleukin (IL)-10 and IL-6 can be informative in the diagnosis of PVRL. B-lymphoma cells secrete IL-10, an immunosuppressive TH2-cytokine of growth and differentiation [59–61]. IL-10 simultaneously stimulates tumor cell proliferation and shields tumor cells from the immune response. Elevated IL-10 levels correlate with shorter event-free survival (EFS) and high levels are found in the vitreous in PVRL patients. As a result, IL-10 levels can be used for PVRL screening to support its diagnosis or for indirect biomarker analysis to determine remission [34, 60, 62–65]. Whereas PVRL B-lymphoid cells produce high levels of IL-10, normal lymphocytes and macrophages produce the proinflammatory cytokine IL-6 during inflammatory states, including uveitis [4, 60, 66]. An IL-10 level >100 pg/mL in combination with IL-10:IL-6 ratio of >1 is beneficial for diagnosing PVRL [31]. Vitreal IL-10:IL-6 ratio less than 1.0 may be due to early stage disease [67]. A retrospective study comparing IL-10/IL-6 ratio greater than 1.0, IgH rearrangements, and cytology in the vitreous specimens of 217 patients found that IL-10/IL-6 ratio had the highest detection rate (91.7%, 80.6%, and 44.5%, respectively) [68]. Both vitreous and aqueous humor levels can be used for IL-10 detection, but aqueous IL-10 levels are variable and cannot alone be used to confirm a PVRL diagnosis.

Patients diagnosed with PVRL should undergo further evaluation with magnetic resonance imaging (MRI) to assess for CNS involvement and a lumbar puncture with CSF studies to assess for leptomeningeal involvement [4, 7, 66]. Since PVRL is a subgroup of PCNSL, diagnosis can be made with a less invasive lumbar puncture with CSF findings of lymphoma cells, sparing the patient from a more invasive diagnostic biopsy or vitrectomy [4, 48, 62, 69]. Oculocerebral lymphoma with a positive brain biopsy may also preclude the requirement for an intraocular biopsy [64]. Brain MRI should then be performed every 3 months for 2 years, then every 6 months [43].

6 Treatment

Management of PVRL requires close surveillance and a multidisciplinary team approach consisting of an ophthalmologist, a neuro-oncologist or hemato-oncologist, and a pathologist [4]. Due to its rarity, there is no consensus on the optimal treatment for PVRL [4, 25]. In 2011, the International PCNSL Collaborative Group (IPCG) recommended dedicated local therapy with intravitreal (IVT) chemotherapy (CT) or irradiation for unilateral isolated PVRL, local or systemic therapy for bilateral PVRL, and systemic with local therapy for concurrent CNS disease [7]. Others have also recommended deferring systemic treatment for CNS involvement to minimize toxicities [16, 70]. At the same time, the British Neuro-Oncology Society recommended systemic therapy with high-dose methotrexate (HD-MTX) followed by ocular and cranial irradiation (www.bnos.org.uk, June 2011). The French Oculocerebral Lymphoma (LOC) Network, which was established in 2011, recommended treating patients with isolated PVRL in good medical condition with intravenous HD-MTX-based therapy and those in poor condition with local therapy. More recently in 2021, they published results from a European survey and updated their guidelines to include additional consolidative low-dose bilateral ocular radiation [71].

There are challenges to the treatment of PVRL. Two blood-ocular barriers, the blood-aqueous and blood-retinal barriers, can limit drug penetration and lead to insufficient drug levels within the eye. The blood-retinal barrier is of key importance given that intraocular lymphoma primarily affects the posterior eye, including optic nerve, vitreous, and retina. To circumvent these barriers, numerous delivery methods have been developed, including the use of both local and systemic treatment modalities [17]. Local therapy includes intravitreal (IVT) chemotherapy (CT) and ocular radiation therapy (ORT), whole-brain radiation therapy (WBRT), and intrathecal (IT) CT. Systemic therapy consists of intravenous CT and autologous stem cell transplantation (ASCT).

6.1 Local Therapy

For isolated PVRL restricted to one eye, local therapies with external beam radiotherapy (EBRT), intravitreal methotrexate (IVT-M), or intravitreal rituximab (IVT-R) are effective therapies [7, 14, 43, 72, 73]. No studies have been conducted to compare these local therapies, but there are no apparent significant differences in local control or visual outcomes among these therapies. Often, the choice of first-line therapy is driven by the specialist involved [6, 24, 43].

6.2 Ocular Radiation Therapy

ORT was previously the mainstay treatment for PVRL [74]. Given the high incidence of bilateral eye involvement, it is typically delivered to both eyes [7, 20]. EBRT to a total of 35–40 Gy delivered in 15 fractions provides good local control rates [20, 22, 75, 76]. One retrospective study showed no relapse in 58% (7/12) of PVRL patients who received radiation therapy (RT; six patients with combined CT and one patient with RT alone). Nevertheless, disease often recurs and progresses to CNSL. Radiation toxicities occur in up to 70% of patients including retinopathy, optic neuropathy, cataract, dry eye, conjunctivitis, and vitreous hemorrhage [77, 78]. While unusual in doses less than 36 Gy, radiation retinopathy can occur even at reduced levels of 20 Gy, particularly in patients with comorbidities such as diabetes and other systemic vascular diseases [79]. Re-treating recurrent disease is a challenge with RT due to the issue of overlapping treatment fields, which may limit the future use of WBRT for CNS disease [74, 80, 81]. CyberKnife has some advantages over EBRT, including shorter treatment time and decreased risk of radiation retinopathy, but experience with this technique is limited by short follow-up [82].

6.3 Intravitreal Therapy

Intravitreal treatment (IVT-M and IVT-R) offers an alternative therapy to overcome the disadvantages of ocular RT [80]. Turaka et al. reported that 58.3% (7/12) PVRL patients treated with either IVT-M or rituximab (RTX) monotherapy achieved complete response (CR) at a median follow-up of 33.5 months [72]. However, as with ocular RT, intravitreal therapy is a focal treatment that does not address concurrent brain disease and is associated with a CNS recurrence risk [70].

Methotrexate (MTX), a dihydrofolate reductase inhibitor, used intravitreally, has shown long-term success in studies and provides good local control without severe toxicity [26, 72, 80, 83]. One 10-year single-institution study of 44 eyes in 26 patients treated with IVT-M showed no intraocular recurrence in the 8 surviving patients after >3 years [26]. MTX can also provide prolonged local remission in recurrent disease after RT and systemic CT [27, 84]. Resistance to IVT-M in PVRL patients may be caused by the simultaneous increased efflux of MTX by multidrug resistance-related protein and decreased influx of MTX by reduced expression of reduced folate carrier and folate binding protein [85]. One disadvantage to IVT-M is the number of injections that must be administered over an extended period of time [43, 83, 86]. In addition, toxicities can develop, including cataract (73%), corneal epitheliopathy (58%), maculopathy (42%), vitreous hemorrhage (8%), optic atrophy (4%), and sterile endophthalmitis (4%) [83]. Nevertheless, IVT-M remains a frequent frontline option for PVRL in the newly diagnosed or recurrent setting.

Rituximab (RTX), a humanized chimeric anti-CD20 monoclonal antibody, is used for treatment of PCNSL and PVRL [87]. RTX induces apoptosis, complement-mediated cytolysis, and antibody-dependent cytotoxicity although its exact role in PCNSL is unclear. IVT-R has been investigated both as a single agent and in combination with IVT-M [72, 87–90]. Kitzmann et al. found no toxicities in five treated eyes [87]. In a prospective case series of 20 patients, Hashida et al. showed improvement with a single course of IVT-R in PVRL patients who previously developed toxicity to IVT-M [88]. Similar to recurrence rates with ocular RT and IVT-M, disease recurrence rates with IVT-R were relatively high and occurred in 55% (11/20) of patients [88]. However, a second remission can be achieved with an additional course of injections [88]. In a retrospective study conducted by Larkin et al., 48 eyes of 34 PVRL patients treated with IVT-R achieved 64.6% (31/48) CR and 22.9% (11/48) partial response (PR) [90]. RTX toxicities include transient elevated intraocular pressure (IOP), keratic precipitates, cataract, vitreous hemorrhage, and retinal detachment [88, 90].

6.4 Systemic Chemotherapy

Some experts follow the PCNSL treatment strategies for PVRL patients [43, 91]. Systemic chemotherapy penetrates the blood-ocular barrier and achieves therapeutic intraocular fluid levels, but the levels in the vitreous humor can be unreliable [48, 92].

Ara-C is a pyrimidine analogue used in the treatment of PCNSL. In 1986, Bauman et al. were the first to report CR with high-dose Ara-C (HiDAC) in a case report of PVRL treated with 3 g/m^2 every 12 h [93]. Therapeutic intraocular levels with 2 g/m^2 were sustained. While promising results were observed in a subsequent study of 3 patients with isolated PVRL, another case series of 6 PVRL patients showed CR in only 20% (1/5) of patients treated with single-agent HiDAC [94, 95]. Toxicities associated with HiDAC include conjunctivitis, keratitis, ocular irritation, myelosuppression, nausea, and vomiting.

Similar to HiDAC, HD-MTX (8 g/m^2) produces sustained drug levels in the vitreous and aqueous humor [24, 92, 96, 97]. In a case series of 9 patients (2 patients with isolated PVRL and 7 patients with PCNSL with vitreoretinal (VR) involvement), Bachelor et al. demonstrated 78% CR in the eye and 100% CR in the brain with HD-MTX 8 g/m^2 every 2 weeks until CR followed by consolidation MTX for 2 doses then maintenance every 4 weeks for 11 doses [92]. In a phase 2 study conducted by the New Approaches to Brain Tumor Therapy (NABTT) 96–07 CNS Consortium, 20% (5/25) of patients with newly diagnosed PCNSL had concurrent ocular lymphoma [98]. Following HD-MTX, CR and partial response (PR) were achieved in 80% and 20%, respectively, suggesting HD-MTX may be effective for patients with PCNSL and concomitant PVRL. Deficient levels or short duration of cytotoxic levels may contribute to HD-MTX resistance [92]. HD-MTX carries a risk of delayed neurotoxicity (NT) and leukoencephalopathy [99]. The optimal dose of HD-MTX and the best combination of chemotherapy agents for PVRL have not been defined.

Temozolomide, an oral alkylating agent, has been shown to be effective in a retrospective study of 21 patients with relapsed/refractory (R/R) PVRL with a CR rate of 71% and median PFS of 12 months [100]. CNS relapses were noted in 24% (5) of the patients.

7 Combined Systemic and Local Treatment

Treatment goals of combined therapy center on both eradication of lymphoma in the eye and preventing subsequent CNS relapse, but evidence for prophylactic therapy to prevent CNS dissemination is conflicting given various modalities have been used. Margolis et al. reported CNS dissemination in 89% (8/9) patients during their disease course and clinical improvement after 7 of the affected patients were treated with CNS irradiation [20]. De la Fuente et al. reported in a retrospective study that combined bilateral ocular RT followed by MTX-based chemotherapy provides effective local control, prevention of CNS relapse, and prolonged survival [101]. Of 12 patients with isolated bilateral PVRL, 10 patients were treated with ORT followed by systemic CT, 1 patient was treated with RT, and 1 patient was treated with IVT-M [101]. Complete response (CR) was achieved in all patients and PFS and overall survival (OS) were not reached at a median follow-up of 68 months. The cumulative incidence of CNS relapse was 37.5%, lower than the previously reported incidence, ranging from 56 to 85%. Moreover, in a prospective study, Kaburaki et al. reported that CNS prophylaxis with combination systemic CT and reduced dose (rd)-WBRT (rituximab, methotrexate, procarbazine, vincristine (R-MPV), rd-WBRT, and HiDAC) significantly decreased CNS relapse in 17 patients, of whom 65% (11/17) had isolated intraocular disease [17]. CNS relapse was noted in 1 (of 11) patient with isolated PVRL and ocular relapse occurred in 3. Four-year PFS and OS were 72.4% and 88.9%, respectively, in isolated PVRL patients. In a retrospective study of 31 isolated PVRL patients, Hormigo et al. reported that CNS prophylaxis with systemic CT, combined CT and RT, or RT alone significantly improves survival compared to treatment after CNS progression [22]. Of these 31 patients, 17 patients received CNS prophylaxis and 14 patients received CNS treatment at the time of progression [22]. The prophylactically treated patients had significantly improved median survival of 60 months compared to the non-prophylactically treated group with a median survival of 35 months. However, CNS progression rates were similar, 53% (9/17) in the prophylactically treated patients and 50% (7/14) in the non-prophylactically treated group, thus raising the question of whether or not treatment modality compromises risk of CNS progression.

In contrast to the reports above, multiple studies have found that treatment modality does not appear to compromise disease control or risk of CNS progression or OS [7, 16, 22, 64, 70, 102]. In a large multicenter retrospective study conducted by Riemens et al., 78 isolated PVRL patients were evaluated. Seventy-five patients were treated with either local therapy alone (31 patients), extensive systemic therapy (21 patients), or combination local and extensive therapy (23 patients). Three patients were not treated. At median follow-up of 49 months, CNSL developed in 36% (28/78) of patients. Progression to CNSL did not differ between patients receiving local therapy alone compared to aggressive systemic therapy with CNSL developing with local therapy alone in 32% (10/31), extensive systemic therapy in 43% (9/21), and combination ocular and extensive treatment in 39% (9/23) [16]. Moreover, in a retrospective study of 26 isolated PVRL patients conducted by Hashida et al., prophylactic therapy did not prevent progression to CNS disease [102]. Fifteen patients received local therapy (IVT-M with 8 patients additionally receiving IVT-R) and 11 patients received prophylactic therapy (6 received HD-MTX and 5 received IT-MTX). CNSL developed in 54% (14/26) of patients at mean follow-up of 44.0 ± 18.7 months, with 40% (6/15) in the local therapy alone group and 73% (8/11) in the prophylactic treatment group. However, the time to onset of CNS progression was significantly prolonged in the prophylactically treated patients compared to the patients who did not receive prophylactic treatment, 42.8 ± 13.8 months and 10.2 ± 2.0 months, respectively. HD-MTX in particular had significantly prolonged time to CNS progression compared to IT-MTX or local therapy. In an IPCG (International PCNSL Collaborative Group) Report, Grimm et al. compared local therapy (23 patients) to extensive therapy (53 patients treated with combinations of systemic CT, ocular CT, WBRT, and ocular RT) [70]. Local therapy alone did not increase relapse risk compared to extensive therapy: 56% and 60%, respectively. Relapse occurred in 47 patients at a median of 19 months, with 47% (22/47) in the brain, 30% (14/47) in the eyes, 15% (7/47) in the eyes and brain, and 8% (4/47) systemically. Further, more toxicities have been reported with systemic CT [16]. Therefore, in the absence of CNS disease, systemic therapy or combination intravitreal and systemic chemotherapy remains controversial [7, 27, 64]. Local therapy remains a reasonable approach for patients with contraindications to systemic chemotherapy, elderly patients, or local recurrence.

8 High-Dose Chemotherapy (HDT) and Autologous Stem Cell Transplant (ASCT)

Thiotepa-based high-dose chemotherapy (HDT) and ASCT is used for consolidation in newly diagnosed PCNSL. In PVRL, it has been investigated in the R/R setting. A prospective pilot study, 11 refractory PVRL patients were treated with HD-MTX and HiDAC; 5 of these patients were treated with ASCT and demonstrated promising results [103]. The conditioning regimen for ASCT consisted of thiotepa 750 mg/m^2, busulfan 10 mg/kg, and cyclophosphamide 120 mg/kg (TBC), all of which are good brain penetrants. All 5 patients had a CR, and 3 remained in CR between 14 and 15 months. Two patients relapsed at 6 months. Encouraged by these results, a study was conducted by Soussain et al. investigating the feasibility of the cytarabine and etoposide (CYVE) followed by TBC-ASCT in R/R patients [104]. In this study, 12 (out of 22) patients had eye involvement (isolated or in conjunction with brain or CSF involvement). Eleven patients had a response after ASCT; ten CR, one PR, and one had systemic progression, although two in CR progressed at 3 and 5 months, respectively. Apparent longer survival times were observed in patients with isolated VRL compared to patients with brain parenchyma involvement, with median survival time not reached and 5.5 months, respectively [104]. However, in a phase 2 prospective study of CYVE and TBC-ASCT in patients with recurrent or primary refractory IOL or PCNSL, there was no significant difference in median PFS or OS in those patients who had VRL (isolated or with brain/CSF disease) compared to those who did not [105]. Soussain et al. also reported on the largest retrospective series of 79 R/R PCNSL and VRL patients [106]. All patients had VRL with or without brain or CSF involvement and CR was achieved in 83.5% (66/79), PR in 5% (4/79), stable disease (SD) in 2.5% (2/79), and progressive disease (PD) in 4% (3/79) of patients. Following ASCT, 35% (28/79) patients relapsed; 68% in the CNS, 11% in the eye, 7% in both the eye and CNS, 3.5% in the CSF, 7% systemically, and 3.5% unknown. Durable CR between 9 and 124 months was achieved in 4 patients. In general, the role of HDT-ASCT is at present restricted to younger and fit R/R patients.

9 Emerging Therapies

Bruton tyrosine kinase (BTK) inhibitors and immunomodulatory drugs (IMiDs) have been investigated in prospective trials in R/R PVRL. Additionally, novel agents including other targeted therapies and immunotherapies are currently under investigation for PCNSL, although many of these have not specifically included PVRL. A checkpoint inhibitor, pembrolizumab, has been studied in a phase 2 trial in R/R PCNSL and PVRL, although the final results are pending (NCT03012620).

9.1 BTK Inhibitors

Constitutive Nuclear factor kappa-light-chain-enhancer of activated B cells (NF-κB) activity is thought to contribute to the poor prognosis of patients with activated B cell-like (ABC) subtype of DLBCL, including PCNSL [107]. PCNSL patients harbor mutations in B-cell antigen receptor (BCR) and toll-like receptor (TLR) signaling pathways that enhance NF-κB activity [108]. Cluster of Differentiation *(CD)79B* and *MYD88* activate the BCR and TLR signaling pathways, respectively. CD79B is a BCR-associated protein, and gene alterations are found in 64% of PCNSL tumors [109]. MYD88 is a cytosolic adapter protein, and gene alterations are found in 71.7–86.7% of PCNSL including PVRL tumors [109, 110]. Drugs targeting the NF-κB pathway both upstream and downstream are under investigation. Upstream, Bruton tyrosine kinase (BTK) links BCR and TLR signaling and BTK inhibition is one of the emerging therapies under investigation.

Ibrutinib is an oral irreversible inhibitor of BTK with good blood–brain barrier penetration. Ibrutinib has demonstrated activity in PVRL and PCNSL [111, 112]. In a retrospective case series of 14 patients with R/R PCNSL treated with ibrutinib monotherapy, Chamoun et al. reported 50% ORR and 2 patients with CR >8 months [113]. Of these 14 patients, 4 patients had VRL. Two phase 1 studies in R/R PCNSL patients showed objective responses to ibrutinib monotherapy and in combination with chemotherapy [111, 114]. The promising results of these retrospective and prospective phase 1 studies led to the first large, multicenter phase 2 proof-of-concept study of ibrutinib (560 mg/day in 28-day cycle) in R/R PVRL and PCNSL patients conducted by the Lymphoma Study Association (LYSA) and the French LOC Network [112]. Of these 52 patients, 14 patients had PVRL, 2 of which had CSF involvement. Responses were achieved in all compartments; 19% (10/52) CR, 33% (17/52) PR, and 10% (5/52) SD. Of the 14 PVRL patients, CR and PR were achieved in 71% (10/14) and 29% (4/14), respectively. The median PFS was longer for patients with PVRL with or without CSF involvement compared to patients with brain or spinal cord lymphoma: 22.7 months vs. 2 months, respectively. Patients without brain involvement also had longer median OS (not reached) compared to with brain involvement (4.3 months). Minimal or undetectable IL-10 anterior chamber levels correlated with clinical CR in 15 evaluable patients and increasing IL-10 levels correlated with progressive disease (PD).

In a phase 1/2 study of second-generation BTK inhibitor, tirabrutinib, partial responses were noted in 3/3 patients [115].

9.2 Immunomodulatory Drugs

Lenalidomide and pomalidomide are IMiDs that suppress NF-κB activity and simultaneously augment interferon beta (IFNβ) production [116]. ABC DLBCL maintains its viability through the regulation of the BCR signaling pathway by SPIB/interferon regulatory factor (IRF4) heterodimers. IMiDs target both IRF4 and mucosa-associated lymphoid tissue lymphoma translocation protein 1 (MALT1) in the NF-κB pathway [108]. IMiDs have demonstrated activity in R/R PCNSL and PVRL.

Lenalidomide has been studied in PVRL and PCNSL in combination with RTX in the R/R setting and as maintenance therapy [117, 118]. Lenalidomide has been shown to have good CNS penetration, and detectable CSF drug levels are observed without blood brain barrier (BBB) disruption [117]. The addition of lenalidomide to RTX may aid in overcoming RTX resistance by augmenting the antibody-dependent cytotoxicity effects of RTX. In a phase 1 study, 14 R/R PCNSL and secondary central nervous system lymphoma (SCNSL) patients (5 with intraocular involvement) were treated with lenalidomide in combination with intraventricular or intravenous RTX [117]. Durable responses were observed in 6 patients for ≥9 months and in 4 for ≥18 months. The PVRL patient had a prolonged CR of ≥25 months. The LYSA and French LOC Network conducted a phase 2 proof-of-concept clinical trial that evaluated lenalidomide and RTX REVlimid RItuximab (REVRI) followed by maintenance lenalidomide in R/R PVRL or PCNSL patients [118]. Induction therapy consisted of lenalidomide at 20 mg daily for 21/28-day cycle combined with RTX at 375 mg/m^2 on day 1. Of a total 45 patients, 17 patients had VRL involvement (9 with isolated PVRL, 2 with PVRL and CSF involvement, and 6 with both CNS and VRL involvement). Responders were treated with maintenance lenalidomide at 10 mg daily for 21/28-day cycle. The median PFS of the PVRL and PCNSL patients was 9.2 and 3.9 months, respectively, and 35% (6/17) of patients with VRL had a CR. Both studies showed clinical activity in the eye, brain, and CSF. The median PFS and OS for the entire group were 7.8 months and 17.7 months, respectively.

Pomalidomide was studied in combination with dexamethasone in a phase 1 study and was found to have activity in R/R PCNSL and PVRL [119].

10 Perspective

PVRL is rare and commonly mimics other diseases. In suspected cases, particularly in elderly or immunocompromised individuals with new onset "uveitis," evaluation by an experienced ophthalmologist is important in order to avoid diagnostic delay. It can be a challenge to diagnose due to its rarity and also as vitreous fluid samples can be paucicellular due to lymphoma cell fragility. Recent advances in cytokine assays and genomic testing have led to increased diagnostic sensitivity of the vitreous fluid. The Study Group for the VitreoRetinal Lymphoma Diagnostics recommends diagnostic vitrectomy as the gold standard for diagnosis [120]. In the absence of positive cytology or flow cytometry, IL-10:IL-6 ratio >1, positive mutation for MYD88, or monoclonality by PCR to identify IgH gene rearrangement is highly suggestive of VRL. Multimodal imaging including optical coherence tomography (OCT), autofluorescence, and angiography can also be helpful in establishing diagnosis. Determining the extent of disease involvement is essential. Additionally, if vitrectomy or retinal biopsy is not revealing/possible, CSF sampling, brain biopsy, or biopsy of systemic lesions, if present, should be utilized for diagnosis.

Treatment modalities include both local and systemic therapies, although there are no standard of care guidelines. While there have been recommendations over the years from various groups, including the IPCG, British Neuro-Oncology Society, and more recently the LOC Network and European Reference Network (ERN)- EuroBloodNet, the treatment typically offered in clinical practice depends on the favored approach of the treating physician and varies between ophthalmologists, oncologists, and neuro-oncologists. Collaboration from a multidisciplinary team of an ophthalmologist, oncologist/neuro-oncologist, and pathologist is critical for diagnostic accuracy and initiation of appropriate treatment. It is important to evaluate the risk of the specific therapeutic modality while considering the best option. In general, we recommend an approach similar to treatment of newly diagnosed PCNSL and consideration of systemic chemotherapy in conjunction with local therapy (with IVT-M or IVT-R and/or ORT) in a young, healthy patient who is able to tolerate systemic treatment with the goal of achieving CR and reducing the risk of CNS relapse. In elderly frail patients, local treatment is suggested to prevent morbidity from systemic chemotherapy. The choice between IVT-M and ORT should depend on patient characteristics and feasibility as there does not appear to be a difference in efficacy. For persistent disease following systemic and/or IVT treatment, ORT is recommended. The role of ASCT in newly diagnosed PVRL remains to be elucidated, although it is a reasonable approach in the R/R setting in an appropriate patient. Comparative studies with ASCT are lacking. If possible and available, clinical trials should be offered to patients with R/R PVRL. Re-treatment with IVT-M can be considered in R/R PVRL. Novel agents like ibrutinib and lenalidomide can be considered as well. Assessment of therapeutic response is an area that also requires standardization. At this time, assessment of ocular response is performed by a clinical ophthalmological examination. Per IPCG guidelines, absence of vitreous cells and resolution of previously seen retinal or optic nerve infiltrates are indicative of ocular CR. However, in clinical practice CR can be difficult to determine on a clinical examination. Biomarker evaluation is ongoing, but there is no definitive correlation between levels of IL-10 and presence or absence of MYD88 mutation in the context of response, progression, or overall survival. It is clear that international and multidisciplinary collaborations are essential. Given the rarity of this disease, much remains to be elucidated, but progress has been made in the last decade and future therapies appear promising.

References

1. Cassoux N. Primary vitreous and retinal lymphoma (PVRL): risk factor and prognosis. Acta Ophthalmol. 2019;97(S263)
2. Chukwueke UN, Nayak L. Central nervous system lymphoma. Hematol Oncol Clin North Am. 2019;33(4):597–611.
3. Cooper EL, Riker JL. Malignant lymphoma of the uveal tract. Am J Ophthalmol. 1951;34(8):1153–8.
4. Chan CC, Sen HN. Current concepts in diagnosing and managing primary vitreoretinal (intraocular) lymphoma. Discov Med. 2013;15(81):93–100.
5. Char DH, Ljung BM, Miller T, Phillips T. Primary intraocular lymphoma (ocular reticulum cell sarcoma) diagnosis and management. Ophthalmology. 1988;95(5):625–30.
6. Pe'er J, Hochberg FH, Foster CS. Clinical review: treatment of vitreoretinal lymphoma. Ocul Immunol Inflamm. 2009;17(5):299–306.
7. Chan CC, Rubenstein JL, Coupland SE, et al. Primary vitreoretinal lymphoma: a report from an international primary central nervous system lymphoma collaborative group symposium. Oncologist. 2011;16(11):1589–99.
8. Bardenstein DS. Intraocular lymphoma. Cancer Control. 1998;5(4):317–25.
9. Kadan-Lottick NS, Skluzacek MC, Gurney JG. Decreasing incidence rates of primary central nervous system lymphoma. Cancer. 2002;95(1):193–202.
10. Olson JE, Janney CA, Rao RD, et al. The continuing increase in the incidence of primary central nervous system non-Hodgkin lymphoma: a surveillance, epidemiology, and end results analysis. Cancer. 2002;95(7):1504–10.
11. Mendez JS, Ostrom QT, Gittleman H, et al. The elderly left behind-changes in survival trends of primary central nervous system lymphoma over the past 4 decades. Neuro-Oncology. 2018;20(5):687–94.
12. Abrey LE, Ben-Porat L, Panageas KS, et al. Primary central nervous system lymphoma: the Memorial Sloan-Kettering Cancer Center prognostic model. J Clin Oncol. 2006;24(36):5711–5.
13. Ferreri AJ, Blay JY, Reni M, et al. Prognostic scoring system for primary CNS lymphomas: the International Extranodal Lymphoma Study Group experience. J Clin Oncol. 2003;21(2):266–72.
14. Kim MM, Dabaja BS, Medeiros J, et al. Survival outcomes of primary intraocular lymphoma: a single-institution experience. Am J Clin Oncol. 2016;39(2):109–13.
15. Levasseur SD, Wittenberg LA, White VA. Vitreoretinal lymphoma: a 20-year review of incidence, clinical and cytologic features, treatment, and outcomes. JAMA Ophthalmol. 2013;131(1):50–5.
16. Riemens A, Bromberg J, Touitou V, et al. Treatment strategies in primary vitreoretinal lymphoma: a 17-center European collaborative study. JAMA Ophthalmol. 2015;133(2):191–7.
17. Kaburaki T, Taoka K, Matsuda J, et al. Combined intravitreal methotrexate and immunochemotherapy followed by reduced-dose whole-brain radiotherapy for newly diagnosed B-cell primary intraocular lymphoma. Br J Haematol. 2017;179(2):246–55.
18. Gavrilovic IT, Hormigo A, Yahalom J, DeAngelis LM, Abrey LE. Long-term follow-up of high-dose methotrexate-based therapy with and without whole brain irradiation for newly diagnosed primary CNS lymphoma. J Clin Oncol. 2006;24(28):4570–4.
19. Abrey LE, Yahalom J, DeAngelis LM. Treatment for primary CNS lymphoma: the next step. J Clin Oncol. 2000;18(17):3144–50.
20. Margolis L, Fraser R, Lichter A, Char DH. The role of radiation therapy in the management of ocular reticulum cell sarcoma. Cancer. 1980;45(4):688–92.
21. Coupland SE, Heimann H, Bechrakis NE. Primary intraocular lymphoma: a review of the clinical, histopathological and molecular biological features. Graefes Arch Clin Exp Ophthalmol. 2004;242(11):901–13.
22. Hormigo A, Abrey L, Heinemann MH, DeAngelis LM. Ocular presentation of primary central nervous system lymphoma: diagnosis and treatment. Br J Haematol. 2004;126(2):202–8.
23. Nussenblatt RB, Chan CC, Wilson WH, Hochman J, Gottesman M, Group CaOLW. International central nervous system and ocular lymphoma workshop: recommendations for the future. Ocul Immunol Inflamm. 2006;14(3):139–44.
24. Plotkin SR, Batchelor TT. Advances in the therapy of primary central nervous system lymphoma. Clin Lymphoma. 2001;1(4):263–75; discussion 276-267.
25. Grimm SA, McCannel CA, Omuro AM, et al. Primary CNS lymphoma with intraocular involvement: International PCNSL Collaborative Group Report. Neurology. 2008;71(17):1355–60.
26. Frenkel S, Hendler K, Siegal T, Shalom E, Pe'er J. Intravitreal methotrexate for treating vitreoretinal lymphoma: 10 years of experience. Br J Ophthalmol. 2008;92(3):383–8.
27. Davis JL. Intraocular lymphoma: a clinical perspective. Eye (Lond). 2013;27(2):153–62.
28. Mochizuki M, Singh AD. Epidemiology and clinical features of intraocular lymphoma. Ocul Immunol Inflamm. 2009;17(2):69–72.
29. Zaldivar RA, Martin DF, Holden JT, Grossniklaus HE. Primary intraocular lymphoma: clinical, cytologic, and flow cytometric analysis. Ophthalmology. 2004;111(9):1762–7.
30. Faia LJ, Chan CC. Primary intraocular lymphoma. Arch Pathol Lab Med. 2009;133(8):1228–32.
31. Whitcup SM, de Smet MD, Rubin BI, et al. Intraocular lymphoma. Clinical and histopathologic diagnosis. Ophthalmology. 1993;100(9):1399–406.
32. Coupland SE, Perez-Canto A, Hummel M, Stein H, Heimann H. Assessment of HOPE fixation in vitrectomy specimens in patients with chronic bilateral uveitis (masquerade syndrome). Graefes Arch Clin Exp Ophthalmol. 2005;243(9):847–52.

33. Vogel MH, Font RL, Zimmerman LE, Levine RA. Reticulum cell sarcoma of the retina and uvea. Report of six cases and review of the literature. Am J Ophthalmol. 1968;66(2):205–15.
34. Wittenberg LA, Maberley DA, Ma PE, Wade NK, Gill H, White VA. Contribution of vitreous cytology to final clinical diagnosis fifteen-year review of vitreous cytology specimens from one institution. Ophthalmology. 2008;115(11):1944–50.
35. Parikh AH, Khan SH, Wright JD, Oh KT. Systemic non-Hodgkin's lymphoma simulating primary intraocular lymphoma. Am J Ophthalmol. 2005;139(3):573–4.
36. Salomão DR, Pulido JS, Johnston PB, Canal-Fontcuberta I, Feldman AL. Vitreoretinal presentation of secondary large B-cell lymphoma in patients with systemic lymphoma. JAMA Ophthalmol. 2013;131(9):1151–8.
37. Char DH, Ljung BM, Deschênes J, Miller TR. Intraocular lymphoma: immunological and cytological analysis. Br J Ophthalmol. 1988;72(12):905–11.
38. Chan CC, Shen D, Hackett JJ, Buggage RR, Tuaillon N. Expression of chemokine receptors, CXCR4 and CXCR5, and chemokines, BLC and SDF-1, in the eyes of patients with primary intraocular lymphoma. Ophthalmology. 2003;110(2):421–6.
39. Coupland SE, Damato B. Understanding intraocular lymphomas. Clin Exp Ophthalmol. 2008;36(6):564–78.
40. Mashayekhi A, Shukla SY, Shields JA, Shields CL. Choroidal lymphoma: clinical features and association with systemic lymphoma. Ophthalmology. 2014;121(1):342–51.
41. Barry RJ, Tasiopoulou A, Murray PI, et al. Characteristic optical coherence tomography findings in patients with primary vitreoretinal lymphoma: a novel aid to early diagnosis. Br J Ophthalmol. 2018;102(10):1362–6.
42. Velez G, Chan CC, Csaky KG. Fluorescein angiographic findings in primary intraocular lymphoma. Retina. 2002;22(1):37–43.
43. Pulido JS, Johnston PB, Nowakowski GS, Castellino A, Raja H. The diagnosis and treatment of primary vitreoretinal lymphoma: a review. Int J Retina Vitreous. 2018;4:18.
44. Iaccheri B, Fiore T, Cerquaglia A, Lupidi M, Cagini C. Transient therapeutic effect of vitrectomy in primary intraocular lymphoma. Int Ophthalmol. 2017;37(6):1333–5.
45. Venkatesh P, Gogia V, Khanduja S, Gupta S, Kumar L, Garg S. Therapeutic vitrectomy for vitreal recurrence of intraocular lymphoma resistant to intravitreal methotrexate post systemic chemotherapy. J Cancer Res Ther. 2015;11(3):668.
46. Coupland SE. Vitreous biopsy: specimen preparation and interpretation. Monogr Clin Cytol. 2012;21:61–71.
47. Chan CC. Molecular pathology of primary intraocular lymphoma. Trans Am Ophthalmol Soc. 2003;101:275–92.
48. Chan CC, Wallace DJ. Intraocular lymphoma: update on diagnosis and management. Cancer Control. 2004;11(5):285–95.
49. Yonese I, Takase H, Yoshimori M, et al. CD79B mutations in primary vitreoretinal lymphoma: diagnostic and prognostic potential. Eur J Haematol. 2019;102(2):191–6.
50. Davis JL, Solomon D, Nussenblatt RB, Palestine AG, Chan CC. Immunocytochemical staining of vitreous cells. Indications, techniques, and results. Ophthalmology. 1992;99(2):250–6.
51. Davis JL, Viciana AL, Ruiz P. Diagnosis of intraocular lymphoma by flow cytometry. Am J Ophthalmol. 1997;124(3):362–72.
52. White VA, Gascoyne RD, Paton KE. Use of the polymerase chain reaction to detect B- and T-cell gene rearrangements in vitreous specimens from patients with intraocular lymphoma. Arch Ophthalmol. 1999;117(6):761–5.
53. Cani AK, Hovelson DH, Demirci H, Johnson MW, Tomlins SA, Rao RC. Next generation sequencing of vitreoretinal lymphomas from small-volume intraocular liquid biopsies: new routes to targeted therapies. Oncotarget. 2017;8(5):7989–98.
54. Bruno A, Boisselier B, Labreche K, et al. Mutational analysis of primary central nervous system lymphoma. Oncotarget. 2014;5(13):5065–75.
55. Gonzalez-Aguilar A, Idbaih A, Boisselier B, et al. Recurrent mutations of MYD88 and TBL1XR1 in primary central nervous system lymphomas. Clin Cancer Res. 2012;18(19):5203–11.
56. Bonzheim I, Giese S, Deuter C, et al. High frequency of MYD88 mutations in vitreoretinal B-cell lymphoma: a valuable tool to improve diagnostic yield of vitreous aspirates. Blood. 2015;126(1):76–9.
57. Montesinos-Rongen M, Godlewska E, Brunn A, Wiestler OD, Siebert R, Deckert M. Activating L265P mutations of the MYD88 gene are common in primary central nervous system lymphoma. Acta Neuropathol. 2011;122(6):791–2.
58. Hiemcke-Jiwa LS, Ten Dam-van Loon NH, Leguit RJ, et al. Potential diagnosis of vitreoretinal lymphoma by detection of MYD88 mutation in aqueous humor with ultrasensitive droplet digital polymerase chain reaction. JAMA Ophthalmol. 2018;136(10):1098–104.
59. Raja H, Snyder MR, Johnston PB, et al. Effect of intravitreal methotrexate and rituximab on interleukin-10 levels in aqueous humor of treated eyes with vitreoretinal lymphoma. PLoS One. 2013;8(6):e65627.
60. Wolf LA, Reed GF, Buggage RR, Nussenblatt RB, Chan CC. Vitreous cytokine levels. Ophthalmology. 2003;110(8):1671–2.
61. Benjamin D, Park CD, Sharma V. Human B cell interleukin 10. Leuk Lymphoma. 1994;12(3–4):205–10.
62. Merle-Béral H, Davi F, Cassoux N, et al. Biological diagnosis of primary intraocular lymphoma. Br J Haematol. 2004;124(4):469–73.
63. Costopoulos M, Touitou V, Golmard JL, et al. ISOLD: a new highly sensitive interleukin score for intraocular lymphoma diagnosis. Ophthalmology. 2016;123(7):1626–8.
64. Fend F, Ferreri AJ, Coupland SE. How we diagnose and treat vitreoretinal lymphoma. Br J Haematol. 2016;173(5):680–92.
65. Buggage RR, Chan CC, Nussenblatt RB. Ocular manifestations of central nervous system lymphoma. Curr Opin Oncol. 2001;13(3):137–42.
66. Sen HN, Bodaghi B, Hoang PL, Nussenblatt R. Primary intraocular lymphoma: diagnosis and differential diagnosis. Ocul Immunol Inflamm. 2009;17(3):133–41.
67. Buggage RR, Velez G, Myers-Powell B, Shen D, Whitcup SM, Chan CC. Primary intraocular lymphoma with a low interleukin 10 to interleukin 6 ratio and heterogeneous IgH gene rearrangement. Arch Ophthalmol. 1999;117(9):1239–42.
68. Kimura K, Usui Y, Goto H, Group JILS. Clinical features and diagnostic significance of the intraocular fluid of 217 patients with intraocular lymphoma. Jpn J Ophthalmol. 2012;56(4):383–9.
69. Chan CC, Buggage RR, Nussenblatt RB. Intraocular lymphoma. Curr Opin Ophthalmol. 2002;13(6):411–8.
70. Grimm SA, Pulido JS, Jahnke K, et al. Primary intraocular lymphoma: an international primary central nervous system lymphoma collaborative group report. Ann Oncol. 2007;18(11):1851–5.
71. Malaise D, Houillier C, Touitou V, et al. Primary vitreoretinal lymphoma: short review of the literature, results of a European survey and French guidelines of the LOC network for diagnosis, treatment and follow-up. Curr Opin Oncol. 2021;33(5):420–31.
72. Turaka K, Bryan JS, De Souza S, et al. Vitreoretinal lymphoma: changing trends in diagnosis and local treatment modalities at a single institution. Clin Lymphoma Myeloma Leuk. 2012;12(6):412–7.
73. Abu Samra K, Oray M, Ebrahimiadib N, Lee S, Anesi S, Foster CS. Intraocular lymphoma: descriptive data of 26 patients includ-

ing clinico-pathologic features, vitreous findings, and treatment outcomes. Ocul Immunol Inflamm. 2018;26(3):347–52.
74. Reichstein D. Primary vitreoretinal lymphoma: an update on pathogenesis, diagnosis and treatment. Curr Opin Ophthalmol. 2016;27(3):177–84.
75. Berenbom A, Davila RM, Lin HS, Harbour JW. Treatment outcomes for primary intraocular lymphoma: implications for external beam radiotherapy. Eye (Lond). 2007;21(9):1198–201.
76. Isobe K, Ejima Y, Tokumaru S, et al. Treatment of primary intraocular lymphoma with radiation therapy: a multi-institutional survey in Japan. Leuk Lymphoma. 2006;47(9):1800–5.
77. Hoffman PM, McKelvie P, Hall AJ, Stawell RJ, Santamaria JD. Intraocular lymphoma: a series of 14 patients with clinicopathological features and treatment outcomes. Eye (Lond). 2003;17(4):513–21.
78. Witmer MT. Primary vitreoretinal lymphoma: management of isolated ocular disease. Cancer Control. 2016;23(2):110–6.
79. Kaushik M, Pulido JS, Schild SE, Stafford S. Risk of radiation retinopathy in patients with orbital and ocular lymphoma. Int J Radiat Oncol Biol Phys. 2012;84(5):1145–50.
80. Fishburne BC, Wilson DJ, Rosenbaum JT, Neuwelt EA. Intravitreal methotrexate as an adjunctive treatment of intraocular lymphoma. Arch Ophthalmol. 1997;115(9):1152–6.
81. Helbig H, Cerny T, de Smet MD. Intravitreal chemotherapy for intraocular lymphoma. Ophthalmologe. 2003;100(2):145–9.
82. Bianciotto C, Shields CL, Lally SE, Freire J, Shields JA. CyberKnife radiosurgery for the treatment of intraocular and periocular lymphoma. Arch Ophthalmol. 2010;128(12):1561–7.
83. Smith JR, Rosenbaum JT, Wilson DJ, et al. Role of intravitreal methotrexate in the management of primary central nervous system lymphoma with ocular involvement. Ophthalmology. 2002;109(9):1709–16.
84. de Smet MD, Vancs VS, Kohler D, Solomon D, Chan CC. Intravitreal chemotherapy for the treatment of recurrent intraocular lymphoma. Br J Ophthalmol. 1999;83(4):448–51.
85. Sen HN, Chan CC, Byrnes G, Fariss RN, Nussenblatt RB, Buggage RR. Intravitreal methotrexate resistance in a patient with primary intraocular lymphoma. Ocul Immunol Inflamm. 2008;16(1):29–33.
86. Mason JO, Fischer DH. Intrathecal chemotherapy for recurrent central nervous system intraocular lymphoma. Ophthalmology. 2003;110(6):1241–4.
87. Kitzmann AS, Pulido JS, Mohney BG, et al. Intraocular use of rituximab. Eye (Lond). 2007;21(12):1524–7.
88. Hashida N, Ohguro N, Nishida K. Efficacy and complications of intravitreal rituximab injection for treating primary vitreoretinal lymphoma. Transl Vis Sci Technol. 2012;1(3):1.
89. Ohguro N, Hashida N, Tano Y. Effect of intravitreous rituximab injections in patients with recurrent ocular lesions associated with central nervous system lymphoma. Arch Ophthalmol. 2008;126(7):1002–3.
90. Larkin KL, Saboo US, Comer GM, et al. Use of intravitreal rituximab for treatment of vitreoretinal lymphoma. Br J Ophthalmol. 2014;98(1):99–103.
91. Hoang-Xuan K, Bessell E, Bromberg J, et al. Diagnosis and treatment of primary CNS lymphoma in immunocompetent patients: guidelines from the European Association for Neuro-Oncology. Lancet Oncol. 2015;16(7):e322–32.
92. Batchelor TT, Kolak G, Ciordia R, Foster CS, Henson JW. High-dose methotrexate for intraocular lymphoma. Clin Cancer Res. 2003;9(2):711–5.
93. Baumann MA, Ritch PS, Hande KR, Williams GA, Topping TM, Anderson T. Treatment of intraocular lymphoma with high-dose Ara-C. Cancer. 1986;57(7):1273–5.
94. Siegel MJ, Dalton J, Friedman AH, Strauchen J, Watson C. Ten-year experience with primary ocular 'reticulum cell sarcoma' (large cell non-Hodgkin's lymphoma). Br J Ophthalmol. 1989;73(5):342–6.
95. Strauchen JA, Dalton J, Friedman AH. Chemotherapy in the management of intraocular lymphoma. Cancer. 1989;63(10):1918–21.
96. DeAngelis LM, Seiferheld W, Schold SC, Fisher B, Schultz CJ. 93-10 RTOGS. Combination chemotherapy and radiotherapy for primary central nervous system lymphoma: Radiation Therapy Oncology Group Study 93-10. J Clin Oncol. 2002;20(24):4643–8.
97. Henson JW, Yang J, Batchelor T. Intraocular methotrexate level after high-dose intravenous infusion. J Clin Oncol. 1999;17(4):1329.
98. Batchelor T, Carson K, O'Neill A, et al. Treatment of primary CNS lymphoma with methotrexate and deferred radiotherapy: a report of NABTT 96-07. J Clin Oncol. 2003;21(6):1044–9.
99. Herrlinger U, Küker W, Uhl M, et al. NOA-03 trial of high-dose methotrexate in primary central nervous system lymphoma: final report. Ann Neurol. 2005;57(6):843–7.
100. Baron M, Belin L, Cassoux N, et al. Temozolomide is effective and well tolerated in patients with primary vitreoretinal lymphoma. Blood. 2020;135(20):1811–5.
101. de la Fuente MI, Alderuccio JP, Reis IM, et al. Bilateral radiation therapy followed by methotrexate-based chemotherapy for primary vitreoretinal lymphoma. Am J Hematol. 2019;94(4):455–60.
102. Hashida N, Nakai K, Saitoh N, Nishida K. Association between ocular findings and preventive therapy with onset of central nervous system involvement in patients with primary vitreoretinal lymphoma. Graefes Arch Clin Exp Ophthalmol. 2014;252(4):687–93.
103. Soussain C, Merle-Béral H, Reux I, et al. A single-center study of 11 patients with intraocular lymphoma treated with conventional chemotherapy followed by high-dose chemotherapy and autologous bone marrow transplantation in 5 cases. Leuk Lymphoma. 1996;23(3–4):339–45.
104. Soussain C, Suzan F, Hoang-Xuan K, et al. Results of intensive chemotherapy followed by hematopoietic stem-cell rescue in 22 patients with refractory or recurrent primary CNS lymphoma or intraocular lymphoma. J Clin Oncol. 2001;19(3):742–9.
105. Soussain C, Hoang-Xuan K, Taillandier L, et al. Intensive chemotherapy followed by hematopoietic stem-cell rescue for refractory and recurrent primary CNS and intraocular lymphoma: Société Française de Greffe de Moëlle Osseuse-Thérapie Cellulaire. J Clin Oncol. 2008;26(15):2512–8.
106. Soussain C, Choquet S, Fourme E, et al. Intensive chemotherapy with thiotepa, busulfan and cyclophosphamide and hematopoietic stem cell rescue in relapsed or refractory primary central nervous system lymphoma and intraocular lymphoma: a retrospective study of 79 cases. Haematologica. 2012;97(11):1751–6.
107. Davis RE, Brown KD, Siebenlist U, Staudt LM. Constitutive nuclear factor kappaB activity is required for survival of activated B cell-like diffuse large B cell lymphoma cells. J Exp Med. 2001;194(12):1861–74.
108. Grommes C, Nayak L, Tun HW, Batchelor TT. Introduction of novel agents in the treatment of primary CNS lymphoma. Neuro-Oncology. 2019;21(3):306–13.
109. Nakamura T, Tateishi K, Niwa T, et al. Recurrent mutations of CD79B and MYD88 are the hallmark of primary central nervous system lymphomas. Neuropathol Appl Neurobiol. 2016;42(3):279–90.

110. Raja H, Salomão DR, Viswanatha DS, Pulido JS. Prevalence of MYD88 L265P mutation in histologically proven, diffuse large b-cell vitreoretinal lymphoma. Retina. 2016;36(3):624–8.
111. Grommes C, Pastore A, Palaskas N, et al. Ibrutinib unmasks critical role of Bruton tyrosine kinase in primary CNS lymphoma. Cancer Discov. 2017;7(9):1018–29.
112. Soussain C, Choquet S, Blonski M, et al. Ibrutinib monotherapy for relapse or refractory primary CNS lymphoma and primary vitreoretinal lymphoma: final analysis of the phase II 'proof-of-concept' iLOC study by the lymphoma study association (LYSA) and the French oculo-cerebral lymphoma (LOC) network. Eur J Cancer. 2019;117:121–30.
113. Chamoun K, Choquet S, Boyle E, et al. Ibrutinib monotherapy in relapsed/refractory CNS lymphoma: a retrospective case series. Neurology. 2017;88(1):101–2.
114. Lionakis MS, Dunleavy K, Roschewski M, et al. Inhibition of B cell receptor signaling by Ibrutinib in primary CNS lymphoma. Cancer Cell. 2017;31(6):833–843.e835.
115. Narita Y, Nagane M, Mishima K, et al. Phase I/II study of tirabrutinib, a second-generation Bruton's tyrosine kinase inhibitor, in relapsed/refractory primary central nervous system lymphoma. Neuro-Oncology. 2021;23(1):122–33.
116. Yang Y, Shaffer AL, Emre NC, et al. Exploiting synthetic lethality for the therapy of ABC diffuse large B cell lymphoma. Cancer Cell. 2012;21(6):723–37.
117. Rubenstein JL, Geng H, Fraser EJ, et al. Phase 1 investigation of lenalidomide/rituximab plus outcomes of lenalidomide maintenance in relapsed CNS lymphoma. Blood Adv. 2018;2(13):1595–607.
118. Ghesquieres H, Chevrier M, Laadhari M, et al. Lenalidomide in combination with intravenous rituximab (REVRI) in relapsed/refractory primary CNS lymphoma or primary intraocular lymphoma: a multicenter prospective 'proof of concept' phase II study of the French Oculo-Cerebral lymphoma (LOC) Network and the Lymphoma Study Association (LYSA)†. Ann Oncol. 2019;30(4):621–8.
119. Tun HW, Johnston PB, DeAngelis LM, et al. Phase 1 study of pomalidomide and dexamethasone for relapsed/refractory primary CNS or vitreoretinal lymphoma. Blood. 2018;132(21):2240–8.
120. Carbonell D, Mahajan S, Chee SP, et al. Consensus recommendations for the diagnosis of vitreoretinal lymphoma. Ocul Immunol Inflamm. 2021;29(3):507–20.

Advances in Imaging in Ocular Oncology: A Radiologist's Perspective

Pim de Graaf, Robin W. Jansen, Paolo Galluzzi, and Marcus C. de Jong

Abbreviations

ADC	Apparent Diffusion Coefficient
CISS	Constructive Interference in Steady State
CT	Computed Tomography
DCE	Dynamic Contrast Enhanced
DRIVE	Driven Equilibrium
DWI	Diffusion Weighted Imaging
FIESTA	Fast Imaging Employing Steady-state Acquisition
MR	Magnetic Resonance
MRI	Magnetic Resonance Imaging
RESOLVE	Readout Segmentation of Long Variable Echo Trains
TIC	Time-Intensity Curve

1 Introduction

Over the last few decades, surgical treatment options for intraocular tumors have shifted toward conservative treatment. Therefore, often no tumor tissue will be available for histopathological analysis, increasing the importance of radiological imaging for diagnosis and staging. Simultaneously, the availability and quality of imaging have increased, allowing for more detailed depiction of ocular structures providing better support for clinical decision-making. Imaging nowadays contributes significantly to the multidisciplinary approach in ocular oncology in middle- and high-income countries. The main diseases analyzed by a radiologist specialized in ocular imaging are primary ocular tumors (i.e., retinoblastoma, uveal melanoma, medulloepithelioma) and their simulating lesions, as well as intraocular metastases.

P. de Graaf (✉) · R. W. Jansen · M. C. de Jong
Department of Radiology and Nuclear Medicine, Amsterdam UMC, Vrije Universiteit Amsterdam, Cancer Center Amsterdam, Amsterdam, The Netherlands
e-mail: p.degraaf@amsterdamumc.nl; r.jansen1@amsterdamumc.nl; mc.dejong@amsterdamumc.nl

P. Galluzzi
Department of Neuroimaging and Neurointervention, Siena University Hospital, Siena, Italy
e-mail: galluzzip@libero.it

2 Radiological Imaging Techniques in Ocular Oncology

Although many intraocular tumors are diagnosed by ophthalmological examination alone, imaging studies are used in almost all patients to confirm the diagnosis; to determine the intraocular disease extent; and to detect extraocular spread, metastasis, or associated lesions (e.g., trilateral retinoblastoma). B-scan ultrasound is usually performed by the ophthalmologist in an outpatient setting to evaluate the intraocular lesions. High-resolution techniques, such as ultrasound biomicroscopy and optical coherence tomography, are valuable additions to the spectrum of imaging tools applied by the ophthalmologist that can help in the diagnosis of anterior segment lesions and retinal pathology. Cross-sectional imaging with CT and especially MRI provides complementary information to the imaging techniques employed by the ophthalmologist. In ocular oncology, MRI is the modality of choice and allows for a detailed tumor classification and staging not only intraocularly but also outside of the confines of the globe [1].

Beyond anatomical information, modern MRI techniques can also provide quantitative information regarding physiological characteristics of tissues, such as tissue perfusion, vascular leakage, and water diffusion. Such parameters can help not only with tumor characterization, but also with treatment susceptibility and treatment response.

In general, MRI is favored over CT imaging for ocular lesions. MRI offers more information than CT because of the increased soft tissue representation and, especially important in children, there is no radiation exposure from MRI. However, should an MR machine not be available,

B. V. Chawla, M. E. Aronow (eds.), *Global Perspectives in Ocular Oncology*, https://doi.org/10.1007/978-3-031-08250-4_10

which is the case in many lower-income countries, a CT scan can still provide valuable information [2]. Ocular MRI is challenging because motion artifacts and susceptibility artifacts due to air-tissue and bone-tissue interfaces cause magnetic field inhomogeneities. Artifacts may also occur as a result of eye cosmetics, with focal distortion of the skin contour of the eyelids and the anterior eye chamber. Ocular imaging in both adults and children have their own challenges. To prevent motion artifacts, young children need to be sedated (preferably with general anesthesia), whereas in adults, eye movements and eye blinking significantly reduce image quality [3]. The patients should be instructed to focus on a fixation-target during the scan and avoid blinking as much as possible. Scanning with eyes closed is an alternative strategy although unintentional eye movements cannot be completely avoided.

Over the years, the quality of MR images in general and specifically of the eyes has increased substantially (Fig. 1). With the advent of high-field MR systems, improvements in imaging coils, and better imaging sequences, high-resolution images with isotropic submillimeter resolution can be created depicting very small anatomical details and disturbances [4].

Ocular MRI is not part of the routine in most MRI units. However, it is crucial for the patient to obtain high-quality images and these examinations must be performed by dedicated teams of MR technicians and radiologists. High-quality examinations providing detailed images of small anatomical structures can only be obtained when a high signal-to-noise ratio is guaranteed. On 1.5 T MR systems, it is advisable to use small surface coils for acquiring high-resolution MR images of the eyes, whereas multi-channel (usually >16 channels) head volume RF coils can be used on 3 T systems.

Although individual examinations should be tailored to the problem of each patient, there is a set of minimal requirements for imaging ocular lesions. These include acquisition of 2D T2- and T1-weighted MR images combined with contrast-enhanced T1-weighted images with fat-suppression. Many centers also obtain contrast-enhanced T1-weighted images without fat suppression to be able to generate additional subtraction images and depict the foci of enhancement, which can be obscured in the presence of an intraocular hemorrhage. These sequences must be obtained at least in the axial plane with a slice thickness ≤2 mm (ref guideline). Additional coronal or sagittal contrast-enhanced T1-weighted images can be obtained to analyze the ocular wall (choroid, scleral) or extrascleral invasion. The axial image plane should be precisely aligned at the middle of the optic disk and the distal (at least 1 cm) end of the optic nerve to increase the diagnostic accuracy for detection of optic nerve tumor invasion (Fig. 2) [4, 5].

The 2D MRI sequences have the highest in-plane resolution, being the most suited for lesion characterization and evaluation of local tumor extension. In the last decade, 3D sequences were developed and improved rapidly, and have become more popular in the imaging protocol for intraocular lesions. Isotropic T2 or contrast enhanced T1 3D sequences

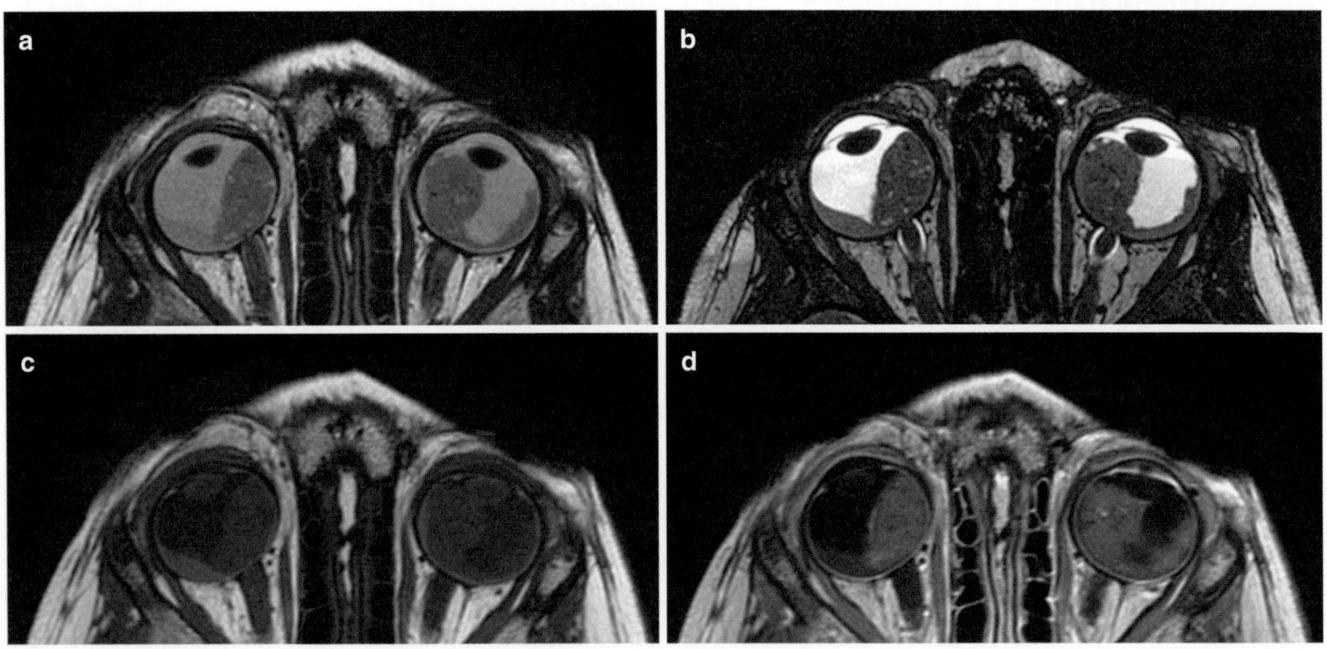

Fig. 1 High-resolution MRI of bilateral retinoblastoma. (**a**) An example of high-resolution MR images obtained on a 3 T MR system combined with a 32-channel head coil, with a T2-weighted image, (**b**) a heavily weighted T2 image (FIESTA), (**c**) a native T1-weighted image and (**d**) a T1-weighted image after administration of a gadolinium contrast agent

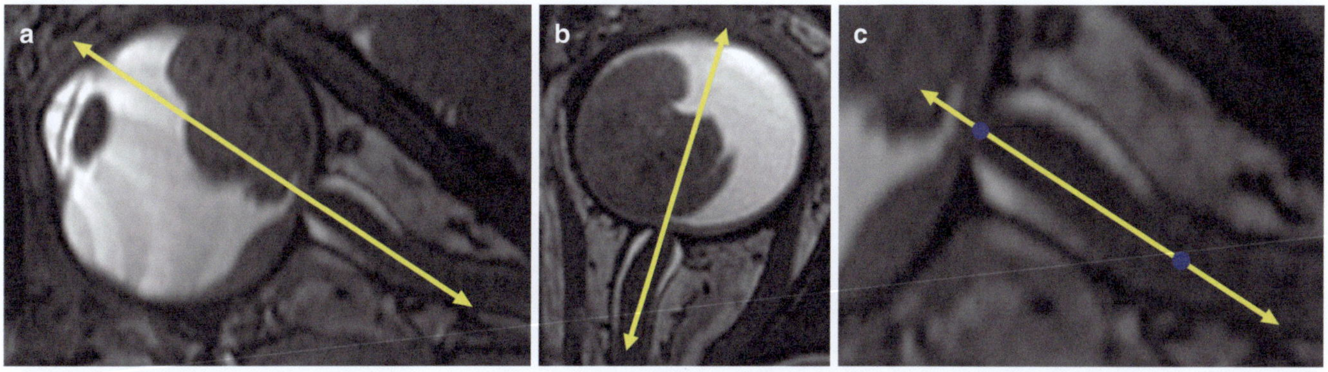

Fig. 2 Planning of slice positions to obtain high-resolution axial MR sequences for optic nerve tumor invasion detection. (**a**) First, a high-resolution heavy T2-weighted sequence is reconstructed in the oblique sagittal and (**b**) axial plane. Subsequently, the planning of the high-resolution axial 2D T1-weighted is aligned exactly in the middle of the optic disc and at least 1 cm posteriorly in the distal optic nerve (**c** between the blue dots) so that the obtained T1-weighted images allow an accurate assessment of optic nerve tumor invasion

allow for multiplanar reconstructions in all directions, allowing the radiologists to perform accurate measurements of the largest basal tumor diameter and tumor prominence perpendicular to the ocular wall independent from tumor location. In uveal melanoma, these measurements are important for choosing an adequate treatment, in particular to decide between enucleation and an eye-preserving therapy [6]. Furthermore, accurate tumor size measurements and availability of a 3D model of the tumor are important for the planning of various forms of radiotherapy, such as brachytherapy, stereotactic radiotherapy, and proton-beam radiotherapy [6]. However, the value of 2D versus 3D sequences in the detection of local tumor extent does not always yield a better diagnostic accuracy. Especially for tumor invasion of the optic nerve, a well-angulated 2D sequence is usually more sensitive than a 3D sequence. However, 3D sequences with heavy T2 weighting (i.e., CISS, FIESTA, DRIVE) outperform 2D T2-weighted sequences in determining the exact three-dimensional tumor extension within the globe. Due to a very high spatial resolution and the high contrast resolution between a solid tumor mass with low T2 signal intensity and the high signal intensity of the vitreous fluid, very small intraocular tumors and even vitreous or subretinal tumor seeding can easily be depicted (Fig. 3).

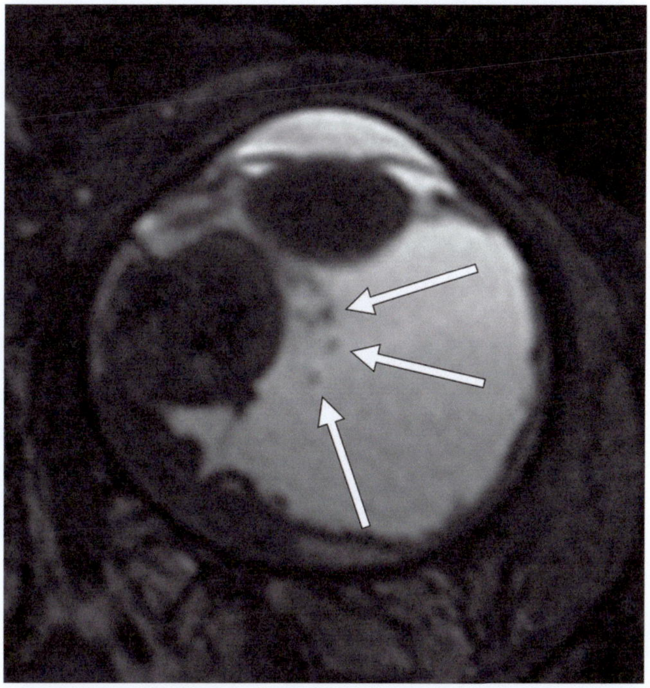

Fig. 3 Vitreous seeding in retinoblastoma. A FIESTA image of retinoblastoma in the left eye with extensive retinal tumoral infiltration especially nasally, combined with partial retinal detachment and extensive tumor seeding into the vitreous (arrows point at some of the free-floating tumor seedings)

Advanced MRI sequences such as diffusion weighted imaging (DWI) with quantitative apparent water diffusion coefficient (ADC) mapping and dynamic contrast enhanced-(DCE) MRI can provide additional information on functional tissue characteristics (Fig. 4). DWI probes the diffusivity of water molecules on a microscopic level and free movement of water is restricted in tissues with high cellular density such as malignant tumors. Magnetic field inhomogeneities due to air and soft-tissue interfaces superficially within the orbit can significantly reduce image quality because of image distortion. However, non-EPI diffusion or newer multishot techniques such as read-out segmented DWI (RESOLVE) can improve image quality significantly [7]. In DCE MR images, the rate of uptake and clearance of contrast media is reflected in the time intensity curve (TIC), which can be quantified, providing many parameters related to tissue vascularity, such as K^{trans} (a measure of capillary permeability); v_e (reflects the volume of the extravascular extracellular space); peak enhancement, time to maximum enhancement, wash-in rate, wash-out rate, and many others (Fig. 5). Benign lesions tend to have a slower enhancement

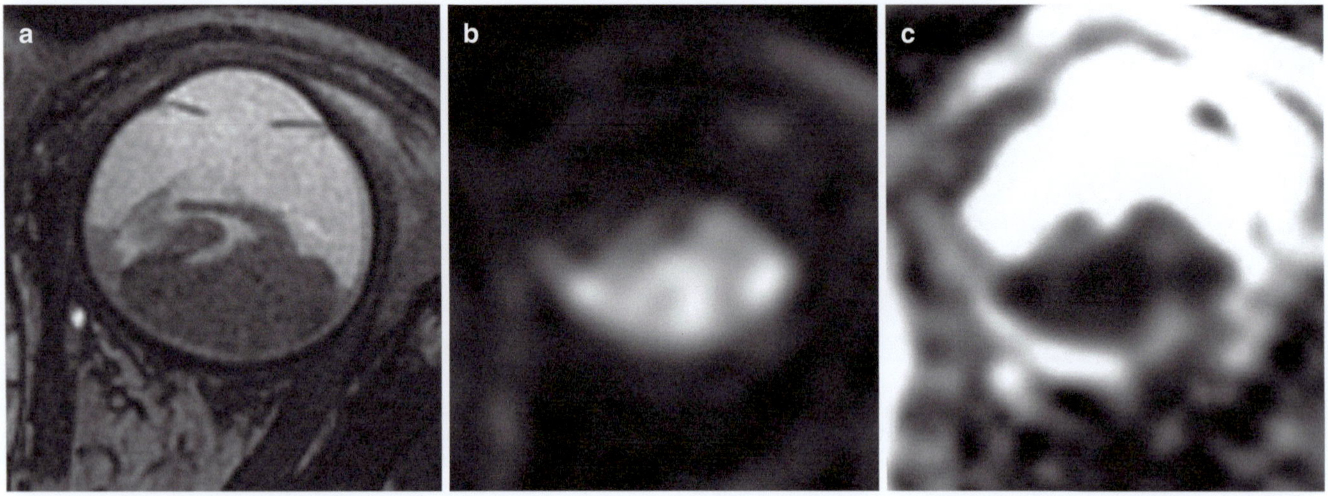

Fig. 4 Diffusion weighted imaging in retinoblastoma. (**a–c**) An example of a heavily T2-weighted image (**a** FIESTA) (**b**) of an eye with a large mass posteriorly in the left eye and a lens luxation showing increased b1000 signal in the mass on the diffusion weighted image and (**c**) a lowered ADC values (<0.9 10^{-3} mm²/s)

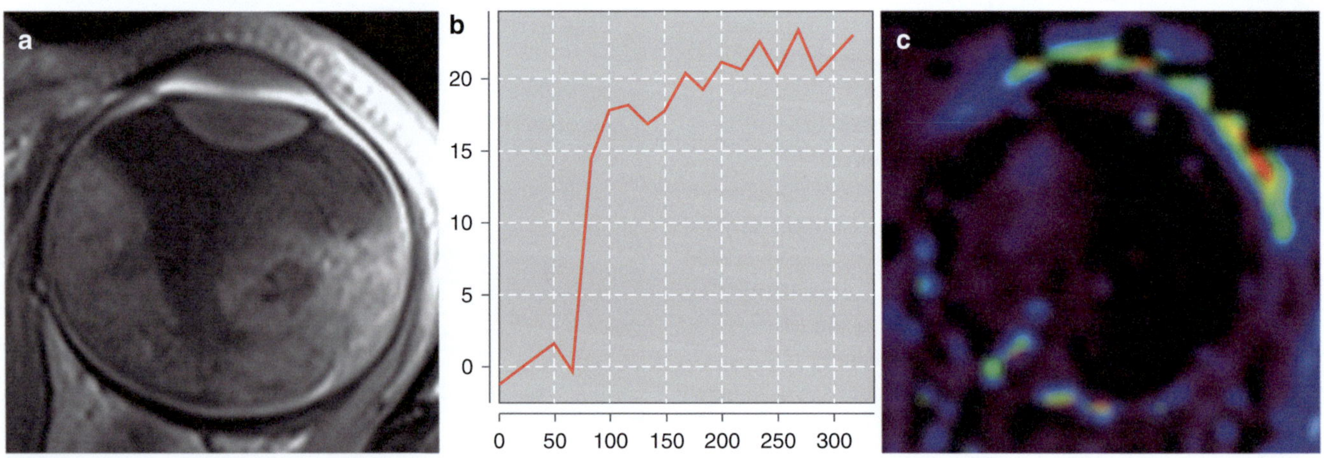

Fig. 5 Perfusion imaging in retinoblastoma. (**a**) Extensive retinoblastoma in the left eye (**b**) with in (**c**) the uptake of contrast agent depicted as a time intensity curve and in a DCE MRI derived map of the K^{trans}

(increase in T1-signal) after contrast injection, reaching a plateau, whereas malignant lesions (especially high-grade tumors) tend to show fast contrast enhancement, and after reaching a peak, a fast drop in T1-signal can be observed (washout phenomenon) [6, 8–10]. The quantitative analysis of DCE parameters may help us in lesion characterization. Nevertheless, some benign lesions may have a very fast contrast uptake (e.g., vascular lesions), and the contrast uptake in the early phase is usually not that fast in retinoblastoma, in which a progressive increase is more common (Fig. 6). Therefore, data from the functional MRI sequences must always be analyzed in combination with the clinical parameters and a detailed analysis of anatomical images. The combined use of DWI and DCE is a valuable tool in oncological imaging for the purpose of response prediction in organ-sparing treatment (Fig. 7).

3 Imaging in the Initial Workup for Ocular Tumors: Diagnosis and Staging

3.1 Radiological Imaging Aiding diagnosis in a Child with Suspected Retinoblastoma

Retinoblastoma is generally diagnosed through extensive ophthalmologic examination including fundoscopy and ultrasonography. MR imaging is usually requested to support the diagnosis, to depict the extent of disease, and to screen the CNS for metastasis and midline tumors (TRB). For retinoblastoma and other pediatric conditions presenting with leukocoria, the diagnosis can, however, generally be made by ophthalmologic assessments. Sometimes MR imaging

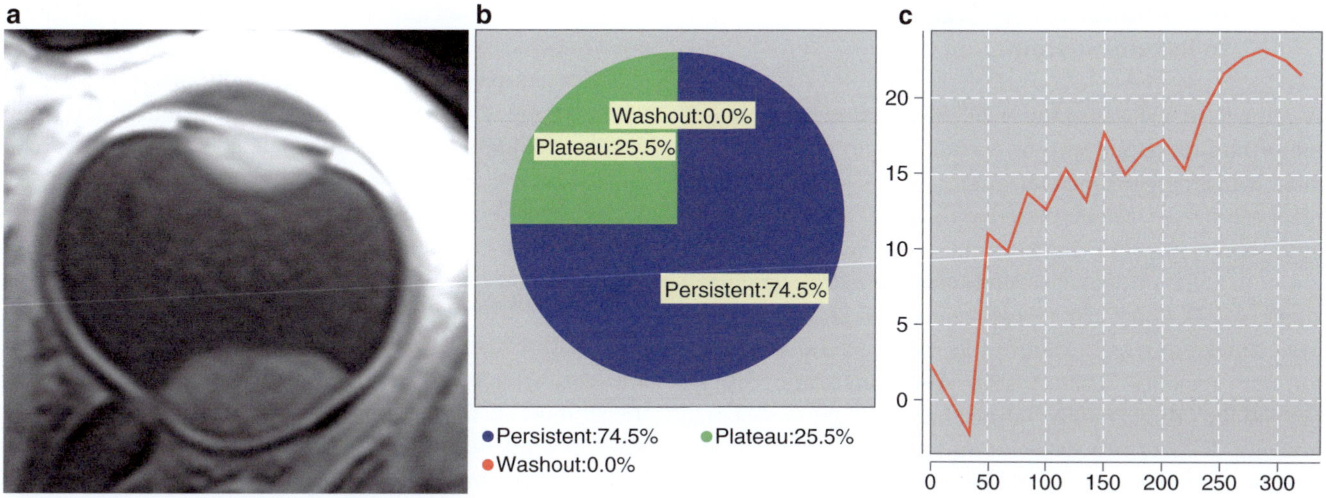

Fig. 6 Persistent increase in contrast medium uptake in retinoblastoma. (**a**) A small exophytic retinoblastoma in the left eye (**b**) showing that the majority of voxels increasingly take up contrast medium (**c**) also depicted in the time intensity curve

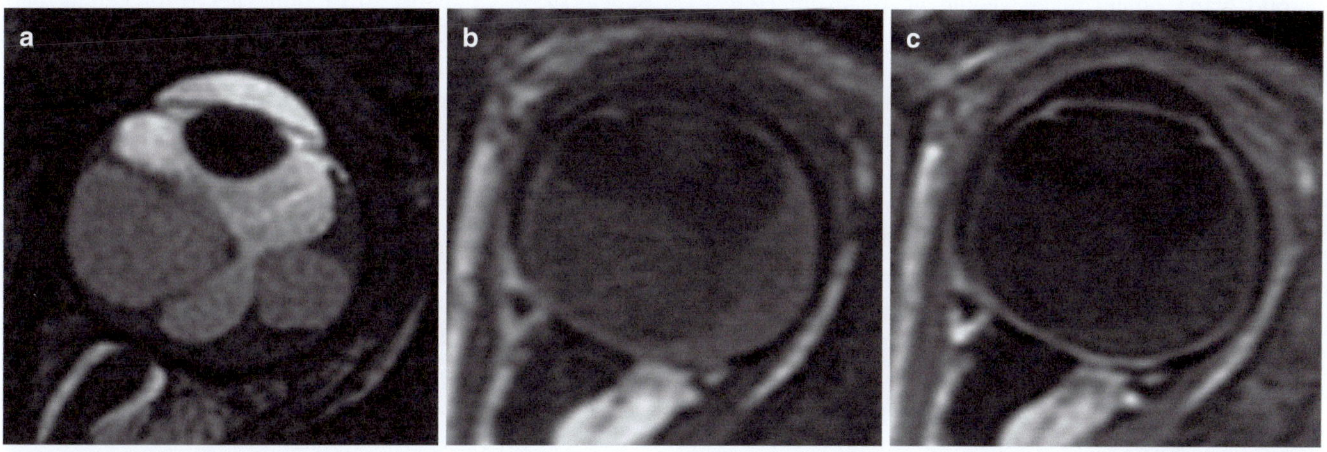

Fig. 7 Coats disease. (**a**) A patient with Coats disease in the left eye as shown on a heavily T2-weighted image, and (**b** and **c**) T1-weighted images before and after administration of contrast agent. Total retinal detachment with retinal thickening combined with retinal proteinaceous fluid. Intraretinal cysts are highly specific at ruling out retinoblastoma with a specificity of 100% (95% confidence interval [CI]: 90–100%) [13]

can be helpful in making the final diagnosis in difficult cases. The most common retinoblastoma mimickers or also known as "pseudo-retinoblastoma" are developmental vascular ocular disorders: Coats' disease and persistent fetal vasculature. A typical feature of retinoblastoma is the presence of calcifications, which can be detected on fundoscopy, ultrasonography, and are also encountered upon histopathologic examination. Increasing MR imaging detail has enabled correct detection of calcifications [11]. Additionally, eye size can be an important discriminatory factor, ranging from (often) severe microphthalmia in persistent fetal vasculature eyes to smaller eyes in Coats' disease. Retinoblastoma-affected eyes tend to be smaller than normal eyes; however, a large tumor volume can also expand the globe with a somewhat larger eye in advanced retinoblastoma as a result [12, 13]. Recently, new imaging findings were identified aiding disease classification. Retinal detachments are common in both retinoblastoma and retinoblastoma mimickers, but a sharp-V-shaped retinal detachment supports retinoblastoma diagnosis, while a Y-shaped detachment supports the diagnosis of retinoblastoma mimickers. A new feature that can probably be better detected using state-of-the-art MR images is the vitreous seeding supporting retinoblastoma diagnosis. Furthermore, different enhancement patterns differentiate between diseases, because in retinoblastoma, the enhancement is usually confined to the solid tumor lesion, whereas in retinoblastoma mimickers, enhancement can be lacking in the solid lesion area or leaking from pathologic vessels outside the solid lesion area. Furthermore, in Coats' disease specifically, intraretinal cysts (Fig. 7) and subretinal enhancing nodules can be seen close to the fovea, which could provide the key to diagnosis in difficult cases [13].

3.2 Imaging for Tumor Staging in Retinoblastoma

A reliable in vivo assessment of the invasion or spread of tumor into the globe wall or outside the globe can only be done with cross-sectional imaging. The generally recognized metastatic risk factors in retinoblastoma are postlaminar optic nerve invasion, massive choroidal invasion (at least 3 mm in width or diameter), and scleral or extrascleral invasion [14–23]. Some also recognize invasion into the anterior eye chamber as a risk factor, but its importance as a risk factor still remains debated [24]. Also, metastatic disease beyond the orbit can only be visualized with cross-sectional imaging. If there is a suspicion of leptomeningeal metastases, the entire neuraxis should be imaged after the administration of a contrast agent containing gadolinium. In case of extensive anterior eye segment involvement with conjunctival tumor invasion, potential lymphogenic metastasis to the parotid gland lymph nodes should be ruled out (Fig. 8). Different classification systems exist for the staging of retinoblastoma, including the AJCC TNM classification (version 8) that explicitly includes the role of cross-sectional imaging for depicting the higher T stages and of course, for the N and M stages [25].

In cases with extensive tumor invasion of the optic nerve beyond the lamina cribrosa, the diagnostic accuracy of MRI is near perfect and will show an enhancing and thickened optic nerve, which can extend all the way into the chiasm. Unlike peripheral nerves, the optic nerve is covered with meninges and with increasing invasion of the optic nerve, the risk of leptomeningeal metastatic spread increases as well. The risk of leptomeningeal metastases is especially large in case of extensive optic nerve invasion (e.g., surgical cut-end involvement, obvious nerve thickening) [26], but are also seen in patients with limited postlaminar optic nerve invasion as presented by De Jong et al. [27] with a case of postlaminar optic nerve invasion that reached the meninges at baseline that developed leptomeningeal metastases later on. After the neoadjuvant systemic treatment for extensive postlaminar optic nerve invasion, MR examinations can be a valuable tool in determining residual tumor in postlaminar optic nerve tumor invasion [28]. Chawla et al. [28] showed a sensitivity of 100% (95% confidence interval [CI] 61–100%) and a specificity of 82.4% (95% CI 67–92%) of optic nerve thickening and enhancement combined for the restaging of postlaminar optic nerve invasion.

Diagnostic accuracy of MRI for limited postlaminar optic nerve invasion is reasonable (Fig. 9a–c), but not perfect [29]. In a meta-analysis, MRI showed a good specificity for postlaminar optic nerve invasion at 94% (95% CI 84–98%), but the sensitivity only reached 59% (95% CI 37–78%) with an

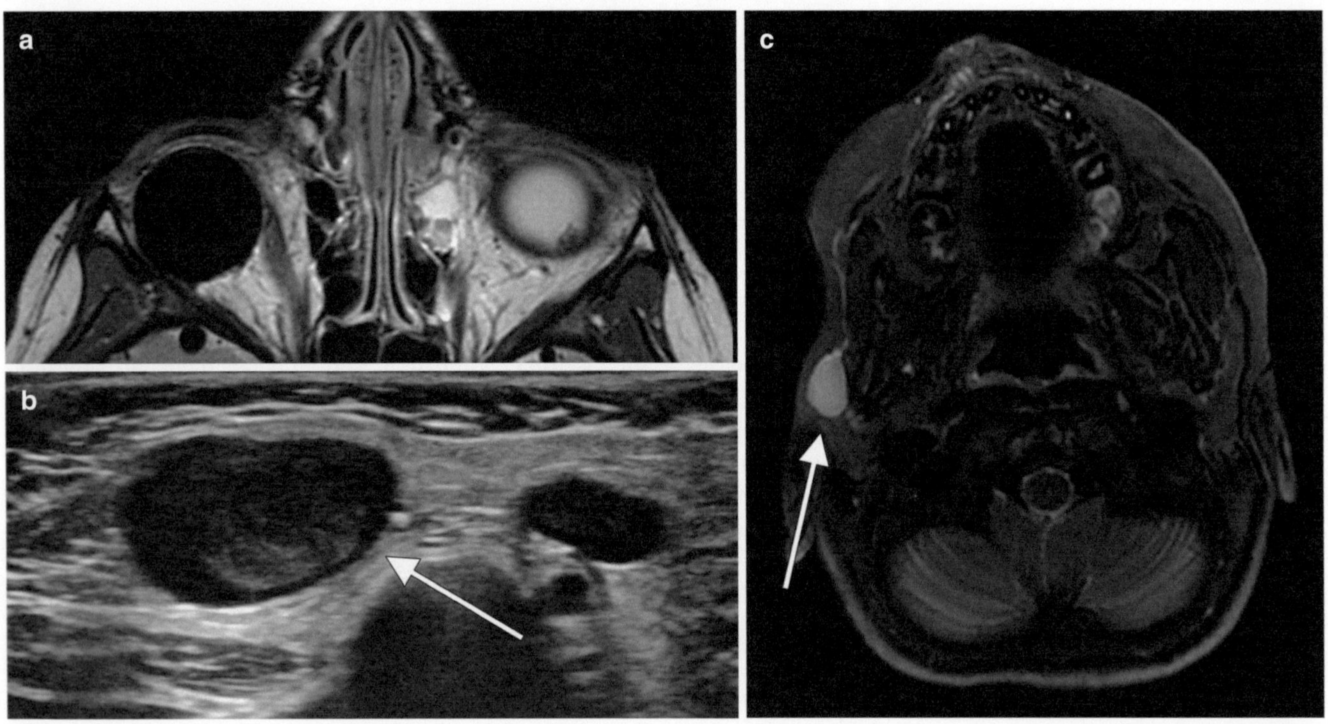

Fig. 8 Locoregional lymph node metastases in retinoblastoma. (**a**) A patient with bilateral retinoblastoma after enucleation of the right eye and insertion of a prosthesis and post-treatment changes in the left eye (**b** and **c**) who presented with an enlarged lymph node (arrows) in the parotid gland with a rounded aspect and lacking a normal fatty hilum. Histopathologic analysis after Ultrasound-guided fine needle aspiration cytology showed that this lymph node was a metastasis of retinoblastoma

upward potential to 76% (95% CI 45–93%) for high-quality MRI [29]. Several characteristics of the enhancement will help differentiate postlaminar enhancement from mimickers, such as posterior bulging of the lamina cribrosa and inflammation. In some instances, MRI can also help in differentiating between retinoblastoma-associated orbital inflammation and extra-ocular tumor spread [30].

It is unlikely to pick up limited postlaminar optic nerve invasion with CT [31], but CT did show good accuracy when it comes to substantial postlaminar optic nerve invasion and extraocular extension and associated intracranial tumors [32].

Tumor invasion into the choroid can be detected as an interruption of the strong linear choroidal enhancement pattern by a segment of less strong enhancement of the retino-

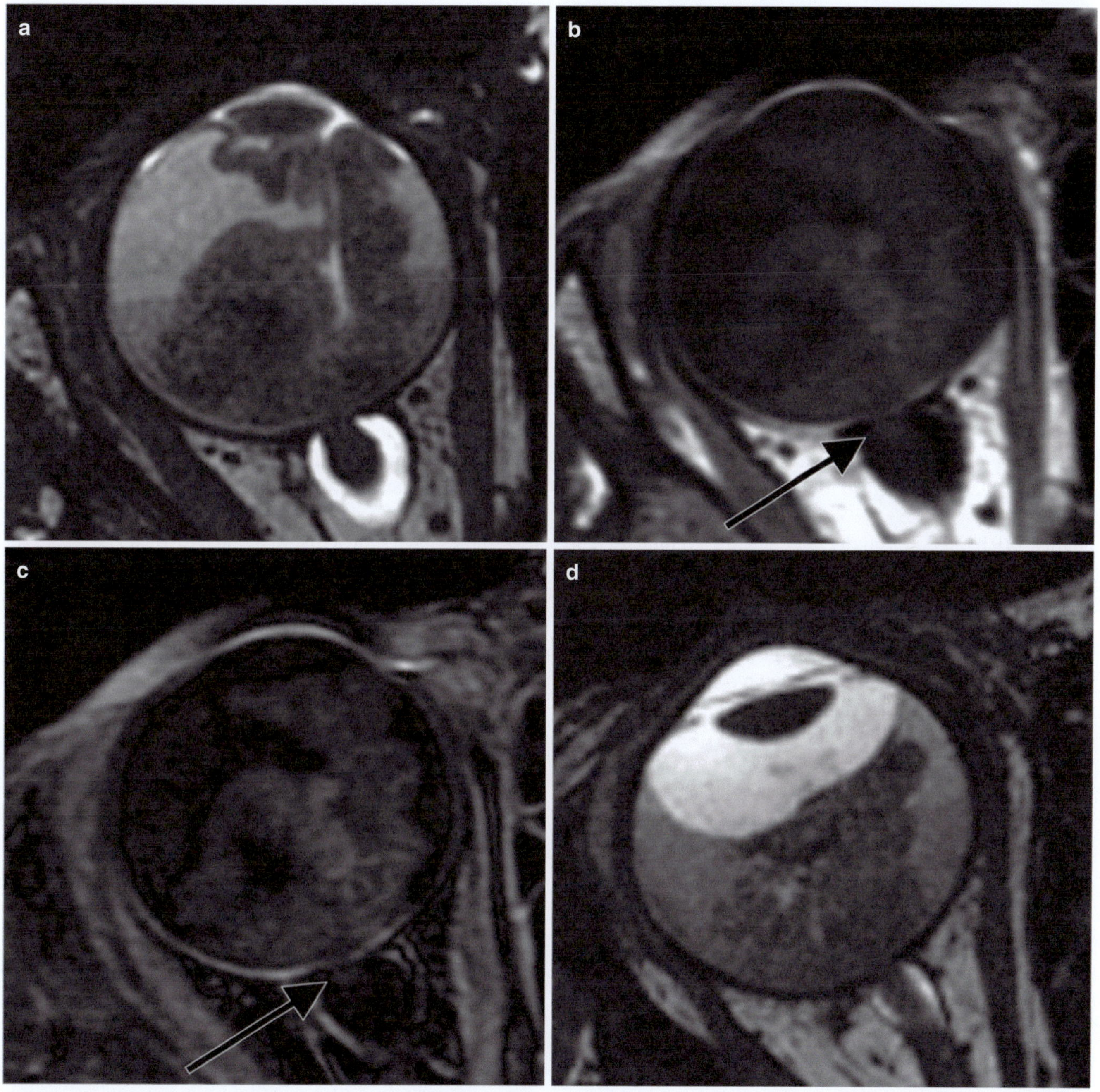

Fig. 9 Tumor invasion in retinoblastoma. (**a–c**) Postlaminar optic nerve invasion and (**d–f**) massive choroidal invasion. (**a**) A heavy T2-weighted (FIESTA) image shows an exophytic retinoblastoma with total retinal detachment and subretinal hemorrhage. The distal optic nerve shows focal postlaminar contrast enhancement (**b** black arrows on a contrast enhanced T1-weighted image and **c** on a subtraction image in), continuous with the intraocular mass, indicative of postlaminar tumor invasion. (**d**) A heavy T2-weighted (FIESTA) image, (**e**) a native T1-weighted image, and (**f**) a contrast enhanced T1-weighted image of an eye with massive choroidal tumor invasion and a discontinuity of the choroid (split choroid), (**f**) see white arrows on the contrast enhanced T1-weighted image

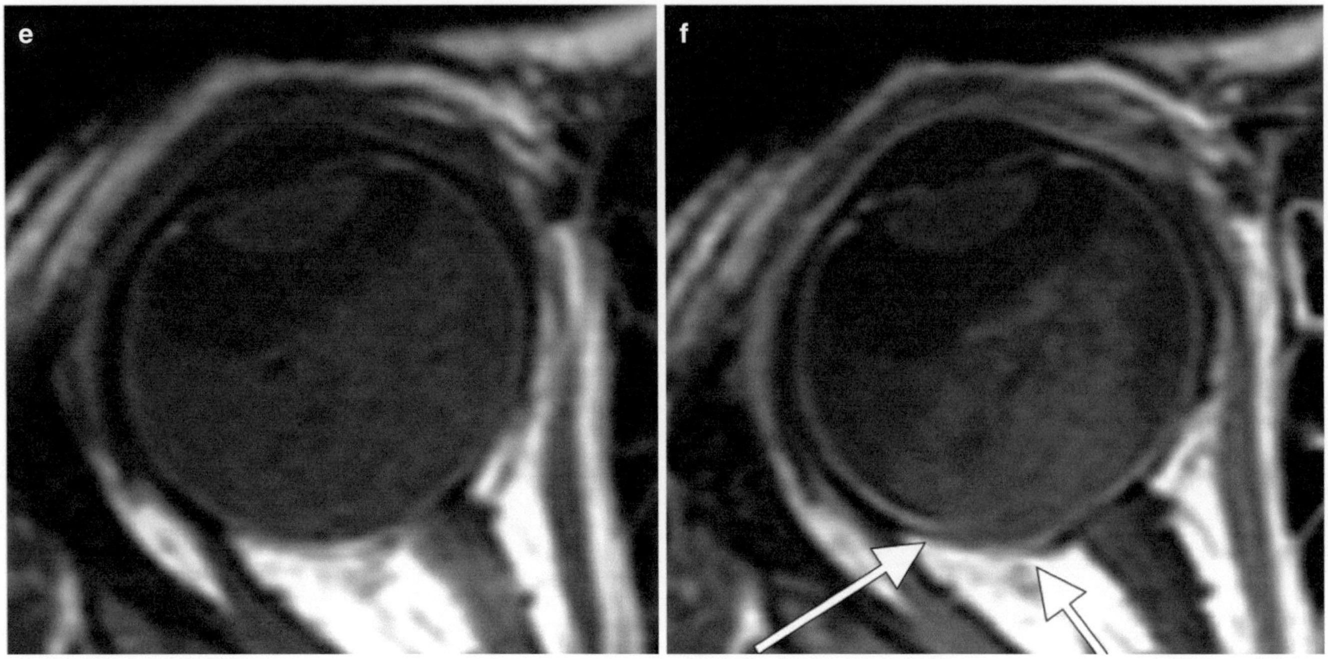

Fig. 9 (continued)

blastoma tumor tissue [33]. A "split choroid sign" can be depicted in cases of massive choroidal invasion (Fig. 9d–f). Also for the detection of choroidal invasion, MRI is valuable but not perfect with a sensitivity of 74% (95% CI 52–88%) and specificity of 72% (95% CI 31–94%). Including high-quality MRI only, sensitivity and specificity increased to respectively 72% (95% CI 31–94%) and 72% (95% CI 31–94%). Limited evidence suggests a good sensitivity of 88% (95% CI 20–100%) and specificity of 99% (95% CI 86–100%) for scleral tumor invasion [29]. Sirin et al. [34] showed promising results that using two orbital surface coils might improve overall diagnostic accuracy of the detection of metastatic risk factors.

Additionally tumor size has been shown to predict postlaminar invasion and massive choroidal invasion [35]. Combining several predictors like tumor size and a postlaminar optic nerve enhancement pattern suspicious for tumor invasion or MRI features of massive choroidal invasion has been shown to increase the diagnostic accuracy of the detection of postlaminar tumor invasion and massive choroidal invasion [36]. Future research might identify additional imaging predictors and combining them might further increase diagnostic accuracy (e.g., with the help of artificial intelligence and deep learning algorithms).

3.3 Imaging for Diagnosis of Uveal Melanoma

Unlike in retinoblastoma, biopsies can be obtained in uveal melanoma, but these can be non-representative due to genetic variability of the tumor. The value of MRI in uveal melanoma is increasingly being recognized. In the traditional standard work-up of melanoma diagnosis, ultrasound is performed, allowing a correct diagnosis of uveal melanoma in most cases; however, MRI might be more accurate [37]. A few studies have shown that functional MRI can be useful [6, 10, 38–40]. In uveal melanoma, perfusion and diffusion can help differentiate between benign and malignant tumors [6, 40]. Furthermore, several studies have shown promising results for treatment follow-up [38, 41] and have shown the ability to give prognostic information such as K^{trans}, which correlated with the presence of monosomy 3 resulting in a worse prognosis [10].

3.4 Imaging for Tumor Staging in Uveal Melanoma

Extrascleral tumor extension is an important factor in uveal melanoma associated with worse patient outcomes. Both MRI and ultrasound are modalities used for evaluating extrascleral extension in uveal melanoma [42–45]. Both have high sensitivities and specificities, but there were only a few small studies. Typical MRI signal characteristics (low on T2-weighted, high on T1-weighted images and enhancing after administration of a gadolinium-based contrast agent) help differentiate the tumor from surrounding tissue [42], even though the T1-signal intensity varies with the melanin content of the tumor (Fig. 10). On MRI, inflammation and vascular structures are sometimes mistaken for tumor extent, but high-resolution MRI might help differentiate between

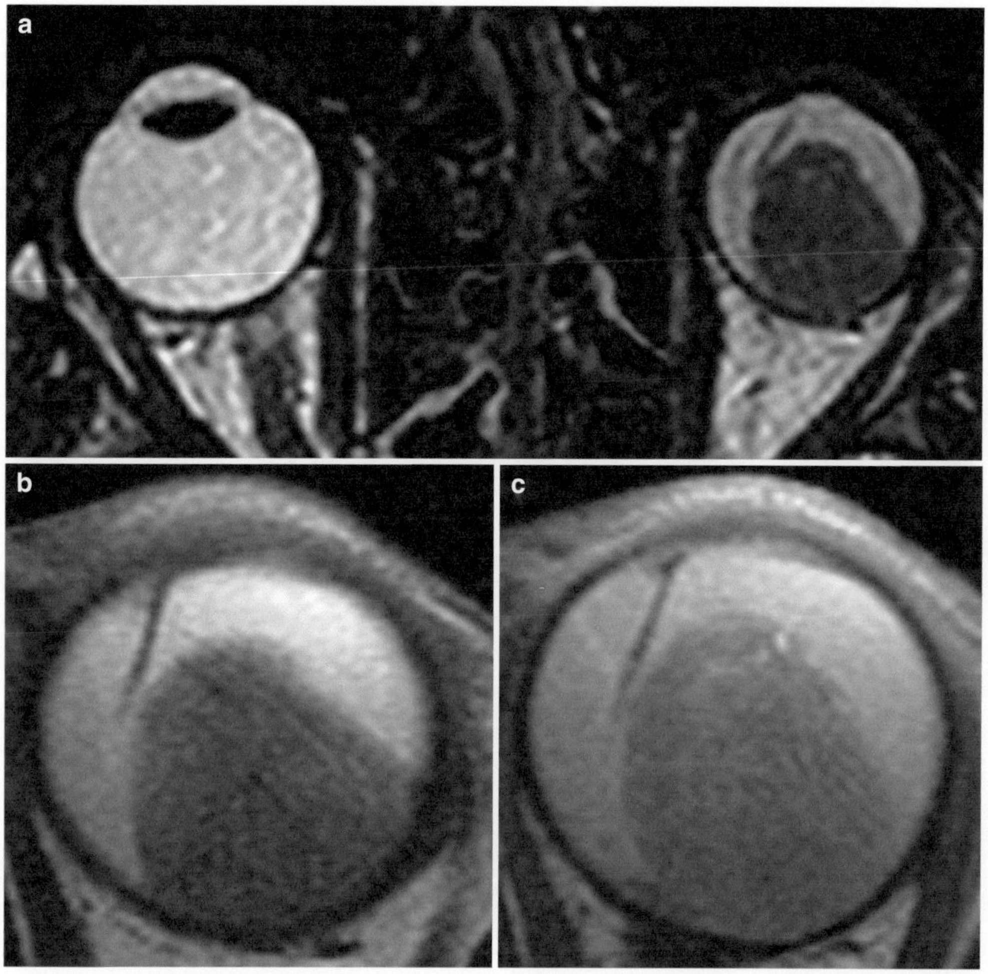

Fig. 10 (**a**) An example of uveal melanoma in the left eye showing a large enhancing intraocular tumor shown on a heavily T2-weighted, (**b**) a T1-weighted before and (**c**) after administration of a contrast agent

the tumor and other tissue [6]. Less often, in up to 5% of patients, uveal melanoma infiltrates the optic nerve [46]. There are hardly any studies about MRI for the detection of optic nerve invasion in uveal melanoma, but its appearance is similar to optic nerve invasion in retinoblastoma [46].

MRI is much more accurate for the determination of tumor thickness in small uveal melanomas than ultrasound, which often suffers from overestimation and a high interobserver variability [47, 48]. Accurate determination of the exact thickness is important because tumors with a thickness of less than 8 mm are usually treated with local brachytherapy, whereas larger tumors usually require proton therapy, external beam radiotherapy, or enucleation [1]. Most commonly uveal melanoma metastasizes to the liver, which can be diagnosed with ultrasound, MRI, or (PET-)CT.

3.5 Imaging of Other Intraocular Tumors

Although much rarer than retinoblastoma, medulloepithelioma constitutes the second most common intraocular tumor in children. Only case reports and small case series, but no population data, are available [49]. These patients generally present later than retinoblastoma, with their tumor at an average of 5 years of age, whereas retinoblastoma usually presents before the age of 2 years. On ultrasound imaging, medulloepithelioma presents as an echogenic mass. Internal cysts, when present, may aid in the diagnosis [50]. On CT imaging, the mass is usually heterogeneous with cystic components and calcifications can appear in the teratoid type [51].

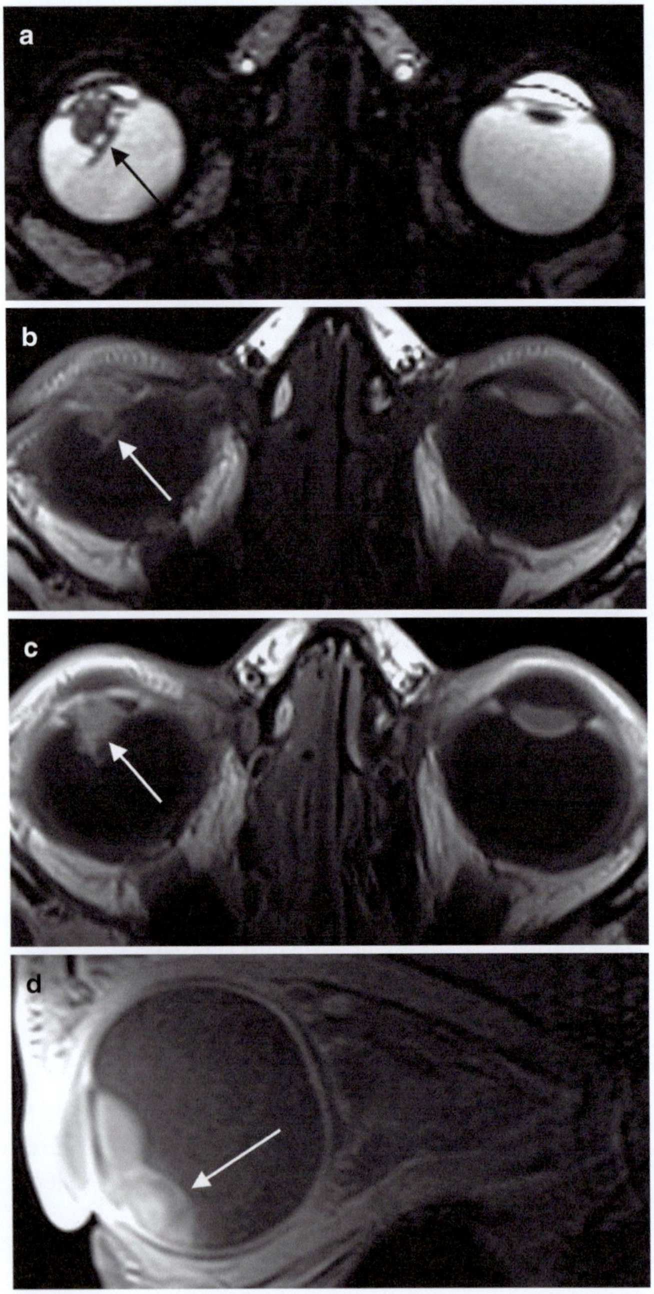

Fig. 11 A patient with medulloepithelioma in the right eye. (**a**) An axial heavily T2-weighted image, (**b**) T1-weighted images before and (**c**) after contrast and (**d**) a sagittal T1-weighted image after contrast (**c** and **d**) showing a typical anteriorly situated mass (arrow) closely related with the ciliary body and a homogeneous enhancement after contrast

On native T1-weighted images, medulloepithelioma is slightly hyperintense to the vitreous and after administration of gadolinium, the tumor shows a homogeneous moderate to strong enhancement of the crescent-shaped mass confined to the ciliary body region [50, 52] (Figs. 11 and 12). The retina is not involved but a secondary retinal detachment can occur [52] (Fig. 13). The mass is hypointense on T2-weighted images and can show areas of hyperintensity when cysts are present [50, 51]. Functional MRI can help in the differential diagnosis since the mean ADC values obtained from DWI in medulloepithioma are usually $>1.1 \times 10^{-3}$ mm^2/s, whereas the mean ADC values in retinoblastoma are $<1.0 \times 10^{-3}$ mm^2/s [7, 49, 53]. On DCE-MRI in medulloepithelioma, the time-intensity curve shows a more rapid increase in enhancement in the early phase followed by a plateau in the late phase, whereas retinoblastoma is usually characterized by a slower increase in the early phase that persists in the late phase (Fig. 14). Also, the mean time to maximum enhancement (TME) is higher in medulloepithelioma than in retinoblastoma. The K^{trans}, area under the contrast concentration curve (AUC), v_e, and TME are higher in teratoid medulloepithelioma, whereas non-teratoid medulloepithelioma shows a slower increase in enhancement [49].

Ocular metastases are the most common intraocular mass lesions in adults and are usually from a primary tumor located in the breast or the lungs (Fig. 15). Less common sites of origin are renal, prostate, thyroid, or gastro-intestinal tumors, and hematologic diseases (lymphoma and leukemia) may also involve the globe [54, 55]. Metastases will present as a mass lesion within the uvea, of which the posterior choroid is most commonly affected. Various signal intensities on T1 and T2 can be present as a result of the site of origin and intralesional hemorrhage [56]. Differentiating metastases from uveal melanoma on MRI can be difficult. The shape of the lesion can help, since metastases are predominantly plaque- or flat shaped or lentiform, whereas uveal melanoma frequently shows a dome or mushroom shape [56]. When there is suspicion of intraocular lymphoma or metastatic breast cancer, it is important to consider MRI of the brain because intraocular and cerebral tumors often appear at the same time [57].

4 Prognosis and Treatment Follow-Up

Up to years after enucleation, the orbit can show changes (such as inflammation and fibrosis) on MRI that can be confused with tumor recurrence [58] (Fig. 16). In cases with tumor recurrence, one would expect to be able to see a lesion with mass-effect, whereas post-therapeutic effects usually present as contrast enhancement without mass-effect. However, especially in the early stages of a recurrence and on low-quality images, this might be hard to differentiate. Sirin et al. [58] have shown that with the use of high-

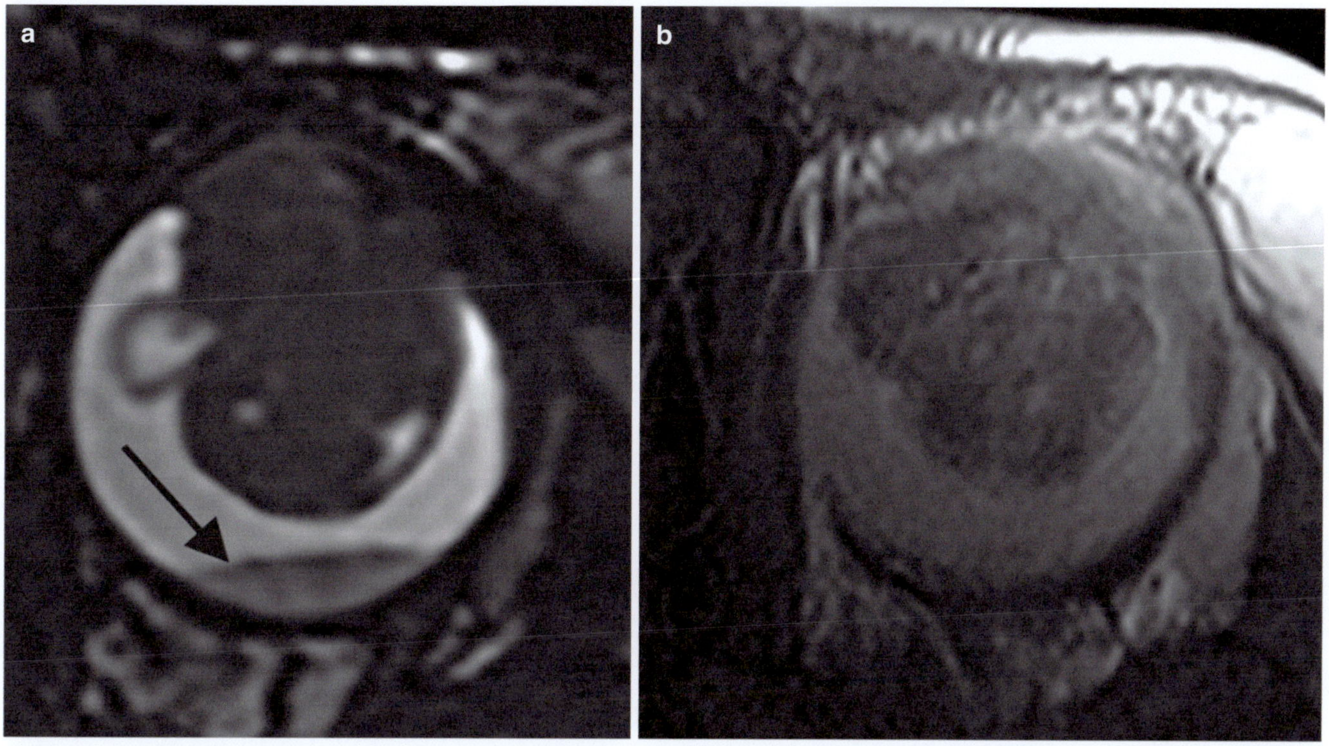

Fig. 12 Example of a large medulloepithelioma in the left eye. (**a**) Axial heavily T2-weighted and (**b**) T1-weighted images showing an anteriorly situated mass closely related to the ciliary body with invasion in the anterior chamber and a vitreous hemorrhage (arrow)

resolution MRI, an accurate distinction between post-treatment effects and tumor recurrence can be made. Also, it is important to consider the time after enucleation as enhancement of the optic nerve and meningeal sheath gradually decrease over time, with enhancement of the optic nerve at 70% just after enucleation (<3 months) to under 10% after 3 years.

The emerging conservative treatment options in ocular oncology, in particular intra-arterial and intravitreal chemotherapy in retinoblastoma but also brachy- and proton beam radiotherapy in uveal melanoma, necessitate new assessment strategies for follow-up. Similar to ophthalmologic reports, MR imaging of eyes treated with intra-arterial chemotherapy shows retinal detachment with subretinal fluid, choroidal ischemia, and extraocular muscle inflammation. Additionally, eyes can show shrinkage after IAC treatment [59]. Multiparametric imaging, in particular DWI and DCE-MRI might have value in follow-up to evaluate the effect of the treatment, especially in ruling out residual vital tumor tissue after curative therapy. In DWI, low ADC values correlate with viable tumor tissue, whereas necrosis shows more facilitated diffusion reflected by high ADC values [7]. Furthermore, ADC values are lower in patients with undifferentiated retinoblastoma and are inversely correlated with the proliferation rate of the tumor (Ki-67 index) [53]. In multiparametric imaging in oncology, an increase in ADC values during therapy is predictive of local control. DCE imaging can be used in retinoblastoma to evaluate and to quantify tumor angiogenesis, and an analysis of the time-intensity curve reflects tissue vitality (Rodjan et al. 2012) [9] (Fig. 17). Perfusion and diffusion imaging also have shown promising results in the follow-up of uveal melanoma [6]. The role of MRI becomes more important for the ocular oncologist when the ocular media is opacified as a result of lens cataract, in the presence of an intraocular hemorrhage or when the vitreous is replaced by silicone oil after a vitrectomy or retinal detachment [60].

5 Detection of Associated Brain Tumors in Retinoblastoma

Up to 5% of heritable retinoblastoma patients develop an associated midline tumor (trilateral retinoblastoma) [61]. About three-quarters constitute a tumor in the pineal gland, that is, pineoblastoma, and about one-quarter develop in the supra- or parasellar region. Even though considerable progress has been made in terms of survival after trilateral retinoblastoma over the years in the form of early detection, followed by high-dose chemotherapy regimens, still about 50% of patients do not survive [62]. Early detection is especially important for pineoblastomas. The radiologist has an important role when it comes to early detection. At the time of retinoblastoma diagnosis, it is advisable to combine the baseline imaging of the intraocular tumor with a scan of the midline structures of the brain. On MRI, this is performed

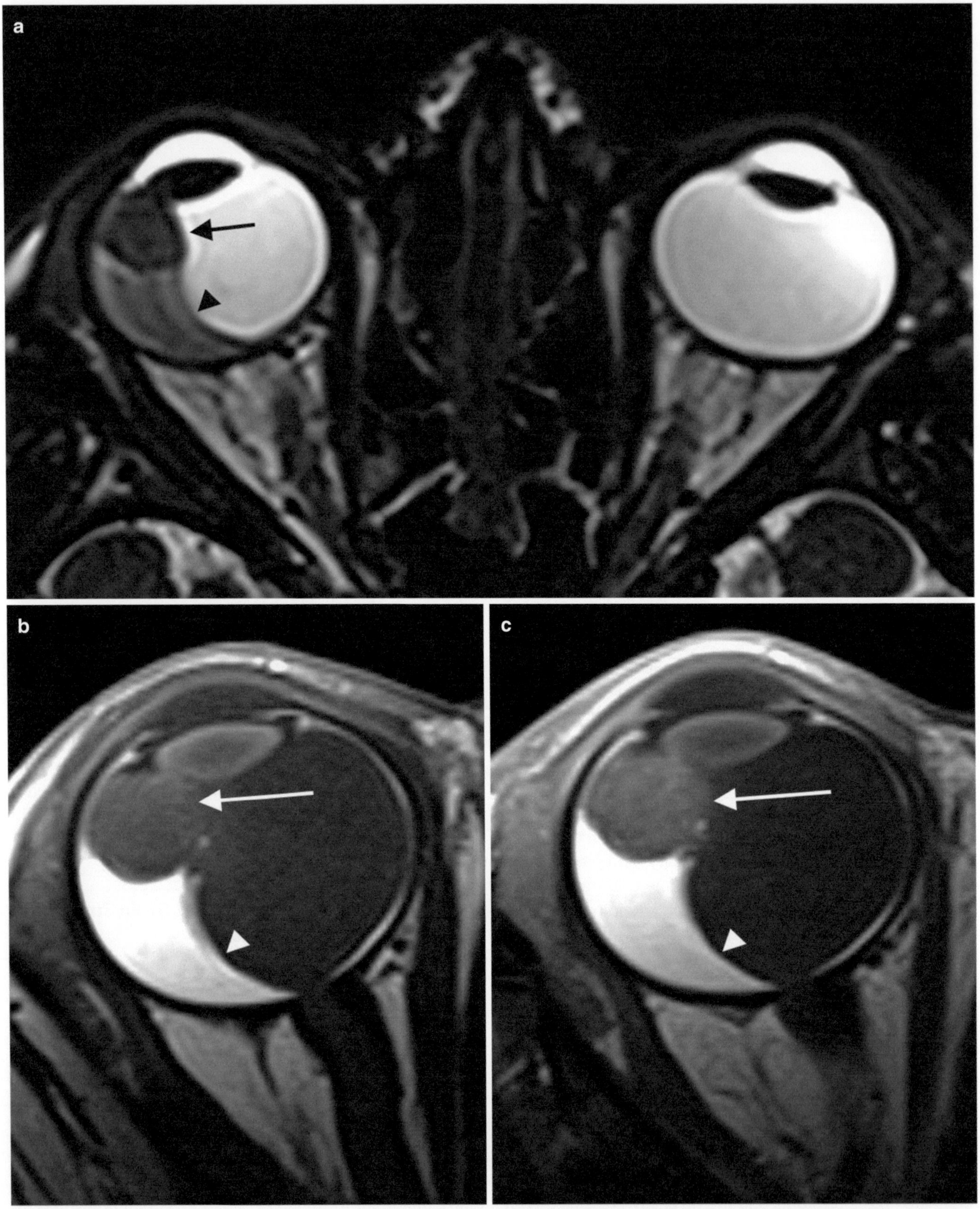

Fig. 13 Medulloepithelioma in the right eye causing a partial retinal detachment. (**a**) An axial heavily T2-weighted image and (**b**) T1-weighted images before and (**c**) after contrast showing a typical anteriorly situated mass (arrow) with a secondary retinal detachment (arrowhead)

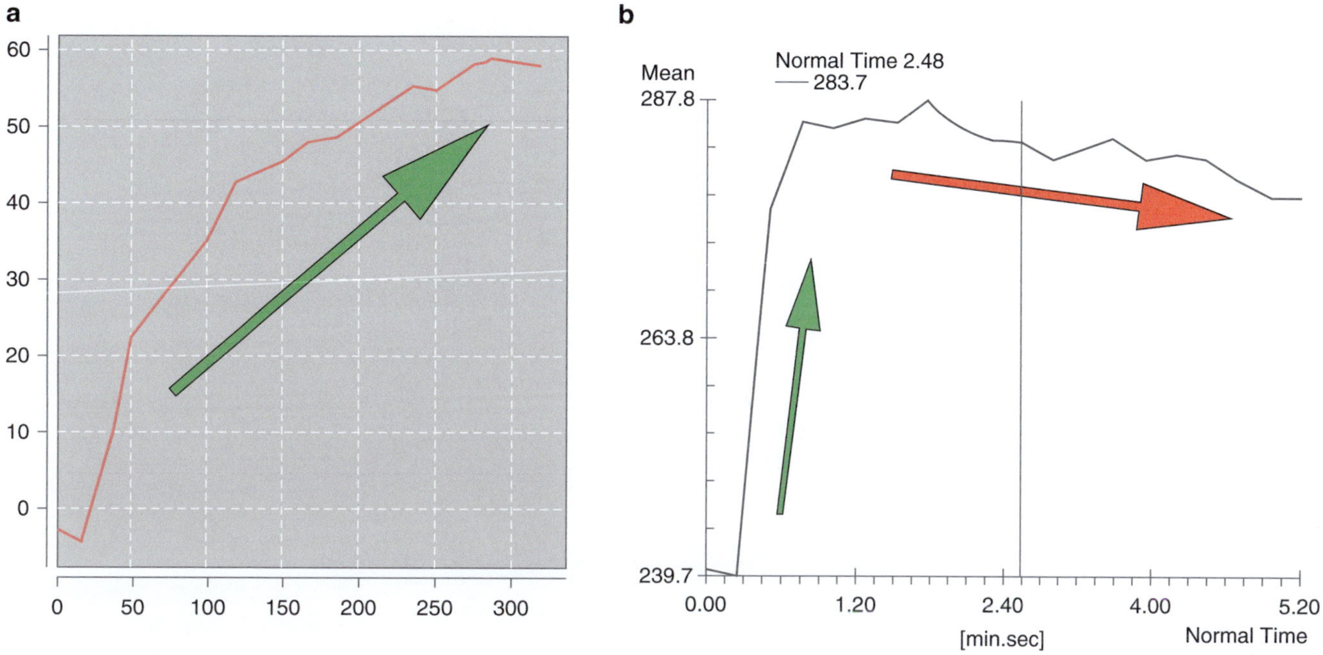

Fig. 14 (**a**) DCE-MRI Time-intensity curve retinoblastoma (**b**) versus medulloepithelioma. (**a**) Time intensity curves showing a persistent increase of contrast medium uptake in retinoblastoma (**b**) versus a rapid initial increase of uptake in early phase and prevalence of plateau in late phase in medulloepithelioma

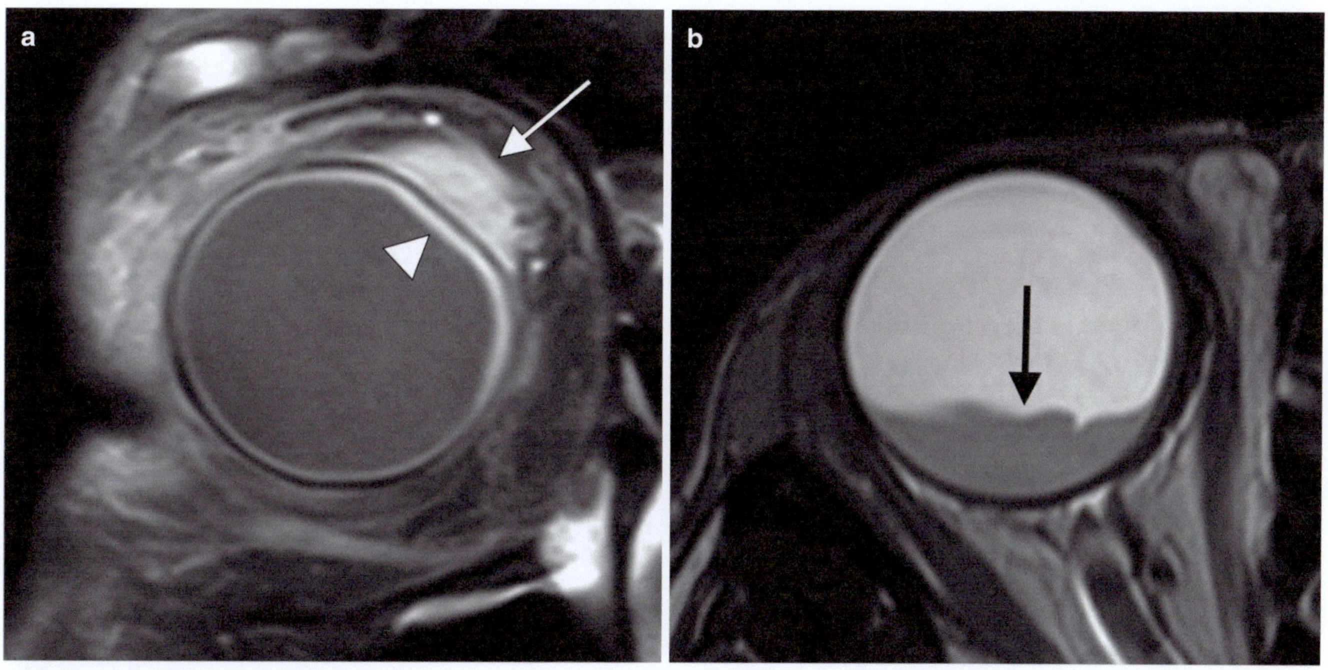

Fig. 15 Ocular metastasis of breast cancer. (**a**) Even though choroidal metastases are more common, tumors can also metastasize into the subtenon space, as can be seen in the right eye of a patient with breast cancer on a coronal contrast-enhanced fat-suppressed T1-weighted image (white arrow in **a**) (**b**) with reactive thickening and increased enhancement of the adjacent choroid (white arrow head in **a**) and secondary partial retinal detachment with subretinal effusion, as can be seen on a T2-weighted image (black arrow in **b**)

with a thin-slice T2-weighted sequence in sagittal direction, combined with a contrast-enhanced sagittal T1-weighted sequence. Because the age at which retinoblastoma is diagnosed appears to be independent of the age when pineoblastoma is diagnosed [63] and because pineoblastoma usually develops at a later age than intraocular retinoblastoma, treating physicians should be aware that at the time of the baseline brain scan, most pineoblastomas will probably not be

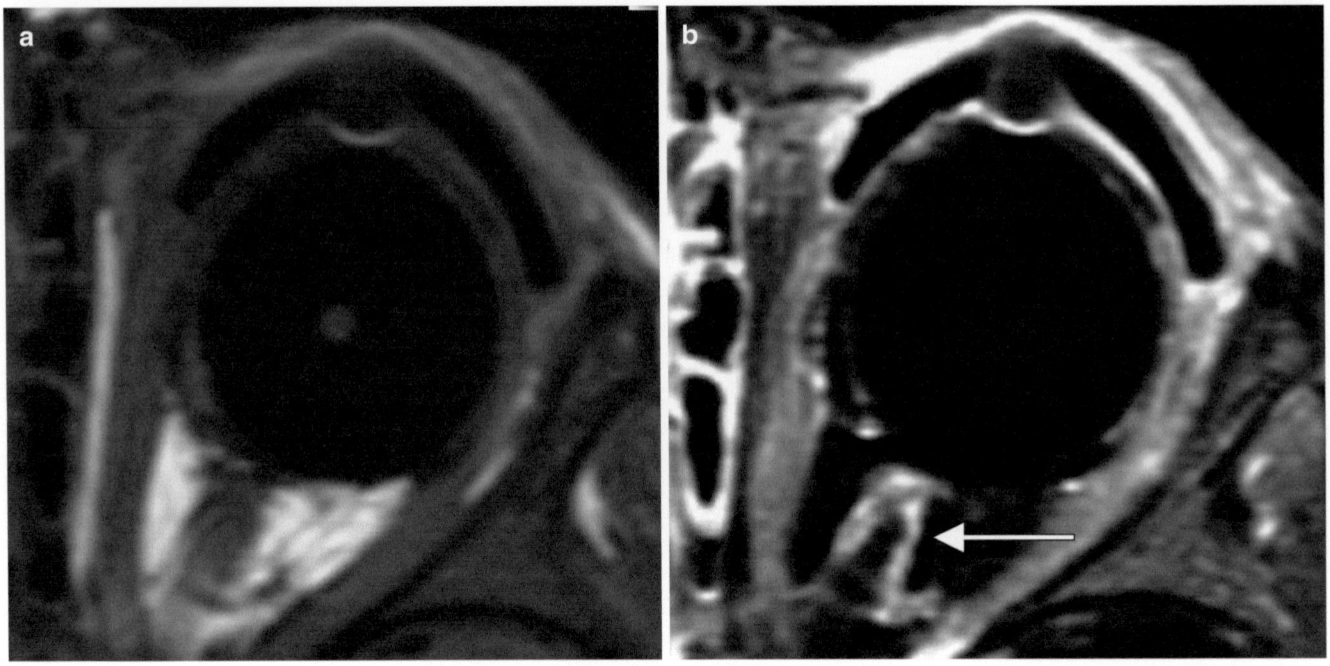

Fig. 16 Postenucleation optic nerve enhancement. (**a**) A native T1-weighted image (**b**) showing a postenucleation orbit with an implant, a prosthesis and a remaining distal end of the optic nerve which after contrast agent administration, enhances vividly at the edges as can be seen on a subtraction image (arrow in **b**)

detected [64]. Perhaps one or more additional MRI scans at a later age are needed to be able to detect pineoblastoma in an early stage. Even though many pineoblastomas might be missed at baseline, the baseline brain scan at the time of retinoblastoma diagnosis is still important to diagnose non-pineal trilateral retinoblastoma that usually present at a younger age than pineoblastoma.

6 Imaging as Screening Tool in Ocular Oncology

Imaging has a limited role for screening in current ocular oncology practice. Although retinoblastoma can be a heritable oncologic disease for which extensive screening programs are in place, the screening is based on ophthalmologic examination, including fundoscopy under anesthesia. For screening for midline tumors associated with an RB1 mutation (TRB), screening has been postulated [62–64] but has not been found cost-effective for implementation. In second primary tumors associated with a heritable RB1 mutation, the incidence is too low and the period at risk too long to be able to implement an effective imaging tool for screening. Therefore, routine screening with (whole-body) MRI is currently not recommended [65].

Among patients treated for uveal melanoma, 50% will develop fatal metastatic disease, which is largely dependent on clinical tumor characteristics (i.e., tumor thickness, tumor diameter) and genomic alterations (i.e., monosomy chromosome 3, chromosome 8q gain). The liver is the initial site of metastasis in the vast majority of patients. Routine screening of the liver with ultrasound or liver MRI is currently recommended [66–68].

7 Future Perspectives

The imaging phenotype of ocular oncology lesions can be studied in several ways and in several layers. Conventionally, radiology was compared to histopathology to assess its accuracy in depicting anatomical structures. However, MR imaging probably contains more information than the sole depiction of anatomical changes and mass lesions. Recently, exploratory investigations looked into deciphering genotype-phenotype correlations. Potentially, MR imaging can be informative of genetic tumor subtypes that require distinct treatment. The study area of radiogenomics investigates the relations between tumor genotype and imaging phenotype (qualitative and quantitative) in an effort to develop imaging biomarkers for genomics. Radiogenomics has been deployed extensively in different fields of oncology, often for areas in which biopsies are unavailable or difficult to obtain, such as glioma [69]. In ocular oncology, the first attempts were successful in the area of uveal melanoma in which the quantitative DCE-MRI derived perfusion metrics (K^{trans}, v_e) showed statistically significant higher values in tumors with the

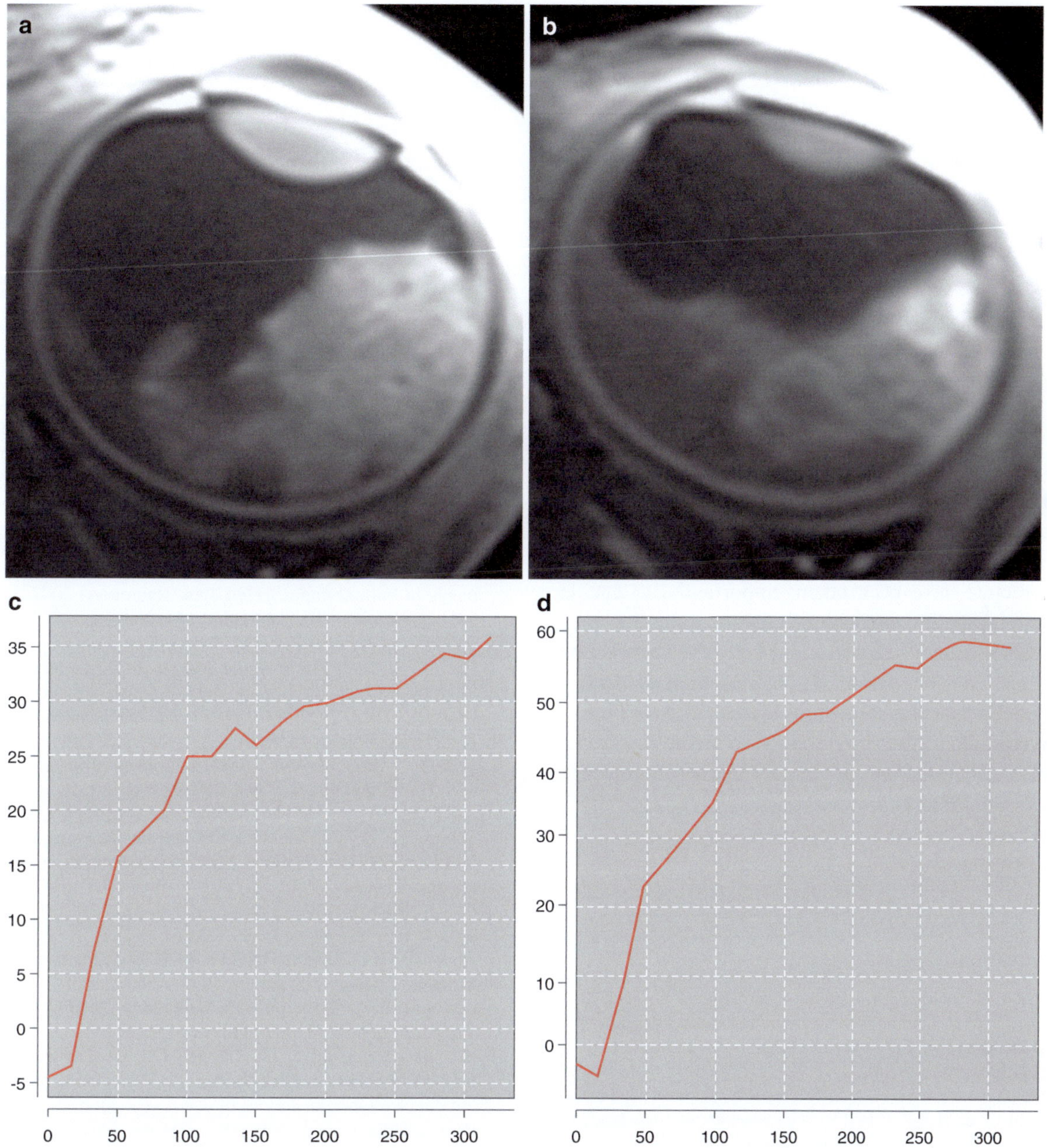

Fig. 17 The effect of intra-arterial chemotherapy on perfusion characteristics in retinoblastoma. (**a**) Contrast enhanced T1-weighted images in a patient with retinoblastoma in the left eye before treatment and (**b**) more than 1 year later. The tumor relapsed despite 4 intra-arterial chemotherapy treatments. (**c**) The pretreatment and (**d**) post-treatment time intensity curves have a very similar shape and behavior

prognostically unfavorable monosomy 3 compared with disomy 3 [10].

Recently, unravelling of imaging phenotype-genotype relations was also initiated for retinoblastoma by combining radiologist-assessed MR imaging features with RNA expression data. A more advanced tumor (more lesions filling the whole globe or retina) on MR imaging correlated with a lower "photoreceptorness" gene expression profile, which was concordant with previous clinical and histopathologic findings for this gene expression profile [70].

Potentially, these efforts could lead to useful MR imaging biomarkers for genetic subtypes in ocular oncology, guiding future clinical decision-making. However, although the increased resolution of MR imaging created a wealth of data that can be explored by the radiologist, it is likely that not all the information of the digital images is correctly deducted from the "on-screen" representation by the human eye. Radiologists' imaging assessments inherently have limitations given their human nature. Imaging interpretation is time-consuming, reproducibility and interreader agreement can be low, and the learning curve of the interpreter is limited to one life-time's experience. In contrast, software interpretation of images could be rapid, reproducible, and self-innovating through the analysis of vast amounts of cases over long periods of time. The quantitative, software-enabled interpretation is usually referred to as radiomics, in which algorithms extract information from clinical imaging. The full potential of radiomics has not yet been explored for ocular oncology. However, initial steps toward radiomics-guided clinical practice have been taken. Importantly, to enable a time-efficient pipeline, algorithms must be trained to recognize the tumor (tumor segmentation) before the actual imaging features can be extracted [71]. Advanced software including deep learning algorithms are suitable for performing these complex tasks. Even though in medicine, artificial intelligence still does not have many clinical applications, research in this field is growing exponentially over the last couple of years.

References

1. Niendorf T, Beenakker JM, Langner S, Erb-Eigner K, Bach Cuadra M, Beller E, et al. Ophthalmic magnetic resonance imaging: where are we (heading to)? Curr Eye Res. 2021:1–20. https://doi.org/10.1080/02713683.2021.1874021.
2. Chantada G, Luna-Fineman S, Sitorus RS, Kruger M, Israels T, Leal-Leal C, et al. SIOP-PODC recommendations for graduated-intensity treatment of retinoblastoma in developing countries. Pediatr Blood Cancer. 2013;60(5):719–27. https://doi.org/10.1002/pbc.24468.
3. Beenakker JW, van Rijn GA, Luyten GP, Webb AG. High-resolution MRI of uveal melanoma using a microcoil phased array at 7 T. NMR Biomed. 2013;26(12):1864–9. https://doi.org/10.1002/nbm.3041.
4. de Graaf P, Goricke S, Rodjan F, Galluzzi P, Maeder P, Castelijns JA, et al. Guidelines for imaging retinoblastoma: imaging principles and MRI standardization. Pediatr Radiol. 2012;42(1):2–14. https://doi.org/10.1007/s00247-011-2201-5.
5. Erb-Eigner K, Warmuth C, Taupitz M, Willerding G, Bertelmann E, Asbach P. Impact of magnetic field strength and receiver coil in ocular MRI: a phantom and patient study. Rofo. 2013;185(9):830–7. https://doi.org/10.1055/s-0033-1335796.
6. Ferreira TA, Grech Fonk L, Jaarsma-Coes MG, van Haren GGR, Marinkovic M, Beenakker JM. MRI of uveal melanoma. Cancers (Basel). 2019;11(3) https://doi.org/10.3390/cancers11030377.
7. de Graaf P, Pouwels PJ, Rodjan F, Moll AC, Imhof SM, Knol DL, et al. Single-shot turbo spin-echo diffusion-weighted imaging for retinoblastoma: initial experience. AJNR Am J Neuroradiol. 2012;33(1):110–8. https://doi.org/10.3174/ajnr.A2729.
8. Ro SR, Asbach P, Siebert E, Bertelmann E, Hamm B, Erb-Eigner K. Characterization of orbital masses by multiparametric MRI. Eur J Radiol. 2016;85(2):324–36. https://doi.org/10.1016/j.ejrad.2015.11.041.
9. Rodjan F, de Graaf P, van der Valk P, Moll AC, Kuijer JP, Knol DL, et al. Retinoblastoma: value of dynamic contrast-enhanced MR imaging and correlation with tumor angiogenesis. AJNR Am J Neuroradiol. 2012;33(11):2129–35. https://doi.org/10.3174/ajnr.A3119.
10. Kamrava M, Sepahdari AR, Leu K, Wang PC, Roberts K, Demanes DJ, et al. Quantitative multiparametric MRI in uveal melanoma: increased tumor permeability may predict monosomy 3. Neuroradiology. 2015;57(8):833–40. https://doi.org/10.1007/s00234-015-1546-0.
11. Rodjan F, de Graaf P, van der Valk P, Hadjistilianou T, Cerase A, Toti P, et al. Detection of calcifications in retinoblastoma using gradient-echo MR imaging sequences: comparative study between in vivo MR imaging and ex vivo high-resolution CT. AJNR Am J Neuroradiol. 2015;36(2):355–60. https://doi.org/10.3174/ajnr.A4163.
12. de Graaf P, Knol DL, Moll AC, Imhof SM, Schouten-van Meeteren AY, Castelijns JA. Eye size in retinoblastoma: MR imaging measurements in normal and affected eyes. Radiology. 2007;244(1):273–80. https://doi.org/10.1148/radiol.2441060456.
13. Jansen RW, de Bloeme CM, Brisse HJ, Galluzzi P, Cardoen L, Goricke S, et al. MR imaging features to differentiate retinoblastoma from Coats' disease and persistent fetal vasculature. Cancers (Basel). 2020;12(12) https://doi.org/10.3390/cancers12123592.
14. Shields CL, Shields JA, Baez KA, Cater J, De Potter PV. Choroidal invasion of retinoblastoma: metastatic potential and clinical risk factors. Br J Ophthalmol. 1993;77(9):544–8. https://doi.org/10.1136/bjo.77.9.544.
15. Shields CL, Shields JA, Baez K, Cater JR, De Potter P. Optic nerve invasion of retinoblastoma. Metastatic potential and clinical risk factors. Cancer. 1994;73(3):692–8. https://doi.org/10.1002/1097-0142(19940201)73:3<692::aid-cncr2820730331>3.0.co;2-8.
16. Chantada GL, Casco F, Fandino AC, Galli S, Manzitti J, Scopinaro M, et al. Outcome of patients with retinoblastoma and postlaminar optic nerve invasion. Ophthalmology. 2007;114(11):2083–9. https://doi.org/10.1016/j.ophtha.2007.01.012.
17. Chantada GL, Dunkel IJ, Antoneli CB, de Davila MT, Arias V, Beaverson K, et al. Risk factors for extraocular relapse following enucleation after failure of chemoreduction in retinoblastoma. Pediatr Blood Cancer. 2007;49(3):256–60. https://doi.org/10.1002/pbc.21067.
18. Uusitalo MS, Van Quill KR, Scott IU, Matthay KK, Murray TG, O'Brien JM. Evaluation of chemoprophylaxis in patients with unilateral retinoblastoma with high-risk features on histopathologic examination. Arch Ophthalmol. 2001;119(1):41–8.
19. Honavar SG, Singh AD, Shields CL, Meadows AT, Demirci H, Cater J, et al. Postenucleation adjuvant therapy in high-risk retinoblastoma. Arch Ophthalmol. 2002;120(7):923–31.
20. Bosaleh A, Sampor C, Solernou V, Fandino A, Dominguez J, de Davila MT, et al. Outcome of children with retinoblastoma and isolated choroidal invasion. Arch Ophthalmol. 2012;130(6):724–9. https://doi.org/10.1001/archophthalmol.2012.567.
21. Kaliki S, Shields CL, Rojanaporn D, Al-Dahmash S, McLaughlin JP, Shields JA, et al. High-risk retinoblastoma based on international classification of retinoblastoma: analysis of 519 enucleated eyes. Ophthalmology. 2013;120(5):997–1003. https://doi.org/10.1016/j.ophtha.2012.10.044.
22. Khelfaoui F, Validire P, Auperin A, Quintana E, Michon J, Pacquement H, et al. Histopathologic risk factors in retinoblastoma:

a retrospective study of 172 patients treated in a single institution. Cancer. 1996;77(6):1206–13.
23. Chevez-Barrios P, Eagle RC Jr, Krailo M, Piao J, Albert DM, Gao Y, et al. Study of unilateral retinoblastoma with and without histopathologic high-risk features and the role of adjuvant chemotherapy: a Children's oncology group study. J Clin Oncol. 2019;37(31):2883–91. https://doi.org/10.1200/JCO.18.01808.
24. Baroni LV, Sampor C, Fandino A, Solernou V, Demirdjian G, de Davila MT, et al. Anterior segment invasion in retinoblastoma: is it a risk factor for extraocular relapse? J Pediatr Hematol Oncol. 2014;36(8):e509–12. https://doi.org/10.1097/MPH.0000000000000167.
25. Mallipatna ACGB, Chéves Barrios P, et al. In: Amin MB, Edge SB, Greene FL, et al., editors. AJCC cancer staging manual. 8th ed. New York: Springer; 2017. p. 819–31.
26. Hu H, Zhang W, Wang Y, Huang D, Shi J, Li B, et al. Characterization, treatment and prognosis of retinoblastoma with central nervous system metastasis. BMC Ophthalmol. 2018;18(1):107. https://doi.org/10.1186/s12886-018-0772-8.
27. de Jong MC, Van Der Valk P, Jansen RW, Abbink F, Bosscha M, Castelijns JA, et al. Full-width postlaminar optic nerve tumor invasion of retinoblastoma as risk-factor for leptomeningeal spread of retinoblastoma. A case report and review of the literature. Ophthalmic Genet. 2020:1–4. https://doi.org/10.1080/13816810.2020.1727535.
28. Chawla B, Chaurasia S, Sharma S, Pattebahadur R, Hasan F, Seth R, et al. Magnetic resonance imaging for tumor restaging after chemotherapy in retinoblastoma with optic nerve invasion. Ophthalmic Genet. 2018;39(5):584–8. https://doi.org/10.1080/13816810.2018.1502790.
29. de Jong MC, de Graaf P, Noij DP, Goricke S, Maeder P, Galluzzi P, et al. Diagnostic performance of magnetic resonance imaging and computed tomography for advanced retinoblastoma: a systematic review and meta-analysis. Ophthalmology. 2014;121(5):1109–18. https://doi.org/10.1016/j.ophtha.2013.11.021.
30. Chawla B, Duraipandi K, Sharma S. MRI in retinoblastoma with orbital cellulitis. Ophthalmology. 2013;120(6):1308–9 e1–4. https://doi.org/10.1016/j.ophtha.2013.01.008.
31. Brisse HJ, Guesmi M, Aerts I, Sastre-Garau X, Savignoni A, Lumbroso-Le Rouic L, et al. Relevance of CT and MRI in retinoblastoma for the diagnosis of postlaminar invasion with normal-size optic nerve: a retrospective study of 150 patients with histological comparison. Pediatr Radiol. 2007;37(7):649–56. https://doi.org/10.1007/s00247-007-0491-4.
32. Sow AS, Ndiaye JMM, Ka AM, Sacramento DGT, Kane H, Nguer M, et al. Role of CT in diagnosis and monitoring of retinoblastoma in Senegal. J Fr Ophtalmol. 2019;42(10):1085–9. https://doi.org/10.1016/j.jfo.2019.06.003.
33. de Graaf P, Barkhof F, Moll AC, Imhof SM, Knol DL, van der Valk P, et al. Retinoblastoma: MR imaging parameters in detection of tumor extent. Radiology. 2005;235(1):197–207. https://doi.org/10.1148/radiol.2351031301.
34. Sirin S, Schlamann M, Metz KA, Bornfeld N, Schweiger B, Holdt M, et al. High-resolution MRI using orbit surface coils for the evaluation of metastatic risk factors in 143 children with retinoblastoma: part 2: new vs. old imaging concept. Neuroradiology. 2015;57(8):815–24. https://doi.org/10.1007/s00234-015-1538-0.
35. de Jong MC, van der Meer FJ, Goricke SL, Brisse HJ, Galluzzi P, Maeder P, et al. Diagnostic accuracy of intraocular tumor size measured with MR imaging in the prediction of postlaminar optic nerve invasion and massive choroidal invasion of retinoblastoma. Radiology. 2016;279(3):817–26. https://doi.org/10.1148/radiol.2015151213.
36. de Jong MC. Epidemiology and imaging of retinoblastoma. PhD. Vrije Universiteit Amsterdam; 2017.
37. Serras-Pereira R, Morais T, Vieira L, Batalha C, Ramalho J, Duarte A, et al. The role of magnetic resonance imaging in diagnosis of uveal melanoma. Acta Ophthalmol. 2019;97(S263) https://doi.org/10.1111/j.1755-3768.2019.5372.
38. Foti PV, Longo A, Reibaldi M, Russo A, Privitera G, Spatola C, et al. Uveal melanoma: quantitative evaluation of diffusion-weighted MR imaging in the response assessment after proton-beam therapy, long-term follow-up. Radiol Med. 2017;122(2):131–9. https://doi.org/10.1007/s11547-016-0697-3.
39. Jiang X, Asbach P, Willerding G, Dulce M, Xu K, Taupitz M, et al. Dynamic contrast-enhanced MRI of ocular melanoma. Melanoma Res. 2015;25(2):149–56. https://doi.org/10.1097/CMR.0000000000000142.
40. Yuan Y, Kuai XP, Chen XS, Tao XF. Assessment of dynamic contrast-enhanced magnetic resonance imaging in the differentiation of malignant from benign orbital masses. Eur J Radiol. 2013;82(9):1506–11. https://doi.org/10.1016/j.ejrad.2013.03.001.
41. Buerk BM, Pulido JS, Chiong I, Folberg R, Edward DP, Duffy MT, et al. Vascular perfusion of choroidal melanoma by 3.0 tesla magnetic resonance imaging. Trans Am Ophthalmol Soc. 2004;102:209–15; discussion 15-7.
42. Tartaglione T, Pagliara MM, Sciandra M, Caputo CG, Calandrelli R, Fabrizi G, et al. Uveal melanoma: evaluation of extrascleral extension using thin-section MR of the eye with surface coils. Radiol Med. 2014;119(10):775–83. https://doi.org/10.1007/s11547-014-0388-x.
43. Recsan Z, Karlinger K, Fodor M, Zalatnai A, Papp M, Salacz G. MRI for the evaluation of scleral invasion and extrascleral extension of uveal melanomas. Clin Radiol. 2002;57(5):371–6. https://doi.org/10.1053/crad.2001.0859.
44. Scott IU, Murray TG, Hughes JR. Evaluation of imaging techniques for detection of extraocular extension of choroidal melanoma. Arch Ophthalmol. 1998;116(7):897–9. https://doi.org/10.1001/archopht.116.7.897.
45. Burris CKH, Papastefanou VP, Thaung C, Restori M, Arora AK, Sagoo MS, et al. Detection of extrascleral extension in uveal melanoma with histopathological correlation. Orbit. 2018;37(4):287–92. https://doi.org/10.1080/01676830.2017.1423083.
46. Lindegaard J, Isager P, Prause JU, Heegaard S. Optic nerve invasion of uveal melanoma: clinical characteristics and metastatic pattern. Invest Ophthalmol Vis Sci. 2006;47(8):3268–75. https://doi.org/10.1167/iovs.05-1435.
47. Beenakker JW, Ferreira TA, Soemarwoto KP, Genders SW, Teeuwisse WM, Webb AG, et al. Clinical evaluation of ultra-high-field MRI for three-dimensional visualisation of tumour size in uveal melanoma patients, with direct relevance to treatment planning. MAGMA. 2016;29(3):571–7. https://doi.org/10.1007/s10334-016-0529-4.
48. Char DH, Kroll S, Stone RD, Harrie R, Kerman B. Ultrasonographic measurement of uveal melanoma thickness: interobserver variability. Br J Ophthalmol. 1990;74(3):183–5. https://doi.org/10.1136/bjo.74.3.183.
49. Galluzzi P, Casseri T, Cerase A, Guglielmucci D, Toti P, Hadjistilianou T. Conventional, diffusion, and permeability MR findings in ocular medulloepithelioma. Neuroradiology. 2018;60(11):1213–22. https://doi.org/10.1007/s00234-018-2094-1.
50. Sansgiri RK, Wilson M, McCarville MB, Helton KJ. Imaging features of medulloepithelioma: report of four cases and review of the literature. Pediatr Radiol. 2013;43(10):1344–56. https://doi.org/10.1007/s00247-013-2718-x.
51. Gupta SRKS. Intraocular medulloepithelioma. In: Rojanaporn D, editor. Ocular oncology retina atlas. Singapore: Springer; 2019.
52. Ashour OZ, Stalling M, Ramsey J, Straka DG, Pierson CR, Martin LC. Intraocular medulloepithelioma: AIRP best cases in radiologic-pathologic correlation. Radiographics. 2018;38(1):194–9. https://doi.org/10.1148/rg.2018170160.

53. Cui Y, Luo R, Wang R, Liu H, Zhang C, Zhang Z, et al. Correlation between conventional MR imaging combined with diffusion-weighted imaging and histopathologic findings in eyes primarily enucleated for advanced retinoblastoma: a retrospective study. Eur Radiol. 2018;28(2):620–9. https://doi.org/10.1007/s00330-017-4993-7.
54. Shields CL, Shields JA, Gross NE, Schwartz GP, Lally SE. Survey of 520 eyes with uveal metastases. Ophthalmology. 1997;104(8):1265–76. https://doi.org/10.1016/s0161-6420(97)30148-1.
55. Jardel P, Sauerwein W, Olivier T, Bensoussan E, Maschi C, Lanza F, et al. Management of choroidal metastases. Cancer Treat Rev. 2014;40(10):1119–28. https://doi.org/10.1016/j.ctrv.2014.09.006.
56. Lemke AJ, Hosten N, Wiegel T, Prinz RD, Richter M, Bechrakis NE, et al. Intraocular metastases: differential diagnosis from uveal melanomas with high-resolution MRI using a surface coil. Eur Radiol. 2001;11(12):2593–601. https://doi.org/10.1007/s003300100936.
57. Cohen VM. Ocular metastases. Eye (Lond). 2013;27(2):137–41. https://doi.org/10.1038/eye.2012.252.
58. Sirin S, de Jong MC, de Graaf P, Brisse HJ, Galluzzi P, Maeder P, et al. High-resolution magnetic resonance imaging can reliably detect orbital tumor recurrence after enucleation in children with retinoblastoma. Ophthalmology. 2016;123(3):635–45. https://doi.org/10.1016/j.ophtha.2015.10.054.
59. Chen S, Ji X, Liu M, Xia Z, Zheng H, Yin Q, et al. The value of MRI in evaluating the efficacy and complications with the treatment of intra-arterial chemotherapy for retinoblastoma. Oncotarget. 2017;8(24):38413–25. https://doi.org/10.18632/oncotarget.16423.
60. Jaarsma-Coes MG, Goncalves Ferreira TA, van Haren GR, Marinkovic M, Beenakker JM. MRI enables accurate diagnosis and follow-up in uveal melanoma patients after vitrectomy. Melanoma Res. 2019;29(6):655–9. https://doi.org/10.1097/CMR.0000000000000568.
61. de Jong MC, Kors WA, de Graaf P, Castelijns JA, Moll AC, Kivelä T. The incidence of trilateral retinoblastoma: a systematic review and meta-analysis. Am J Ophthalmol. 2015;160(6):1116–26 e5. https://doi.org/10.1016/j.ajo.2015.09.009.
62. de Jong MC, Kors WA, de Graaf P, Castelijns JA, Kivelä T, Moll AC. Trilateral retinoblastoma: a systematic review and meta-analysis. Lancet Oncol. 2014;15(10):1157–67. https://doi.org/10.1016/S1470-2045(14)70336-5.
63. de Jong MC, Kors WA, Moll AC, de Graaf P, Castelijns JA, Jansen RW, et al. Screening for pineal trilateral retinoblastoma revisited: a meta-analysis. Ophthalmology. 2020;127(5):601–7. https://doi.org/10.1016/j.ophtha.2019.10.040.
64. de Jong MC, Shaikh F, Gallie B, Kors WA, Jansen RW, Dommering C, et al. Asynchronous pineoblastoma is more likely after early diagnosis of retinoblastoma: a meta-analysis. Acta Ophthalmol. 2021; https://doi.org/10.1111/aos.14855.
65. Tonorezos ES, Friedman DN, Barnea D, Bosscha MI, Chantada G, Dommering CJ, et al. Recommendations for long-term follow-up of adults with heritable retinoblastoma. Ophthalmology. 2020;127(11):1549–57. https://doi.org/10.1016/j.ophtha.2020.05.024.
66. Diener-West M, Reynolds SM, Agugliaro DJ, Caldwell R, Cumming K, Earle JD, et al. Screening for metastasis from choroidal melanoma: the collaborative ocular melanoma study group report 23. J Clin Oncol. 2004;22(12):2438–44. https://doi.org/10.1200/JCO.2004.08.194.
67. Francis JH, Catalanotti F, Landa J, Barker CA, Shoushtari AN, Abramson DH. Hepatic abnormalities identified by staging MRI and accuracy of MRI of patients with uveal melanoma. Br J Ophthalmol. 2019;103(9):1266–71. https://doi.org/10.1136/bjophthalmol-2018-312612.
68. Mariani P, Dureau S, Savignoni A, Rouic LL, Levy-Gabriel C, Piperno-Neumann S, et al. Development of a prognostic nomogram for liver metastasis of uveal melanoma patients selected by liver MRI. Cancers (Basel). 2019;11(6) https://doi.org/10.3390/cancers11060863.
69. Jansen RW, van Amstel P, Martens RM, Kooi IE, Wesseling P, de Langen AJ, et al. Non-invasive tumor genotyping using radiogenomic biomarkers, a systematic review and oncology-wide pathway analysis. Oncotarget. 2018;9(28):20134–55. https://doi.org/10.18632/oncotarget.24893.
70. Jansen RW, de Jong MC, Kooi IE, Sirin S, Goricke S, Brisse HJ, et al. MR imaging features of retinoblastoma: association with gene expression profiles. Radiology. 2018;288(2):506–15. https://doi.org/10.1148/radiol.2018172000.
71. Strijbis VIJ, de Bloeme CM, Jansen RW, Kebiri H, Nguyen HG, de Jong MC, et al. Multi-view convolutional neural networks for automated ocular structure and tumor segmentation in retinoblastoma. Sci Rep. 2021;11(1):14590. https://doi.org/10.1038/s41598-021-93905-2.

Systemic and Genetic Associations of Ocular and Ocular Adnexal Neoplasms

Gangadhara Sundar

Ophthalmic oncology is a rapidly evolving ophthalmic subspecialty that has developed both independently and in association with advances in basic and translational research in systemic oncology. Ocular and ocular adnexal oncology, historically neglected and considered a rarity, is increasingly being recognized as a more common condition affecting all age groups—from the newborn to the elderly. Thus, a detailed yet comprehensive approach is essential for the complete diagnosis, staging, and management of the patient.

While most cases do not pose a diagnostic or therapeutic dilemma, the occasional patient, even if not diagnostically challenging, may be difficult to manage or occasionally may have significant systemic implications [1]. This may prompt the astute clinician not only to counsel the patient appropriately, but also to ensure proper systemic screening is performed either at diagnosis or while management is underway. An additional necessary step in the patient's long-term management, when indicated, is to provide or refer for genetic testing and genetic counseling, which is likely to affect the family members and the succeeding generations. Medical genetics nowadays is no longer restricted to broad genetic counseling based on karyotypic analysis and known inheritance patterns of the tumors [2]. Newer advances include immunophenotyping, mutational analysis, and identification of specific molecules that can serve as biomarkers, not just for the diagnosis and guide targeted therapy, but also aid prognostication. In addition, some distinctive molecules closely related to the growth profiles of different tumors can serve as valuable indicators of prognosis and for survival analysis.

Broadly, ocular and ocular adnexal tumors may be classified into primary and secondary tumors. Primary tumors may be benign or malignant, the latter arising either de novo or from premalignant lesions. Secondary tumors may be tumor spread by contiguity from adjacent structures or from distant known or unknown (occult) primary sites—metastatic lesions. Not infrequently, mass and infiltrative lesions are misdiagnosed as neoplasms and patients counselled when, in fact, they may be developmental anomalies, reactive, or other. These tumor-like conditions include hamartomas, choristomas, vascular malformations, and inflammatory disorders such as granulomas. An overview of some common and uncommon benign, premalignant, and malignant eyelid, lacrimal drainage, and orbital neoplasms is presented in Table 1.

Several adnexal tumors have genetic etiology, often with systemic association. It thus has implications for ophthalmic and systemic clinical evaluation with embryologic correlations and genetic association, which aid and guide prognostication, systemic screening, and family counseling. In general, tumors of genetic origin present much earlier compared to sporadic tumors, may be bilateral, and are often associated with multiple neoplasms—systemic and visceral.

There are several important considerations in looking for underlying syndromes which may involve more than one organ system. Apart from performing a more complete clinical examination and appropriate imaging, the awareness may prompt complete systemic screening of the patient and their family members to detect potential life-threatening conditions early, offering management and finally, prompt regular systemic screening for such conditions (Table 2).

We herewith provide an overview of the spectrum of common and less common systemic features and associations related to ocular and ocular adnexal tumors and tumor-like conditions of interest to the ophthalmologist. Where relevant, their genetic correlations are also mentioned.

G. Sundar (✉)
Orbit and Oculofacial Surgery, Ophthalmic Oncology, Department of Ophthalmology, National University Hospital, National University of Singapore, Singapore, Singapore
e-mail: Gangadhara_sundar@nuhs.edu.sg

B. V. Chawla, M. E. Aronow (eds.), *Global Perspectives in Ocular Oncology*, https://doi.org/10.1007/978-3-031-08250-4_11

Table 1 Overview of common eyelid, lacrimal drainage system, and orbital neoplasms

	Eyelid neoplasms	Lacrimal drainage neoplasms	Orbital neoplasms
Benign	Nevi, papilloma	**Tumor like conditions:** Granulomas, granulomatous disorders, e.g., sarcoidosis, tuberculosis, granulomatosis with polyangiitis (GPA), rhinosporidiosis, amyloidosis. **True tumors:** Papillomas, cystadenomas, pleomorphic adenoma, adenoacanthoma, etc.	**Lacrimal gland:** Pleomorphic adenoma **Optic nerve/nerve sheath:** Optic nerve glioma, optic nerve sheath meningioma Sphenoid wing meningioma **Orbital nerves:** Neurilemmoma (schwannoma), neurofibroma, granular cell tumor **Vascular**: Tumor like conditions: Venous malformation ('orbital varix'), lymphatic malformation ('lymphangioma'), veno-lymphatic malformations, etc. True tumors: Capillary hemangioma (congenital, infantile—Rapidly involuting (RICH) or partially involuting (PICH). **Fibrous connective tissue:** Fibroma, myxoma, fibrous histiocytoma, solitary fibrous tumor, fibro-osseous lesions **Bone:** Osteoma
Pre-malignant	Actinic keratosis, Intraepithelial neoplasia, Sebaceous nevus of Jadassohn, Xeroderma pigmentosa, Congenital dysplastic nevus, Lentigo maligna (Hutchison's melanocytic freckle)	Inverted papilloma, Viral papilloma	Pleomorphic adenoma (long-standing, inadequately, or partially excised) Fibrous dysplasia
Malignant	Keratoacanthoma Basal cell carcinoma Squamous cell carcinoma Sebaceous gland carcinoma Melanoma Merkel cell carcinoma	**Primary:** Transitional cell carcinoma, squamous cell carcinoma, epidermoid carcinoma, mucoepidermoid carcinoma, oncocytic adenocarcinoma, lymphoma, melanoma, etc. **Secondary:** Sebaceous gland carcinoma, melanoma, nasopharyngeal carcinoma, metastasis, etc.	**Lacrimal gland:** Adenoid cystic carcinoma, adenocarcinoma, mixed malignant tumor, mucoepidermoid carcinoma, lymphoproliferative disorders Optic nerve/nerve sheath: Malignant astrocytoma **Orbital fat:** Liposarcoma **Orbital nerves:** Alveolar soft part sarcoma, malignant peripheral nerve sheath tumor, primitive neuroectodermal tumors, Ewing sarcoma, esthesioneuroblastoma **Orbital vessels:** Angiosarcoma **Fibrous connective tissue:** Malignant solitary fibrous tumor **Bone:** Osteosarcoma Miscellaneous: Melanoma, carcinoid tumors **Secondary tumors:** Metastatic disorders: Leukemia, neuroblastoma, breast carcinoma, lung carcinoma, prostatic carcinoma, plasmacytoma, etc.

1. Leser-Trelat syndrome/sign

   Seborrheic keratosis, otherwise termed "basal cell papillomas" or senile warts, are common age-related benign degenerative skin lesions that may be seen in the periorbital region and elsewhere on the face. They may be flat or elevated (stuck on appearance) with varying degrees of pigmentation. Patients may be reassured, and lesions may either be observed or have simple excision. Occasionally, *new onset eruptive form of multiple seborrheic keratosis* may be a hallmark of underlying systemic malignancy, typically adenocarcinoma of the stomach, colon, breast, or other visceral organs [3]. Ophthalmologists should be aware of the same and refer patients for systemic evaluation.
2. Cowden syndrome, also termed *multiple hamartoma syndrome*, is a rare autosomal dominant genodermatosis characterized by multiple nonmalignant hamartomas [4]. Phosphatase and Tensin Homolog deletion on Chromosome 10 (PTEN) is the affected tumor suppressor gene located on chromosome 10q. Periorbitally, they may present as *inverted follicular keratosis or multiple tricholemmomas*, typically in young adults. Systemic malignancies associated with such lesions include breast, thyroid, and endometrial carcinomas.

Table 2 Ocular adnexal neoplasms with systemic assocations

Eyelid neoplasms	Neurofibromatosis, Capillary hemangioma (congenital & infantile), Nevus flammeus & Sturge Weber syndrome, Gardner syndrome, Gorlin-Goltz (basal cell nevus) syndrome, Cowden syndrome, Carney complex (NAME syndrome, LAMB syndrome), Muir-Torre syndrome, Xeroderma pigmentosa
Ocular surface neoplasms	Peutz-Jegher's syndrome, sebaceous nevus syndrome of Jadassohn, Goldenhar (Oculo-auriculo-vertebral) syndrome, Proteus syndrome, MEN syndromes (type IIb), xeroderma pigmentosa, amyloidosis, lymphoma
Orbital neoplasms	Lymphoma (T cell, B cell, Burkitt's lymphoma), neuroblastoma, Ewing sarcoma, Langerhans cell histiocytosis, xanthogranulomas, (necrobiotic xanthogranuloma (NBX), adult-onset asthma with periocular xanthogranuloma (AAPOX), Erdheim-Chester disease, adult onset xanthogranuloma (AOX), Rosai-Dorfman disease, McCune-Albright syndrome

3. Sweet syndrome is a rare neutrophilic dermatosis characterized by a sudden onset of *periorbital and facial skin/subcutaneous nodules* although they may also occur elsewhere. Occasionally mimicking pseudoepitheliomatous or pseudocarcinomatous hyperplasia, which may also present as eyelid and facial nodules, they may be associated with underlying hematologic malignancies [5], typically leukemia, and thus should be referred for systemic work-up in suspected cases.
4. Nevus sebaceous of Jadassohn is a form of epidermal nevus syndrome [6, 7]. Described in 1895, this is a congenital hamartoma of dermal and dermal adnexal origin which includes the epidermis, hair follicles, and sebaceous and apocrine glands. It is characterized by *smooth or velvety yellow-orange well-circumscribed plaques of the face or scalp* (Fig. 1). Slowly enlarging with age, a significant proportion of affected patients may develop benign tumors within the lesion in adulthood—typically trichoblastomas—which histologically may be misdiagnosed sometimes as basal cell carcinoma. Malignant transformation is rare and includes most commonly basal cell carcinomas. Other malignancies that may develop include sebaceous gland carcinoma, squamous cell carcinoma, and keratoacanthoma. While most lesions are stable and may be conservatively managed, there is a strong case for early excision with clear margins if feasible and desired by the parents/children [8].
5. Schimmelpenning syndrome is a distinct subtype of epidermal nevus syndrome characterized by *multiple sebaceous nevi* associated with defects of the brain, eyes, and bone [9]. Although present at birth affecting the scalp and the midface, they may not be noticed until much later, from progressive growth and prominence. Ophthalmic associations include epibulbar lipodermoids, iris, and choroidal colobomas, occasionally causing retinal detachment. Systemic features include craniofacial defects, seizures, and developmental delays from intracranial abnormalities and skeletal associations, which include abnormal spinal curvature, dislocation of the hips, and deformities of the limbs.
6. Xeroderma pigmentosa is an autosomal recessive inherited disorder characterized by increased sensitivity to sunlight, premature skin aging, and predisposition to skin cancers [10]. The spectrum of cancers includes *multiple recurrent basal cell carcinoma, squamous cell carcinoma* (Fig. 2), *and cutaneous melanoma* from cellular

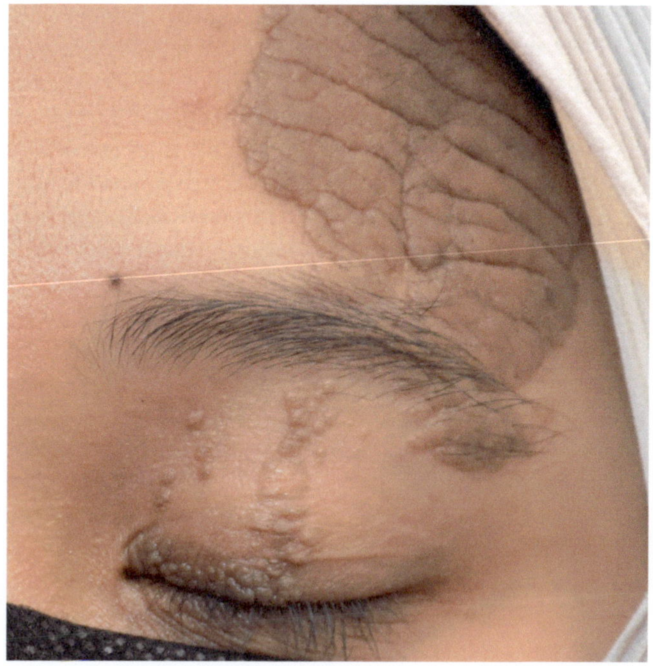

Fig. 1 Nevus sebaceous of Jadassohn

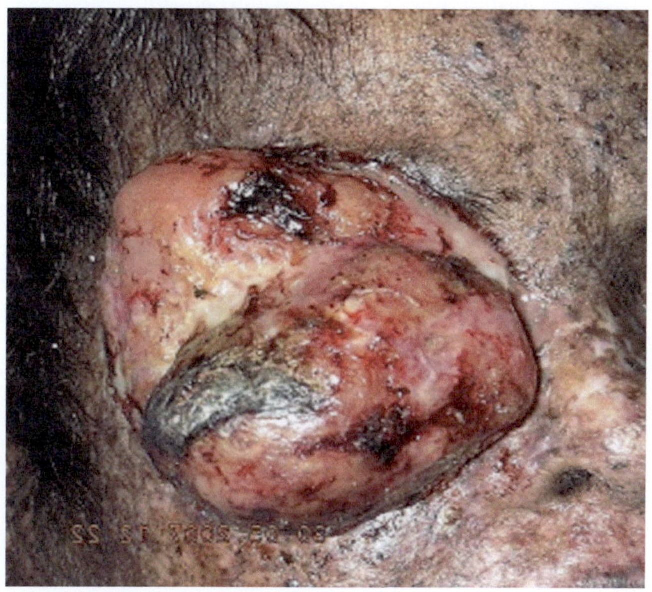

Fig. 2 Xeroderma pigmentosa with recurrent extensive squamous cell carcinoma

hypersensitivity to ultraviolet radiation. Pathogenetic mechanisms include impaired DNA repair of UV-related cell damage along with immunosuppressive effects such as from the depletion of Langerhans cells in the epidermis. Patients are symptomatic not just from periorbital and facial lesions but also from neoplastic lesions arising from the ocular surface. While there is no definitive or permanent cure, sun protection, protective clothing, isotretinoin application to minimize development of neoplasms, and routine screening to diagnose and manage lesions early are recommended. Patients often need multiple periocular facial and ocular surface neoplasm treatment, either surgically or by topical chemotherapeutic applications, with reduced mortality in most patients from recurrent skin cancers.

7. Nevoid basal cell carcinoma syndrome (Gorlin-Goltz syndrome, Hermans-Herzberg phakomatosis) is a rare complex genetic disorder with an approximate prevalence of 1 in 30,000. It manifests as a wide variety of multisystem developmental abnormalities sometimes noted even at infancy [11]. The term nevoid, however, reflects more on the multiplicity of the lesions rather than on nevoid characteristics. In affected individuals, 90% develop *multiple recurrent basal cell carcinomas* with recurrent keratocystic odontogenic tumors of the jaw, typically the mandible, palmar and plantar pits, bifid ribs, vertebral anomalies, and CNS lesions including calcifications of the falx cerebri (Fig. 3a–e) [12]. Autosomal dominantly inherited with complete penetrance, most cases are caused by mutation in the tumor suppressor PTCH1 gene that involves the sonic hedgehog pathway, although those in the SUFU and the PTCH 2 genes may also have similar phenotypes.
8. Rombo syndrome is a rare dominantly inherited disorder of unknown etiology which often manifest in the first decade of life. It may be sporadic or inherited. Clinical features include *milia, hypotrichosis, trichoepitheliomas*, peripheral vasodilatation with cyanosis vermicular atrophoderma, and basal cell carcinomas, along with *abnormal eyebrow and eyelash* morphology.
9. Bazex-Dupre-Christol syndrome is a rare X-linked dominant inherited disorder of the hair follicle characterized by *multiple basal cell carcinomas of the face*, follicular atrophoderma of the extremities with *localized or generalized hypohidrosis, hypotrichosis, and milia* [13]. Differentiating features from Gorlin-Goltz syndrome include facial but not palmar or plantar pits or skeletal abnormalities.
10. Ferguson-Smith syndrome, also called multiple self-healing squamous epithelioma (MSSE), is another extremely rare inherited disorder caused by mutations in the TGFBR1 gene. Clinical characteristics include *spontaneously resolving keratoacanthoma or squamous cell carcinoma-like lesions of the face* (although less common on the eyelids), arms, and legs with resultant flat or pitted scars. Caused by an autosomal dominantly inherited mutation of the 9q22-q31 gene, lesions are reported to go through a precursor/follicle phase followed by invasion and then regression.
11. Oculocutaneous albinism (OCA) is an autosomal recessive disorder characterized by defective melanin synthesis, thus affecting the skin, eyes, ears, and hair [14]. The absence or deficiency of melanin predisposes individuals to ultraviolet-related damage inducing actinic keratosis, which in turn predisposes the affected individuals to *squamous cell carcinoma, basal cell carcinoma, and even malignant melanoma.*
12. Oculodermal melanocytosis (nevus of Ota) is a congenital, mostly benign, mesodermal melanocytosis occurring more commonly in Asians and Africans, and in women, and is less common in Caucasians. Variable degree of cutaneous, ocular surface, and intraocular involvement may be present (Fig. 4). The presence of scleral pigmentation suggests increased risk of glaucoma. From an oncologic perspective, there is a higher incidence of malignancy on the ipsilateral side [15], more so in the Caucasian population. Associated malignancies include the development of melanoma within the cutaneous pigmented lesion, intraocularly [16] and rarely intraorbitally. Ipsilateral intracranial meningeal involvement has also been reported [17] and hence magnetic resonance imaging may be indicated. *Nevus of Ito* represents a similar lesion with hyperpigmented lesions involving the neck shoulders, axilla, and the extremities. *Nevus of Hori* is a similar lesion where there is bilateral involvement.
13. Familial atypical multiple mole melanoma syndrome (FAMMM syndrome) is usually an autosomal dominant inherited condition manifested by appearance of multiple "atypical moles." These are indeed *dysplastic nevi* which are predisposed to the development of melanoma [18]. While in 60% of cases, the cause is unknown, in other cases it is caused by mutation in the CDKN2A gene or, in rare cases, the CDK4 gene. The diagnostic criteria include the presence of *atypical multiple moles along with a first or second degree relative with a melanoma.* Oncologic associations in addition to melanoma include pancreatic adenocarcinoma. Management of melanoma is surgical and family members should be regularly screened for development of malignant lesions.
14. Muir-Torre syndrome is a variant of a more common condition called Lynch syndrome, the most common inherited cancer-predisposing syndrome. Muir-Torre syndrome is characterized by the development of single

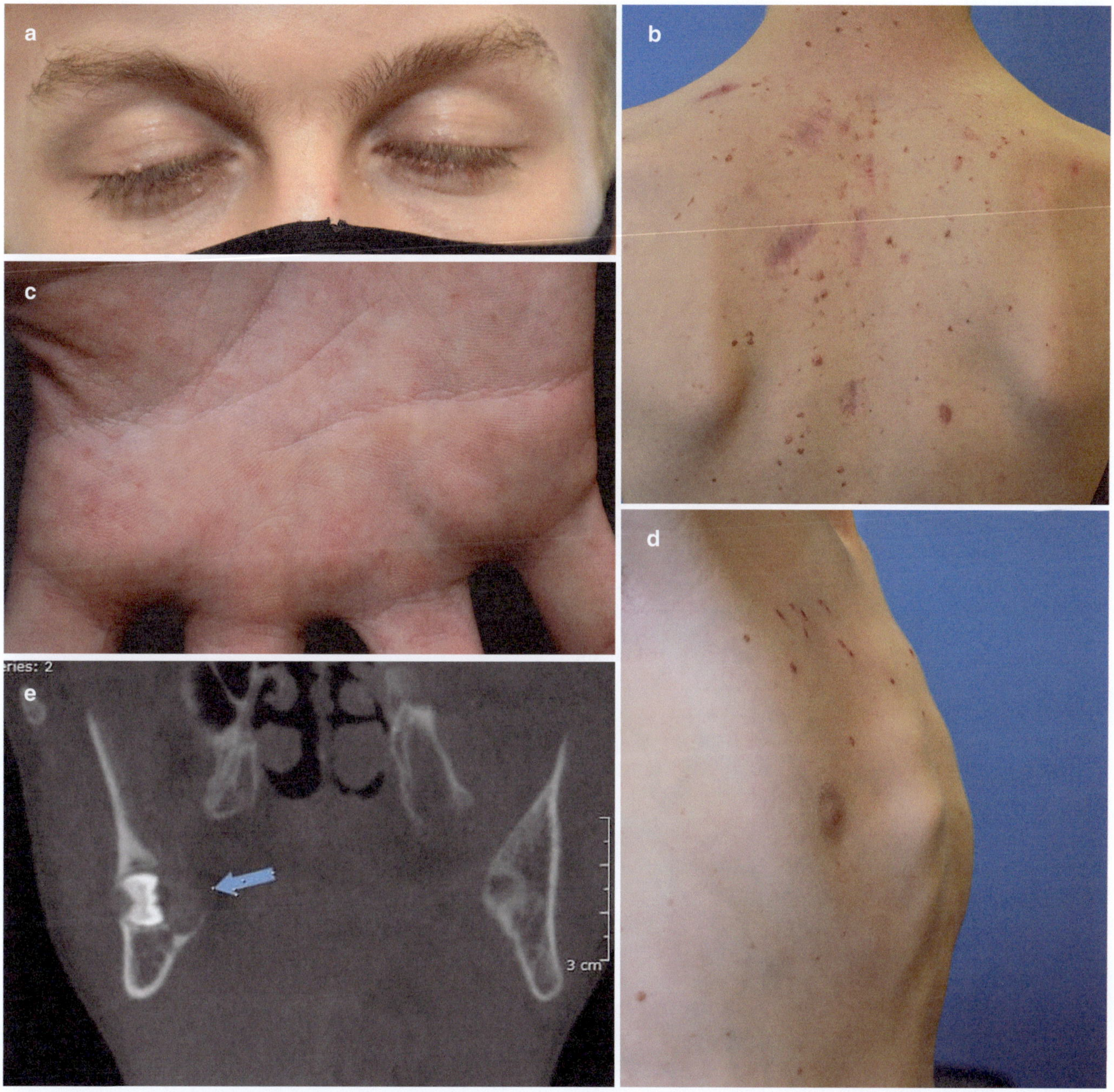

Fig. 3 Gorlin-Goltz Syndrome. (**a–b**). Periocular and truncal basal cell carcinomas with scars following multiple excisions. (**c**) Palmar pits, (**d**) Pectus carinatum, (**e**) Odontogenic keratocyst on Cone Beam CT Scan

or multiple *sebaceous gland tumors associated with systemic malignancies*—primary gastrointestinal and less commonly genitourinary. It has an autosomal dominant inheritance in about 60% of afflicted individuals with high penetrance, albeit with variable expression, from an inherited defect in one copy of a DNA repair mismatch repair (MMR) gene. *Periocular sebaceous adenomas* are typical. Other conditions include *sebaceous epitheliomas, sebaceous gland carcinoma, and even keratoacanthoma* [19]. The most common gastrointestinal malignancy is colorectal carcinoma, occurring in about half the affected individuals, and thus patients should be screened following the initial diagnosis and at regular intervals.

15. Pilomatrixoma can be syndromic. Isolated pilomatrixomas (calcifying epithelioma of Malherbe) are common benign solid tumors seen in children and young adults arising from the matrix of the hair follicles. Caused by a mutation in the beta catenin gene, isolated lesions do not have any systemic significance. However, *multiple pilomatrixomas* may be associated with several systemic conditions. These include myotonic dystrophy, familial

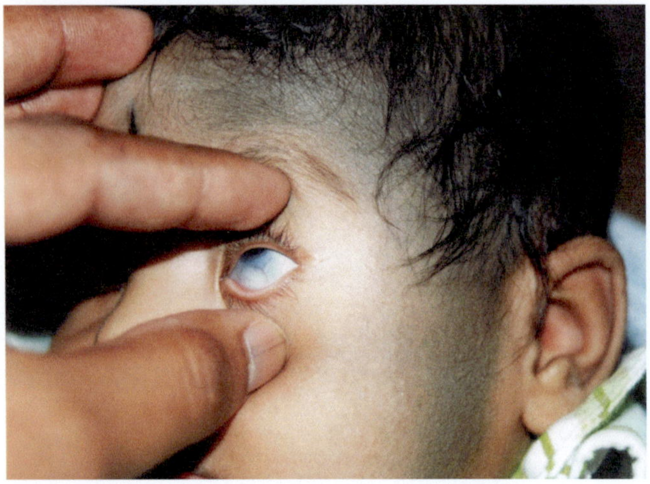

Fig. 4 Child with oculodermal melanocytosis

adenomatous polyposis-related syndromes including Gardner syndrome, Turner syndrome, and Rubinstein-Taybi syndrome. The presence of 6 or more pilomatrixoma should prompt a more extensive assessment to rule out any of the associated systemic syndromes [20].

Vascular anomalies are uncommon and challenging space-occupying lesions of the periorbita, the orbit, and the face. While most are sporadic, occasional syndromic association may be present, which is of great significance from the management perspective. Broadly, they are classified into tumors and malformations [21].

16. Capillary hemangiomas are vascular tumors that may be either congenital or infantile. Rarely, infantile hemangioma, which typically presents after birth and more commonly after In vitro fertilization (IVF) conception, may have systemic involvement—skin, liver, and so on. They may involve the eyelids, the periorbital and facial regions, or the orbit (Fig. 5). A rare sporadic syndrome associated with infantile hemangioma is the PHACES syndrome [22]. The components of this syndrome include posterior fossa abnormalities in the brain, hemangioma of the face, scalp, or neck, abnormal arterial lesions of the head and neck, congenital cardiac abnormalities including heart defects or coarctation of the aorta, eye, or endocrine abnormalities, and sternal abnormalities. These are best managed by a multidisciplinary team comprising an ophthalmologist, a pediatric oncologist, a pediatric surgeon, an interventional radiologist, and a geneticist.

    Kasabach-Merritt syndrome is a triad of vascular tumors, thrombocytopenia, and hemorrhagic diathesis typically seen in infants and young children, which can potentially be life threatening. Historically associated with congenital or infantile hemangiomas, it is now recognized to be associated with Kaposiform hemangioendothelioma or tufted angiomas. Coagulopathy reported is either from the sequestration of platelets or from consumption coagulopathy.

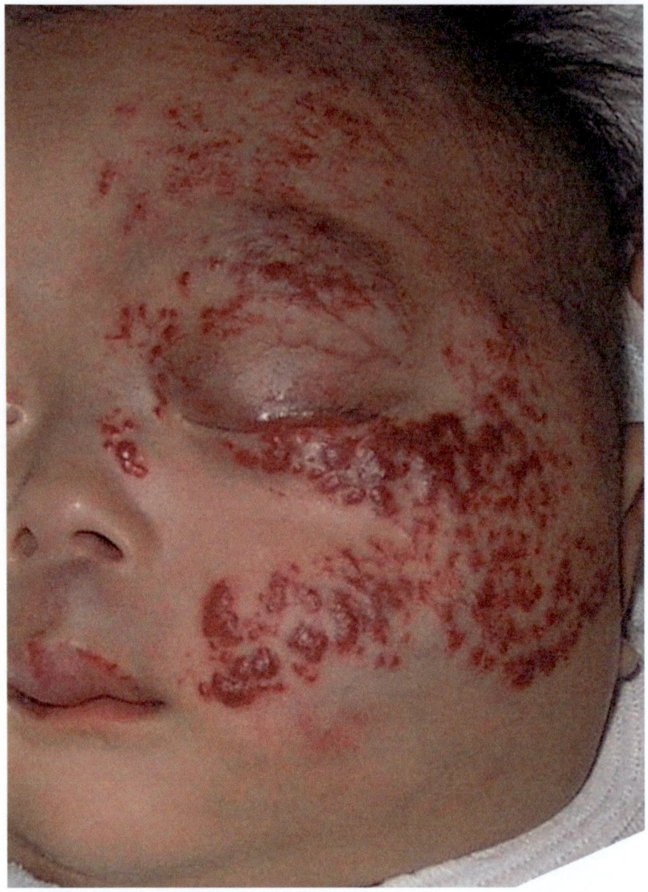

Fig. 5 Infant with extensive palpebrofacial capillary hemangiomatosis

17. Vascular malformations may be classified based on the nature of vessels: arteries, capillaries, and veins, or based on their flow characteristics. Initially presenting in childhood or adolescence either as a gradual or acute proptosis (Fig. 6), these low-flow malformations may be associated with Klippel-Trenaunay syndrome, Proteus syndrome, Cutis marmorata telangiectasia congenita, Adams-Oliver syndrome, Blue rubber nevus or Bean syndrome, Maffucci syndrome, Graham-Stout syndrome, or more commonly Sturge-Weber syndrome. High-flow malformations may be associated with Wyburn-Mason syndrome, Rendu-Osler-Weber syndrome (hereditary hemorrhagic telangiectasia), Cobb syndrome, Cowden syndrome, and Ehlers-Danlos syndrome (Type4) [23].
18. Sturge-Weber Syndrome is a rare neurocutaneous syndrome characterized by the association of a facial/peri-

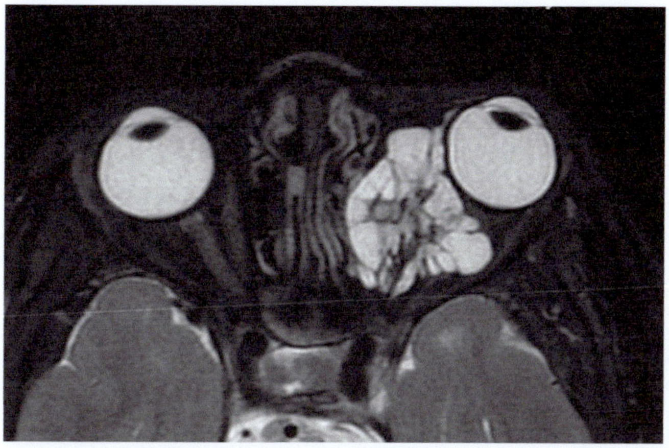

Fig. 6 T2 Axial MRI showing extensive involvement of left orbit with a venolymphatic malformation

orbital birth mark (port wine stain) with ipsilateral intraocular and intracranial vascular abnormalities [24]. It is caused by a somatic mutation of the GNAQ gene. Affected patients may have either skin alone, skin and eye, or skin, eye, and brain involvement. Characteristic and clinically significant ophthalmic findings include *periocular and ipsilateral facial capillary malformation* (Fig. 7), *ipsilateral iris heterochromia, choroidal hemangioma, and secondary glaucoma*, typically seen in Type II disease. Glaucoma may present at birth or manifest anytime later and is often challenging to manage both medically and surgically. Intracranial involvement of angiomas of the leptomeninges may manifest as seizures, which is not uncommon, making imaging and referral to a pediatric neurologist important.

19. Blue rubber nevus syndrome, also called Bean syndrome, is a rare vascular abnormality characterized by venous malformations and hemangiomas affecting the skin and visceral organs, especially the gastrointestinal system causing bleeds [25]. These lesions are *soft, elevated compressible lesions* involving the skin or subcutaneous tissues, may be tender to touch, and generally increase in size over time. Ophthalmologic associations include vascular lesions of the *periorbital region including the eyelids, conjunctiva, iris, retina, and the orbit*. The latter may either be cavernous venous malformation ("orbital varix or cavernous hemangioma"). Ocular adnexal and intraocular lesions may be managed conservatively unless visually symptomatic. Thus, management is expectant and can be challenging, especially those of the GI system with a combination of vascular agents or surgical management.
20. Neurofibromatosis is a common group of phakomatoses which have ophthalmic, facial, and occasionally intracranial implications. Arising sporadically, they are typically inherited as an autosomal dominant trait. Three distinct types have been described.

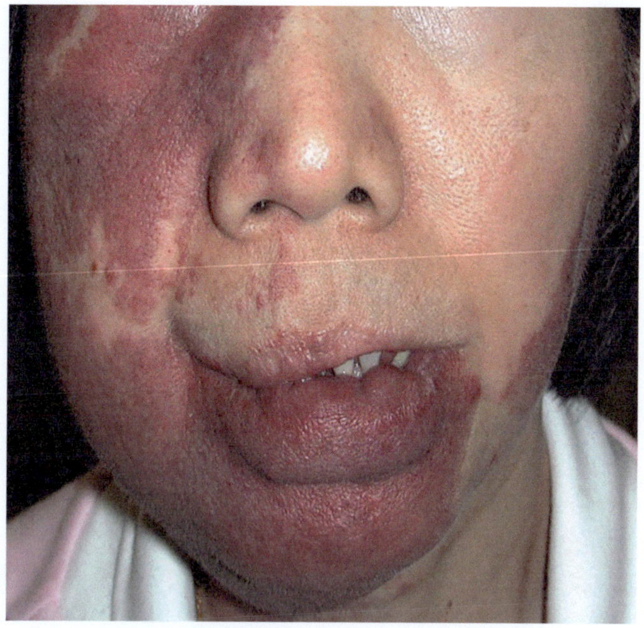

Fig. 7 Sturge-Weber syndrome

(a) Neurofibromatosis Type I is a tumor predisposition syndrome seen in 1 in 3000 births, caused by a mutation on chromosome 17 encoding a cytoplasmic protein neurofibrin, a tumor suppressor gene. It manifests as *café-au-lait patches, axillary and groin freckling, nodular or plexiform neurofibromas in one or more dermatomal distributions of the face* (Fig. 8), which increase in size and numbers over the years, and scoliosis [26]. Functionally, there may be learning or behavioral problems. Ophthalmic features may include eyelid and/or orbital neurofibromatosis with S-shaped mechanical ptosis, pulsatile proptosis from direct transmission of intracranial pulsations due to sphenoidal wing dysplasia, iris hamartomas (Lisch nodules), secondary glaucoma, and optic nerve glioma. Clinical diagnosis typically requires at least 2 of the 7 criteria mentioned below, some of which may manifest later in life.

- Six or more café-au-lait spots or hyperpigmented macules greater than 5 mm in diameter in prepubertal children and greater than 15 mm in postpubertal children
- Axillary or inguinal freckles (>2)
- Two or more typical neurofibromas or one plexiform neurofibroma
- Optic nerve glioma
- Two or more iris hamartomas (Lisch nodules)

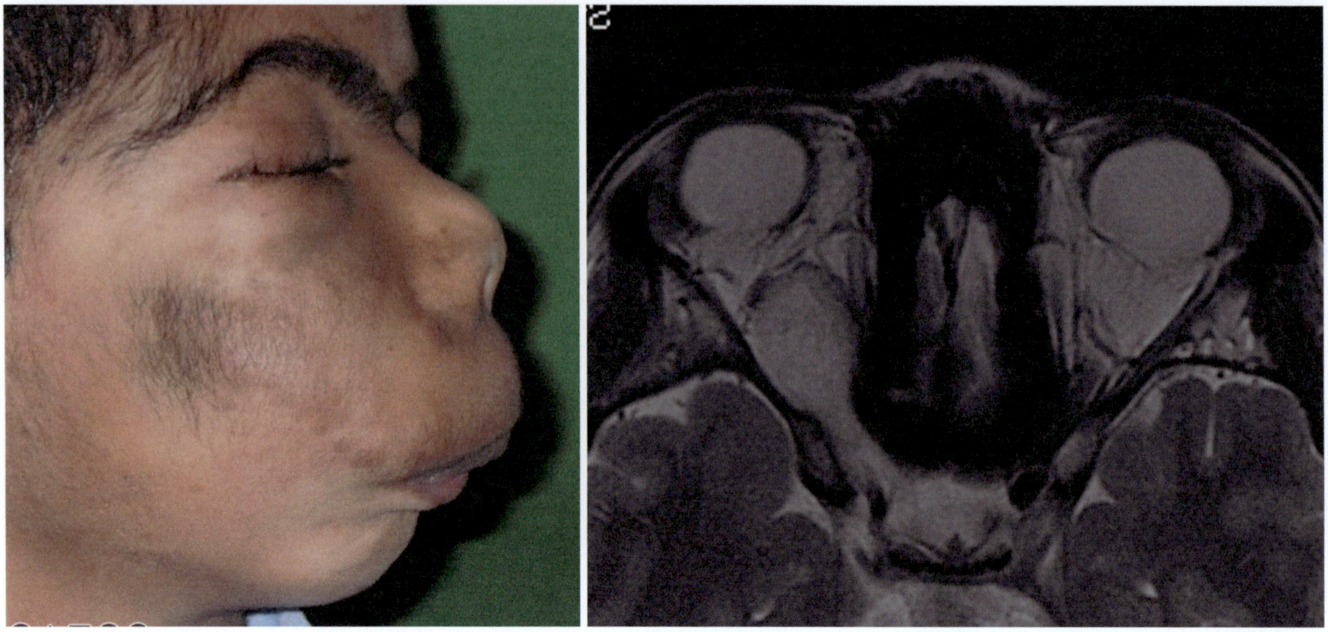

Fig. 8 Child with orbitofacial neurofibromatosis with optic pathway glioma

- Sphenoid dysplasia or typical long-bone abnormalities such as pseudarthrosis
- First-degree relative (e.g., mother, father, sister, brother) with NF1

(b) Type II neurofibromatosis, seen in 1 in 25,000, births is caused by a mutation on Chromosome 22 that encodes a cytoplasmic protein merlin. It is associated with cataracts, hearing loss from unilateral or *bilateral acoustic schwannomas*, flesh-colored skin flaps (schwannomas), problems with maintaining balance, and muscle wasting. It is considered confirmed in cases with bilateral vestibular schwannomas and probable when a unilateral vestibular schwannoma or any 2 of the following tumor types—meningioma, glioma, schwannoma, *juvenile cortical or posterior subcapsular catarac*t—are present along with a positive family history.

(c) Type III is also called *Schwannomatosis* and is associated with various mutations on the SMARCB1 gene and often presents as multiple painful lesions along the peripheral and spinal cord.

21. Gardner syndrome is a dominantly inherited familial cancer syndrome, a subgroup of familial adenomatous polyposis (FAP), characterized by colorectal polyps with extracolonic manifestations including benign and malignant tumors elsewhere. Because this syndrome results from a mutation in the APC gene, patients have a 100% risk of malignancy sometime in adulthood. Apart from early onset colorectal carcinoma, other FAP-related cancers include those of the small bowel, stomach, pancreas, thyroid, CNS, liver, bile ducts, and/or adrenal glands. Ophthalmic findings that may suggest systemic work-up includes *multiple pigmented ocular fundus lesions,* [27] which can resemble but are clinically distinct from more typical congenital hypertrophy of retinal pigment epithelium (CHRPE). Associated periocular lesions may include *epidermoid tumors, fibromas, lipomas, osteomas, and desmoid tumors*. Thus, screening and prophylactic surgical intervention remain the mainstay of management.
22. Carney complex is yet another rare hereditary genetic disorder from mutations in the PRKAR1A gene. Either sporadic or inherited (60–70%) as an autosomal dominant disorder, it is characterized by lentigines and blue nevi, which may be associated with multiple benign tumors affecting the heart (myxoma) and the endocrine system—pituitary and adrenals (primary pigmented nodular adrenocortical disease [PPNAD]). Apart from myxomas of the skin and peripheral nerves, cardiac myxomas may cause life-threatening complications such as stroke, valvular obstruction, or heart failure. *Lentigines may affect the eyelids, conjunctiva including caruncle,* lips, ears, and the genital region. It has also been labelled as NAME syndrome (Nevi, Atrial myxoma, Myxoid neurofibromas, and Ephelides [freckles]) and LAMB syndrome (Lentigines, Atrial Myxoma, and Blue nevi) with a reported case of uveal melanoma [28].
23. Peutz-Jeghers syndrome is an inherited condition characterized by the development of hamartomatous polyps of the digestive tract in addition to cancers of the breast, colon, rectum, pancreas, stomach, lung, cervix, and testicles/ovaries [29]. Periorbital features include *mucocu-*

taneous pigmented lesions that may also be present around the lips, and pigmented lesions of the mouth, fingers, or toes. The diagnosis is confirmed by the presence of such characteristic freckling, at least 2 Peutz-Jeghers type of hamartomatous polyps of the small intestine and at least 1 relative with PJS. Given the autosomal dominant transmission, all family members are advised to have genetic testing for mutation in the STK11/LKB1 gene and genetic counseling.

24. Goldenhar syndrome, also called a facio-auriculo-vertebral syndrome, is a craniofacial disorder that occurs sporadically, caused by a dysgenesis of the first and second branchial arches in utero. Although there is no known genetic mutation, 1–2% of patients do have a family history, from autosomal dominant transmission. Mostly unilateral, 10–25% of patients may have a variable component of bilateral facial involvement [30]. Ophthalmic features include *epibulbar tumors (angular or limbal lipodermoids), anophthalmia /microphthalmia, eyelid, and ocular colobomas* (Fig. 9). Facial features include microtia/anotia, hemifacial microsomia with underdeveloped facial bones (temporal, zygoma and maxilla), cleft lip/palate, macrostomia, and dental abnormalities. Systemic association includes abnormalities of the heart, lungs, kidneys, central nervous system, and the spine. Apart from referral to a pediatrician and a geneticist, principles of management include surgical intervention for visually significant, symptomatic, or esthetically significant epibulbar dermoids, colobomas, and microphthalmos/anophthalmic sockets including amblyopia management as indicated [31].
25. Multiple endocrine neoplasia (MEN) syndrome, specifically MEN Type 2b, is associated with various ophthalmic lesions. In this rare autosomal dominant tumor syndrome, ophthalmic features include *prominent corneal nerves, conjunctiva mucosal neuromas*, secondary open angle glaucoma, and dry eyes.
26. Amyloidosis is a disorder of diverse etiologies involving the synthesis and extracellular deposition of abnormal misfolded proteins. They may be classified into primary amyloidosis, which is more common, and secondary amyloidosis. Primary amyloidosis, now termed amyloid light chain (AL) amyloidosis, is caused by the proliferation of bone marrow residing plasma cell clones resulting in unstable immunoglobulin light chain proteins which infiltrate various organ systems. Apart from *conjunctival and eyelid involvement* (Fig. 10a), which may occasionally clinically misdiagnosed as lymphoproliferative disorders, other organ systems which may be affected include the kidneys, heart (Fig. 10b, c), the GI tract including liver, and the nervous system [32]. Principles of management include early diagnosis, and systemic evaluation to effectively manage plasma cell

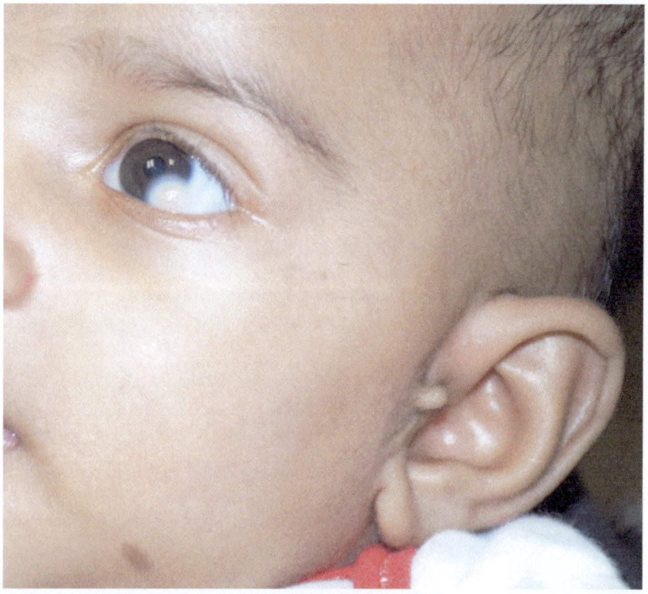

Fig. 9 Goldenhar syndrome with limbal dermoid and preauricular tag

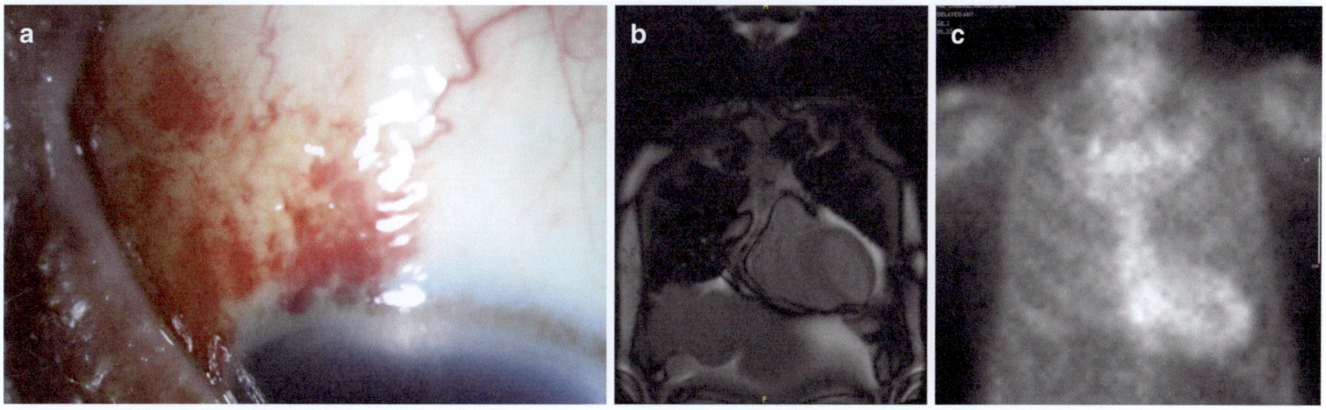

Fig. 10 (**a**) Systemic amyloidosis presenting with conjunctival infiltration and hemorrhages. (**b**) MRI showing cardiomegaly from infiltration. (**c**) Technetium 99 isotope scan diagnostic of cardiac amyloidosis

dyscrasia, and to prevent or halt organ damage with autologous stem cell transplant (ASCT) as the definitive treatment.

27. Lymphomas are a diverse group of proliferative and infiltrative lesions that may affect the conjunctiva, the eyelids, and the orbits. Broadly they may be classified into Hodgkin and non-Hodgkin lymphomas. The latter may be classified into more common B-cell and far less common T-cell lymphomas. Lymphomas are now classified not only based on morphology but also by immunophenotype, genetic and molecular profiles, cellular derivation, and clinical features. While the most indolent are the mucosa-associated lymphoid tissue (MALT) lymphomas, the more aggressive forms are mantle cell lymphoma (MCL) and the diffuse large B-cell lymphomas (DLBCLs) [33]. Lesions may present as *proptosis from orbital infiltration (lacrimal gland, orbital fat, extraocular muscles) and conjunctival lesions appearing as salmon-patches or eyelid involvement* (Fig. 11a). Morphologically, based on the ocular adnexal structure involved, the presence of systemic disease varies. In the increasing order of systemic involvement are the conjunctiva (least), followed by the orbits and finally the eyelids (highest). All suspected cases should be biopsied, immunophenotyped, staged (Fig. 11b), and counselled regarding prognosis. Treatment options include observation for indolent minimally symptomatic lymphomas, for example, MALT Lymphoma, to more aggressive chemotherapeutic and targeted therapeutic interventions with close follow-up [34].
28. Burkitt's lymphomas are a rare yet aggressive type of non-Hodgkin B-cell lymphoma that is typically seen in children, is rapidly growing, and is potentially lethal if poorly managed [35]. Although encountered more commonly in the African continent, it has also been reported elsewhere in the world. The three main types recognized include the African type, which typically affects the orbits and the maxilla, and is reportedly related to the Epstein-Barr virus; the non-African or American type, which involves the lymph nodes, bone marrow, and the viscera and finally the even more aggressive type, which typically involves the CNS and is reportedly associated with human immunodeficiency virus-acquired immunodeficiency syndrome (HIV-AIDS). The tumor has been reported to be due to a translocation between chromosomes 8 and 14 affecting c-myc. Based on a high degree of suspicion, diagnosis is established by early biopsy, followed by systemic evaluation and aggressive chemo-

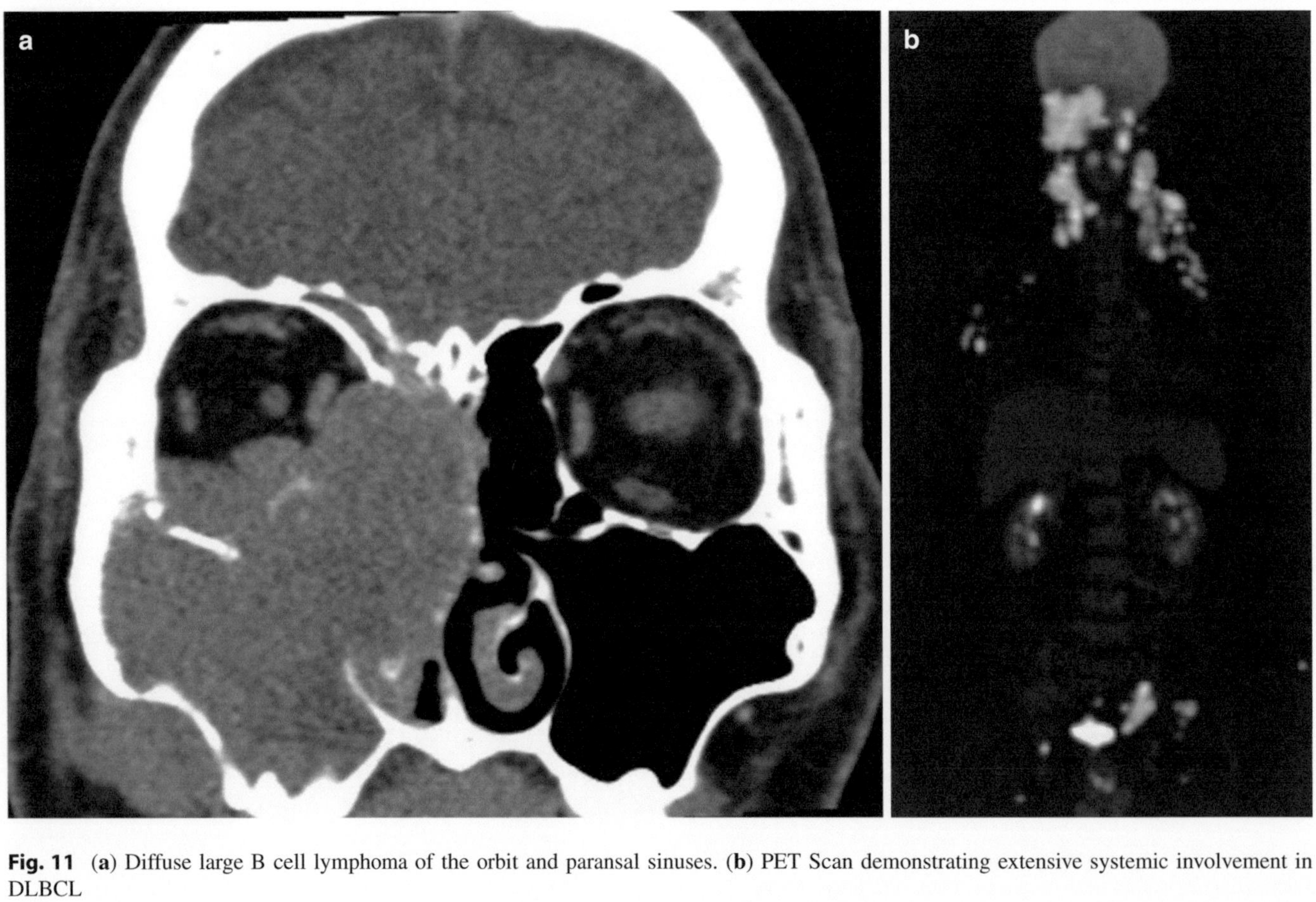

Fig. 11 (**a**) Diffuse large B cell lymphoma of the orbit and paransal sinuses. (**b**) PET Scan demonstrating extensive systemic involvement in DLBCL

therapy. Other adjuvant modalities that may be required include rituximab (monoclonal antibody therapy), radiation therapy, and ASCT in rare situations.

29. Neuroblastoma is a common type of neuroendocrine tumor that is typically seen in young children, has a high propensity for metastasis, and interestingly, albeit rarely, has a tendency for spontaneous regression in infancy. They are typically seen in children between 2 and 7 years of age presenting as an *acute unilateral or bilateral proptosis, with periorbital ecchymosis*-like appearance (Fig. 12a). It may be either sporadic or inherited, with mutations reported both in the ALK and PHOX2B genes. The presence of myc-n amplification usually portrays an aggressive type of neuroblastoma. CT scans typically reveal a soft tissue mass with a spiculated bony involvement with a "hair on end" appearance (Fig. 12b). While general management is chemotherapy, a risk-stratified approach is used for low- and intermediate-risk disease. High-risk disease is treated with intense induction and myeloablative chemotherapy, followed by the treatment of minimal residual disease using differentiation therapy and immunotherapy [36].
30. Langerhans cell histiocytosis comprises a spectrum of histiocytic conditions characterized by ERK pathway activation including BRAF V600E mutations, which may be either unifocal or multifocal, or have multiorgan involvement. Typically seen in young children, they commonly present as an *upper eyelid mass or superior/superotemporal lytic orbital bone* involvement which are often mistaken for metastasis. The organ systems involved include the bone, skin, lung, and the pituitary gland [37]. Three forms of the disease have been described: a localized Eosinophilic granu-

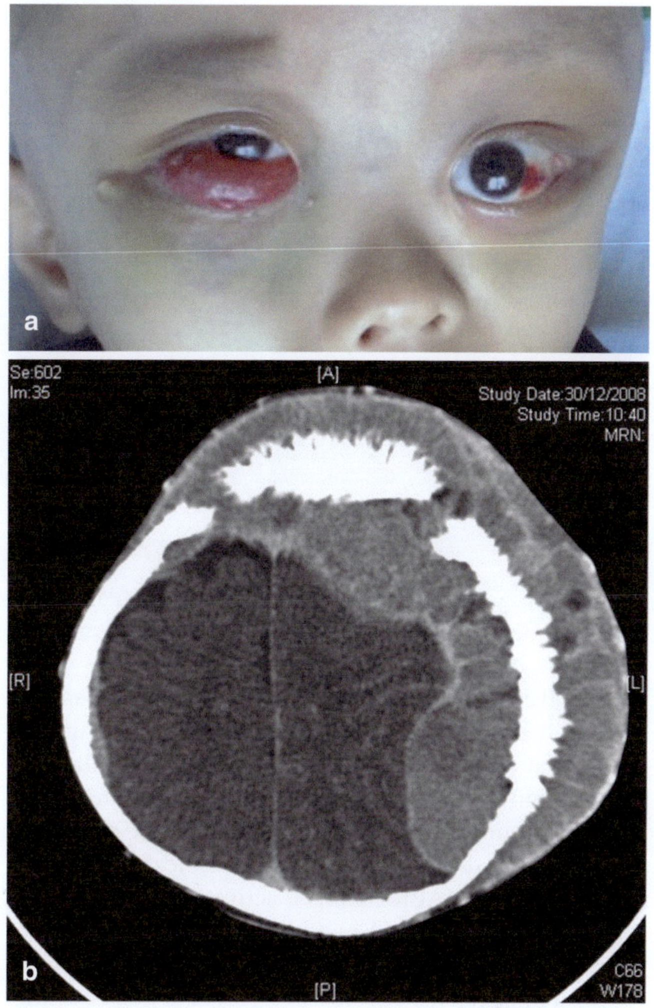

Fig. 12 (**a**) Bilateral proptosis with periorbtial 'ecchymosis' in metastatic neuroblastoma. (**b**) CT scan showing spicular 'hair on end' appearance

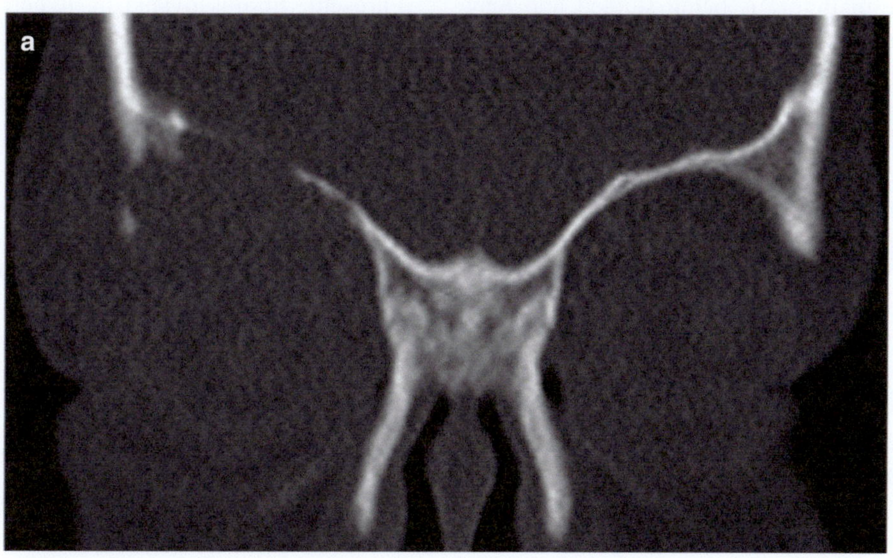

Fig. 13 (**a**) Langerhan cell histiocytosis. Coronal CT Bone window showing lytic lesion of the right superotemporal orbit in LCH. (**b–d**) Skeletal survey with lytic lesions of the temporal bone, lumbar spine and iliac bone

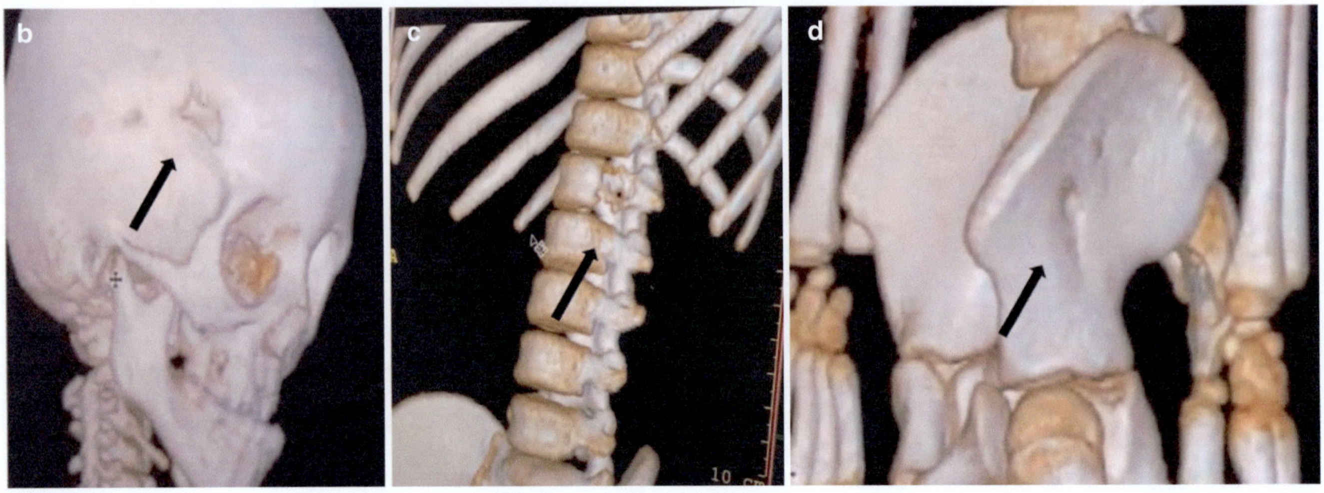

Fig. 13 (continued)

loma (Fig. 13a), Hand-Schuller-Christian disease (triad of orbital involvement with bony lytic lesions and diabetes insipidus) and Letterer-Siwe disease (with involvement of the skin, bones, brain, lungs, spleen, and liver) (Fig. 13b–d). While the features of inflammation (CD207+ cells with accompanying inflammatory infiltration with a local or systemic cytokine storm) may be misleading, features supportive of a myeloid neoplastic disorder include clonality and gene mutations in the MAPK (mitogen activated protein kinase) pathway with shared mutation of hematopoietic precursors. Isolated orbital lesions may be curetted out with intralesional steroids with resultant bony healing. The multifocal and symptomatic systemic disease may warrant conventional chemotherapeutic regimens (vinblastine, 6-mercaptopurine, prednisone). Targeted therapy with vemurafenib (a small molecule BRAF (V600E) kinase inhibitor) is being studied and may hold promise in patients with this mutation.

31. Rosai-Dorfman disease, previously termed sinus histiocytosis with massive lymphadenopathy, is a non-malignant proliferation and accumulation of histiocytes. Typically, it presents with a painless progressive mass usually with lymphadenopathy. Occasional cases of *unilateral or bilateral proptosis* without systemic involvement have been reported [38]. Of unknown etiology, it is diagnosed by histopathology based on characteristic features. Most patients may warrant some form of treatment, which includes corticosteroid therapy, surgical debulking, or even chemotherapy [39]. Occasional cases may resolve spontaneously, although over months to years.
32. Xanthogranulomas are a group of non-Langerhans cell histiocytic granulomatous disorders similar in their predominant cell type but diverse in their prognosis, which ranges from benign self-limited conditions to malignant and ultimately fatal lesions. Distinct clinical syndromes but with considerable overlap suggest a continuum. The spectrum includes juvenile xanthogranuloma (JXG) seen in children and adult orbital xanthogranuloma (AOX), adult-onset asthma and periocular xanthogranuloma (AAPOX) [40], necrobiotic xanthogranuloma (NXG), and Erdheim-Chester disease (ECD), all seen in adults. Lesions typically present as unilateral or bilateral *infiltrative eyelid or orbital lesions*, responsive to corticosteroid treatment, warranting a tissue diagnosis and appropriate management [41].
33. McCune-Albright syndrome, described in 1937, is a multisystem genetic disorder affecting the bone, skin, and endocrine organs [42]. A mosaic disease from the action of somatic mutations in GNAS, it is often varied in clinical presentation. The disease is suspected when two or more of the following conditions are present: fibrous dysplasia, hyperpigmented macules along the midline with a jagged "coast of Maine" appearance, and endocrinopathies. The latter may present as precocious puberty, testicular abnormalities, hyperthyroidism, growth hormone excess, Cushing's syndrome, and hypophosphatemia. Fibrous dysplasia of the orbit or the skull is suspected during puberty or beyond when *bony thickening results in globe dystopia*, usually without visual loss. Characteristic CT scan findings of cortical and cancellous bone of a ground glass appearance are diagnostic. Principles of management include addressing systemic endocrine abnormalities, expectant management, and, when indicated, surgical management with reconstruction. Bisphosphonates were historically used but are no longer thought to stabilize the disease. Denosumab is postulated to stabilize growth and relieve bone pain, but safety data is limited.

Ocular and ocular adnexal tumors and tumor-like lesions may be the presenting feature of a systemic or genetic disorder. A detailed history, a complete ophthalmic examination with review of systems, a high degree of suspicion, tissue diagnosis when indicated, prompt referral to the pediatrician or adult physician, genetic testing followed by counseling go a long way in the complete management of afflicted patients and their families.

References

1. McNab AA. The 2017 Doyne Lecture: the orbit as a window to systemic disease. Eye (Lond). 2018;32(2):248–61. https://doi.org/10.1038/eye.2017.224. Epub 2017 Nov 10.
2. Khong JJ, Moore S, Prabhakaran VC, Selva D. Genetic testing in orbital tumors. Orbit. 2009;28(2–3):88–97. https://doi.org/10.1080/08820530802506094.
3. Bernett CN, Schmieder GJ. Leser Trelat Sign. In: StatPearls [Internet]. Treasure Island (FL): StatPearls Publishing; 2020; 2021 Jan.
4. Pilarski R, Burt R, Kohlman W, Pho L, Shannon KM, Swisher E. Cowden syndrome and the PTEN hamartoma tumor syndrome: systematic review and revised diagnostic criteria. J Natl Cancer Inst. 2013;105(21):1607–16. https://doi.org/10.1093/jnci/djt277. Epub 2013 Oct 17.
5. Villarreal-Villarreal CD, Ocampo-Candiani J, Villarreal-Martínez A. Sweet syndrome: a review and update. Actas Dermosifiliogr. 2016;107(5):369–78. https://doi.org/10.1016/j.ad.2015.12.001. English, Spanish. Epub 2016 Jan 27.
6. Asch S, Sugarman JL. Epidermal nevus syndromes: new insights into whorls and swirls. Pediatr Dermatol. 2018;35(1):21–9. https://doi.org/10.1111/pde.13273. Epub 2017 Oct 16.
7. Menascu S, Donner EJ. Linear nevus sebaceous syndrome: case reports and review of the literature. Pediatr Neurol. 2008;38(3):207–10. https://doi.org/10.1016/j.pediatrneurol.2007.10.012.
8. Moody MN, Landau JM, Goldberg LH. Nevus sebaceous revisited. Pediatr Dermatol. 2012;29(1):15–23. https://doi.org/10.1111/j.1525-1470.2011.01562.x. Epub 2011 Oct 13.
9. Dwiyana RF, Hazari MN, Diana IA, Gondokaryono SP, Effendi RMRA, Gunawan H. Schimmelpenning syndrome with large nevus sebaceous and multiple epidermal nevi. Case Rep Dermatol. 2020;12(3):186–91. https://doi.org/10.1159/000509992.
10. Karass M, Naguib MM, Elawabdeh N, Cundiff CA, Thomason J, Steelman CK, Cone R, Schwenkter A, Jordan C, Shehata BM. Xeroderma pigmentosa: three new cases with an in depth review of the genetic and clinical characteristics of the disease. Fetal Pediatr Pathol. 2015;34(2):120–7. https://doi.org/10.3109/15513815.2014.982336. Epub 2014 Dec 2.
11. Bresler SC, Padwa BL, Granter SR. Nevoid basal cell carcinoma syndrome (Gorlin syndrome). Head Neck Pathol. 2016;10(2):119–24. https://doi.org/10.1007/s12105-016-0706-9. Epub 2016 Mar 14.
12. Schierbeck J, Vestergaard T, Bygum A. Skin cancer associated genodermatoses: a literature review. Acta Derm Venereol. 2019;99(4):360–9. https://doi.org/10.2340/00015555-3123.
13. Glaessl A, Hohenlautner U, Landthaler M, Vogt T. Sporadic Bazex-Dupré-Christol-like syndrome: early onset basal cell carcinoma, hypohidrosis, hypotrichosis, and prominent milia. Dermatol Surg. 2000;26(2):152–4. https://doi.org/10.1046/j.1524-4725.2000.99146.x.
14. Marçon CR, Maia M. Albinism: epidemiology, genetics, cutaneous characterization, psychosocial factors. An Bras Dermatol. 2019;94(5):503–20. https://doi.org/10.1016/j.abd.2019.09.023. Epub 2019 Sep 30.
15. Patel BC, Egan CA, Lucius RW, Gerwels JW, Mamalis N, Anderson RL. Cutaneous malignant melanoma and oculodermal melanocytosis (nevus of Ota): report of a case and review of the literature. J Am Acad Dermatol. 1998;38(5 Pt 2):862–5. https://doi.org/10.1016/s0190-9622(98)70477-3.
16. Pan X, Zheng S. Clinical and genetic characteristics of nevus of Ota with choroidal melanoma in Chinese. Ophthalmic Genet. 2019;40(4):338–41. https://doi.org/10.1080/13816810.2019.1650073. Epub 2019 Aug 13.
17. Kuo KL, Lin CL, Wu CH, Chang CH, Tsai HP, Loh JK, Lieu AS, Su YF. Meningeal melanocytoma associated with nevus of Ota: analysis of twelve reported cases. World Neurosurg. 2019;127:e311–20. https://doi.org/10.1016/j.wneu.2019.03.113. Epub 2019 Mar 21.
18. Czajkowski R, Placek W, Drewa G, Czajkowska A, Uchańska G. FAMMM syndrome: pathogenesis and management. Dermatol Surg. 2004;30(2 Pt 2):291–6. https://doi.org/10.1111/j.1524-4725.2004.30088.x.
19. Eiger-Moscovich M, Eagle RC Jr, Shields CL, Racher H, Lally SE, Silkiss RZ, Shields JA, Milman T. Muir-Torre syndrome associated periocular sebaceous neoplasms: screening patterns in the literature and in clinical practice. Ocul Oncol Pathol. 2020;6(4):226–37. https://doi.org/10.1159/000504984. Epub 2020 Jan 15.
20. Ciriacks K, Knabel D, Waite MB. Syndromes associated with multiple pilomatricomas: when should clinicians be concerned? Pediatr Dermatol. 2020;37(1):9–17. https://doi.org/10.1111/pde.13947. Epub 2019 Oct 16.
21. Sundar G. Vascular lesions of the orbit: conceptual approach and recent advances. Indian J Ophthalmol. 2018;66(1):3–6. https://doi.org/10.4103/ijo.IJO_1272_17.
22. Garzon MC, Epstein LG, Heyer GL, Frommelt PC, Orbach DB, Baylis AL, Blei F, Burrows PE, Chamlin SL, Chun RH, Hess CP, Joachim S, Johnson K, Kim W, Liang MG, Maheshwari M, McCoy GN, Metry DW, Monrad PA, Pope E, Powell J, Shwayder TA, Siegel DH, Tollefson MM, Vadivelu S, Lew SM, Frieden IJ, Drolet BA. PHACE syndrome: consensus-derived diagnosis and care recommendations. J Pediatr. 2016;178:24–33.e2. https://doi.org/10.1016/j.jpeds.2016.07.054. Epub 2016 Sep 19.
23. Martinez-Lopez A, Salvador-Rodriguez L, Montero-Vilchez T, Molina-Leyva A, Tercedor-Sanchez J, Arias-Santiago S. Vascular malformations syndromes: an update. Curr Opin Pediatr. 2019;31(6):747–53. https://doi.org/10.1097/MOP.0000000000000812.
24. Higueros E, Roe E, Granell E, Baselga E. Sturge-Weber syndrome: a review. Actas Dermosifiliogr. 2017;108(5):407–17. https://doi.org/10.1016/j.ad.2016.09.022. English, Spanish. Epub 2017 Jan 23.
25. Baigrie D, Rice AS, An IC. Blue rubber bleb nevus syndrome. In: StatPearls [Internet]. Treasure Island (FL): StatPearls Publishing; 2021.
26. Karaconji T, Whist E, Jamieson RV, Flaherty MP, Grigg JRB. Neurofibromatosis type 1: review and update on emerging therapies. Asia Pac J Ophthalmol (Phila). 2019;8(1):62–72. https://doi.org/10.22608/APO.2018182. Epub 2018 Nov 2.
27. Traboulsi EI, Krush AJ, Gardner EJ, Booker SV, Offerhaus GJ, Yardley JH, Hamilton SR, Luk GD, Giardiello FM, Welsh SB, et al. Prevalence and importance of pigmented ocular fundus lesions in Gardner's syndrome. N Engl J Med. 1987;316(11):661–7. https://doi.org/10.1056/NEJM198703123161104.
28. Salomão DR, Ida CM, Greipp PT, Carney JA. Case report with review of the literature: uveal melanoma in a patient with carney complex—another rare component of the syndrome? Ocul Oncol Pathol. 2020;6(5):311–7. https://doi.org/10.1159/000506205. Epub 2020 Apr 21

29. Patel LM, Lambert PJ, Gagna CE, Maghari A, Lambert WC. Cutaneous signs of systemic disease. Clin Dermatol. 2011;29(5):511–22. https://doi.org/10.1016/j.clindermatol.2011.01.019.
30. Beleza-Meireles A, Clayton-Smith J, Saraiva JM, Tassabehji M. Oculo-auriculo-vertebral spectrum: a review of the literature and genetic update. J Med Genet. 2014;51(10):635–45. https://doi.org/10.1136/jmedgenet-2014-102476. Epub 2014 Aug 12.
31. Schmitzer S, Burcel M, Dăscălescu D, Popteanu IC. Goldenhar syndrome—ophthalmologist's perspective. Rom J Ophthalmol. 2018;62(2):96–104.
32. Al-Nuaimi D, Bhatt PR, Steeples L, Irion L, Bonshek R, Leatherbarrow B. Amyloidosis of the orbit and adnexae. Orbit. 2012;31(5):287–98. https://doi.org/10.3109/01676830.2012.707740. Epub 2012 Sep 4.
33. Olsen TG, Holm F, Mikkelsen LH, Rasmussen PK, Coupland SE, Esmaeli B, Finger PT, Graue GF, Grossniklaus HE, Honavar SG, Khong JJ, McKelvie PA, Mulay K, Sjö LD, Vemuganti GK, Thuro BA, Heegaard S. Orbital lymphoma-an international multicenter retrospective study. Am J Ophthalmol. 2019;199:44–57. https://doi.org/10.1016/j.ajo.2018.11.002. Epub 2018 Nov 10.
34. Poon LM. Lymphoproliferative disorders—overview. In: Amrith S, Sundar G, Young S, editors. Ocular adnexal lesions. Singapore: Springer; 2019. https://doi.org/10.1007/978-981-13-3798-7_14.
35. Gupta R, Yadav JS, Yadav S, Wadood A. Orbital involvement in nonendemic Burkitts lymphoma. Orbit. 2012;31(6):441–5. https://doi.org/10.3109/01676830.2012.711886.
36. Mallepalli S, Gupta MK, Vadde R. Neuroblastoma: an updated review on biology and treatment. Curr Drug Metab. 2019;20(13):1014–22. https://doi.org/10.2174/1389200221666191226102231.
37. Lakatos K, Sterlich K, Pötschger U, Thiem E, Hutter C, Prosch H, Minkov M. Langerhans cell histiocytosis of the orbit: spectrum of clinical and imaging findings. J Pediatr. 2021;230:174–181.e1. https://doi.org/10.1016/j.jpeds.2020.10.056. Epub 2020 Nov 4.
38. Tan JJ, Narang S, Purewal B, Langer PD, Blaydon S, Schwarcz RM, McCormick SA, Kim JY, Walrath JD, Burt BO, Shinder R. Extranodal rosai-dorfman disease of the orbit: clinical features of 8 cases. Ophthalmic Plast Reconstr Surg. 2016;32(6):458–61. https://doi.org/10.1097/IOP.0000000000000589.
39. Abla O, Jacobsen E, Picarsic J, Krenova Z, Jaffe R, Emile JF, Durham BH, Braier J, Charlotte F, Donadieu J, Cohen-Aubart F, Rodriguez-Galindo C, Allen C, Whitlock JA, Weitzman S, McClain KL, Haroche J, Diamond EL. Consensus recommendations for the diagnosis and clinical management of Rosai-Dorfman-Destombes disease. Blood. 2018;131(26):2877–90. https://doi.org/10.1182/blood-2018-03-839753. Epub 2018 May 2.
40. Sivak-Callcott JA, Rootman J, Rasmussen SL, Nugent RA, White VA, Paridaens D, Currie Z, Rose G, Clark B, McNab AA, Buffam FV, Neigel JM, Kazim M. Adult xanthogranulomatous disease of the orbit and ocular adnexa: new immunohistochemical findings and clinical review. Br J Ophthalmol. 2006;90(5):602–8. https://doi.org/10.1136/bjo.2005.085894.
41. Amrith S, Young SM, Goh PS, Wu B, Nga ME, Sundar G. Xanthogranuloma. In: Amrith S, Sundar G, Young S, editors. Ocular adnexal lesions. Singapore: Springer; 2019. https://doi.org/10.1007/978-981-13-3798-7_14.
42. Holbrook L, Brady R. McCune Albright syndrome. In: StatPearls [Internet]. Treasure Island (FL): StatPearls Publishing; 2021.

A Singular View: The Ocularist's Role in Eye Loss Restoration and Rehabilitation

Michael O. Hughes and Neill Hughes

1 The Fourth "O" in Eye Care: Ocularists

The successful rehabilitation of an individual who has lost an eye requires the attention of several eye care specialists: ophthalmologists, optometrists, opticians, and ocularists. Ocularists are eye care professionals whose task is to restore the appearance of a patient who has lost an eye to disease, trauma, or congenital malformation. Of course, eye removal is considered only after all vision-saving procedures are exhausted. Patients are generally referred by the surgeon who operated on the affected eye; they can tell the patients what to expect from the ocularist's art.

While the ocularist's work has long been considered an art form, the eye-maker's role in health care has rarely been clearly defined. An artificial eye maker creates custom ocular prostheses, or prosthetic eyes, but what we give patients can be much more: improved self-image and the confidence necessary to return to independent, productive living.

2 Introduction

The injury or surgery is the first of many challenges for a patient who loses an eye. The newly monocular may stumble when walking, have difficulty doing other everyday activities, and feel disoriented. These difficulties can last up to a year or more. Coday notes the challenges of eye loss as follows:

> Loss of a sighted eye results in loss of depth perception and a decrease in peripheral visual field. The sudden loss of vision in one eye can also result in psychological trauma and cosmetic deformity. The annual incidence of enucleation is 4.3 per 100,000. Although it has been estimated that 50,000 patients lose a sighted eye each year, the annual incidence of acquired monocular vision is probably much higher since any patient who has no light perception vision in one eye is monocularly blind. Patients who become blind in one eye as a result of glaucoma, optic neuropathies, proliferative diabetic retinopathy, intraocular tumors, expulsive choroidal hemorrhage, endophthalmitis, and chronic uveitis could all be considered to have acquired monocular vision if their other eye functions relatively well [1].

Ocularists are dedicated to caring mainly for monocular patients (Fig. 1). Members of the profession spend many hours with each patient in the course of designing, fitting, and maintaining prosthetic eyes. Patients often visit the ocularist just 4–6 weeks after eye removal surgery, when they are just beginning to adjust to the eye loss. Newly monocular patients and even many health care providers are unaware of the specific challenges of losing an eye.

3 The Main Visual Challenges of Monocularity

The sense of proprioception (knowing where one's limbs are) is unchanged after eye loss. However, monocular patients have lost an important source of spatial cues that those with binocular vision use constantly: stereopsis (depth perception). People who have never had stereopsis are adept at judging distance from monocular clues, according to neuro-ophthalmologist Steven A. Newman, M.D. He notes "Playing squash with a 1-eyed patient was not a problem, as he never had stereopsis and could easily judge the ball's distance. I also took care of one [individual] of the centers of UVA [University of Virginia] basketball who had no stereopsis, and it did not keep him from putting the ball through the hoop" [Personal communication, April 4, 2014].

Newly monocular patients, however, notice the loss of stereopsis the first time they reach for an object and miss it. Newman observes, "There is no question that patients who have become acutely monocular or have been used to stereopsis will have difficulties at the length of their arms, particularly with reaching for objects, pouring objects, etc., although, over time, this will gradually improve" [Personal communication, April 4, 2014]. It takes practice to reconcile objects' physical locations with monocular perception.

M. O. Hughes (✉) · N. Hughes
Artificial Eye Clinic, Vienna, VA, USA
e-mail: eye226@aol.com

B. V. Chawla, M. E. Aronow (eds.), *Global Perspectives in Ocular Oncology*, https://doi.org/10.1007/978-3-031-08250-4_12

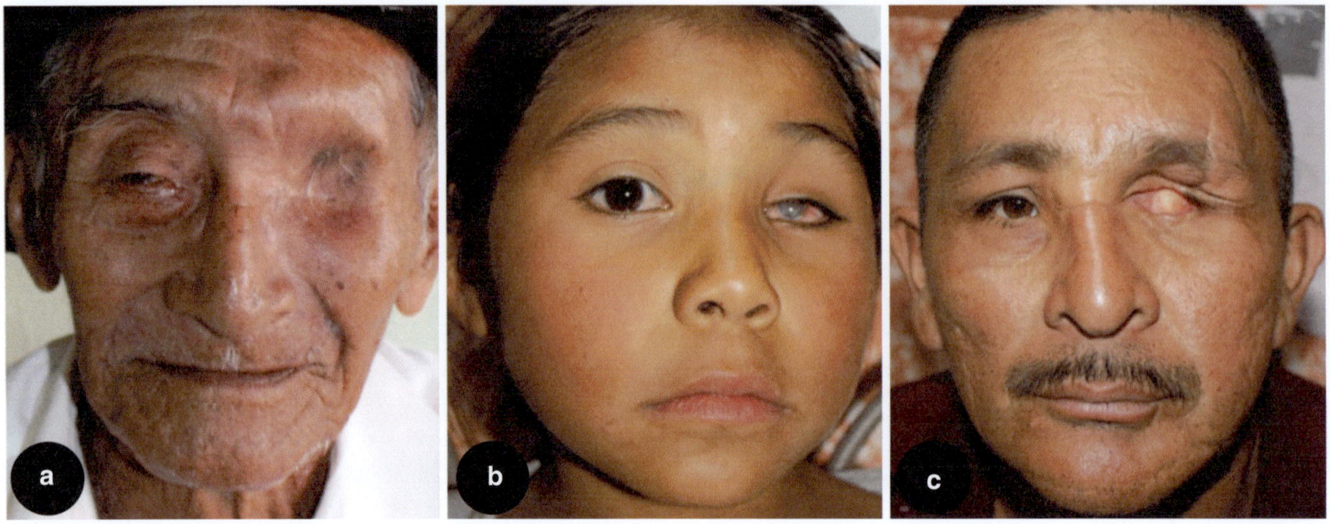

Fig. 1 Typical causes of eye loss include: (**a**) exenteration, (**b**) blindness, and (**c**) enucleation. Patients with all these conditions require prosthetic restoration. Of course, the cause of eye loss is not always as obvious as shown here

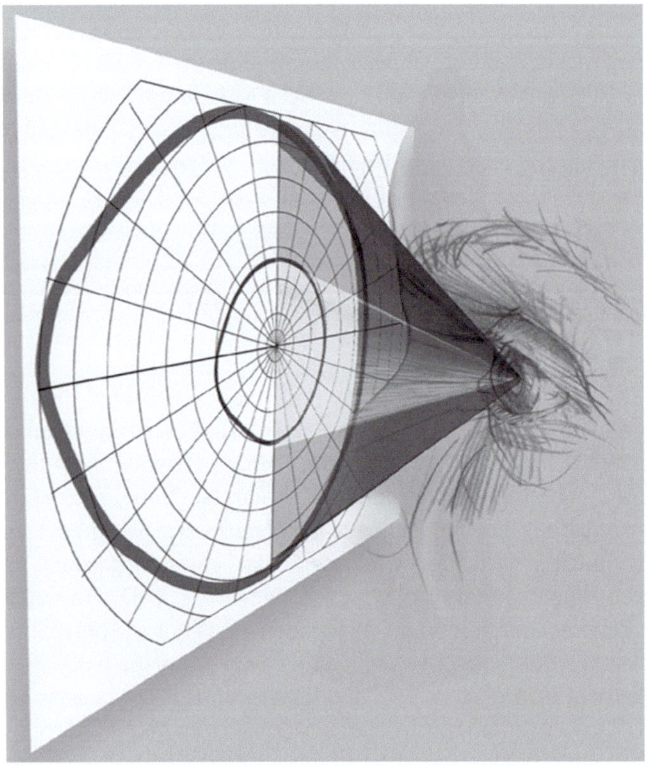

Fig. 2 The central and peripheral visual fields may be different shapes

In his book A Singular View, written long after his own adjustment to monocularity, Frank B. Brady includes tips and advice on compensating for these losses. Brady found he could engage in most of the activities he had done with both eyes once he compensated for depth of field. He coped so well that, using modern instruments, he was able to pursue his passion for aviation and even fly solo again [2]. Brady was not alone; aviator Wiley Post adjusted to eye loss so well that he made the first solo flight around the world and set many other aviation records [3].

4 Visual Field Loss

A binocular field of vision includes information from the area where the eyes' visual fields overlap. As all eye care providers know, the brain assembles images from signals sent by the eye. When 2 synchronized fields are presented to the visual pathways, the brain will construct a 3-dimensional experience from the combined fields (Fig. 2) [4]. As Brady points out, the normal horizontal visual field is 180°, but a monocular person has only up to 160° because the nose gets in the way of the single working eye (Fig. 3) [4]. With these deficits, the patient with one eye sees as if they are looking through a window at a 2-dimensional picture, rather than experiencing it in 3 dimensions.

A newly monocular person may experience the world as if surrounded by optical illusions. They do not receive all the visual cues that a binocular person does because the eyes normally work together. (Some 15%–18% of binocular people do have limited depth perception) [5]. For example, the brain usually processes the difference in field signals from both retinas to alert a person that something is approaching [6]. For monocular people, although the functional eye sends a signal to the brain, there is no longer any difference to pick up [5]. Thus, monocular people are at risk of injuries that people with both eyes can easily avoid.

The monocular patient must learn to identify risks by training and experiment. Moving the remaining eye can also help the brain adapt by sending it more than one image of the

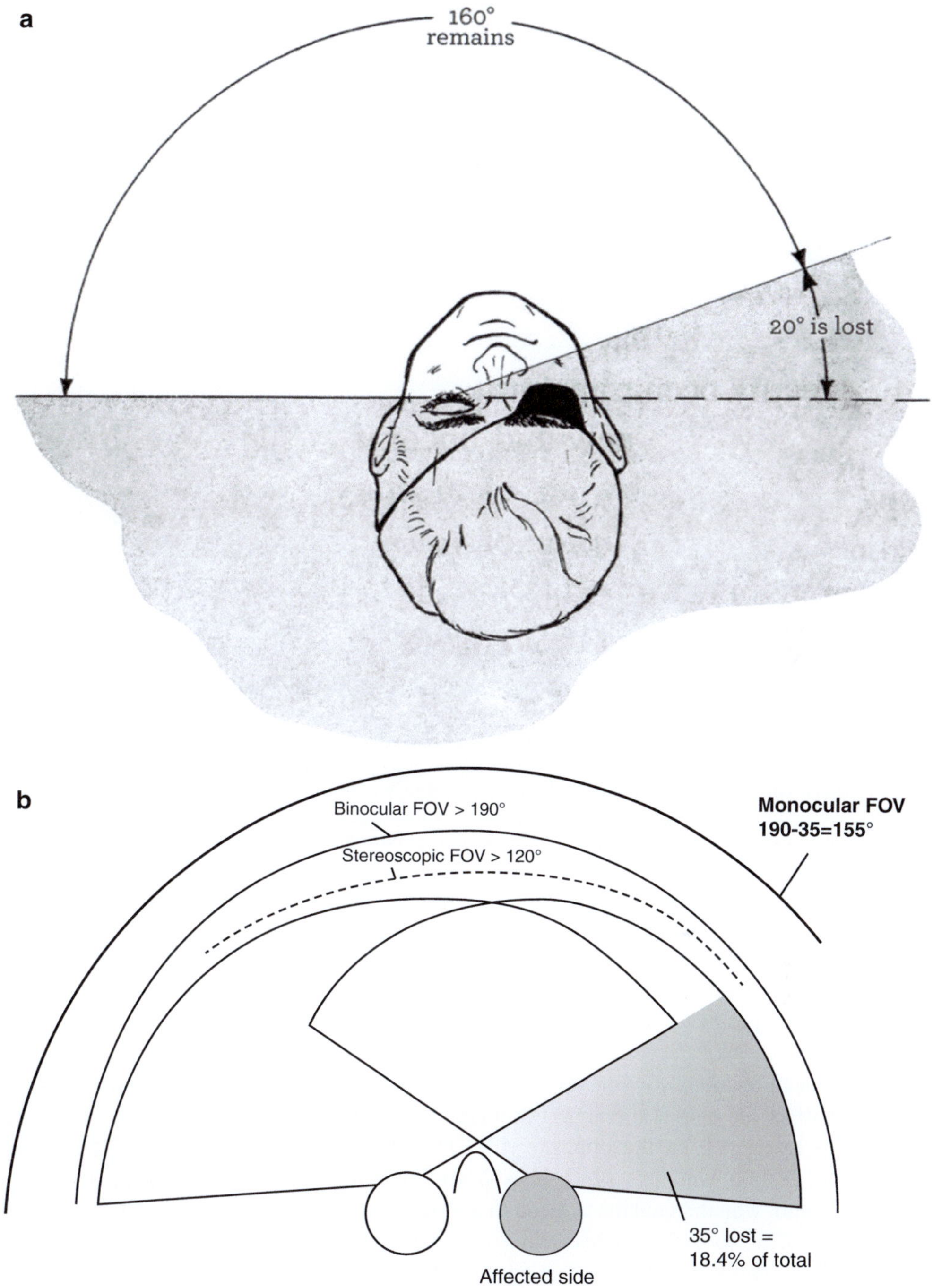

Fig. 3 The field of view (FOV) is the area visible to the eye. Binocular humans have an FOV of about 190° and can see about 120° in stereo using both eyes. Each eye sees about 60° toward the nose and 95° to the side. Monocular FOV is 35° less than binocular FOV (95–60 = 35). This means that 35°, or 18.4% of total binocular FOV, is lost on the side of the eye loss. While the FOV is sometimes simplified to 180°, it is reasonable to conclude that maximum FOV of 190° is only available at the straight lateral, not at cheek or brow

surrounding environment [2]. This can be done by moving the head. Movement in any direction will help, but because this movement can be hard to do subtly, a vertical movement may be less obvious and appear more positive (Fig. 4).

5 Areas of Visual Field Limitation

The normal monocular visual field (VF) can be imagined as a cone extending beyond potential barriers, such as the bridge of the nose. The central visual field (what is viewed directly in the macula) accounts for only 15° of total vision [6]. Peripheral vision (normally 160–180°) (Fig. 5a) is most affected in monocular patients. It is impinged by the surrounding anatomical structures of the nose, brow, and cheek (Fig. 5b). The most central occlusion is the eyelids and lashes, which present a blurred outline. While the lower eyelid can flatten the inferior VF in down-gaze, both the upper and lower eyelids and lashes are usually seen; they also function to dispel reflected glare. As visual fields are usually tested, the area of the face that is visible defines the outer extent of the VF. In our practice, we refer to this as the facial

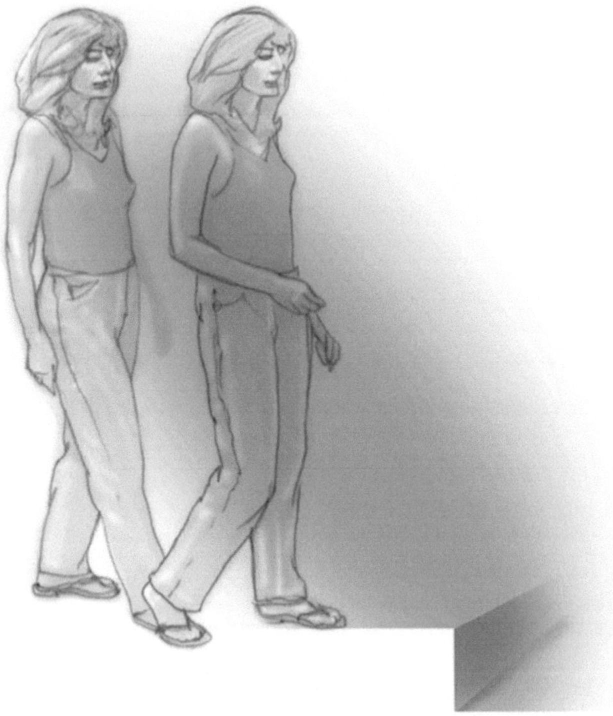

Fig. 4 Moving the eyes is the best way to gather subjective information about the environment. Monocular people can add movement by moving their heads. This figure shows a monocular person raising her chin slightly as she approaches a step. Depending on cultural norms, vertical head movement may be more socially acceptable and more subtle than moving the head back and forth horizontally

visual field deficit (FVFD) (Fig. 5c). It may be a different shape from the tested visual fields because it is determined by a dynamic, moving eye rather than a fixed central position, as in static perimetry. Figure 5d shows an example of the FVFD, which varies according to the shape and size of individual facial features.

In the FVFD, the nose is the largest problem area, as the sole barrier to the VF on the opposite side. The extreme example of dealing with this obstacle is from Frederico, Duke of Urbino, who directed his surgeon to remove the glabellar region of his nose after the loss of his right eye (Fig. 6). Newman notes that while VF loss has more to do with the location of retinal receptors in the remaining eye than with facial anatomy, it is possible that anatomical features, such as the nose, prominent brows, or sunken eyes, can reduce the visual field if the lids or the brow impinges close to the visual axis [Personal communication, April 4, 2014]. How much anatomical features impinge on VF depends on individual anatomy, and it is rare that patients are aware of this impingement.

6 Solutions to Visual Field Limitations

While anatomical visual field barriers are unavoidable, ocularists can avoid adding to the monocular patient's burden by helping patients find appliances that avoid further obstruction. Eyeglasses or facial prostheses that impinge on the visual fields are simply a new obstacle to monocular patients.

Some monocular patients may also wear facial prostheses. Patients may wear eyeglasses with these prostheses to disguise the seams of the appliance or help to hold it in place. Figure 7 shows both standard ocular prostheses in various materials [a–c] and oculofacial prostheses [d–f]. For monocular patients, eyeglasses also help protect the remaining natural eye. However, both the glasses and any facial prostheses are also VF barriers, so it is important to select frames for minimal interference with the patient's VF.

Unfortunately, most eyeglass frames are designed primarily for fashion or fit (Fig. 8), not to minimize VF limitations. Tips for choosing eyeglasses include limiting frame elements that fall within the FVFD (usually in the nasal inferior area). Though some elements of the eyeglass frames will be within the FVFD (usually nasal-inferior), those elements in the VF should be limited. (Figure 7e shows bulky eyeglass frames that help hide the margins of the prosthesis but may also limit the VF). The brain unconsciously fills in most of the details from the blocked area, just as it does in the blind spot over the optic disk.

Most tests of vision and VFs are done to reveal changes in the visual fields over time, rather than to demarcate the FVFD. It may be necessary to refer the patient to an ophthalmologist or optometrist to delineate the full VF. Perimetry (the demarcation of VFs) can now be performed by an automated instrument in less than 3 min, though full VF testing takes much longer. Alternatively, the patient's FVFD may be evaluated and drawn directly on the face with a temporary water-soluble marker, as shown in Fig. 5d.

Ocularists and other eye care professionals may also share practical guidance to help monocular patients compensate for visual field deficits, as shown in Fig. 9. Monocular patients and those with other visual impairments may find digital media more challenging than audio or large print instructions. This is not necessarily caused by monocularity itself. In our practice, we have observed that patients with eye loss often belong to older age groups that may use digital media less frequently than the young or working-age populations.

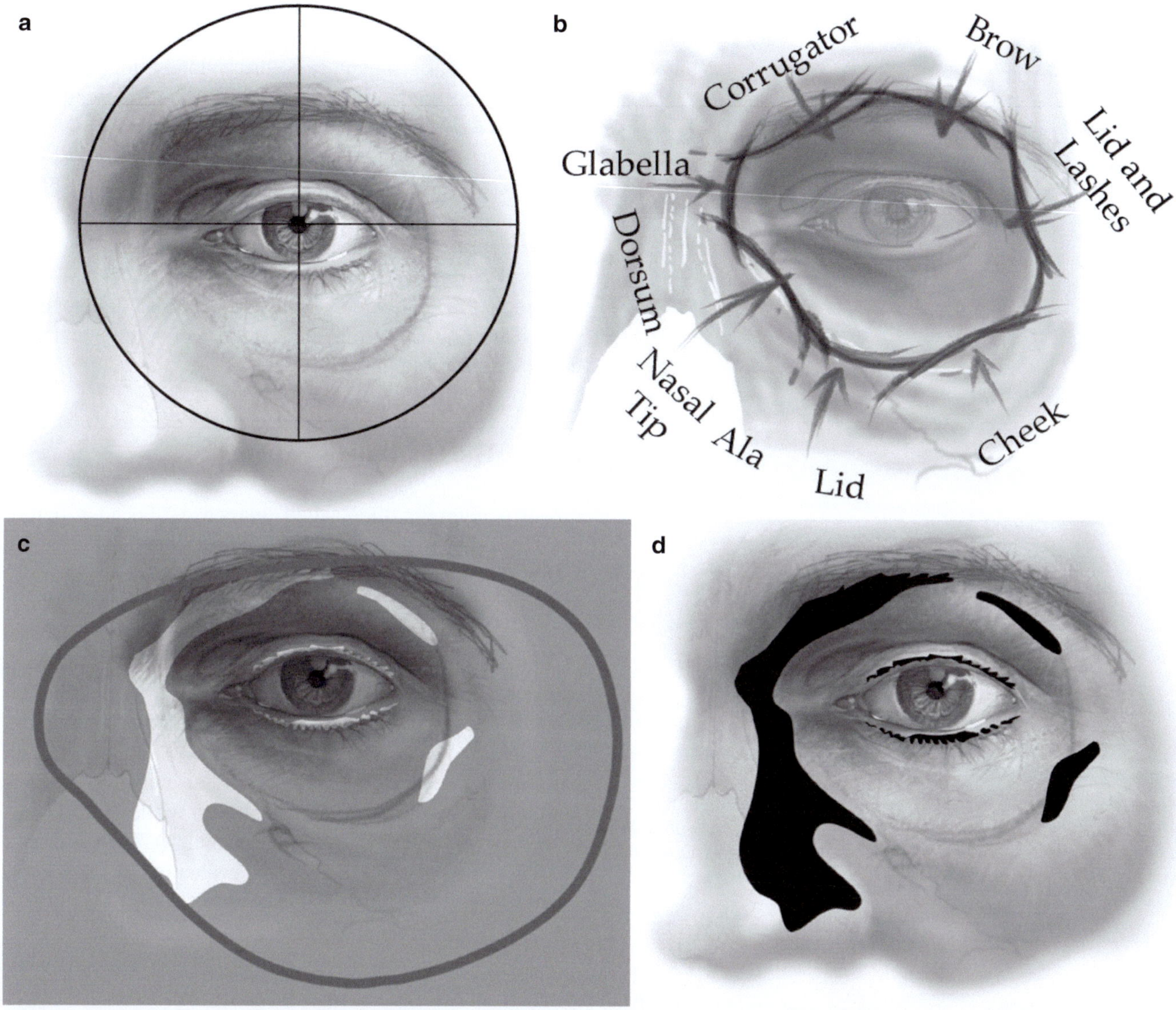

Fig. 5 The visual field (VF) and facial visual field deficits (FVFD). (**a**) The theoretical cone of the VF as centered on the pupil. (**b**) The anatomical structures shown impinge on the VF of a single eye. (**c**) Facial visual field deficits (FVFD) are caused by anatomical barriers inside the visual field. (**d**) FVFD mapped on the skin. The deficits are different for each patient. Ocularists, anaplastologists, and optometrists should avoid prosthetics or appliances that enlarge these deficits, if possible. The area of the eyeglass frame is subtracted from the FVFD shown

A surprising observation is that quite often, even surrounding a difficult diagnosis and treatment, many individuals are more concerned with their appearance following eye loss (evisceration, enucleation, exenteration) surgery than their medical condition.

7 Reconstruction Following Eye Loss

While evisceration, enucleation, and exenteration all entail the removal of eye tissue, enucleation, the removal of the eyeball from the orbit, remains the most common procedure. Evisceration and enucleation are generally followed by insertion of an ocular implant. To be effective, the implant must reasonably reproduce the volume, position, and motility of the natural eye; it must retain a covering suitable for lubrication, and it must neither migrate nor extrude.

The size, material, and placement of the implant depend on the surgeon's work and the patient's needs. Generally, a smaller implant is used when it is placed within the eyeball or its fascial capsule (Tenon's capsule) or when it is wrapped in another material. To increase covering tissue thickness, the implant is often placed behind the posterior Tenon's capsule (see Fig. 10).

Proper sizing of the implant is crucial: too small an implant will cause possible migration, enophthalmos, or a

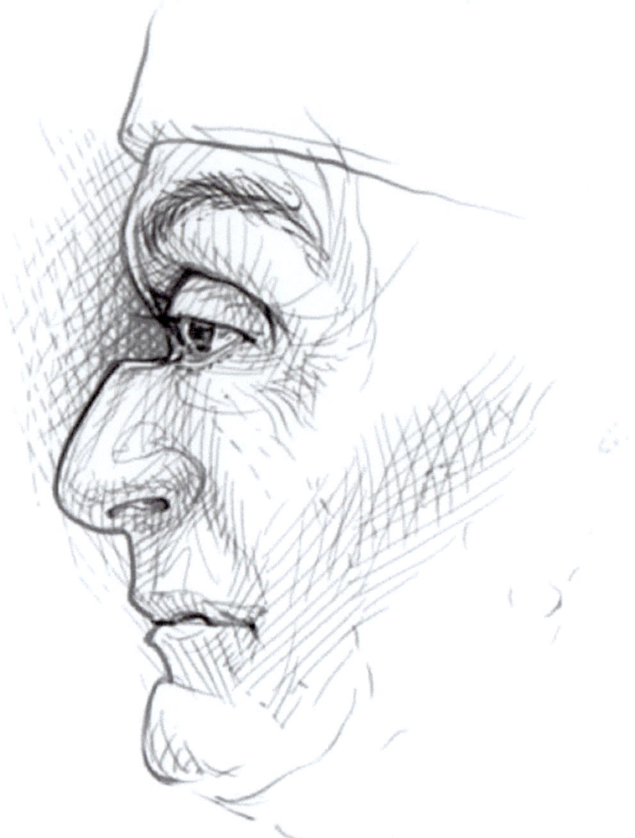

Fig. 6 Frederic, Duke of Urbino, had the glabellar portion of his nose removed to reduce the visual field deficit caused by his eye loss. We cannot recommend this elective procedure. (Illustration by C.A. Luce based on four known portraits)

deep sulcus. If too large an implant is used, pressure on the front of the implant may increase the risk of wound dehiscence, erosion, or implant exposure and infection. It is ideal for the ocular implant to provide 65–70% of the volume of the lost eye, with the remaining volume taken up by the ocular prosthesis.

In evisceration, the sclera remains, while in enucleation, the extraocular eye muscles are either attached to the implant or cross-sutured and the anterior tissues (Tenon's and conjunctiva) closed without tension. Two of the more difficult challenges for ophthalmologists and ocularists are superior sulcus deformities from inadequate orbital volume and eyelid ptosis or laxity.

8 The Ocularist's Work

Prosthetic eyes are often called "glass eyes" because, before the development of polymethyl-methacrylate plastics in the 1940s, prosthetic eyes and ocular implants were generally made of hand-blown glass, a technique that dates to the mid-1800s. (Cryolite glass is still used in parts of Eastern Europe).

The initial visit to the ocularist usually takes place 6 weeks after surgery. Most ocularists begin by obtaining an alginate (gel) impression of the eye socket, the sensitive tissue which will house the prosthetic eye. (Although this is a painless procedure, some younger patients may find the one-minute setting time uncomfortably long.) While careful post-surgery observation by other professional "Os" in eye care is often assumed to provide adequate evaluation of the socket,

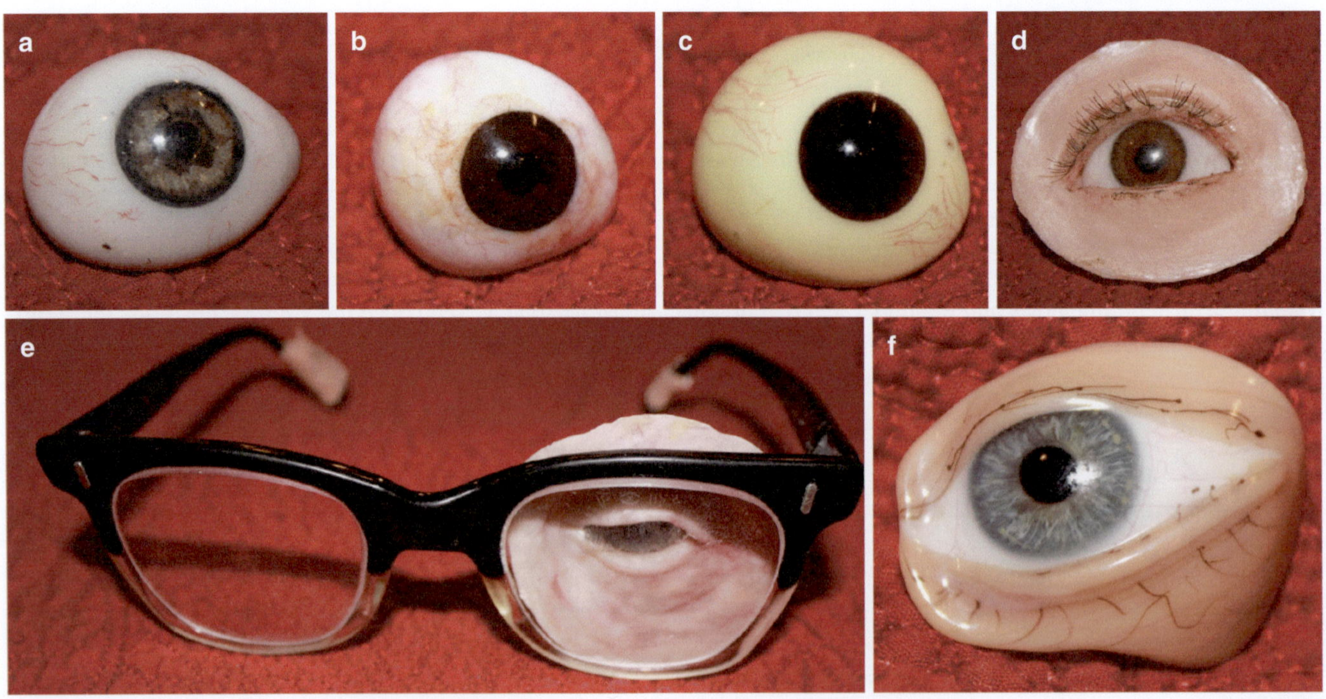

Fig. 7 Common prostheses and materials, including: (**a**) silicone ocular prosthesis, (**b**) acrylic (PMMA) ocular prosthesis, (**c**) glass (cryolite) prosthesis, (**d**) silicone orbital prosthesis, (**e**) acrylic orbital prosthesis attached to eyeglasses, and (**f**) glass orbital prosthesis

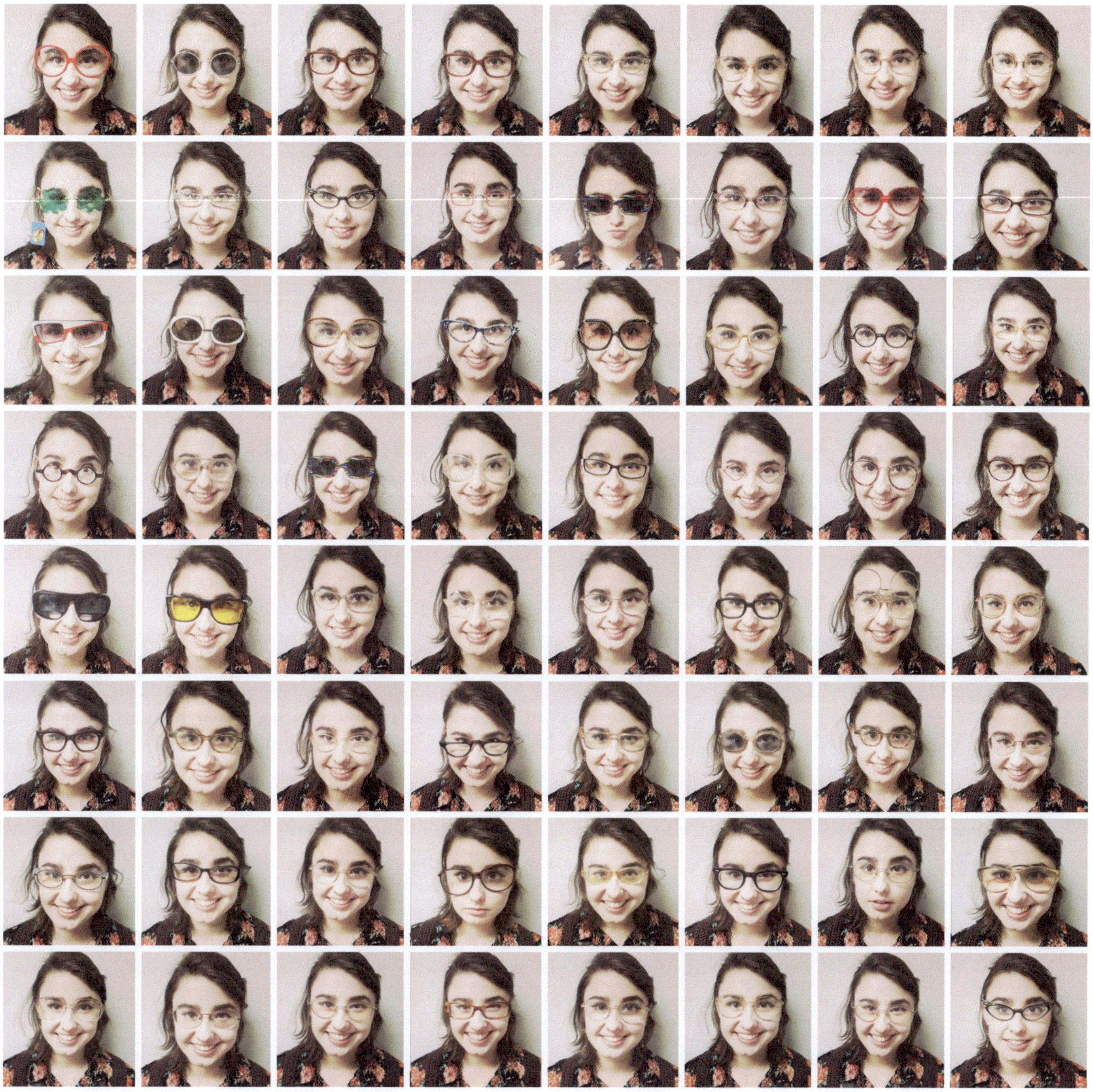

Fig. 8 This collage shows a patient with a prosthetic right eye wearing some of the many eyeglass styles available. As the photos show, eyeglasses can complement a patient's appearance and camouflage eye conditions, including ptosis and superior sulcus problems, but frames can also obstruct peripheral vision. Style may take priority over function, especially for younger patients. The ocularist and optometrist can help the patient balance these priorities

many irregularities are only discovered when the alginate mold (or "impression") of the healed socket made in the ocularist's office is examined. Though most swelling has usually subsided by this time, only after 3 or 4 months is the healed socket's shape stabilized.

Duplicating the socket shape precisely reduces irritation of the conjunctiva and maximizes the movement of the finished eye. When the proper fit is achieved, the lubricating tear system often operates normally. After the impression and fitting of a wax pattern, the resulting shape is cast in plastic.

Several factors are important in successfully fitting a patient with a prosthetic eye. For the most natural appearance, it is essential to simulate the iris of the companion eye.

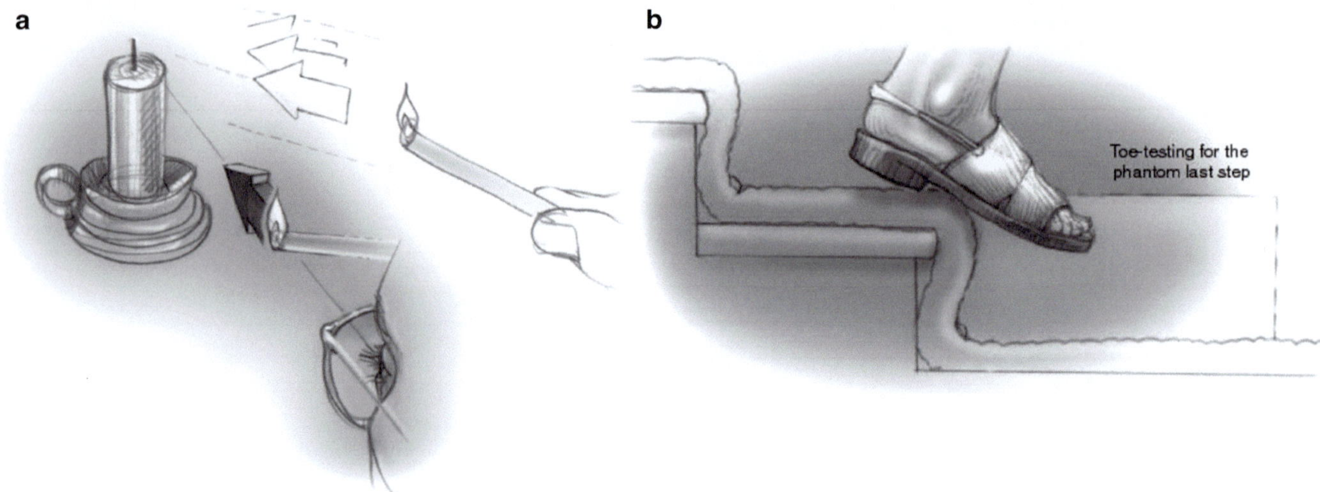

Fig. 9 The ocularist is a source of practical guidance on learning to live with one eye. For example, (**a**) Lining up the working eye with a target like the candle shown here can help a monocular person reach that target correctly. (**b**) Monocular people must learn new ways to navigate even familiar spaces, such as using the feet to feel for the end of a staircase

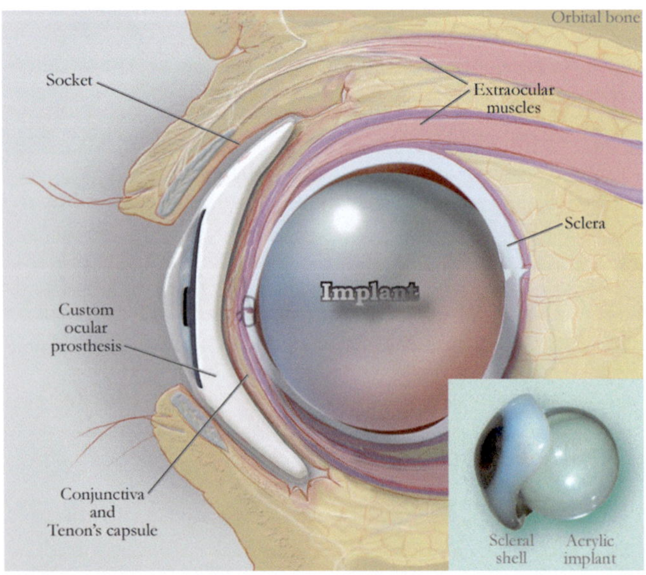

Fig. 10 Illustration depicts a left post-evisceration eye socket in the parasagittal section. The implant replacing the volume of the eye is placed inside the sclera. In front of the repositioned conjunctiva, the custom-made prosthesis is placed under the eyelids

This requires a 3-dimensional effect. Because the human iris is living tissue, bathed with ocular fluids and moving naturally, the ocularist can only aim to simulate its appearance, not duplicate it completely. Hand painting both the iris and sclera using a combination of pigments and liquid plastics is the most common practice in replicating the eye with a prosthesis.

After fitting the eye, the ocularist hand-paints the iris and sclera using direct observation of the patient's unaffected eye, mixing a variety of pigments, lacquers, or oils onto the acrylic shape bonded with liquid acrylic (see Fig. 11). The painting is sealed with acrylic, and a cornea of clear plastic is cast and cured under heat and pressure. Polishing the eye to a flawless surface ensures there will be smooth eyelid movement and no recesses to accommodate flora.

Mass-produced, digitally printed eyes with painted or digitally printed irises have become increasingly popular in recent years. While digital printing is not new, the quality has improved greatly from its earliest days. While it is virtually impossible to create a mirror image of the companion eye due to the infinite array of iris colors and textures, digital irises provide excellent approximate matches. Minimal touch-up and overpainting allow an even closer match while saving time for the practitioner. Digital iris buttons may be most appreciated in cases where patients need bilateral ocular prostheses and 2 matched irises are needed.

When the finished eye is inserted, the patient is given a mirror to see the restored image (see Fig. 12). Care of the prosthetic eye is simple; new patients are often surprised to learn that they need not remove it for routine washing. A cleaning and polishing by the ocularist during each annual examination are sufficient.

Refinements in surgical procedures, ocular implants (including materials) and custom hand-painted prostheses have made great improvements in the cosmesis and comfort of prosthetic eye wearers.

9 Conclusion

Patients with acquired monocular vision often experience a lengthy process of adjustment to monocularity and prosthetic restoration. Health care professionals must accom-

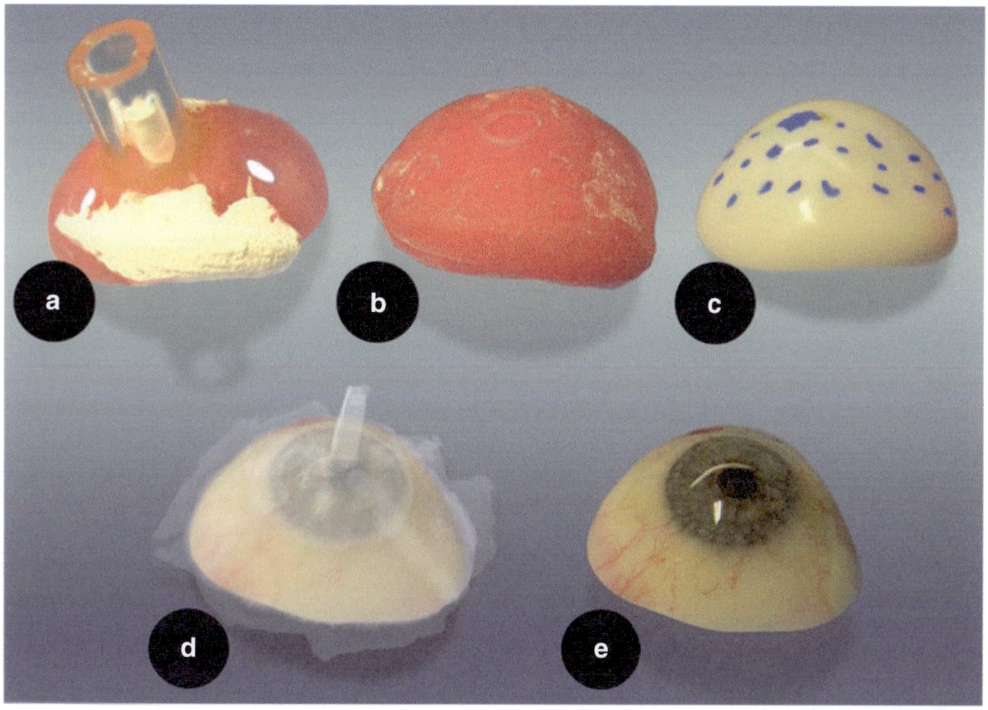

Fig. 11 The process of fabricating an artificial eye in acrylic, as seen in stages: (**a**) The gel impression (negative) of the socket. (**b**) The wax pattern cast from the impression and fitted further. (**c**) An acrylic shape sized to the socket and refined as to gaze. (**d**) The painted prosthesis just out of the mold and before polishing. (**e**) The final prosthesis ready to insert

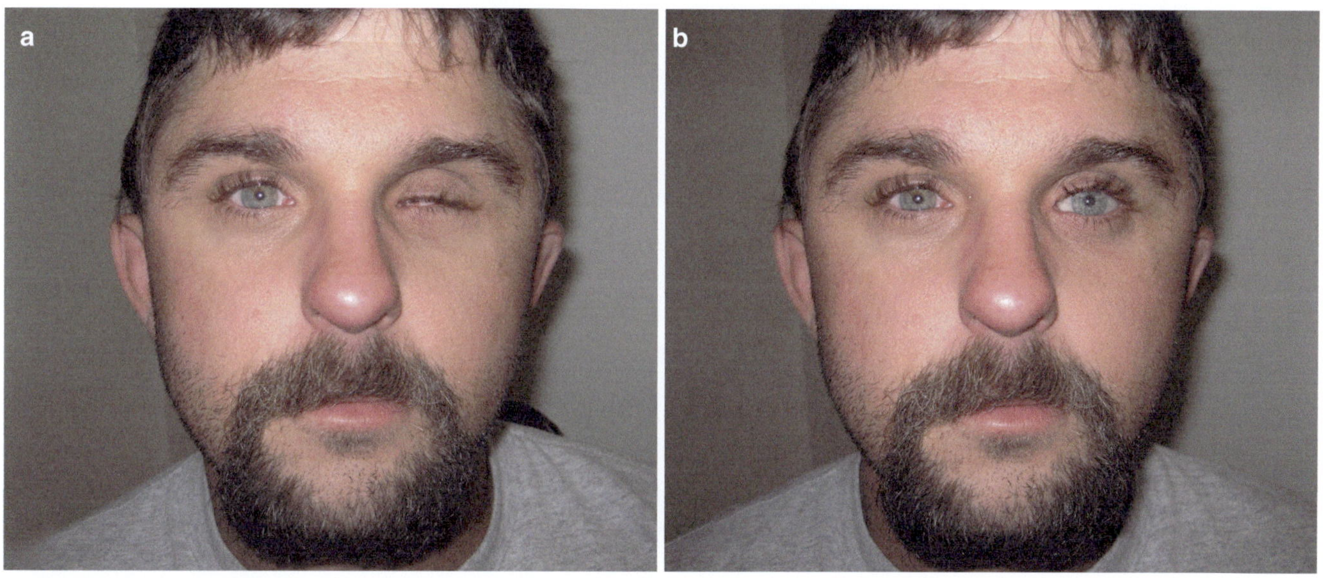

Fig. 12 Monocular patient with a successful OS prosthesis

modate these patients' needs as they prescribe and create appliances for functional and cosmetic rehabilitation, including ocular and maxillofacial prostheses and eyeglasses. Anything applied to the face must limit the visual field as little as possible, whether it is an appliance or a necessary eyeglass frame. As formal studies may never be published, it is suggested that any appliance that might impinge on a monocular patient's visual field should be tested, possibly in consultation with an eye care provider, documented directly on the face, or both. With time, attention to detail, and awareness of educational resources, anaplastologists and ocularists can serve patients' needs for as complete a functional and cosmetic recovery as possible.

References

1. Coday MP, Warner MA, Jahrling KV, Rubin PAD. Acquired monocular vision: functional consequences from the patient's perspective. Ophth Plast Reconstr Surg. 2002;18:56–63.
2. Newman SA. Wiley post and visual standards for pilots. Surv Ophthalmol. 2014;59(3):373–4. https://doi.org/10.1016/j.survophthal.2013.08.004. Epub 2013 Dec 22.
3. Brady F. A singular view: the art of seeing with one eye. 1st ed. Oradell, NJ: Medical Economics Co.; 1972.
4. Montés-Micó R. Prevalence of general dysfunctions in binocular vision. Ann Ophthalmol. 2001;33:205–8.
5. Kandel E, Schwartz J, Jessell T. Principles of neural science. 4th ed. New York: McGraw-Hill; 2000. p. 515–20.
6. Journal of Ocular Prosthetics. American Society of Ocularists. http://www.ocularist.org/resources_journal.asp. Accessed 9 November 2010.

Part III

Current Concepts in Ocular Oncology

Guidelines and Recommendations for Retinoblastoma Screening

Doaa Elfadaly, Mandeep S. Sagoo, and M. Ashwin Reddy

1 Introduction

Retinoblastoma is the most common intraocular cancer in childhood. The incidence is estimated to range from 1 in 13,915 to 18,000 live births [1–3]. There are two forms of the disease: heritable and non-heritable.

Approximately 15% of the unilateral [4] and all bilateral cases have the heritable form. Only a minority of the heritable cases will have a family history and it appears that most of the heritable cases are the result of de novo mutations (pathogenic variants) [5]. Clinically, it is difficult to distinguish between the heritable and non-heritable forms, though, high-penetrant germline carriers of *RB1* pathogenic variants have an earlier age of onset and more tumors than the one tumor in one eye associated with non-germline carriers of *RB1* pathogenic variants [6].

Children with a family history of retinoblastoma are at elevated risk for retinoblastoma and require surveillance for the development of retinoblastoma tumors [7]. Early diagnosis, when the tumors are small, maximizes survival and vision outcomes and reduces the need for chemotherapy, enucleation, and radiotherapy [8]. Screening for retinoblastoma in at-risk individuals (offspring or siblings of the proband) takes two forms: genetic and clinical screening. Results from the former inform the need for the latter.

D. Elfadaly
Retinoblastoma Service, Royal London Hospital, London, UK

Department of Ophthalmology, Faculty of Medicine, Minia University, Minia, Egypt
e-mail: doaa.elfadaly@nhs.net

M. S. Sagoo
Retinoblastoma Service, Royal London Hospital, London, UK

National Institute for Health Research Biomedical Research Centre at Moorfields Eye Hospital NHS Foundation Trust and UCL Institute of Opthalmology, London, UK
e-mail: mandeep.sagoo1@nhs.net

M. A. Reddy (✉)
Retinoblastoma Service, Royal London Hospital, London, UK

Queen Mary University of London, London, UK
e-mail: Ashwin.reddy4@nhs.net

2 Genetic Testing

Genetic testing allows for the identification of the child who needs to be assessed, thus saving children who will never develop tumors from multiple examinations under anesthesia and the potential risks from anesthetic agents on the developing brain [9–11]. In addition, tumors can be detected early so that focal therapies such as laser and cryotherapy can be used to treat small tumors.

This starts with performing comprehensive *RB1* genetic testing of a family member with retinoblastoma (the proband) to identify heritability; if it is heritable, the causative pathogenic variant is specifically evaluated in at-risk relatives [8]. At-risk relatives who do not carry the *RB1* pathogenic variant found in their parent or sibling require no further specific retinoblastoma screening, as their risk status can be modified to population risk. Moreover, the average savings in direct costs from these avoided clinical examinations substantially exceed the cost of genetic testing [12]. However, in cases where the pathogenetic *Rb1* variant is found in a relative or where genetic testing is non-contributory, clinical screening should be undertaken. Genetic testing can give prognostic information about the number of tumors in each eye [6] with a median of 3 tumors per eye noted in carriers of high-penetrant *RB1* pathogenic variants.

3 Risks for Each Individual Depend on Genetic Testing and Clinical Presentation

All bilaterally affected children carry an RB1 pathogenic variant (even in the event that no RB1 pathogenic variant is found in blood due to limitations of genetic testing) and are consid-

B. V. Chawla, M. E. Aronow (eds.), *Global Perspectives in Ocular Oncology*, https://doi.org/10.1007/978-3-031-08250-4_13

ered high risk. In addition to the treatment of their bilateral disease, they benefit from surveillance of the retinae to detect more developing retinoblastoma tumors in infancy, and lifelong surveillance for second cancers. Unilaterally affected children without a close family history have 15–19% [13] likelihood of carrying an underlying RB1 pathogenic variant.

Highly sensitive genetic testing can determine which of the at-risk children are at a high risk of developing retinoblastoma. If no RB1 pathogenic variant is found, there is <1% residual risk of an unidentified RB1 pathogenic variant or undetectable mosaicism.

Once the *RB1* pathogenic variant is known in a proband with bilateral or unilateral retinoblastoma, their offspring or siblings who test positive for that specific *RB1* pathogenic variant have a high risk of manifesting disease depending on the penetrance for retinoblastoma, as well as a lifelong risk for second cancers [14]. Probands with unilateral retinoblastoma where no *RB1* pathogenic variant is found in blood and with no tumor available for testing carry a residual risk of undetectable mosaicism. Surveillance protocols to monitor for retinoblastoma development in the other eye, and in siblings and offspring, are guided by these calculations [15, 16].

When the blood test is negative for both the *RB1* pathogenic variants identified in the tumor of unilateral probands, the proband still has residual small risk of undetected mosaicism. However, since mosaicism cannot be inherited, the proband's parents, siblings, and offspring who test negative for the two specific *RB1* pathogenic variants detected in the proband's tumor require no additional ophthalmic cancer surveillance [17].

4 Screening Protocols

A consensus statement about retinoblastoma screening was published in 2018 and it was agreed that early and frequent clinical screening is required for babies at elevated risk, and the examinations may be spaced out over time as children grow older [15]. They recommended screening for at-risk children from birth up to the age of 7 years. After the age of 7 years, no further screening of asymptomatic children is recommended.

Screening strategies are determined by the accuracy of the genetics laboratory that performs the testing. As a result, low accuracy will require more screening under anesthesia compared to units that have a higher accuracy. At our unit at the Royal London Hospital [16], a screening program based on genetic testing was developed based on genetic risk stratification into high- and low-risk groups. High frequency of screening early in life is recommended and the schedule differs for low- and high-risk individuals. Cessation of screening is also different according to the genetic risk: in low-risk patients, clinical screening is not required beyond 3 years of age, while high-risk patients continue to be seen initially by a retinoblastoma specialist but can be followed by a local ophthalmologist. Once out of the peak period, the latter can be annual until the age of 16. This was found appropriate for all children as the current molecular genetic screening techniques can detect up to 96.6% of *RB1* pathogenic variants in bilateral/heritable retinoblastoma and it was shown that 18% of sporadic, unilateral patients carried detectable mutations [18]. Shared care of children until that age of 16 allows for genetic counselling to be given to children as they transition to adulthood and advice regarding the risks of their own children developing retinoblastoma. Other centers adopt prenatal molecular diagnosis with early-term delivery if the *RB1* pathogenic variant is identified by amniocentesis [17].

Table 1 Clinical screening protocols for offspring or siblings of probands with retinoblastoma, stratified by genetic testing into high risk and low risk

Age of sibling or offspring	High risk (or RB1 pathogenic variant carrier)	Low risk
2 weeks	Awake/examination under anaesthesia screening by 2 weeks	
4 weeks		Awake screening by 4 weeks
Up to 6 months	4 weekly	6 weekly
6–12 months	Every 4–6 weeks	9 and 12 months
1–2 years	Every 2 months until 18 months Then 21 months and 24 months	16 and 22 months
2–3 years	Every 4 months	Every 6 months
After 3 years	Stop, unless family history of late onset	Stop

At our center, children are divided into high-risk (>1% risk) and low-risk (1% or less) categories, and our current screening protocols are summarized in (Table 1). Figure 1 shows a flow chart for screening children at risk based on the laterality of their relative with retinoblastoma. It is essential to audit the findings on a regular basis to ensure that no child is missed. In low-risk cases, it is possible to downgrade clinical screening from examinations under anesthesia to awake examinations, depending on the preference of the clinical team.

5 Examination Under Anesthesia Versus Non-Sedated Office Examination

The risk of continuing examinations under anesthesia should be weighed against the risk of developing retinoblastoma. Parents are sometimes concerned that screening under anesthesia might be associated with neuro-development sequelae [11]. A parent whose older children previously may have been screened without any tumors being found may be skeptical about the number of examinations that are necessary, though

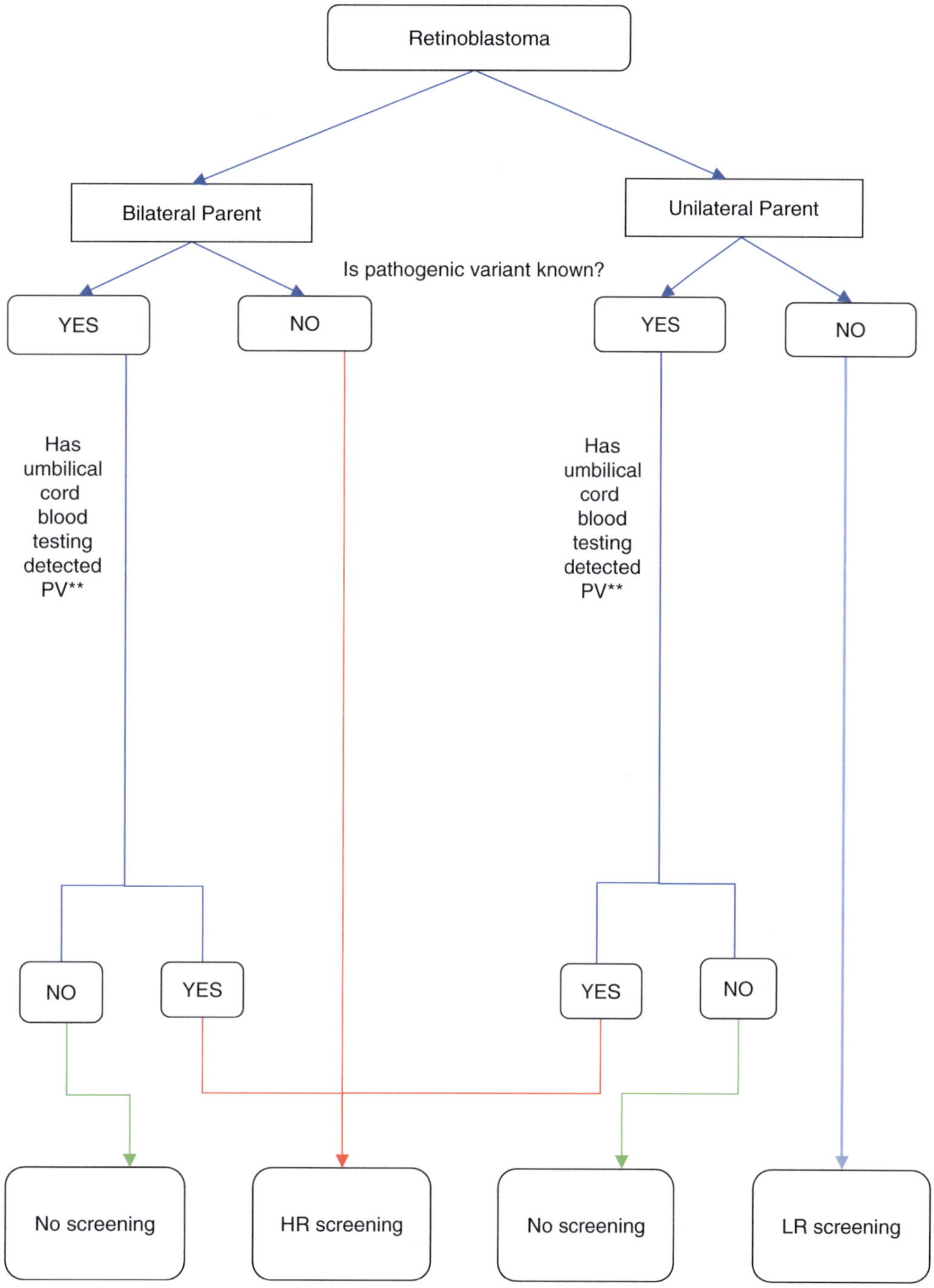

Fig. 1 Flow diagram showing screening protocol based on laterality. *PV* Pathogenic variant, *HR* High risk, *LR* Low risk. **Umbilical cord blood testing for neonate at risk

having an unaffected older sibling is no guarantee that the younger sibling will not develop the disease. Therefore, knowing the exact number of screening examinations is important.

The decision regarding the examination method (examinations under anesthesia versus non-sedated office examination) is debatable and best decided by the clinician in discussion with the patient's family. Skalet et al. in 2018 [15] published management guidelines for childhood screening for retinoblastoma (Fig. 2), where office examinations were recommended early in life with anesthetic examinations after 8 weeks of age.

6 Risks of Developing Retinoblastoma in the Absence of Genetic Testing

Genetic testing is not always available in many low-income countries. In this situation, clinicians should evaluate the likelihood that a child has heritable retinoblastoma, based on clinical presentation and family history.

In this context, a patient "at risk" is defined as a person with a family history of retinoblastoma in a parent, sibling, or first- or second-degree relative. While risk status can be stratified as high risk or low risk [16], another stratification

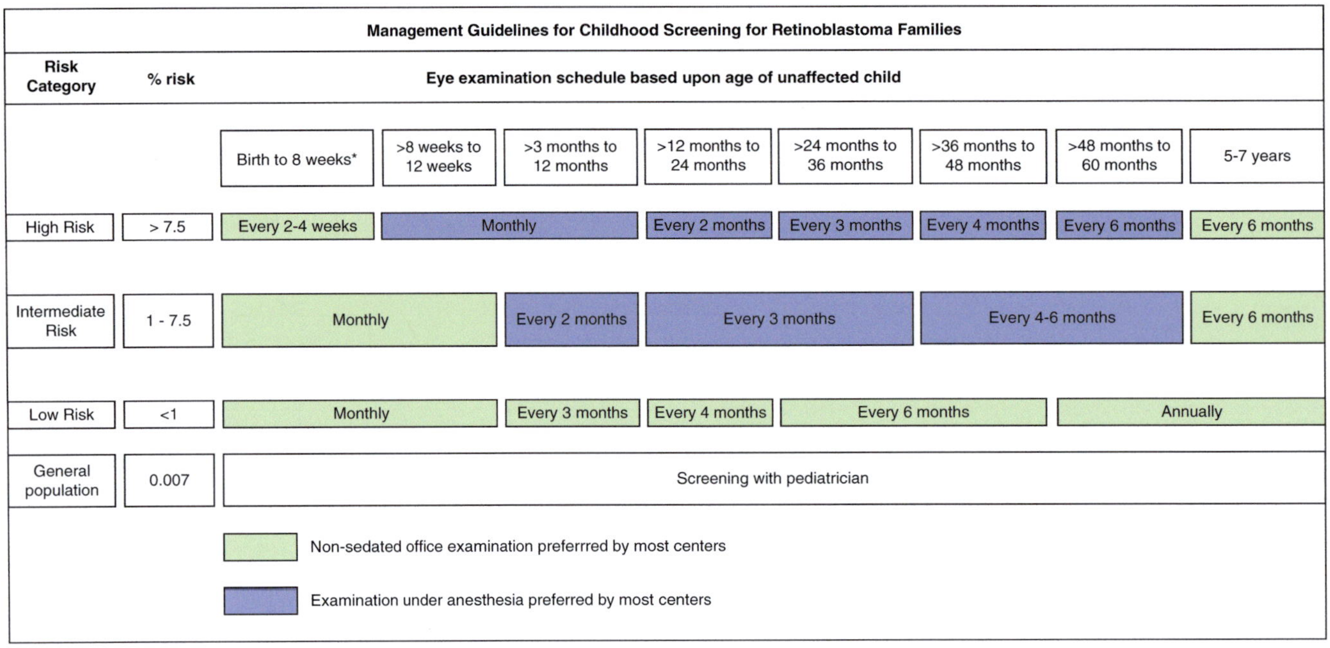

Fig. 2 Management guidelines for childhood screening for retinoblastoma suggested by a consensus group [15]

Table 2 Empiric risks of developing retinoblastoma in siblings and offspring of probands with retinoblastoma

	More than one affected person in family	One person with bilateral or multifocal retinoblastoma	One person with unilateral unifocal retinoblastoma
Siblings	50%	5%	1%
Offspring	50%	50%	5–10%
More distant relatives	Need to assess pedigree, may be at risk	Not at increased risk	Not at risk

1% = low risk; >1% = high risk

was adopted by a large consensus group of pediatric oncologists and ophthalmologists [15], where they stratified the risk into high, intermediate, and low risk, and calculated a pretest risk for RB1 pathogenic variants in family members of the affected child with retinoblastoma. If genetic testing is not possible, empiric risks are given in (Table 2). These figures can be used for genetic advice to families.

Clues to heritable retinoblastoma include age (median of 15 months), bilaterality, being multifocal, a family history of retinoblastoma, and the presence of retinoma on examination of parents or siblings in addition to a family history of childhood enucleation [16]. Important factors are whether more than one person in the family has retinoblastoma and, if there is no one else affected in the family, whether the affected person has multifocal/bilateral or unilateral retinoblastoma. The categories are grouped by the level of risk, with more than 1% being considered "high risk" and 1% or less considered "low risk." The other algorithm for risk detection was explained by the consensus group where they divided the risk to be high, intermediate, and low according to whether the proband has unilateral versus bilateral disease. All offspring of bilateral patients are considered high risk, while siblings are considered at intermediate risk. The offspring of unilateral patients have intermediate risk and siblings have low risk of developing retinoblastoma. These risk detection data reflect the *RB1* mutation detection rates based on a large data set of molecular genetics results for retinoblastoma patients and their family members [13, 15].

7 Conclusion

All offspring and siblings of an individual with retinoblastoma are considered to be at increased risk of developing retinoblastoma. Genetic testing can reduce the numbers needed to be screened. Frequent examinations under anesthesia provide early detection of the disease in at-risk individuals. Lack of genetic information might influence reproductive decisions, so it is important for families to understand genetic implications of retinoblastoma and risks in their children and siblings [19]. As genetic testing becomes more widely available, screening protocols will need to take these advances into account.

References

1. MacCarthy A, Draper GJ, Steliarova-Foucher E, Kingston JE. Retinoblastoma incidence and survival in European children (1978-1997). Report from the Automated Childhood Cancer Information System project. Eur J Cancer. 2006;42(13):2092–102.
2. Bishop JO, Madson EC. Retinoblastoma. Review of the current status. Surv Ophthalmol. 1975;19(6):342–66.
3. Stacey AW, Bowman R, Foster A, Kivelä TT, Munier FL, Cassoux N, et al. Incidence of retinoblastoma has increased: results from 40 European countries. Ophthalmology. 2021;
4. Lohmann DR, Gerick M, Brandt B, Oelschläger U, Lorenz B, Passarge E, et al. Constitutional RB1-gene mutations in patients with isolated unilateral retinoblastoma. Am J Hum Genet. 1997;61(2):282–94.
5. Yandell DW, Campbell TA, Dayton SH, Petersen R, Walton D, Little JB, et al. Oncogenic point mutations in the human retinoblastoma gene: their application to genetic counseling. N Engl J Med. 1989;321(25):1689–95.
6. Reddy MA, Butt M, Hinds AM, Duncan C, Price EA, Sagoo MS, et al. Prognostic information for known genetic carriers of RB1 pathogenic variants (germline and mosaic). Ophthalmol Retina. 2021;5(4):381–7.
7. Dhar SU, Chintagumpala M, Noll C, Chévez-Barrios P, Paysse EA, Plon SE. Outcomes of integrating genetics in management of patients with retinoblastoma. Arch Ophthalmol. 2011;129(11):1428–34.
8. Al-Nawaiseh I, Ghanem AQ, Yousef YA. Familial retinoblastoma: raised awareness improves early diagnosis and outcome. J Ophthalmol. 2017;2017:5053961.
9. Stargatt R, Davidson AJ, Huang GH, Czarnecki C, Gibson MA, Stewart SA, et al. A cohort study of the incidence and risk factors for negative behavior changes in children after general anesthesia. Paediatr Anaesth. 2006;16(8):846–59.
10. Stratmann G, Lee J, Sall JW, Lee BH, Alvi RS, Shih J, et al. Effect of general anesthesia in infancy on long-term recognition memory in humans and rats. Neuropsychopharmacology. 2014;39(10):2275–87.
11. Loepke AW, Soriano SG. An assessment of the effects of general anesthetics on developing brain structure and neurocognitive function. Anesth Analg. 2008;106(6):1681–707.
12. Richter S, Vandezande K, Chen N, Zhang K, Sutherland J, Anderson J, et al. Sensitive and efficient detection of RB1 gene mutations enhances care for families with retinoblastoma. Am J Hum Genet. 2003;72(2):253–69.
13. Soliman SE, Racher H, Zhang C, MacDonald H, Gallie BL. Genetics and molecular diagnostics in retinoblastoma—an update. Asia Pac J Ophthalmol (Phila). 2017;6(2):197–207.
14. MacCarthy A, Bayne AM, Brownbill PA, Bunch KJ, Diggens NL, Draper GJ, et al. Second and subsequent tumours among 1927 retinoblastoma patients diagnosed in Britain 1951-2004. Br J Cancer. 2013;108(12):2455–63.
15. Skalet AH, Gombos DS, Gallie BL, Kim JW, Shields CL, Marr BP, et al. Screening children at risk for retinoblastoma: consensus report from the American Association of Ophthalmic Oncologists and Pathologists. Ophthalmology. 2018;125(3):453–8.
16. Rosser E, Sagoo MS. Germline retinoblastoma: estimating risk and counselling the family. Community Eye Health. 2018;31(101):8–9.
17. Soliman SE, Dimaras H, Khetan V, Gardiner JA, Chan HS, Héon E, et al. Prenatal versus postnatal screening for familial retinoblastoma. Ophthalmology. 2016;123(12):2610–7.
18. Price EA, Price K, Kolkiewicz K, Hack S, Reddy MA, Hungerford JL, et al. Spectrum of RB1 mutations identified in 403 retinoblastoma patients. J Med Genet. 2014;51(3):208–14.
19. Foster A, Boyes L, Burgess L, Carless S, Bowyer V, Jenkinson H, et al. Patient understanding of genetic information influences reproductive decision making in retinoblastoma. Clin Genet. 2017;92(6):587–93.

Orbital and Metastatic Retinoblastoma: Conquests and Challenges

Abdul Wajid Moothedath, Rachna Seth, and Bhavna V. Chawla

1 Introduction

Retinoblastoma (RB) is the most common intraocular malignancy in children with an annual incidence rate of approximately 11.8 per million children below 5 years of age [1]. It has got an excellent prognosis in the developed world, but unfortunately, the visual prognosis in the developing world lags behind mainly due to late presentation. Orbital and metastatic retinoblastoma are an advanced stage of retinoblastoma seen relatively more commonly in developing countries. This is attributed mostly due to late presentations, lack of sensitization or awareness among caregivers and healthcare professionals, poor socioeconomic factors, and lack of standard treatment protocols. The presence of orbital extension increases the risk of metastasis 10–27 times compared to eyes without orbital extension and is associated with an inferior outcome [2–4]. This chapter provides an update on the current concepts in the management of orbital and metastatic RB.

2 Orbital Retinoblastoma

2.1 Definition and Classification

Retinoblastoma extending outside the confines of the eye clinically, radiologically or with histopathological evidence, is termed orbital retinoblastoma. The reported incidence in developed countries ranges from 5 to 8%, whereas in developing countries, it varies between 20 and 40% [5–9], where it is a major cause of mortality from retinoblastoma. It is classified based on clinical, radiological, and histopathological characteristics. According to the ***Children's Cancer Study Group Classification criteria* (CCSG)** [10], classes 1 to 3 are used to denote orbital retinoblastoma, while in the ***International Retinoblastoma Staging System*** [11], Stages 2 and 3 define orbital retinoblastoma (Table 1). The most recent ***2017 American Joint Commission on Cancers' TNMH*** staging (Table 2) included orbital retinoblastoma in **cT4** (clinical) and **pT4** categories (pathological) [12].

Table 1 The International Retinoblastoma Staging System (IRSS) [11]

Stage 0	Patients treated conservatively
Stage I	Eye enucleated, completely resected histologically
Stage II	Eye enucleated, microscopic residual tumor
Stage III	Regional extension (a) Overt orbital disease (b) Preauricular or cervical lymph node extension
Stage IV	Metastatic disease (a) Hematogenous metastasis (without CNS involvement) 1. Single lesion 2. Multiple lesions (b) CNS extension (with or without any other site of regional or metastatic disease) 1. Pre-chiasmatic lesion 2. CNS mass 3. Leptomeningeal and CSF disease

2.2 Routes of Spread

Orbital disease results from the invasion of retinoblastoma directly through the sclera or via the scleral canals (areas within the sclera where ciliary vessels, nerves, and vortex veins enter or exit the eye). It can also spread anteriorly through the sclera into the conjunctiva and via the lymphatics into the preauricular, submandibular, and cervical lymph nodes. It is important to know about the anatomy of the optic

A. W. Moothedath · R. Seth (✉)
Division of Pediatric Oncology, Department of Pediatrics, All India Institute of Medical Sciences, New Delhi, India

B. V. Chawla
Ocular Oncology Service, Rajendra Prasad Centre for Ophthalmic Sciences, All India Institute of Medical Sciences, New Delhi, India
e-mail: bhavna2424@aiims.edu

B. V. Chawla, M. E. Aronow (eds.), *Global Perspectives in Ocular Oncology*, https://doi.org/10.1007/978-3-031-08250-4_14

Table 2 AJCC TNMH classification [12]

• **Definitions for Primary Tumor Staging (cT)**		
cTX		Unknown evidence of intraocular tumor
cT0		No evidence of intraocular tumor
cT1		Intraocular tumor(s) with subretinal fluid ≤5 mm from the base of any tumor
	cT1a	Tumors ≤3 mm and farther than 1.5 mm from the disc and fovea
	cT1b	Tumors >3 mm or closer than 1.5 mm to the disc and fovea
cT2		Intraocular tumor(s) with retinal detachment, vitreous seeding, or subretinal seeding
	cT2a	Subretinal fluid >5 mm from the base of any tumor
	cT2b	Tumors with vitreous seeding or subretinal seeding
cT3		Advanced intraocular tumor(s)
	cT3a	Phthisis or pre-phthisis bulbi
	cT3b	Tumor invasion of the pars plana, ciliary body, lens, zonules, iris, or anterior chamber
	cT3c	Raised intraocular pressure with neovascularization or buphthalmos
	cT3d	Hyphema or massive vitreous hemorrhage
	cT3e	Aseptic orbital cellulitis
cT4		**Extraocular tumor(s) involving the orbit, including the optic nerve**
	cT4a	**Radiologic evidence of retrobulbar optic nerve involvement or thickening of the optic nerve or involvement of the orbital tissues**
	cT4b	**Extraocular tumor clinically evident with proptosis and orbital mass**
• **Definitions for Regional Lymph Node Staging (cN)**		
cNX		Regional lymph nodes cannot be assessed
cN0		No regional lymph node involvement
cN1		**Evidence of preauricular, submandibular, and cervical lymph node involvement**
• **Definitions for Distant Metastasis Staging (M)**		
cM0		No signs or symptoms of intracranial or distant metastasis
cM1		Distant metastasis without microscopic confirmation
	cM1a	Tumor(s) involving any distant site (e.g., bone marrow, liver) on clinical or radiologic tests
	cM1b	Tumor involving the CNS on radiologic imaging (not including trilateral RB)
pM1		Distant metastasis with microscopic confirmation
	pM1a	Histopathologic confirmation of tumor at any distant site (e.g., bone marrow, liver, or other)
	pM1b	Histopathologic confirmation of tumor in the cerebrospinal fluid or CNS parenchyma
• **Definitions for Heritable Trait Staging (H)**		
HX		Unknown or insufficient evidence of a constitutional RB1 gene mutation
H0		Normal RB1 alleles in blood tested with demonstrated high sensitivity assays
H1		Bilateral RB, RB with an intracranial CNS midline embryonic tumor (i.e., trilateral RB), patient with family history of RB, or molecular definition of constitutional RB1 gene mutation
• **Definitions for Pathological Tumor Staging (pT)**		
pTX		Unknown evidence of intraocular tumor
pT0		No evidence of intraocular tumor
pT1		Intraocular tumor(s) without any local invasion, focal choroidal invasion, or pre- or intralaminar involvement of the optic nerve head
pT2		Intraocular tumor(s) with local invasion
	pT2a	Concomitant focal choroidal invasion and pre- or intralaminar involvement of the optic nerve head
	pT2b	Tumor invasion of stroma of iris or trabecular meshwork or Schlemm's canal
pT3		Intraocular tumor(s) with significant local invasion
	pT3a	Massive choroidal invasion (>3 mm in largest diameter, or multiple foci of focal choroidal involvement Totaling >3 mm, or any full-thickness choroidal involvement)
	pT3b	Retrolaminar invasion of the optic nerve head, not involving the transected end of the optic nerve
	pT3c	Any partial-thickness involvement of the sclera within the inner two-thirds
	pT3d	Full-thickness invasion into the outer third of the sclera or invasion into or around emissary channels
pT4		**Evidence of extraocular tumor: Tumor at the transected end of the optic nerve, tumor in the meningeal spaces around the optic nerve, full-thickness invasion of the sclera with invasion of the epi-sclera, adjacent adipose tissue, extraocular muscle, bone, conjunctiva, or eyelids**

nerve, which is divided into an intraocular (1 mm), intraorbital (25–30 mm), intracanalicular (5–9 mm), and intracranial (10–16 mm) parts. Involvement of the optic nerve head implies that the disease is still intraocular.

2.3 Clinical Features

Orbital presentation of retinoblastoma occurs late compared to intraocular disease. The average age of diagnosis varied

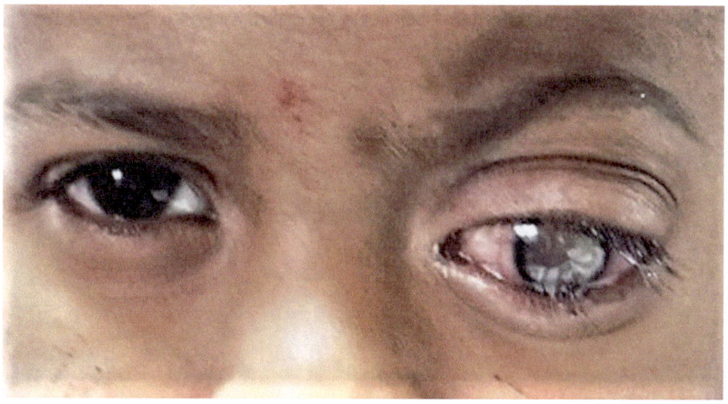

Fig. 1 Clinical presentation of a 3-year-old girl with left orbital retinoblastoma

between 30 and 39 months [9, 13, 14]. The most common presenting feature was proptosis in the majority of the series (Fig. 1), whereas leukocoria predominated in some [9, 13–17]. It is advisable to actively look for subtle proptosis, which is frequently overlooked, especially in cases of advanced intraocular disease. Other clinical presentations of orbital retinoblastoma include a palpable orbital mass, conjunctival or episcleral nodule, and in some cases, a fungating mass [13–17].

Recurrent orbital retinoblastoma can either arise from the viable residual tumor cells in the orbit or from the cut end of the optic nerve after enucleation. Generally agreed risk factors for orbital recurrence include post-laminar invasion of the optic nerve, involvement of the transected end of the optic nerve, and scleral and extra-scleral extension [2]. Orbital recurrence may characteristically present as unexplained displacement, bulging or extrusion of an orbital implant, or a previously well-fitting prosthesis occurring months to years after surgery. Recurrence arising from the cut end of the optic nerve may present as intracranial extension which may be clinically silent unless advanced.

2.4 Diagnostic Evaluation

A clinical history of presenting features including a customary family history, followed by a thorough clinical examination is mandatory. An examination under anesthesia (EUA) helps to rule out intra-ocular disease in the other eye. The imaging modality of choice is a Contrast Enhanced Magnetic Resonance Imaging of the orbit and brain (MRI) to confirm the diagnosis and to detect extraocular spread including optic-nerve infiltration [18]. In resource-limited settings, a Contrast Enhanced Computed Tomography scan (CECT) of the orbit and brain can be done to confirm orbital retinoblastoma, though CECT scan is best avoided due to the risk of radiation exposure. Metastatic workup includes a bilateral bone marrow biopsy from the posterior superior iliac crest, Cerebrospinal fluid examination, and Technetium-99 bone scintigraphy. 18-Fluoro Deoxy Glucose PET-CT may be of help in detecting distant metastasis in stage 3 orbital retinoblastoma. Orbital biopsy may be required in cases when the diagnosis is unclear on clinical and radiological examination or when a child presents with recurrent orbital mass where the primary histopathology is unavailable (Table 3). Preauricular and submandibular chains of lymph nodes are to be palpated and if enlarged, a fine-needle aspiration and cytology are warranted. Baseline complete blood count, renal and liver function tests, viral markers, and a Mantoux test are to be done prior to commencing chemotherapy.

MRI findings of orbital retinoblastoma includes an orbital mass contiguous with the eyeball (Fig. 2) or abnormal enhancement, irregularity, or thickening of the optic nerve. Scleral and extra-scleral extension is visualized as a protruding enhancing tissue through the thickened choroid into or

Table 3 Recommended baseline investigations in orbital RB

Investigations	Comments
CE-MRI of orbit and brain	Confirm diagnosis, define local extent of disease and detection of associated intracranial primitive neuroectodermal tumor
Bilateral bone marrow biopsy	To detect bone marrow metastasis
Cerebrospinal fluid examination (CSF)	To detect neuraxial dissemination
Technetium-99 bone scan	To detect bone metastasis

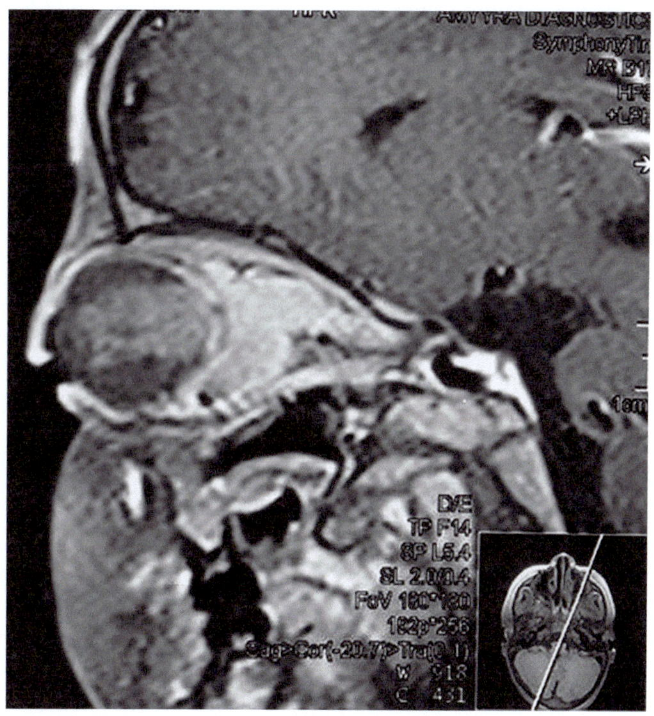

Fig. 2 MRI scan (T1-weighted image) of the orbit showing an intra-ocular mass with orbital extension

outside the sclera [19, 20]. Retinoblastoma metastasis appear as clusters of small round blue malignant cells in the bone/bone marrow biopsy/CSF sample in cases associated with involvement of these areas.

2.5 Treatment

Orbital retinoblastoma is a challenging disease to treat and it requires a multimodal approach. In the past, various investigators have tried treating it with aggressive chemotherapy, orbital exenteration, and external beam radiotherapy, either alone or in combination, but with unsatisfactory outcomes. *Hungerford* et al. found that for orbital recurrence of retinoblastoma, orbital exenteration alone was not an acceptable treatment as none of such patients survived [21]. External beam radiotherapy alone without chemotherapy is less likely to prevent systemic metastasis. These indicate that orbital retinoblastoma requires a combination of chemotherapy, limited surgery, and radiation for better outcomes.

Antoneli et al. treated 83 cases of CCG I,II,III retinoblastoma with combination chemotherapy consisting of cisplatin, teniposide, vincristine, doxorubicin, and cyclophosphamide or cisplatin and teniposide alternating with ifosfamide and etoposide, and reported 5-year overall survival rates of 55 and 59%, respectively [17]. Chantada et al. reported the outcomes of 15 orbital or lymph nodal disease patients treated with a 5-drug combination neoadjuvant chemotherapy regimen comprising vincristine, cyclophosphamide, etoposide, carboplatin/cisplatin, and idarubicin/doxorubicin, followed by appropriate surgery, radiotherapy, and adjuvant chemotherapy. The 5-year event free survival (EFS) was encouraging at 84% [22]. *Honavar and Singh* in 2005 suggested a protocol consisting of 3–6 cycles of neoadjuvant chemotherapy with vincristine, carboplatin, and etoposide (CEV), followed by enucleation of the primary tumor, external beam radiotherapy to the orbit, and adjuvant chemotherapy with the same agents for a total of 12 cycles. Compared to the standard-dose CEV, this alternate regimen has a 50% increased dose of carboplatin and a 20% increased dose of etoposide [23] (Table 4). In a preliminary report of 6 patients treated with this protocol, all of them were free of local recurrence and systemic metastasis after a median follow-up of 32 months [23]. Some centers prefer to use a further higher dose of etoposide (12 mg/kg/day on day 1,2). In majority of the patients, adequate reduction in tumor size can be achieved with 3–6 cycles of chemotherapy to the extent that the eye becomes phthisical. Since the probability of resistance to chemotherapy increases with increase in the number of cycles, efforts should be made to perform enucleation as soon as possible.

Table 4 High-dose CEV for orbital retinoblastoma [23]

Drug	Dose (mg/kg/day)	Day
Vincristine	0.025	1
Carboplatin	28	1
Etoposide	6	1 and 2

Each cycle is repeated every 3–4 weeks.

Authors from our institute published a prospective randomized study on IRSS stage IIIa patients comparing high-dose CEV and the 5-drug combination of carboplatin and etoposide alternating with cyclophosphamide, idarubicin, and vincristine [16]. Twenty-seven patients were randomized into each group. Viable tumor cells after neoadjuvant chemotherapy were found in 50% of enucleated specimens. High-dose CEV-treated patients had better local tumor control as assessed by MRI, and lower post-laminar optic nerve infiltration rates on histopathology. The probability of overall survival at 4 years was significantly better in the high-dose CEV group compared to the 5-drug group (63 vs. 25%). Hematological toxicity, especially grade 4 neutropenia, was significantly higher in the 5-drug group with no cases of second malignancy during the follow-up period reported in both the arms [16]. Currently, we use the 5-drug intensive chemotherapy regimen only for those patients who remain refractory to 3–6 cycles of high-dose CEV (Table 5). Growth factors are used to hasten neutrophil recovery while using this regimen.

The multi-institutional, prospective trial (COG ARET0321) enrolled 20 patients with stage 2 and 3 regional extra-ocular RB to be treated with 4 cycles of intensive conventional chemotherapy *(Vincristine 0.05 mg/kg/day, Cisplatin 3.5 mg/kg/day, Cyclophosphamide 65 mg/kg/day ×2 days, Etoposide 4 mg/kg/day ×2 days)*, followed by involved field RT (4500 cGy) with excellent outcomes. The treatment duration for this protocol is short and lasts around 6 months. Event-free survival at 36 months was 87.7% (90% CI 65.4 to 96.0%) for subjects with stage 2 or 3 disease, although toxicity was significant [24].

Table 5 Augmented chemotherapy regimen for retinoblastoma [16]

Drug	Dose (per day)	Cycles	Day
Vincristine	1.5 mg/m^2 0.05 mg/kg (<3 y)	Weeks 0, 6, 12, and 18	1
Etoposide	100 mg/m^2 3.3 mg/kg (<3 y)	Weeks 3, 9, 15, and 21	1, 2, 3
Carboplatin	560 mg/m^2 18.6 mg/kg (<3 y)	Weeks 3, 9, 15, and 21	1, 2
Cyclophosphamide Mesna	65 mg/kg 60 mg/kg	Weeks 0, 6, 12, and 18	1
Idarubicin/ Doxorubicin	10 mg/m^2 30 mg/m^2	Weeks 0, 6, 12, and 18	1

2.5.1 Management Algorithm

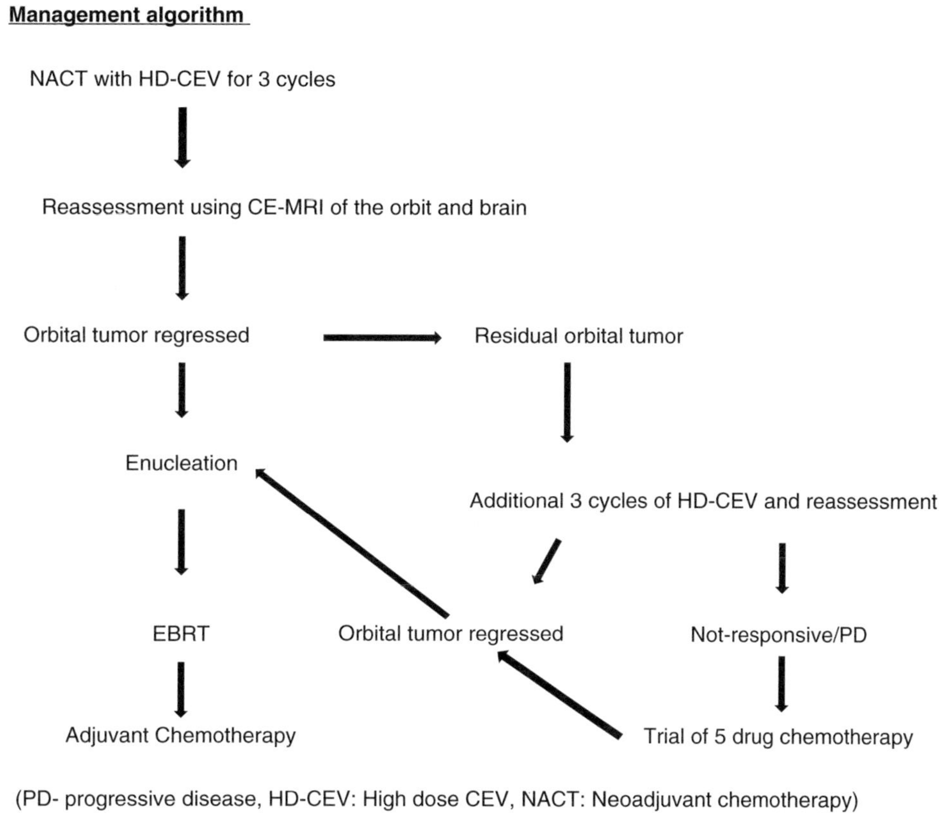

Residual orbital retinoblastoma can be managed in a similar manner as primary orbital RB with neoadjuvant chemotherapy, surgery, and external beam radiotherapy, followed by continuation of chemotherapy for 12 cycles. The difference is in the surgical intervention, which may be limited to excision of the residual orbital mass or orbital exenteration depending on the extent of involvement after NACT [13, 23].

Stage 2 IRSS RB is defined by histopathological evidence of involvement of the transected end of the optic nerve by tumor cells, full-thickness scleral infiltration, and extrascleral extension in the enucleated eye. Such cases are best managed by orbital external beam radiotherapy and 12 cycles of high-dose chemotherapy [13, 23, 25]. We prefer to avoid radiotherapy in cases with only extra-scleral extension, especially in younger patients, due to concerns of late effects. Analysis of our data (unpublished) has shown that all such patients did well without local or distant recurrence.

2.6 Radiotherapy

Adjuvant external beam radiotherapy to the affected orbit is usually administered within 4–6 weeks after enucleation. The dose used is 40 Gy in 20 fractions over 4 weeks as a 2 Gy fraction daily for 5 days per week. Computerized tomography-based, three-dimensional, conformal radiotherapy, usually by noncoplanar beams to cover the entire disease volume, is practiced at our center [16]. Most of the children required sedation during delivery of the radiation dose. Care should be taken to spare organs at risk, like the optic chiasma, brain parenchyma, and the opposite eye (if the disease is not bilateral). Advances in external beam radiotherapy have made it possible to deliver the required dose of radiation more precisely. This further helps to mitigate the late effects associated with EBRT and favors its use in the management of retinoblastoma.

3 Metastatic Retinoblastoma

Metastatic retinoblastoma, like orbital disease, is far more common in the developing countries with an incidence ranging between 5 and 10% [26, 27]. It includes Stage IVa (distant metastatic disease without central nervous system (CNS) involvement) and Stage IVb disease (CNS involvement) as per IRSS (Table 1). Contiguous spread through the optic nerve and/or its meninges can lead to central nervous system disease. It is also hypothesized that the area around the optic nerve is rich in vessels that penetrate the sclera to nourish the choroid and the optic nerve (short ciliary vessels and the circle of Zinn). These vessels have small branches that pierce the sclera into the meninges. There are spaces between the sclera and the meninges, and between the sclera and the choroid through which the tumor cells can invade and reach the meninges from the choroid. Disseminated disease occurs when it gains access to the systemic circulation after massive invasion of the choroid (> 3 mm in any dimension) or through the canal of Schlemm to the aqueous veins. Common sites of metastasis outside the CNS include the bone, bone marrow, and rarely, the liver. It is a highly lethal disease and with conventional chemotherapy, the prognosis is dismal, even in the developed world.

3.1 Risk Factors for Metastatic Disease

The most important prognostic indicators in the enucleated eye for the development of metastasis are the presence of tumor in the optic nerve posterior to the lamina cribrosa (PLONI), massive choroidal invasion (defined as posterior uveal invasion ≥3 mm in largest dimension), anterior chamber invasion, iris and ciliary body invasion, scleral invasion or a combination of focal choroidal with optic nerve invasion (optic nerve head, prelamina, and lamina cribrosa) [3, 4, 28–31]. Apart from these, extra-scleral extension of tumor into the orbit increases the risk of systemic metastasis by 10–27 times [2, 3]. The incidence of metastasis is greatly reduced with the use of six cycles of adjuvant chemotherapy when such high-risk factors (HRF) are present [32]. In a large prospective study for unilateral RB (COG ARET 0332), the prevalence of PLONI and massive choroidal invasion were 16.5 and 13.1%, respectively. Concomitant focal choroid (less than 3 mm) and optic nerve invasion (lamina and prelaminar) were seen in 4.7% of cases, but the combination did not increase the chance of recurrence and hence may not warrant adjuvant chemotherapy. The 2-year EFS for patients with HRFs requiring adjuvant chemotherapy was 96% and those without HRFs for which observation was indicated was 99%. This study also found that the eyes with both massive choroidal invasion in the peripapillary posterior choroid (around the head of the optic nerve) and PLONI particularly conferred a poor prognosis, and a more intensive adjuvant treatment may be required for such cases including orbital radiotherapy [31] (Table 6).

The clinical presentation of metastatic disease depends on the site of involvement. Bone metastasis may present with pain, fever, and cytopenias. CNS involvement usually presents with headache, lethargy, vomiting, and focal neurological deficits. Workup for a suspected metastatic disease includes a complete blood count, CE-MRI of the orbit and brain, bilateral bone marrow biopsies, lumbar puncture and CSF studies for malignant cells, and a bone scan. USG or abdominal CT scan may also be performed depending on the clinical signs.

Table 6 Histopathological risk factors for metastasis based on tumor invasion of ocular structures

Site of involvement	Definition
Choroid	Massive invasion≥ 3 mm in largest dimension
Optic nerve	• Post laminar **(PLONI)** • At surgical margin • Subarachnoid
Anterior segment seeding	
Ciliary body/Iris infiltration	

3.2 Management

Historically, stage 4 disease with distant and/or CNS metastasis had an extremely poor prognosis and was almost incurable with conventional multimodal therapy [17, 22]. The outcome of stage 4a metastatic RB has improved with the incorporation of intensive multimodal therapy including high-dose chemotherapy (HDCT) and autologous stem cell rescue although stage 4b disease is almost always fatal [24, 33–38].

Namouni et al. treated 8 patients of stage 4a disease at relapse with CARBOPEC (carboplatin and etoposide at 350 mg/m^2/day on day 1 to 5 and cyclophosphamide at 1.6 g/m^2/day from day 2 to day 5), followed by autologous stem cell rescue. Radiotherapy was given to the spinal axis and CNS to 3/8 patients after HDCT. Five patients were alive with no evidence of disease and 3 patients relapsed in the CNS. Of the 4 patients with stage 4b relapse, only 1 patient survived [33]. *Dunkel* et al. reported 15 intraocular RB patients who developed stage 4a metastasis at variable time points after enucleation [37]. Treatment consisted of induction chemotherapy with 3–6 cycles of vincristine, cisplatin, cyclophosphamide, and etoposide. Stem cells were collected once the bone marrow was clear of metastasis, followed by conditioning with high-dose carboplatin, thiotepa, and either etoposide or topotecan, and these stem cells were administered. Disease-free survival at 5 year was 67%. Six out of 10 surviving patients received radiotherapy. The main toxicity was hematological and mucositis. Three patients developed secondary osteosarcoma [37]. The same author reported outcomes of eight patients with stage 4b RB [38]. The treatment included induction chemotherapy, followed by HDCT (Carboplatin, thiotepa ± etoposide or CARBOPEC) and stem-cell rescue once the disease was in major or complete remission. Three patients died before ASCT and out of the 5 patients who received HDCT and ASCT, 2 survived [38].

In the multi-institutional, prospective **(COG ARET 0321)** study, 20 patients each with stage 4a and stage 4b were treated with 4 cycles of an intensive chemotherapy backbone. Patients with at least a partial response were then given one cycle of HDCT **(carboplatin, thiotepa, and etoposide),** followed by **autologous stem cell rescue**. Patients with metastatic RB who did not experience an adequate response to chemotherapy also received RT. Event-free survival at 36 months was **79.3 and 8%** for patients with **stage 4a and stage 4b/trilateral disease**, respectively [24].

3.2.1 Management Algorithm for Metastatic Disease

- CE-MRI orbit and brain
- B/L bone marrow biopsy
- Lumbar puncture and CSF examination
- Tc-99 bone scan
- Biopsy of distant metastatic site, if indicated (To differentiate from second malignancy)
- 18-FDG-PET-CT

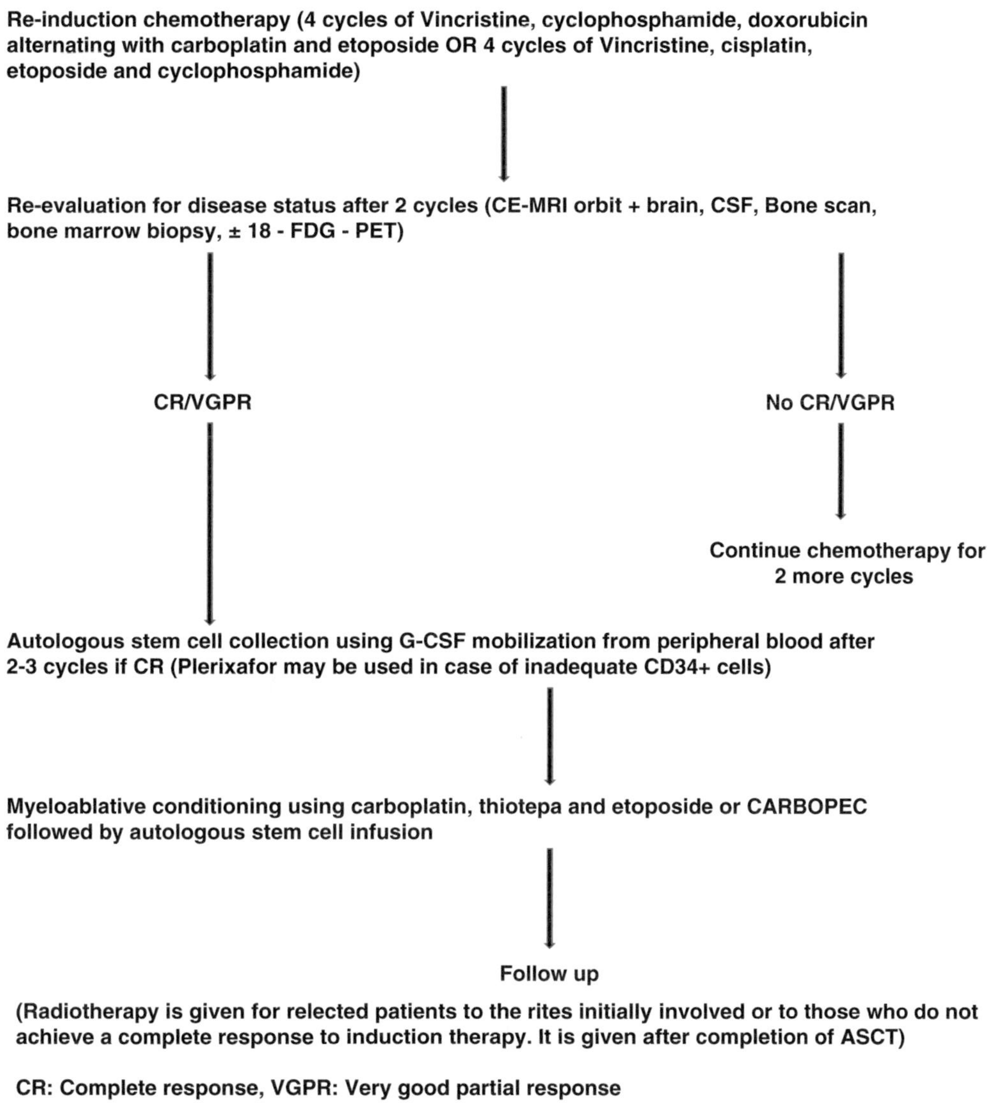

At the authors' institute, two patients with stage 4a relapse were recently managed with HDCT and ASCT. Both of them had bilateral intraocular disease. The first patient relapsed at 6 months follow up in the right maxillary bone and the second patient had a distant bone relapse in the left tibia 10 years after the primary treatment. Second malignancy was ruled out by biopsy in both cases. Our induction regimen consisted of augmented chemotherapy with vincristine, cyclophosphamide, and doxorubicin alternating with carboplatin and etoposide for 3–6 cycles (Tables 5, 7).

At our center, we offer palliation to all of our patients who progress/relapse with stage 4b disease. There are no long-term survivors with stage 4b disease/relapse currently being followed up in our clinic.

To summarize, approximately 60–70% of stage 4a retinoblastoma can be cured with high-dose, marrow-ablative chemotherapy and autologous stem cell rescue. The outcome of stage 4b RB remains dismal despite therapeutic intensification and use of ASCT. Although traditionally practiced, there is no robust evidence to support the use of intrathecal chemotherapy in stage 4b RB. The contribution of radiotherapy to the cure of stage 4a and 4b disease is not clear, and it is usually given to bulky sites of disease at relapse or to those with an inadequate response to induction chemotherapy.

Table 7 Characteristics of patients who underwent stem cell transplant at our center

No	Age at diagnosis (months)	Disease status	Upfront therapy	Time of relapse	Site of relapse	CSF and BMA	Disease status at ASCT	Conditioning	Follow-up (months)	RT
1)	48	Left group E, Right group B	Left enucleation, focal therapy + CEV regimen	6 months	Right maxillary sinus	Negative	CR	CARBOPEC	12	No
2)	3	Right group E, left group B	Right enucleation, focal therapy + CEV regimen	10 years	Left tibia	Negative	CR	Carboplatin, thiotepa, etoposide	6	No

CR Complete remission, *RT* Radiotherapy, *IORB* Intraocular RB, *ASCT* Autologous stem cell transplant

4 Challenges and Future Directions

Although an improvement in outcomes has been achieved in orbital retinoblastoma with the use of multimodal approach, the event-free survival rates are much lower than those for intraocular disease. For stage 4a metastatic disease patients, outcomes without high-dose chemotherapy and autologous stem cell rescue are dismal. Limited access to ASCT and high rates of treatment abandonment further compromise the survival in developing countries. Improving the access to autologous stem cell rescue with high-dose chemotherapy is likely to salvage a greater proportion of patients with distant metastatic disease. For the majority of patients with stage 4b RB, treatment remains largely palliative. More clinical trials incorporating novel multimodal therapies may be required to at least partially improve the outcomes of such patients. Apart from these concerns, monitoring for and management of long-term adverse effects of treatment like visual handicap, prosthesis care, sensorineural hearing loss, development of subsequent malignant neoplasms (SMN), diminished orbital growth following radiotherapy, and impaired neurocognitive functioning should also take priority. The risk of SMN is particularly increased in patients with heritable retinoblastoma and in those who have received radiation therapy [39–41].

Proton beam therapy, because of its unique physical properties and lack of exit dose, may be an excellent option for children who require radiation therapy. It minimizes damage to the normal tissues and may reduce the incidence of radiation-associated second malignancies. Retrospective series of RB patients including those with advanced disease and heavily pretreated eyes have found that proton beam therapy can achieve good local control and ocular salvage with less ocular side effects and second malignancies [42, 43].

From a community point of view, the strategies likely to make the greatest impact in the developing nations are those that will help with early diagnosis when the tumor is still intraocular and in reducing the number of families opting out of treatment/lost to follow-up. There is a high proportion of families who deny enucleation due to associated social stigma. For early diagnosis, the American Academy of Paediatrics recommends a red reflex examination within the first 2 months of life using a direct ophthalmoscope. This can be done in a well baby clinic at the time of routine immunizations. Absence of a normal and symmetrical red reflex should warrant a referral to an ophthalmologist. Creating awareness among primary healthcare providers and the general population through community education programs will help prevent late presentations to the clinic.

References

1. Broaddus E, Topham A, Singh AD. Incidence of retinoblastoma in the United States: 1975–2004. Br J Ophthalmol. 2009;93:21–3.
2. Singh AD, Shields CL, Shields JA. Prognostic factors in retinoblastoma. J Pediatr Ophthalmol Strabismus. 2000;37:134–41.
3. Kopelman JE, McLean IW, Rosenberg SH. Multi-variate analysis of risk factors for metastasis in retinoblastoma treated by enucleation. Ophthalmology. 1987;94(4):371–7.
4. Khelfaoui F, Validire P, Auperin A, Quintana E, Michon J, Pacquement H, et al. Histopathologic risk factors in retinoblastoma: a retrospective study of 172 patients treated in a single institution. Cancer. 1996;77(6):1206–13.
5. Grabowski EF, Abramson DH. Intraocular and extraocular retinoblastoma. Hematol Oncol Clin North Am. 1987;1:721–35.
6. Jubran RF, Erdreich-Epstein A, Butturini A, et al. Approaches to treatment for extraocular retinoblastoma: Children's Hospital Los Angeles experience. J Pediatr Hematol Oncol. 2004;26:31–4.
7. Kao LY, Su WW, Lin YW. Retinoblastoma in Taiwan: survival and clinical characteristics 1978-2000. Jpn J Ophthalmol. 2002;46:577–80.
8. Badhu B, Sah SP, Thakur SK, Dulal S, Kumar S, Sood A, et al. Clinical presentation of retinoblastoma in eastern Nepal. Clin Exp Ophthalmol. 2005;33:386–9.
9. Chawla B, Hasan F, Azad R, et al. Clinical presentation and survival of retinoblastoma in Indian children. Br J Ophthalmol. 2016;100:172–8.
10. Wolff JA, Boesel C, Ellsworth RM. Childrens cancer study group protocol CCSG 962. New York: Children Cancer Group; 1978.
11. Chantada G, Doz F, Antoneli CB, Grundy R, Clare Stannard FF, Dunkel IJ, et al. A proposal for an international retinoblastoma staging system. Pediatr Blood Cancer. 2006;47:801–5.
12. Mallipatna A, Gallie BL, Chevez-Barrios P, et al. AJCC cancer staging manual. 8th ed. New York, NY: Springer; 2017. p. 819–31.
13. Chawla B, Hada M. Orbital retinoblastoma: diagnosis. Clin Ophthal Oncol Retinoblastoma. 2019 Apr;23:239.
14. Menon BS, Reddy SC, Wan Maziah WN, et al. Extra ocular retinoblastoma. Med Pediatr Oncologia. 2000;35:75–6.

15. Chawla B, Singh R. Recent advances and challenges in the management of retinoblastoma. Indian J Ophthalmol. 2017;65(2):133–9.
16. Chawla B, Hasan F, Seth R, Pathy S, Pattebahadur R, Sharma S, Upadhyaya A, Azad R. Multimodal therapy for stage III retinoblastoma (international retinoblastoma staging system): a prospective comparative study. Ophthalmology. 2016 Sep;123(9):1933–9.
17. Antoneli CB, Steinhorst F, de Cassia Braga RK, et al. Extra ocular retinoblastoma a 13-year experience. Cancer. 2003;2003(98):1292–8.
18. Neupane R, Gaudana R, Boddu SHS. Imaging techniques in the diagnosis and management of ocular tumors: prospects and challenges. AAPS J. 2018;20(6):97.
19. Razek AA, Elkhamary S. MRI of retinoblastoma. Br J Radiol. 2011;84(1005):775–84.
20. de Graaf P, Göricke S, Rodjan F, Galluzzi P, Maeder P, Castelijns JA, Brisse HJ. European retinoblastoma imaging collaboration (ERIC). Guidelines for imaging retinoblastoma: imaging principles and MRI standardization. Pediatr Radiol. 2012 Jan;42(1):2–14.
21. Hungerford JL, Kingston JE, Plowman PN. Orbital recurrence of retinoblastoma. Ophthalmic Pediatr Genet. 1987;8:63–8.
22. Chantada GL, Fandino AC, Casak S, et al. Treatment of overt extraocular retinoblastoma. Med Pediatr Oncol. 2003;40:158–61.
23. Honavar SG, Singh AD. Management of advanced retinoblastoma. Ophthalmol Clin N Am. 2005;18:65–73, viii.
24. Dunkel IJ, Krailo MD, Chantada GL, Banerjee A, Abouelnaga S, Buchsbaum J, et al. Intensive multi-modality therapy for extraocular retinoblastoma (RB): a Children's Oncology Group (COG) trial (ARET0321). J Clin Oncol. 2017;35(15_suppl):10,506. (Abstract).
25. Honavar SG, Singh AD, Shields CL, Meadows AT, Demirci H, Cater J, et al. Postenucleation adjuvant therapy in high-risk retinoblastoma. Arch Ophthalmol. 2002;120:923–31.
26. Leal-Leal CA, Rivera-Luna R, Flores-Rojo M, Juárez-Echenique JC, Ordaz JC, Amador-Zarco J. Survival in extra-orbital metastatic retinoblastoma: treatment results. Clin Transl Oncol. 2006;8:39–44.
27. Cozza R, De Ioris MA, Ilari I, Devito R, Fidani P, De Sio L, et al. Metastatic retinoblastoma: single institution experience over two decades. Br J Ophthalmol. 2009;93:1163–6.
28. Shields CL, Shields JA, Baez K, Cater JR, De Potter P. Optic nerve invasion of retinoblastoma. Metastatic potential and clinical risk factors. Cancer. 1994;73(3):692–8.
29. Messmer EP, Heinrich T, Höpping W, et al. Risk factors for metastases in patients with retinoblastoma. Ophthalmology. 1991;98:136–41.
30. Shields CL, Shields JA, Baez KA, et al. Choroidal invasion of retinoblastoma: metastatic potential and clinical risk factors. Br J Ophthalmol. 1993;77:544–8.
31. Chévez-Barrios P, Eagle RC Jr, Krailo M, Piao J, Albert DM, Gao Y, et al. Study of unilateral retinoblastoma with and without histopathologic high-risk features and the role of adjuvant chemotherapy: a Children's Oncology Group Study. J Clin Oncol. 2019;37(31):2883–91.
32. Kaliki S, Shields CL, Shah SU, et al. Postenucleation adjuvant chemotherapy with vincristine, etoposide, and carboplatin for the treatment of high-risk retinoblastoma. Arch Ophthalmol. 2011;129:1422–7.
33. Namouni F, Doz F, Tanguy ML, et al. High-dose chemotherapy with carboplatin, etoposide and cyclophosphamide followed by a haematopoietic stem cell rescue in patients with high-risk retinoblastoma: a SFOP and SFGM study. Eur J Cancer. 1997;33:2368–75.
34. Palma J, Sasso DF, Dufort G, et al. Successful treatment of metastatic retinoblastoma with high-dose chemotherapy and autologous stem cell rescue in South America. Bone Marrow Transplant. 2012;47(4):522–7.
35. Rodriguez-Galindo C, Wilson MW, Haik BG, et al. Treatment of metastatic retinoblastoma. Ophthalmology. 2003;110(6):1237–40.
36. Kremens B, Wieland R, Reinhard H, et al. High-dose chemotherapy with autologous stem cell rescue in children with retinoblastoma. Bone Marrow Transplant. 2003;31(4):281–4.
37. Dunkel IJ, Khakoo Y, Kernan NA, Gershon T, Gilheeney S, Lyden DC, et al. Intensive multimodality therapy for patients with stage 4a metastatic retinoblastoma. Pediatr Blood Cancer. 2010;55(1):55–9.
38. Dunkel IJ, Chan HS, Jubran R, Chantada GL, Goldman S, Chintagumpala M, et al. High-dose chemotherapy with autologous hematopoietic stem cell rescue for stage 4B retinoblastoma. Pediatr Blood Cancer. 2010;55(1):149–52.
39. Dommering CJ, Marees T, van der Hout AH, et al. RB1 mutations and second primary malignancies after hereditary retinoblastoma. Familial Cancer. 2012;11(2):225–33.
40. Temming P, Arendt M, Viehmann A, et al. Incidence of second cancers after radiotherapy and systemic chemotherapy in heritable retinoblastoma survivors: a report from the German reference center. Pediatr Blood Cancer. 2017;64(1):71–80.
41. Kleinerman RA, Schonfeld SJ, Sigel BS, et al. Bone and soft-tissue sarcoma risk in long-term survivors of hereditary retinoblastoma treated with radiation. J Clin Oncol. 2019;37(35):3436–45.
42. Mouw KW, Sethi RV, Yeap BY, MacDonald SM, Chen YL, Tarbell NJ, et al. Proton radiation therapy for the treatment of retinoblastoma. Int J Radiat Oncol Biol Phys. 2014;90(4):863–9.
43. Biewald E, Kiefer T, Geismar D, Schlüter S, Manthey A, Westekemper H, et al. Feasibility of proton beam therapy as a rescue therapy in heavily pre-treated retinoblastoma eyes. Cancers. 2021;13(8):1862.

Metastatic Behavior of Uveal Melanoma: From Biology to Treatment

İrem Koç and Hayyam Kiratli

1 Introduction

Uveal melanoma (UM) is still among the few human cancers with no improvement in survival despite increasingly successful primary ocular tumor treatments. This tumor, which arises from neural-crest-derived melanocytes, is the most common primary intraocular malignancy in adults [1]. While UM represents only 5% of all human melanomas, it accounts for 13% of deaths directly caused by the tumor [2]. The UM-related mortality has been calculated as 31% at 5 years, 45% at 15 years, 49% at 25 years, and 52% at 35 years [3]. Recent estimates suggest a lower risk of metastasis beyond 15 years [4]. The liver is involved in upto 90% of patients in the metastatic process, and liver failure is the leading cause of death. Once liver metastasis is detected, the prognosis is poor with 92% of patients expiring within 2 years [5].

It was Fuchs in 1882 who first convincingly demonstrated that the liver was the most frequent site for UM metastasis based on a systematic review of 229 patients [6]. The author argued that the frequency of metastasis did not change if the patient was treated early or late in the disease course [6]. Later in 1901, this view was challenged by Lagrange who observed that metastases were frequent within the first 2 years after enucleation or exenteration [7]. The author also remarked that the patient should be declared cured if no metastasis developed after 3 years and recommended early intervention in order to prevent metastasis [7]. This controversy was reignited seven decades later by Zimmerman et al. who observed a 2–3 year peak mortality rate following enucleation [8]. This is now known as the Zimmerman effect, and is due to multiple factors, including *BAP1* mutation [9].

İ. Koç · H. Kiratli (✉)
Ocular Oncology Service, Department of Ophthalmology, Hacettepe University School of Medicine, Ankara, Turkey
e-mail: hkiratli@hacettepe.edu.tr

2 Risk Factors for Metastasis

Several clinical (Table 1), histopathological (Table 2), and genetic risk factors have been identified. Recent advances in multi-omics analyses have further refined the risk stratifications and allowed the ability to devise new classification schemes [12, 13]. Onken et al. showed two distinct classes of UM based on specific gene expression profiling by mRNA analysis [14]. The 5-year metastasis risk is 5% for Class 1 tumors, whereas it is 51% for Class 2 tumors [14]. More recently, the cancer genome atlas

Table 1 Clinical risk factors for poor prognosis and metastasis for uveal melanoma

Risk factor	Remarks
Older age	Decreased immune surveillance?
Large tumor size	More tumor cells with mutations
Diffuse tumors	Larger basal diameter, optic nerve invasion
Fast tumor growth	Rapid rates of proliferation, more tumor cells with mutations?
Rapid tumor regression after radiotherapy	Rapid rates of proliferation, more tumor cells with mutations?
Ciliary body location	Larger tumors, more vascularity, higher mortality rate
Extrascleral extension	Larger and more aggressive tumors

Adopted in part from references number [10] and [11]

Table 2 Histopathological risk factors for poor prognosis and metastasis in uveal melanoma

Risk factor	Remarks
Epithelial cell type	More cells with mutations
High mitotic figures	Field area of 0.152 mm^2 must be used
Extravascular matrix "loop or network" patterns	3 back-to-back loops must be observed
High microvascular density	Must be counted in 0.31 mm^2
High number of tumor-infiltrating macrophages and lymphocytes	CD68, CD163

B. V. Chawla, M. E. Aronow (eds.), *Global Perspectives in Ocular Oncology*, https://doi.org/10.1007/978-3-031-08250-4_15

Table 3 Current assessment of poor prognosis and risk of metastasis based on chromosome copy numbers, mutations, and transcriptomics

Risk level	Low	Intermediate	High	
Primary driver mutation	*GNAQ/GNA11*			
Secondary driver mutation	*EIF1AX*	*SF3B1*	*BAP1*	
Chromosome 3	Disomy 3	Disomy 3	Monosomy 3	Monosomy 3
Chromosome 6	+6p	+6p		
Chromosome 8	Normal 8q	Partial +8q	+8q	++8q Loss of 8p
Inflammation	–	–	Variable	Prominent
GEP class (mRNA)	1A	1B	2A	2B
TCGA class (mRNA, miRNA, lncRNA)	1	2	3	4
TCGA class modified by Jager et al. [13]	A	B	C	D

+ increase, – none, *GEP* gene expression profiling, *TCGA* the cancer genome atlas

(TCGA) network defined four groups of UM based on copy numbers, mRNA, miRNA, and DNA methylation (Table 3) [12].

3 Genetic Background

Uveal melanoma has the lowest mutation burden in human cancers, only comparable to that of pediatric malignancies. The neoplastic transformation of uveal melanocytes into a melanoma requires at least two major mutational events. The first is the mutually exclusive *GNAQ/GNA11* gain-of-function mutations, which are found in over 90% of UMs [5]. In a minority of tumors, *CYSLTR2* and *PLCB4* mutations occur [15, 16]. The second major event, called the "BSE mutations," is prognostically significant, and involves *BAP1* (44%), *SF3B1* (21%), and *EIF1AX* (21%) genes, which confer high, intermediate, and low risks of metastasis, respectively [15–17]. Cytogenetic analyses revealed that loss of one copy of chromosome 3 (monosomy 3) is the most common chromosomal change in UM, followed by amplification of 8q, both of which are associated with poor prognosis [5, 17]. Chromosome 3 harbors the *BAP1* gene and monosomy 3 is currently the strongest indicator for the development of metastasis [5]. Isodisomy 3 is also associated with increased metastatic risk [18]. The *MYC* gene is located on 8q, and the amplitude of gain of this chromosome has a direct impact on the metastatic risk and prognosis [18]. However, it is not the *MYC* oncogene that increases the metastatic risk, but the adjacent *PVT1* gene that dysregulates transcriptional miRNA activity [18]. Also found on 8q is the *DDEF* (development and differentiation enhancing factor) oncogene, which increases cell motility and promotes invasiveness [18]. Thirty percent of UM patients may have a deletion of chromosome 1p, which is also associated with a higher risk of metastasis [5]. Loss on 6q and 9p or gain on 1q or 6p are less frequently detected chromosomal aberrations and these do not increase the risk of metastasis [5]. The amplification of 6p, which contains genes for eye development and immunomodulation, is associated with a protective effect [19].

The preferentially expressed antigen in the melanoma (PRAME) gene encodes an antigen that is expressed in human melanomas and recognized by cytotoxic T-cells [20]. PRAME + status independently worsens the prognosis in both class 1 and 2 tumors, shortens the time to metastasis, and is correlated with largest basal diameter and tumor volume [20]. PRAME is overexpressed in the subclass of UM, which has *SF3B1* mutations, and disomy 3 without *BAP1* mutations, which results in late metastasis [21].

Loss of nuclear *BAP1* (*BRCA-1* associated protein 1) expression, a major tumor suppressor gene located on 3p21, leads to a wide array of changes in the tumor microenvironment. In 84% of metastatic UM, only the mutated allele of *BAP1* remains [5]. *BAP1* loss disrupts the maintenance of the differentiated melanocyte phenotype and causes a shift toward a stem cell-like phenotype [5, 18–20]. The highly aggressive course of Class 2 can be explained by gain of neural crest-like migratory behavior, which in turn may be due to alterations in DNA methylation triggered by *BAP1* loss [22]. This dedifferentiation is a prerequisite for epithelial-to-mesenchymal transition leading to metastasis [18–20]. *BAP1* regulates the release of Ca + 2 into the cytosol and controls apoptosis. Loss of *BAP1* results in a reduction of Ca + 2 influx and impedes apoptosis [5, 18–20]. Another consequence of BAP1 loss is the upregulation of several immunosuppressive genes that affect leukocyte, B-cell functions, and antigen presenting patterns, all creating a more tolerogenic microenvironment for the tumor cell [23]. The few genes that are downregulated by *BAP1* loss of function are involved in mounting an anti-tumor immune response [23].

Dysregulation of glycogen storage is a newly described unfavorable prognostic factor attributable to monosomy 3 [24]. Chromosome 3 harbors several genes involved in glycogen metabolism, and loss of these genes results in impaired storage of glucose as glycogen in tumor cells, sustained hyperglycemia, and insulin resistance [24]. The compensatory secretion of insulin-like growth factor by the liver acts as a chemoattractant for liver metastasis [24].

4 Metastasis and Liver Tropism

It has long been recognized that micrometastases commonly develop early during melanoma formation via hematogenous dissemination, but at the time of initial ocular diagnosis, only 4% of patients have detectable metastases [5, 18]. Metastasis is a highly complex process and involves several steps including cellular detachment, migration within the stroma, epithelial-to-mesenchymal transition, intravasation, survival in the circulation, endothelial adhesion, and establishment of tumors at new distant sites all by evading immune detection and destruction. The tumor microenvironment, which is made up of melanoma cells, supporting stromal cells, tumor infiltrating immune cells, and tumor vasculature, has a fundamental role in sustaining tumor growth and promoting metastasis [25]. Tumor-infiltrating immune cells are composed of CD4+ T-cells, CD8+ T-cells, regulatory T cells (Treg), and tumor-associated macrophages (TAM), which are of M2 immunosuppressive phenotype [25, 26]. These cells produce TGF-β, INF-γ, and IL-15, which suppress NK cell activity against tumor cells. INF-γ also upregulates HLA and IDO-1 expressions in tumor cells, which helps them elude NK cell recognition [25, 26]. The presence of VEGF and other angiogenic factors creates an immunosuppressive microenvironment by inhibiting dendritic cell maturation and recruiting suppressive T-cells [27]. This inflammatory tumor microenvironment is most often associated with monosomy 3 and BAP1 loss, and portends a poor prognosis with increased risk of metastasis.

MicroRNAs (miRNAs) are small, non-coding RNAs that regulate gene expression by binding to mRNA. Oncogenic miRNAs, collectively named as oncomirs, are overexpressed in UM [17, 28]. High expression of miRNA-17-5p was shown to promote cellular proliferation, invasion, and metastasis, and miRNA-21-5p and miRNA-151a-3p were associated with epithelial-to-mesenchymal transition [17]. The tumor suppressor miRNA-34 family is downregulated in UM [28]. These oncomirs and many other RNA, DNA, lipids, and proteins are transported in extracellular vesicles (EV), which are nanoparticles released from cancer cells [17, 29]. UM-emitted EVs contain proteins that are involved in cell growth and metastatic organotropism, maintenance of the metastatic niche, and extracellular matrix remodelling [29]. Particularly EVs expressing ITGαvβv and HSBP1 directly influence liver tropism and micrometastasis, respectively [29].

The preferential homing of uveal melanoma cells to the liver is due to the expression of several receptors by the tumor cells including c-MET, IGF-IR, and CXCR4, and their corresponding ligands in the liver including HGF, IGF, and CXCL12, respectively [5, 25]. Moreover, UM arises and grows in an immune-tolerant intraocular environment, which contains MSH, VIP, MIF, TGF-β2, and IDO, all inhibiting cytotoxic T-cell (CTL) and NK cell responses [19, 26]. The liver provides a similar microenvironment that allows metastatic UM cells to survive and proliferate. Additionally, the liver produces tryptophan metabolites and expresses MHC class I antigens, which significantly inhibit NK cell lysis. [5, 19, 25]

Grossniklaus identified two main growth patterns of metastatic uveal melanoma to the liver, and the two may coexist [9]. The first is the more common infiltrative pattern developing in the sinusoidal spaces [9]. The sinusoidal spaces are lined by liver sinusoidal endothelial cells (LSECs), hepatic stellate cells, and Kupffer cells (stellate macrophages), which can express PD-L1 controlling T-cell activation, and secrete IL-10 and PGE2, downregulating MHC class II resulting in less antigen presenting to T-helper cells [26]. Despite its own newly developed vasculature, the infiltrative tumor may become hypoxic, and cMET and CXCR4 may be produced. The second type is the periportal nodular pattern in which tumors lodge in the periportal areas, become hypoxic with ensuing VEGF production and angiogenesis [5, 9]. Melanoma cells may secrete PDGF-BB and TGF-β, which impede hepatic stellate cell functions [5, 15]. It is clear that CD163 + TAMs and tumor-infiltrating lymphocytes expressing TIM-3, LAG-3, and TIGIT in the hepatic tumor microenvironment acquire protumorigenic features and shift the balance toward immune tolerance and resistance [30].

5 Management of Metastatic Disease in Uveal Melanoma

Detection of metastatic disease during uveal melanoma **(UM)** follow-up is a major breakpoint in uveal melanoma management since life expectancy is considerably affected by the presence of metastatic disease. Median overall survival **(OS)** is generally expected not to extend 12 months and 1-year OS is around 40% once the disease is disseminated, even so with appropriate treatment [31, 32]. There exists a lack of standardized treatment algorithm for metastatic UM and the general approach involves case-based treatments. According to the recent Expert Panel review of the American Society of Clinical Oncology guidelines, when results from all adult patients with cutaneous and noncutaneous melanoma in 1 systematic review, 1 meta-analysis, and 34 randomized clinical trials were evaluated, no recommendation for or against metastatic UM in terms of systemic therapy could be made [33]. Briefly, certain biological differences in UM such as low mutational burden and lack of *BRAF* or *KIT* mutations compared to its cutaneous and mucosal counterparts limit the use of B-Raf or KIT inhibitors and immunotherapy in disseminated UM [34]. Palliative measures such as best supportive care in advanced cases of metastatic UM have also been reported where no survival benefit is expected compared with medical intervention [35]. In such a clinical entity as metastatic UM where OS could only be improved to a very limited extent and in a small subset of patients, treatment planning should be preceded by appropriate disease staging and prognostication in order to sensitively predict the candidates who are most likely to benefit from treatment. Consequently, a discussion of management of metastatic UM through this chapter will follow the order stated below with an initial emphasis on staging:

1. Disease staging and nomograms.
2. Best supportive care.
3. Systemic chemotherapy.
4. Local (liver-directed) treatment modalities.
   - Transarterial chemoembolization (TACE)
   - Isolated/percutaneous hepatic perfusion (IHP)
   - Hepatic intra-arterial chemotherapy (HIA)
   - Immunoembolization
   - Radioembolization
   - Surgical resection.
5. Immunotherapy.

5.1 Disease Staging and Nomograms

5.1.1 TNM Classification

According to the most recent American Joint Committee on Cancer Staging Manual, which helps defining prognostic stage groups for UM based on Tumor (T) Node (N) and Metastasis (M) status, all cases of metastatic disease are grouped under Stage IV disease [36]. Metastatic disease (M1) is further divided into three categories (M1a-c) depending on the largest diameter of largest metastasis being ≤3.0 cm, 3.1–8.0 cm, and ≥8.1 cm, and median survival times are reported as 17.5, 9.6, and 5.0 months through a-c categories, respectively. Given that OS is shown to be strongly correlated with not only the largest diameter of largest metastasis, but also substantially with numerous other clinical factors such as performance status and liver function tests, no further substaging for metastatic UM was performed in the current AJCC Cancer Staging guidelines [36]. In the planning management of metastatic UM, one should also note that TNM clinical staging does not differentiate primary treatment, and classifications are based on parameters preceding the initiation of treatment [36].

5.1.2 Helsinki University Hospital Working Formulation

With regard to highlighting the importance of staging in predicting treatment and survival outcomes, a recent study has analyzed the impact of staging based on the Helsinki Working Formulation (HWF) on OS [37]. This model aids in the grouping of metastatic disease in three categories with distinct median overall survivals (Stage IVa: 14.9 months, Stage IVb: 8.9 months, Stage IVc: 2.0 months, respectively), where each group represents combinations of variables that are independently shown to strongly affect survival, namely: Karnofsky index, the largest dimension of the largest metastasis and serum alkaline phosphatase (ALP) [38]. According to the analysis of 216 actively treated metastatic UM patients who were substaged as per HWF, patients treated with chemoimmunotherapy, selective internal radiation, and surgical resection fared better in terms of median survival (13,16, and 24 months, respectively) than those treated with conventional chemotherapy (5.1 months), and substaging additionally proved that surgical resection in Stage IVa resulted in significantly longer median survival (27 months) than with best supportive care (BSC) (12 months) [37]. These results altogether support that disseminated UM comprises cases with various prognoses, and the factors to further improve prognostication thus management remain to be elucidated.

5.1.3 International Rare Cancers Initiative (IRCI) Ocular Melanoma Study

The meta-analysis conducted by the International Rare Cancers Initiative (IRCI) included patient-level progression free survival (PFS) and OS data of 29 clinical trials [32]. In both univariate and multivariate analyses, the factors to be strongly related to shorter OS and lower 6-month PFS rate were found to be elevated serum lactate dehydrogenase (LDH) and ALP. Additionally, liver-directed treatments were shown to result in improved PFS and OS. Even though this study does not suggest a staging system per se, it provides high-level evidence for identifying clinical risk factors such as high serum LDH and ALP for poor PFS and OS, which are in turn candidates to be incorporated in prognostication. The patients receiving liver-directed therapies had longer PFS and OS outcomes; however, it has previously been reported that differences in OS in different modalities would not necessarily imply improvement in survival but rather point to screening, selection, and publication bias [31].

5.1.4 Nomograms

Further stratification of metastatic UM can be aided by prognostic nomograms [39, 40]. These nomograms aim to define objective formulations of survival prediction. It has been previously concluded and externally validated that the percentage of liver involvement (HR 1.6), LDH (HR 1.6), the WHO performance score (HR 1.5 and 4.6 for performance scores 1 and 2–3, respectively) and the time from UM diagnosis to detection of metastasis (HR 0.9) are significant factors that affect survival in metastatic UM. Another set of nomograms consisting of 224 metastatic UM patients detected by liver magnetic resonance imaging defined factors for lower OS as less than 6 months of time from diagnosis of UM to metastasis (HR 3.39), more than 10 liver metastases (HR 3.95), LDH greater than 1.5 (HR 3.72), and greatest metastasis of more than 1000 mm^2 area (HR 2.47). One should note that the former study reports the results of metastasis screening mainly with computed tomography or ultrasound, and the latter with magnetic resonance imaging, which may serve as a source of discrepancy in clinical settings where different imaging modalities are used for liver screening.

5.2 Best Supportive Care

Due to a lack of clear superiority between either surgical or nonsurgical methods of management and the absence of a standard of care in metastatic UM, definitions of survival outcomes in patients who receive no intervention of any kind gain importance. Herein data on patients managed with best supportive care is believed to be able to serve as a natural reference point. In a retrospective multivariate analysis of 48 metastatic UM patients who received either systemic chemotherapy or best supportive care, the median OS were 10.83 and 8.03 months, respectively. This minor difference in OS did not reach statistical significance and the difference was attributable to the significantly higher Eastern Cooperative Oncology Group (ECOG) performance score in the best supportive care group. The area of metastases or the methods of screening were not stated. On multivariate analysis, the ECOG score and the number of hepatic metastases were the only factors found to be significantly affecting OS [41]. More recently, Rantala et al. have elaborated on the factors affecting OS in 108 patients receiving best supportive care [35]. The majority of their cohort (55%) had Stage IVc disease according to HWF and more than half (52%) had ECOG performance status 3–4. The median overall survival was 1.6 months. Even though 1.6 months of OS falls short of previously reported nearly 12 months of OS for metastatic UM in general, it should be noted this study mainly involved the most advanced metastatic cases according to HWF stratification. Even though it is currently generally accepted that OS can not be improved with active treatment in metastatic UM, further subgrouping and prognostication of metastatic UM may yield subcategories which can potentially benefit from active treatment.

5.3 Systemic Chemotherapy

Data on systemic chemotherapy for metastatic UM is mostly derived from either conventional chemotherapy-receiving arms in clinical trials or deduced from advances in cutaneous melanoma treatment, or chemosensitivity assays; all of which proved limited effect of systemic chemotherapy in metastatic UM due to chemoresistance. The agents which are so far reported on include, but are not limited to, dacarbazine, gemcitabine+treosulfan with or without cisplatin, fotemustine, and temozolomide. Conventional chemotherapy has been reported to yield median OS ranging between 4.5 and 17.0 months; however, due to disparities in study designs and patient selection, a comparison of outcomes among these agents could not be made [31]. Given the same limitations, a combination of systemic chemotherapy and an immunomodulating agent such as interferon (IFN) has been shown to result in comparable OS with chemotherapy alone [31].

5.4 Locoregional Therapies

Local therapies for metastatic UM mainly describe the liver-directed treatment options due to the dominance of hepatic metastases in metastatic UM. Of those, transarterial chemotherapy (TACE), isolated hepatic perfusion (IHP), and hepatic intaarterial chemotherapy (HIA) are interventional procedures, which are defined as embolization of the hepatic artery after intra-arterial administration of chemotherapy, surgical isolation and subjection of hepatic perfusion to high concentrations of desired agents, mainly melphalan, and infusion of chemotherapy following selective catheterization of the hepatic artery, respectively [42].

5.4.1 Transarterial Chemoembolization

TACE for liver metastasis of UM with cisplatin has previously been studied, and treatment results with N,N′-bis(2-chloroethyl)-N-*nitrosourea* (*BCNU*) have also been reported. A large-scale pooled analysis of patients with different degrees of tumor burden reported the median OS with this method as ranging between 5.0 and 28.8 months [31]. More recently, it has been suggested that TACE with a lipophilic agent such as BCNU could be superior locoregional therapies to that with a hydrophilic agent, due to the entrapment of higher concentrations of ethiodized oil in a highly vascular liver metastasis, resulting in increasing OS and lower tumor burden [43]. TACE with BCNU is also reported to be a treatment option reserved for cases with more than 50% liver involvement or refractory to radioembolization or systemic treatment with immunotherapy [43].

5.4.2 Isolated/Percutaneous Hepatic Perfusion

The rationale for IHP is to expose the liver to higher concentrations of melphalan while avoiding systemic side-effects. This invasive procedure requires laparotomy and overall yielded a median OS of 8.9–23.9 months [31]. The inherent risks and concerns of mortality are the main limitations for its use. The minimally invasive counterpart of this procedure is percutaneous hepatic perfusion (PHP). Over 80% tumor regression and stabilization rates have been reported with this method; however, OS is found comparable with other liver-directed treatment modalities [43].

5.4.3 Hepatic Intra-Arterial Chemotherapy

With OS ranging between 10 and 24 months, HIA has been performed with several agents including fotemustine, carboplatin, melphalan, or a combination of cisplatin vinblastine and dacarbazine [44]. The comparison of HIA with fotemustine and intravenous fotemustine resulted in longer progression-free survival in HIA with fotemustine than in intravenous fotemustine groups (4.5 vs 3.5 months, respectively, p = 0.002) yet with statistically similar median OS [45]. Overall median survival with this method is considered comparable to conventional chemotherapy [31].

5.4.4 Immunoembolization

Immunoembolization for metastatic UM has been described as the simultaneous application of embolization of the granulocyte-macrophage colony-stimulating factor and liver embolization to enhance the immunologic response and clearance of extrahepatic metastases. This method overall revealed 18.4–21.6 months of median OS and more recently some treatment-related clinical factors: receiving immunoembolization only, a longer period before switching the treatment modality, the type of response after first immunoembolization, have been associated with prolonged OS with immunoembolization [31, 46].

5.4.5 Radioembolization

Selective internal radiation therapy (SIRT) is also known as radioembolization and employs Yttrium-90 microshperes to selectively target tumor tissue sparing healthy liver parenchyma. Both earlier and more recent noncomparative retrospective analyses reveal OS within a 9–24-month range with SIRT. A comparison of SIRT with best supportive care in patients with similar ECOG scores ended up in a prolonged survival with SIRT (19.9 vs. 4.8 months, p < 0.0001) [44, 47]. The first prospective trial for SIRT compared OS in treatment-naive patients to those previously treated with immunoembolization, all of whom had less than 50% tumor burden in the liver. The study resulted in median OS of 18.5 and 19.2 months in the treatment-naive group and the group pre-treated with immunoembolization, respectively. Both groups had a more than 90% rate of extrahepatic disease development or progression. While the rate of extrahepatic disease calls for improvement, targeting the metastatic disease with a burden of less than 50%, the authors suggest SIRT as the first- or second-line treatment, particularly in the absence of extrahepatic disease and less than 10 metastases in the liver [47, 48].

5.4.6 Surgical Resection

When resectable disease is encountered in the liver, surgery with or without other modalities including TACE, HIA, and radiofrequency ablation could be performed with prolonged median OS, ranging from 8.1 to 65.2 months [31]. A recent review of 793 patients undergoing surgery for UM liver metastasis has reported a better median OS (range: 10–35 months) than those receiving chemotherapy or best supportive care (range: 9–15 months) [44]. A retrospective cohort has also shown that surgery is the only treatment modality that significantly prolongs OS beyond that with best supportive care in general and in Stage IVa disease according to HWF (overall median survival: 24 vs. 1.6 months, median survival in Stage IVa: 27 vs. 12 months with surgery vs. best supportive care, respectively) [37].

5.5 Immunotherapy

Over the last decade, the use of immune checkpoint inhibitors such as anti-CTLA-4 (ipilimumab), anti-PD-1 (nivolumab, pembrolizumab), and anti-PD-L1 in metastatic cutaneous melanoma showed survival benefit; nevertheless, OS results for metastatic UM have been disappointing. The underlying biological reasons for this distinction are listed as low mutational burden and thus low PD-L1 expression, immune-privileged environment of the eye which in turn effects the immunological properties of the metastases and immune-modulating function of liver [49]. The median OS with checkpoint inhibitors lays between 4.6 and 12.8 months for metastatic UM even though the interpretation of lower OS is confounded by patient selection or first-line treatment percantage [31]. This is in keeping with the finding that the first-line application of checkpoint inhibitors improved overall survival from 7.8 to 10.0 months in a retrospective cohort of 126 patients [50]. Given that the lower median OS with checkpoint inhibitors compared to other modalities are subject to confounders such as the percentage of first-line therapy, the pursuit of improved OS with immunotherapy has shifted to combination therapies and strategies to enhance the immunogenicity of UM [49]. Additionally, the question whether patients with high risk of metastasis should be assigned to adjuvant immunotherapy still remains unanswered.

In general, in the management of metastatic UM, there is no standard of care. The generally encountered low-mutational burden is held responsible for less-than-expected rates of OS improvement in metastatic UM with immunotherapy. Even though the tumor is not considered mutationally hot, ongoing molecular studies of targeted therapy are shaped around the recurrent molecular characteristics encountered in metastatic UM, such as characteristic copy number alterations, gene expression profile, and common somatic mutations [51]. These factors are also thought to be determinative whether a patient would benefit from immunotherapy for metastatic UM, or would require adjuvant therapy including sunitib or crizotinib in the management of primary disease, or would yield more favorable results with targeted therapy agents such as MAP-Kinase or YAP/TAZ inhibitors [51]. Tebentafusp is a chimeric protein that is included in more recent agents among targeted therapy. It is currently an FDA-approved, highly specific gp100 peptide and CD3 domain-binding protein reported to have promising results in non-treated HLA-A*02:01-positive metastatic UM patients [52]. Both OS at 1 year and PFS were reported to be higher in the tebentafusp group compared to the control group receiving pembrolizumab, ipilimumab, or dacarbazine (73% vs 59% $p < 0.001$ and 31% vs. 19% $p = 0.01$, respectively) [52].

Metastatic UM remains a therapeutic challenge as there is no proven standard treatment that efficiently prolongs OS. Even though comparative data is limited, the liver predominance metastatic dissemination of UM advocates for liver-directed therapies in surgically unresectable cases. Surgery is the prominent beneficial treatment when the tumor is in less advanced stages and resectable with free surgical margins. The numerous ongoing trials will add to the knowledge of management of this condition.

Acknowledgements The authors report no conflicts of interest.

No financial support was received for this submission.

This research did not receive any specific grant from funding agencies in the public, commercial, or not-for-profit sectors.

References

1. Tarlan B, Kiratli H. Uveal melanoma: current trends in diagnosis and management. Turk J Ophthalmol. 2016;46:123–37.
2. Mahendraraj K, Lau CSM, Lee I, Chamberlain RS. Trends in incidence, survival, and management of uveal melanoma: a population-based study of 7516 from the surveillance, epidemiology, and end-results database (1973-2012). Clin Ophthalmol. 2016;10:2113–9.
3. Kujala E, Makitie T, Kivela T. Very long-term prognosis of patients with malignant uveal melanoma. Invest Ophthalmol Vis Sci. 2003;44:4651–9.
4. Singh AD, Zabor EC, Radivoyevitch T. Estimating cured fractions of uveal melanoma. JAMA Ophthalmol. 2021;139:174–81.
5. Bustamente P, Piquet L, Landreville S, Burnier JV. Uveal melanoma pathobiology. Semin Cancer Biol. 2021;71:65–85. https://doi.org/10.1016/j.semcancer.2020.05.003.
6. Fuchs E. Das Sarkom des Uvealtractus. Wien: Wilhelm Braumüller; 1882. p. 197–206.
7. Lagrange F. Traité des tumeurs de l'oeil, de l'orbite et des annexes. Paris: G Steinheil, editeur; 1901. p. 384–8.
8. Zimmerman LE, McLean IW, Foster WD. Does enucleation of the eye containing a malignant melanoma prevent or accelerate the dissemination of tumour cells? Br J Ophthalmol. 1978;62:420–5.
9. Grossniklaus HE. Understanding uveal melanoma metastasis to the liver: the Zimmerman effect and the Zimmerman hypothesis. Ophthalmology. 2019;126:483–7.
10. Pavlick AC, Kujala E, Coupland SE, Finger PT. Uveal melanoma. In: Amin MB, et al., editors. AJCC staging manual. 8th ed. Springer: Switzerland; 2017. p. 805–17.
11. Garg G, Finger PT, Kivela T, et al. Patients presenting with metastases: stage IV uveal melanoma, an international study. Br J Ophthalmol. 2021;106(4):510–7. https://doi.org/10.1136/bjophthalmol-2020-317949.
12. Robertson AG, Shih J, Yau C, et al. Integrative analysis identifies four molecular and clinical subsets in uveal melanoma. Cancer Cell. 2017;32:204–20.
13. Jager MJ, Brouwer NJ, Esmaeli B. The cancer genoma atlas project: an integrated molecular view of uveal melanoma. Ophthalmology. 2018;125:1139–42.
14. Onken MD, Worley LA, Ehlers JP, Harbour JW. Gene expression profiling in uveal melanoma reveals two molecular classes and predicts metastatic death. Cancer Res. 2004;64:7205–9.
15. Violanti SS, Bononi I, Gallenga CE, Martini F, Tognon M, Perri P. New insights into molecular oncogenesis and therapy of uveal melanoma. Cancers. 2019;11(5):694. https://doi.org/10.3390/cancers11050694.
16. Harbour JW. Therapeutic escape in Gαq-mutant uveal melanoma: it's a FAK. Clin Cancer Res. 2021;27(11):2967–9. https://doi.org/10.1158/1078-0432.CCR-21-0567.
17. Smit KN, Chang J, Derks K, Vaarwater J, Brands T, Verdijk RM, Wiemer EAC, Mensink HW, Pothof J, de Klein A, Kılıç E. Aberrant microRNA expression and its implications for uveal melanoma metastasis. Cancers. 2019;11(6):815. https://doi.org/10.3390/cancers11060815.
18. Smit KN, Jager MJ, de Klein A, Kiliç E. Uveal melanoma: towards a molecular understanding. Prog Retin Eye Res. 2020;75:100800. https://doi.org/10.1016/j.preteyeres.2019.100800.
19. Amaro A, Gangemi R, Piaggio F, et al. The biology of uveal melanoma. Cancer Metastasis Rev. 2017;36:109–40.
20. Shain AH, Bagger MM, Yu R, et al. The genetic evolution of metastatic uveal melanoma. Nat Genet. 2019;51:1123–30.
21. Schefler AC, Koca E, Bernicker EH, Correa ZM. Relationship between clinical features, GEP class, and PRAME expression in uveal melanoma. Greafes Arch Clin Exp Ophthalmol. 2019;257:1541–5.
22. Field MG, Kuznetsov JN, Bussies PL, et al. BAP1 loss is associated with DNA methylomic repatterning in highly aggressive class 2 uveal melanomas. Clin Cancer Res. 2019;25:5663–73.
23. Figueiredo CR, Kalirai H, Sacco JJ, et al. Loss of *BAP1* expression is associated with an immunosuppressive microenvironment in uveal melanoma, with implications for immunotherapy development. J Pathol. 2020;250:420–39.
24. Vardanyan S, Brosig A, Merz H, Ranjbar M, Kakkassery V, Grisanti S, Tura A. Metastasis of uveal melanoma with monosomy-3 is associated with less glycogenetic gene expression profile and the dysregulation of glycogen storage. Cancers. 2020;12(8):2101. https://doi.org/10.3390/cancers12082101.
25. Javed A, Milhem M. Role of natural killer cells in uveal melanoma. Cancers. 2020;12(12):3694. https://doi.org/10.3390/cancers12123694.
26. Basile MS, Mazzon E, Fagone P, et al. Immunobiology of uveal melanoma: state of the art and therapeutic targets. Front Oncologia. 2019;9:1145. https://doi.org/10.3389/fonc.2019.01145. eCollection 2019
27. Garcia-Mulero S, Alonso MH, del Caprio LP, Sanz-Pamplona R, Piulats JM. Additive role of immune system infiltration and angiogenesis in uveal melanoma progression. Int J Mol Sci. 2021;22:2669. https://doi.org/10.3390/ijms22052669.
28. Aughton K, Kalirai H, Coupland SE. MicroRNAs and uveal melanoma: understanding the diverse role of these small molecular regulators. Int J Mol Sci. 2020;21(16):5648. https://doi.org/10.3390/ijms21165648.
29. Tsering T, Laskaris A, Abdouh M, et al. Uveal melanoma-derived extracellular vesicles display transforming potential and carry protein cargo involved in metastatic niche preparation. Cancers. 2020;12(10):2923. https://doi.org/10.3390/cancers12102923.

30. Tosi A, Cappellesso R, Tos APD, el. The immune cell landscape of metastatic uveal melanoma correlates with overal survival. J Exp Clin Cancer Res. 2021;40(1):154. https://doi.org/10.1186/s13046-021-01947-1.
31. Rantala ES, Hernberg M, Kivelä TT. Overall survival after treatment for metastatic uveal melanoma: a systematic review and meta-analysis. Melanoma Res. 2019;29:561–8.
32. Khoja L, Atenafu EG, Suciu S, Leyvraz S, Sato T, Marshall E, Keilholz U, Zimmer L, Patel SP, Piperno-Neumann S, Piulats J, Kivelä TT, Pfoehler C, Bhatia S, Huppert P, Van Iersel LBJ, De Vries IJM, Penel N, Vogl T, Cheng T, Fiorentini G, Mouriaux F, Tarhini A, Patel PM, Carvajal R, Joshua AM. Meta-analysis in metastatic uveal melanoma to determine progression free and overall survival benchmarks: an international rare cancers initiative (IRCI) ocular melanoma study. Ann Oncol. 2019;30:1370–80.
33. Seth R, Messersmith H, Kaur V, Kirkwood JM, Kudchadkar R, McQuade JL, Provenzano A, Swami U, Weber J, Alluri KC, Agarwala S, Ascierto PA, Atkins MB, Davis N, Ernstoff MS, Faries MB, Gold JS, Guild S, Gyorki DE, Khushalani NI, Meyers MO, Robert C, Santinami M, Sehdev A, Sondak VK, Spurrier G, Tsai KK, van Akkooi A, Funchain P. Systemic therapy for melanoma: ASCO guideline. J Clin Oncol. 2020;38:3947–70.
34. Rodrigues M, Koning L, Coupland SE, Jochemsen AG, Marais R, Stern MH, Valente A, Barnhill R, Cassoux N, Evans A, Galloway I, Jager MJ, Kapiteijn E, Romanowska-Dixon B, Ryll B, Roman-Roman S, Piperno-Neumann S, UM Cure 2020 Consortium. So close, yet so far: Discrepancies between uveal and other melanomas. A position paper from UM Cure 2020. Cancers (Basel). 2019;11:1032.
35. Rantala ES, Hernberg MM, Lundin M, Lundin J, Kivelä TT. Metastatic uveal melanoma managed with best supportive care. Acta Oncol. 2021;60:135–9.
36. Kivelä T, Simpson ER, Grossniklaus HE, Jager MJ, Singh AD, et al. Uveal melanoma. In: Amin MB, Edge SB, Greene FL, et al., editors. AJCC cancer staging manual. 8th ed. Switzerland: Springer; 2017. p. 805–17.
37. Rantala ES, Kivelä TT, Hernberg MM. Impact of staging on survival outcomes: a nationwide real-world cohort study of metastatic uveal melanoma. Melanoma Res. 2021;31:224–31.
38. Eskelin S, Pyrhönen S, Hahka-Kemppinen M, Tuomaala S, Kivelä T. A prognostic model and staging for metastatic uveal melanoma. Cancer. 2003;97:465–75.
39. Valpione S, Moser JC, Parrozzani R, Bazzi M, Mansfield AS, Mocellin S, Pigozzo J, Midena E, Markovic SN, Aliberti C, Campana LG, Chiarion-Sileni V. Development and external validation of a prognostic nomogram for metastatic uveal melanoma. PLoS One. 2015;10:e0120181.
40. Mariani P, Dureau S, Savignoni A, Rouic LL, Levy-Gabriel C, Piperno-Neumann S, Rodrigues MJ, Desjardins L, Cassoux N, Servois V. Development of a prognostic nomogram for liver metastasis of uveal melanoma patients selected by liver MRI. Cancers (Basel). 2019;11:863.
41. Pons F, Plana M, Caminal JM, Pera J, Fernandes I, Perez J, Garcia-Del-Muro X, Marcoval J, Penin R, Fabra A, Piulats JM. Metastatic uveal melanoma: is there a role for conventional chemotherapy? A single center study based on 58 patients. Melanoma Res. 2011;21:217–22.
42. Brown DB, Gould JE, Gervais DA, Goldberg SN, Murthy R, Millward SF, Rilling WS, Geschwind JF, Salem R, Vedantham S, Cardella JF, Soulen MC, Society of Interventional Radiology Technology Assessment Committee and the International Working Group on Image-Guided Tumor Ablation. Transcatheter therapy for hepatic malignancy: standardization of terminology and reporting criteria. J Vasc Interv Radiol. 2009;20:S425–34.
43. Gonsalves CF, Adamo RD, Eschelman DJ. Locoregional therapies for the treatment of uveal melanoma hepatic metastases. Semin Intervent Radiol. 2020;37:508–17.
44. Rowcroft A, Loveday BPT, Thomson BNJ, Banting S, Knowles B. Systematic review of liver directed therapy for uveal melanoma hepatic metastases. HPB (Oxford). 2020;22:497–505.
45. Leyvraz S, Piperno-Neumann S, Suciu S, Baurain JF, Zdzienicki M, Testori A, Marshall E, Scheulen M, Jouary T, Negrier S, Vermorken JB, Kaempgen E, Durando X, Schadendorf D, Gurunath RK, Keilholz U. Hepatic intra-arterial versus intravenous fotemustine in patients with liver metastases from uveal melanoma (EORTC 18021): a multicentric randomized trial. Ann Oncol. 2014;25:742–6.
46. Ford R, Gonsalves C, Adamo R, Ahmad H, Orloff M, Sato T, Eschelman D. 03:09 PM abstract no. 317 prolonged survival after treatment of hepatic uveal melanoma metastases using immunoembolization. J Vasc Interv Radiol. 2019;30(Supplement):S140.
47. Xing M, Prajapati HJ, Dhanasekaran R, Lawson DH, Kokabi N, Eaton BR, Kim HS. Selective internal Yttrium-90 radioembolization therapy (90Y-SIRT) versus best supportive care in patients with unresectable metastatic melanoma to the liver refractory to systemic therapy: safety and efficacy cohort study. Am J Clin Oncol. 2017;40:27–34.
48. Gonsalves CF, Eschelman DJ, Adamo RD, Anne PR, Orloff MM, Terai M, Hage AN, Yi M, Chervoneva I, Sato T. A prospective phase II trial of radioembolization for treatment of uveal melanoma hepatic metastasis. Radiology. 2019;293:223–31.
49. Wessely A, Steeb T, Erdmann M, Heinzerling L, Vera J, Schlaak M, Berking C, Heppt MV. The role of immune checkpoint blockade in uveal melanoma. Int J Mol Sci. 2020;21:879.
50. Bol KF, Ellebaek E, Hoejberg L, Bagger MM, Larsen MS, Klausen TW, Køhler UH, Schmidt H, Bastholt L, Kiilgaard JF, Donia M, Svane IM. Real-world impact of immune checkpoint inhibitors in metastatic uveal melanoma. Cancers (Basel). 2019;11:1489.
51. Seedor RS, Orloff M, Sato T. Genetic landscape and emerging therapies in uveal melanoma. Cancers (Basel). 2021;13:5503.
52. Nathan P, Hassel JC, Rutkowski P, Baurain JF, Butler MO, Schlaak M, Sullivan RJ, Ochsenreither S, Dummer R, Kirkwood JM, Joshua AM, Sacco JJ, Shoushtari AN, Orloff M, Piulats JM, Milhem M, Salama AKS, Curti B, Demidov L, Gastaud L, Mauch C, Yushak M, Carvajal RD, Hamid O, Abdullah SE, Holland C, Goodall H, Piperno-Neumann S, IMCgp100-202 Investigators. Overall survival benefit with Tebentafusp in metastatic uveal melanoma. N Engl J Med. 2021;385:1196–206.

Intra-vitreal Chemotherapy for Vitreoretinal Lymphoma

Jacob Pe'er and Shahar Frenkel

1 Introduction

Vitreoretinal lymphoma (VRL), although a rare disease, is the most common type of intraocular lymphoma, and may involve the vitreous, retina, sub-retinal space, retinal pigment epithelium, and the optic nerve. These are high-grade, mostly B-cell malignancies that are associated with a poor prognosis, if the patient also develops central nervous system lymphoma (CNSL) [1]. T-cell VRLs are much less common [2]. Three other groups of intraocular lymphomas involve various parts of the uvea and are usually low-grade B-cell lymphomas [1].

VRL is often associated with CNSL, and is considered by specialists as a subgroup of CNSL [3, 4]. It has been reported that 56–90% of VRL patients ultimately develop CNSL, while 11–25% of patients with CNSL develop VRL [3, 5–8]. VRL is commonly diagnosed in patients over 50 years of age, although younger patients are also diagnosed. There is no clear sex predilection [3, 4], although in several studies more women were affected than men [9–11].

The hallmark of VRL is the presence of cells in the vitreous, mainly in clumps, which is often misdiagnosed as a non-responsive uveitis, along with retinal and sub-retinal infiltrates [12]. These findings may reduce the visual acuity, although often the visual acuity is unexpectedly good.

When VRL is suspected clinically, a diagnostic vitrectomy or vitreous tap is performed. The vitreous samples can be analyzed for the presence of malignant cells by cytopathology with possible immunohistochemical staining or flow cytometry to identify the cell type and monoclonality. Other diagnostic methods are the measurement of the levels of interleukins (IL-10 and IL-6) and the ratio between them, which was found to be a very sensitive test, also in aqueous humor samples from the anterior chamber (AC) of the eye; PCR for detection of immunoglobulin heavy chain (IgH) or T-cell receptor (TCR) gene rearrangement which indicates clonality of malignant cells; and a search for an L265P mutation in the myeloid differentiation primary response gene 88 (MYD88) in diffuse large B-cell lymphoma [3, 8, 13–17].

Since intraocular lymphoma was first recognized in 1951 [18, 19], initially as ocular reticulum cell sarcoma, its treatment has evolved from enucleation [19] through radiation therapy, with or without whole-brain radiotherapy, systemic chemotherapy, intrathecal chemotherapy, intra-vitreal chemotherapy, and biological therapy.

The treatment of VRL aims to eradicate the intraocular disease. For years it has been debated whether treatment of VRL may prevent the development of CNSL, or whether patients with VRL without evidence of CNSL should be treated systemically to prevent CNSL [3]. So far, there have been no randomized clinical trials that can lead to a consensus recommendation that will solve this debate. In their report, the International CNSL Collaborative Group recommended on systemic treatment if the disease involves the CNS and local ocular treatment if the disease involves only the eye, with close follow-up and ongoing collaboration between neuro-oncologists and ophthalmologists [3].

Radiation therapy in doses ranged between 30 and 50 Gy was the gold standard for the treatment of intraocular lymphoma in many institutions. However, because of high recurrence rate and ocular complications, radiation is less often considered nowadays for therapy of VRL [7]. Systemic chemotherapy, mainly with high-dose methotrexate (MTX), sometimes combined with rituximab, which is used for treating CNSL, has also been used for treating VRL. However, the limited penetration of systemic drugs into the vitreous is well known, leading to incomplete response [7]. Direct intra-vitreal injection of drugs, including among others, chemotherapeutic and biological drugs, has become routine in the treatment of various infectious, inflammatory, neovascular, and malignant intraocular disease. Intra-vitreal chemother-

J. Pe'er (✉) · S. Frenkel
Ocular Oncology Service, Division of Ophthalmology, Hadassah—Hebrew University Medical Center, Jerusalem, Israel
e-mail: peer@hadassah.org.il; Shahar@hadassah.org.il

B. V. Chawla, M. E. Aronow (eds.), *Global Perspectives in Ocular Oncology*, https://doi.org/10.1007/978-3-031-08250-4_16

apy has become the most common method of treating VRL. In this chapter we review the current status of intraocular chemotherapy for VRL.

2 Intra-vitreal Chemotherapy

Intra-vitreal chemotherapy can be given as primary therapy for VRL, or as adjuvant therapy to other treatment methods, although in recent years the primary intra-vitreal treatment has become the gold standard.

A range of drugs has been used intra-vitreally for treating intraocular malignancies. Already in 1964 Ericson and associates [20] had performed trials of intra-vitreal injections of thiotepa, nitrogen mustard, cyclophosphamide, and methotrexate into rabbits' eyes, finding no significant intraocular toxicity except in those treated with nitrogen mustard. They even treated several patients with retinoblastoma with intra-vitreal injections of thiotepa. Unfortunately, since then, until the recent two to three decades, there were no further investigations of direct intra-vitreal chemotherapy in treating intraocular malignancies.

In the following paragraphs we will describe the main drugs which are currently used in intra-vitreal injections for treating VRL.

2.1 Intra-vitreal Methotrexate

MTX is currently the most commonly used drug for VRL. It is an anti-metabolite that acts by competitive inhibition of the enzyme dihydrofolate reductase, resulting in reduced thymine synthesis, an essential nuclear base in DNA [21].

Fishburne and associates at the Oregon Health & Science University (OHSU, Portland, Oregon, USA) [21] were the first to report in 1997 on the treatment of VRL in seven eyes of four patients with intra-vitreal injections of 400 μg of MTX, injecting 6–11 injections per eye, in conjunction with systemic chemotherapy delivered by hyper-osmotic blood brain-barrier disruption (BBBD). All patients had complete remission without serious ocular toxic effects.

de Smet and associates [22, 23] from the National Eye Institute at the NIH reported two successful cases of treating recurrent VRL with combined intra-vitreal chemotherapy, one case with intra-vitreal MTX and thiotepa and one case with intra-vitreal MTX and dexamethasone, with a full remission.

de Smet and colleagues tested the pharmacokinetics of a single dose of intraocular injection of MTX in a blind eye of a patient with recurrent VRL by injecting 400 μg. This resulted in concentrations that were lymphocytotoxic for 5 days [22]. Velez and associates [24] investigated the pharmacokinetics and toxicity of several intra-vitreal injections of 400 μg MTX in rabbits' eyes, together with single injections of fluorouracil and dexamethasone. They found that MTX vitreous levels remain therapeutic (>0.5 μM) in the rabbit eye for 48–72 h without evidence of toxicity.

In 2002 the OHSU group together with the Hadassah Medical Center group, reported a larger series of 26 eyes of 16 human immunodeficiency virus (HIV)-negative patients with VRL from the two centers, treated by intra-vitreal injections of 400 μg MTX in 0.1 mL [25]. Their protocol included three phases: two injections per week for a month as an induction phase; weekly injections for a month in one center and 2 months in the other center as a consolidation phase; and subsequently a maintenance phase of monthly injections to complete a year of treatment. All eyes achieved remission after a maximum of 12 MTX injections (mean of 8.5 injections). Three patients of one center had relapse in the eye, and were treated again using the same intra-vitreal injections protocol with complete remission. Six of the 16 patients died in follow-up as a result of progressive PCNSL, but without clinical ocular involvement.

Frenkel and associates at the Hadassah Medical Center reported a large series of 44 eyes of 26 patients from a single center, who were treated by the same induction-consolidation-maintenance regimen of intra-vitreal MTX injections [9]. This group of patients also included several patients with T-cell lymphoma. (This group included half of the patients reported by Smith et al. [25]). Clinical remission was reached in all eyes after an average of 6.4 injections with 95% of the eyes needing 13 injections or less to be cleared of lymphoma cells. None of the patients had a relapse. All patients in these reports who had CNSL were also treated for the brain disease by systemic chemotherapy. Sou and colleagues [26] reported similar results in one Japanese center.

Some of the patients had decreased visual acuity during the early stages of the treatment, but most of them preserved their vision or had visual improvement. The most common side effects of the intra-vitreal injections are conjunctival hyperemia and transient keratopathy, ranging from diffuse punctate keratopathy to severe epitheliopathy, which usually subside during the maintenance phase [9, 25, 27]. Other complications are acceleration of existing cataract, which could also be due to diagnostic vitrectomy, neovascular glaucoma, which could have occurred because of the VRL itself, and intraocular inflammation that can be successfully treated by corticosteroids [9, 25, 28]. Patients who were treated by BBBD for CNSL may develop maculopathy without significant effect on their visual acuity [25]. None of the patients who were treated by intra-vitreal injections of MTX but were not treated by BBBD developed maculopathy [29].

There have been some differences in the protocols used in various institutions for intra-vitreal MTX monotherapy for treating VRL. Most treating ophthalmologists inject 400 μg in 0.1 mL, as in the first studies. Only a few inject less than

400 µg, and some, like us, reduced the injection volume to 0.05 mL. However, the number of injections varies widely, and some will inject "according to the clinical behavior of the lymphoma" [30], usually with higher relapse rate.

Combined treatment of intra-vitreal injections with systemic chemotherapy, mostly high-dose MTX, has been used in treating VRL [30–33]. However, there is no evidence that the systemic MTX improves or shortens the time of treatment, or increases the time to relapse and progression of the VRL. In addition, there is no proof that systemic chemotherapy prevents the development of CNSL in VRL patients without CNSL [8, 11]. In our experience and that of others, intra-vitreal MTX injections should be used for treating VRL and systemic chemotherapy for treating CNSL. We recommend avoiding systemic chemotherapy in the treatment of VRL patients when the CNS is not involved. Other combinational treatments for VRL are the use of intra-vitreal MTX and rituximab, sometimes with the addition of systemic chemotherapy or even radiotherapy [34–37].

2.2 Intra-vitreal Rituximab

Rituximab is a humanized monoclonal antibody that targets CD20-postive B-cells in all stages, from a pre-B-cell through a mature B-cell. Thus, CD20 also presents on lymphomatous B-cells in VRL and CNSL. Rituximab was approved in 1997 by the FDA to be used in B-cell lymphomas of various types. Since the vast majority of VRL and CNSL are B-cell in origin, it makes rituximab an ideal drug for intra-vitreal therapy. Obviously, rituximab is not an appropriate drug when the VRL is of T-cell type. The option of using intra-vitreal injections of rituximab for treating VRL was raised in order to overcome MTX-related side effects, to reduce the initially required frequency of intra-vitreal injections of MTX, and to reduce resistance to MTX therapy.

Some animal studies on intra-vitreal injections of rituximab were performed, and showed its effect on VRL. In all these studies the researchers injected 1 mg/0.1 mL rituximab. Kim and associates [38], investigating the pharmacokinetics of intra-vitreal injections of rituximab into rabbit eyes, found a half-life of 4.7 days in both the aqueous and vitreous. Pulido and colleagues [39] found that rituximab penetrated all retinal layers in rabbit eyes, and Kitzmann and associates [40] showed no toxicity to the rabbit eyes. Mineo and colleagues [41] showed eradication of lymphoma in more than half of the animals and significant inhibition of tumor progression in the rest.

The first reported use of intra-vitreal injection of rituximab for treating VRL was in 2007 by Kitzmann and colleagues [40], who published their experience in treating five eyes of three patients. They used 3–4 injections of 1 mg/0.1 mL rituximab with a good response, no toxicity and no evidence of recurrence after a short median follow-up of 3.6 months. Ohguro and associates [42] treated two patients who had VRL relapse after intra-vitreal MTX by 4 weekly injections of 1 mg/0.1 mL rituximab with complete remission and no recurrence after 2 months.

Hoshida and associates [43] reported their experience in treating 20 eyes of 13 patients who had discontinued previous intra-vitreal MTX treatment because of severe corneal epitheliopathy. They used 4 weekly injections of 1 mg/mL rituximab as one-course protocol, and additional injections were administered when VRL recurred in 11 of the eyes. All patients completed 1 year follow-up. Twelve eyes showed transient intraocular pressure elevation. No other significant side effects developed.

In 2014 Larkin and associates [44] presented what is still the largest series of intra-vitreal rituximab-based treatment for treating VRL, including 48 eyes of 34 patients in clinics in five countries. The eyes were treated with a median of 3.5 injections; the most common interval was monthly. About two-third of the eyes were also injected with MTX, usually on the same day with rituximab. Others were treated with more extensive cytotoxic therapies. Complete remission was achieved in 65% of the eyes and 23% showed partial remission. Among eyes that were treated only by intraocular chemotherapy, 53% experienced complete remission and 11 partial remission. After a median follow-up of 18 months, VRL recurred in 23% of the eyes. The main complication in this series was cataract in 19% of eyes.

The use of intra-vitreal rituximab for VRL was also reported in other small series and case reports. It was used mainly as a secondary treatment [45–47] or in combination with other drugs, mainly MTX [34–37]. There is still no significant series of eyes with VRL treated by rituximab alone as primary treatment. Such a study should be considered.

2.3 Other Drugs for Intra-vitreal Chemotherapy

The experience with using drugs other than MTX and rituximab for the treatment of VRL is very limited.

Intra-vitreal injections of **melphalan** have been often used in recent years for treating retinoblastoma. Melphalan is a phenylalanine derivative of nitrogen mustard and an alkylating agent. Shields and associates [48] reported in 2017 their experience in treating three eyes of two patients with VRL by intra-vitreal injections of 10 µg/0.1 mL melphalan. One of the patients with bilateral VRL showed clinical remission within 3 weeks after a single injection. Recurrence in one of the eyes was treated by additional 6 bimonthly injections with a good response and no recurrence after 19 months of follow-up. The other patient with bilateral VRL was treated by intra-vitreal melphalan in one eye and

MTX in the other eye. The VRL in the eye treated with melphalan was cured by one injection. No toxicity was observed. This group expanded their use of melphalan and reported on 12 more patients with encouraging results [49]. Damato and associates [50] reported their good experience in treating one patient with VRL by intra-vitreal melphalan.

Thiotepa is an organophosphorus alkylating agent, which results in crosslinking of the double-stranded DNA helix and interferes with DNA replication. Ericson and associates reported their results of using intra-vitreal thiotepa injections for treating intraocular malignancies in rabbits' eyes already in 1964 [20], finding no significant toxicity. de Smet and associates [22, 23] combined thiotepa (2 mg/0.1 mL) with MTX injections in treating a patient with VRL. However, the thiotepa injection was associated with elevated intraocular pressure and loss of vision. In light of the good results with intra-vitreal MTX alone, thiotepa is no longer being used.

Corticosteroids have lymphotoxic effect; however, the response is usually partial. Thus, corticosteroids are not used as a single agent for treating lymphoma. de Smet used a combination of MTX and dexamethasone in treating one patient with VRL resulting in full remission. Castellino and associates reported the use of intra-vitreal corticosteroids injections with other systemic and intra-vitreal drugs [47]. However, intra-vitreal injections of corticosteroids did not become part of the standard practice in treating VRL.

2.4 Investigational Drugs for Intra-vitreal Injections

During the recent two decades researchers reported their experience using various experimental drugs for intra-vitreal or intra-cameral injections in animal models of VRL. However, none of them have matured for clinical use.

Gregory and associates [51] studied the use of membrane FasL vesicles, the membrane-only form of Fas ligand, to activate innate immunity and terminate the immune privilege of the eye. By a single injection of membrane FasL vesicles into the anterior chamber of mice, they eliminated the lymphoma cells that were previously injected into this site.

Li and associates [52] used recombinant immunotoxin HA22 targeting human B-cell lymphoma in a mouse model of intraocular lymphoma. A single intra-vitreal injection of immunotoxin HA22 resulted in complete regression of the lymphoma, demonstrating B-cell-specific immunotoxin therapy.

Ublituximab is a glycoengineered anti-human-CD20 monoclonal antibody that was developed for treating multiple sclerosis. In 2013 Ben-Abdelwahed and associates [53] reported their results in treating the murine model of VRL by a single intra-vitreal injection of ublituximab with marked effect against the lymphoma B-cells expressing CD20.

Some other monoclonal antibodies such as daclizumab, efalizumab, and alemtuzumab showed positive results in animal models, and have the potential to be a useful adjuvant therapy for intraocular lymphoma [54]. However, as with previous experimental drugs, no further reports are available on their use in treating VRL.

3 Summary

Since intraocular lymphoma was first recognized about 70 years ago, its treatment has gradually evolved. Enucleation was often performed in the early years, when the disease was diagnosed late. When VRL was more frequently diagnosed, and its common association with CNSL was recognized, other methods of treatments have been used, including radiation therapy, systemic chemotherapy using various drugs, or in combination. Because of the limited penetration of drugs administered systemically into the eye and their systemic toxicity, and the local side effects of radiation to the eye, direct intra-vitreal chemotherapy has gained popularity and became a common method of treating VRL in the last two decades.

Intra-vitreal injections of MTX as monotherapy was found to be very effective in inducing intraocular tumor remission with acceptable side effects and rare occurrence of relapse. Additional systemic chemotherapy probably does not add to the cure rate of the VRL, and should be used only when CNS lymphoma is associated with the VRL.

In recent years the use of intra-vitreal injections of rituximab has been carried out in several centers, with or without combining MTX, with encouraging results and no significant adverse effects. However, its use varies markedly among experts and the results are still inferior to MTX. Intra-vitreal injection of melphalan was also proved to be an effective drug, but at this time has been employed only in one ocular oncology center.

Because of the rarity of VRL, international collaboration is needed for defining the role of intra-vitreal chemotherapy in eradicating this disease. The present drugs which are used clinically are effective, and probably a consensus on protocols of using them is needed. It seems that in the future the treatment of VRL will continue to evolve, new drugs will be introduced and new methods of intraocular delivery will be developed.

References

1. Coupland SE, Damato B. Understanding intraocular lymphomas. Clin Exp Ophthalomol. 2008;36:564–78.
2. Chaput F, Amer R, Baglivo E, Touitou V, Kozyreff A, Bron D, Bodaghi B, Lettoang P, Bergstrom C, Grossniklaus HE, Chan CC, Pe'er J, Caspers LE. Intraocular T-cell lymphoma; clinical presen-

tation diagnosis, treatment and outcome. Ocul Immunol Inflamm. 2017;25:644–53.

3. Chan CC, Rubenstein JL, Coupland SE, Davis JL, Harbour JW, Johnston PB, Cassoux N, Touitou V, Smith JR, Batchelor TT, Pulido JS. Primary vitreoretinal lymphoma: a report from an international primary central nervous system lymphoma collaborative group symposium. Oncologist. 2011;16:1589–99.
4. Kvopka M, Lake SR, Smith JR. Intraocular chemotherapy for vitreoretinal lymphoma: a review. Clin Exp Ophthalmol. 2020;48:240–8.
5. Hochberg FH, Miller DC. Primary central nervous system lymphoma. J Neurosurg. 1988;68:835–53.
6. Farall AL, Smith JR. Eye involvement in primary central nervous system lymphoma. Surv Ophthalmol. 2020;65:548–61.
7. Pe'er J, Hochberg FH, Foster CS. Clinical review: treatment of vitreoretinal lymphoma. Ocul Immunol Inflamm. 2009;17:290–306.
8. Grimm SA, Pulido JS, Jahnke K, et al. Primary intraocular lymphoma: an international primary central nervous system lymphoma collaborative group report. Ann Oncol. 2007;18:1851–5.
9. Frenkel S, Hendler K, Siegal T, Shalom E, Pe'er J. Intravitreal methotrexate for treating vitreoretinal lymphoma: 10 years of experience. Br J Ophthalmol. 2008;92:383–8.
10. Kimura K, Usui Y, Goto H, for Japanese Intraocular Lymphoma Study Group. Clinical features and diagnostic significance of the intraocular fluid of 217 patients with intraocular lymphoma. Jpn J Ophthalmol. 2012;56:383–9.
11. Riemens A, Bromberg J, Touitou V, et al. Treatment strategies in primary vitreoretinal lymphoma. A 17-center European colaborative study. JAMA Ophthalmol. 2015;133:191–7.
12. Coupland SE, Heimann H, Bechrakis NE. Primary intraocular lymphoma: a review of the clinical, histopathological and molecular biological features. Graefes Arch Clin Exp Ophthalmol. 2004;242:901–13.
13. Fend F, Ferreri AJ, Coupland SE. How we diagnose and treat vitreoretinal lymphoma. Br J Haematol. 2016;173:680–92.
14. Chan CC, Sen HN. Current concepts in diagnosing and managing primary vitreoretinal (intraocular) lymphoma. Discov Med. 2013;15:93–100.
15. Reichstein D. Primary vitreoretinal lymphoma: an update on pathogenesis, diagnosis and treatment. Curr Opin Ophthalmol. 2016;27:177–84.
16. Frenkel S, Pe'er J, Kaufman R, Maly B, Habot-Wilner Z. The importance of cytokines analysis in the diagnosis of vitreoretinal lymphoma. Acta Ophthalmol. 2020;98:e668–78.
17. Carbonell D, Mahajan S, Chee SP, et al. Consensus recommendations for the diagnosis of vitreoretinal lymphoma. Ocul Immunol Inflamm. 2021;29(3):507–20.
18. Cooper EL, Riker JL. Malignant lymphoma of the uveal tract. Am J Ophthalmol. 1951;34:1153–8.
19. Vogel MH, Font RL, Zimmerman LE, Levine RA. Reticulum cell sarcoma of the retina and uvea. Report of six cases and review of the literature. Am J Ophthalmol. 1968;66:2005–15.
20. Ericson L, Karlberg B, Rosengren BH. Trials of intravitreal injections of chemotherapeutic agents in rabbits. Acta Ophthalmol. 1964;42:721–6.
21. Canellos GP, Lister TA, Skarin AT. Chemotherapy of the non-Hodgkin's lymphomas. Cancer. 1978;42(2 Suppl):932–40.
22. de Smet MD, Vancs VS, Kohler D, Solomon D, Chan CC. Intravitreal chemotherapy for the treatment of recurrent intraocular lymphoma. Br J Ophthalmol. 1999;83:448–51.
23. de Smet MD. Management of non-Hodgkin's intraocular lymphoma with intravitreal methotrexate. Bull Soc Belg Ophthalmol. 2001;279:91–5.
24. Velez G, Yuan P, Sung BC, Tansey G, Reed GF, Chan CC, Nussenblatt RB, Robinson MR. Pharmacokinetics and toxicity of intravitreal chemotherapy for primary intraocular lymphoma. Arch Ophthalmol. 2001;119:1518–24.
25. Smith JR, Rosenbaum JT, Wilson DJ, Doolittle ND, Siegal T, Neuwelt EA, Pe'er J. Role of intravitreal methotrexate in the management of primary central nervous system lymphoma with ocular involvement. Ophthalmology. 2002;109:1709–16.
26. Sou R, Ohguro N, Maeda T, Sainshin Y, Tano Y. Treatment of primary intraocular lymphoma with intravitreal methotrexate. Jpn J Ophthalmol. 2008;52:167–74.
27. Jeong Y, Ryu JS, Park UC, Oh JY. Corneal epithelial toxicity after intravitreal methotrexate injection for vitreoretinal lymphoma: clinical and in-vitro studies. J Clin Med. 2020;18:2672.
28. Goldberg S, Frenkel S, Blumenthal EZ, Solomon A, Pe'er J. Intraocular lymphoma. Ophthalmology. 2007;114:1236–7.
29. Vicuna-Kojchen J, Frenkel S, Siegal T, Shalom E, Chowers I, Pe'er J. Maculopathy in patients with CNS lymphoma treated with chemotherapy in conjunction with blood brain barrier disruption. Br J Ophthalmol. 2008;92:231–5.
30. Klimova A, Heissigerawa J, Rihova E, Brichova M, Pytlik R, Spicka I, Mrazova K, Karolova J, Svozilkova P. Combined treatment of primary vitreoretinal lymphoma significantly prolongs the time to first relapse. Br J Ophthalmol. 2018;102:1579–85.
31. Akiyama H, Takase H, Kubo F, Miki T, Yamamoto M, Tomita M, Mochizuki M, Miura O, Arai A. High-dose methotrexate following intravitreal methotrexate administration in preventing central nervous system involvement of primary intraocular lymphoma. Cancer Sci. 2016;107:1458–64.
32. Ma WL, Hou HA, Hsu YJ, Chen YK, Tang JL, Tsay W, Yeh PT, Yang CM, Lin CP, Tien HF. Clinical outcome of primary intraocular lymphoma patients treated with front-line systemic high-dose methotrexate and intravitreal methotrexate injection. Ann Hematol. 2016;95:593–601.
33. Kaburaki T, Taoka K, Matsuda J, Yamashita H, Matsuda I, Tsuji H, Tanaka R, Nakazaki K, Nakamura F, Kamiya K, Kurokawa M, Ohtomo K, Aihara M. Combined intravitreal methotrexate and immunochemotherapy followed by reduced-dose whole-brain radiotherapy for newly diagnosed B-cell primary intraocular lymphoma. Br J Haematol. 2017;179:246–55.
34. Abu Samra K, Oray M, Ebrahimiadib N, Lee S, Anesi S, Foster CS. Intraocular lymphoma: descriptive data of 26 patients including clinico-pathologic features, vitreous finding, and treatment outcome. Ocul Immunol Inflamm. 2018;26:347–52.
35. Pulido JS, Johnston PB, Nowakowski GS, Castellino A, Raja H. The diagnosis and treatment of primary vitreoretinal lymphoma: a review. Int J Retina Vitreous. 2018;4:18.
36. Castellino A, Pulido JS, Johnston PB, Ristow KM, Bennani NN, Inwards DJ, Macon WR, Michallef IN, King RL, Salomao DR, Witzig TE, Habermann TM, Nowakowski GS. Role of systemic high-dose methotrexate and combined approaches in the management of vitreoretinal lymphoma: a single center experience 1990-2018. Am J Hematol. 2019;94:291–8.
37. Giuffre C, Cicinelli MV, Marchese A, Modorati GM, Brambati M, Ferreri AJM, Calimeri T, Ponzoni M, Bandello F, Miserocchi E. Clinical experience in a large cohort of patients with vitreoretinal lymphoma in a single center. Ocul Immunol Inflamm. 2020;26:1–7.
38. Kim H, Csaky KG, Chan CC, et al. The pharmacokinetics of rituximab following an intravitreal injection. Exp Eye Res. 2006;82:760–6.
39. Pulido JS, Bakri SJ, Valyi-Nagy T, Shukla D. Rituximab penetrates full-thickness retina in contrast to tissue plasminogen activator control. Retina. 2007;27:1071–3.
40. Kitzmann AS, Pulido JS, Mohney BG, Baratz KH, Grube T, Marler RJ, Donaldson MJ, O'Neill BP, Johnston PB, Johnson KM, Dixon LE, Salomao DR, Cameron JD. Intraocular use of rituximab. Eye. 2007;21:1524–7.
41. Mineo JF, Scheffer A, Karkoutly C, Nouvel L, Kerdraon O, Trauet J, Bordron A, Dessaint JP, Labalette M, Berthou C, Labalette P. Using human CD20-transfected murine lymphoma-

tous B cells to evaluate the efficacy of intravitreal and intracerebral rituximab injections in mice. Invest Ophthalmol Vis Sci. 2008;49:4738–45.
42. Ohguro N, Hashida N, Tano Y. Effect of intravitreous rituximab injections in patients with recurrent ocular lesions associated with central nervous system lymphoma. Arch Ophthalmol. 2008;126:1002–3.
43. Hashida N, Ohguro N, Nishida K. Efficacy and complications of intravitreal rituximab injection for treating primary vitreoretinal lymphoma. Transl Vis Sci Technol. 2012;98:99–103.
44. Larkin KL, Saboo US, Comer GM, et al. Use of intravitreal rituximab for treatment of vitreoretinal lymphoma. Br J Ophthalmol. 2014;98:99–103.
45. Echegaray JJ, Llop S, Sepulveda M, Velez-Rosario R, Perez N, Oliver AL. Intravitreal rituximab for the treatment of secondary intraocular relapse of a large B-cell lymphoma. Am J Ophthalmol Case Rep. 2018;9:77–9.
46. Fernandez-Canabate E, Fernandez-Canabate S. Intravitreal rituximab for the treatment of intraocular relapse of non-Hodgkin's lymphoma. Farm Hosp. 2018;42:20–1.
47. Cicinelli MV, Marchese A, Miserocchi E, Giuffre C, Berchicci L, Querques G, Bandello F, Modaroti GM. Retinal and choroidal changes of vitreoretinal lymphoma from active remission phase after intravitreal rituximab. Ocul Immunol Inflamm. 2020;28:637–46.
48. Shields CL, Sioufi K, Masheyeki A, Shields JA. Intravitreal Melphalan for treatment of primary vitreoretinal lymphoma: a new indication for an old drug. JAMA Ophthalmol. 2017;135:815–8.
49. Dalvin LA, Lim LAS, Ancona-Lezama D, Mozloumi M, Chang M, Mashayekhi A, Shields CL. Tumor control and visual acuity outcomes in vitreoretinal lymphoma with and without sub–retinal pigment epithelium infiltration. Ophthalmol Retina. 2019;3:998–1005.
50. Damato B, Bever GJ, Kim DJ, Afshar AR, Rubenstein JL. An audit of retinal lymphoma treatment at the University of California San Francisco. Eye. 2020;34:515–22.
51. Gregory MS, Koh S, Huang E, Saff RR, Marshak-Rothstein A, Mukai S, Ksander BR. A novel treatment for ocular tumors using membrane FasL vesicles to activate innate immunity and terminate immune privilege. Invest Ophthalmol Vis Sci. 2005;46:2495–502.
52. Li Z, Mahesh SP, Shen DF, Liu B, Siu WO, Hwang FS, Wang QC, Chan CC, Pastan I, Nussenblatt RB. Eradication of tumor colonization and invasion by a B cell-specific immunotoxin in a murine model for human primary intraocular lymphoma. Cancer Res. 2006;66:10586–93.
53. Ben-Abdelwahed R, Donnou S, Ouakrim H, et al. Preclinical study of Ublituximab, a glycoengineered anti-human CD20 antibody, in morine models of primary cerebral and intraocular B-cell lymphomas. Invest Ophthalmol Vis Sci. 2013;54:3657–65.
54. Rodrigues EB, Farah ME, Maia M, et al. Therapeutic monoclonal antibodies in ophthalmology. Prog Retin Eye Res. 2009;28:117–44.

Update on Uveal Lymphoma

Arman Mashayekhi

1 Introduction

Neoplastic proliferation of lymphoid cells in the uveal tract is a rare intraocular malignancy. Uveal lymphoma can affect all parts of the uveal tract but the choroid is more commonly affected than the ciliary body or iris.

Uveal lymphomas developing in patients without prior history of systemic lymphoma are classified as primary type and those developing in patients with prior history of systemic lymphoma are considered the secondary type [1–7]. The majority of cases of primary uveal lymphoma are indolent, low-grade, B-cell non-Hodgkin lymphomas, but secondary uveal lymphomas are usually composed of higher grade lymphoma cells.

Uveal lymphoma has distinct features on clinical examination and ancillary imaging, but tissue biopsy may be required for definite diagnosis, especially in atypical cases. Treatment of primary uveal lymphoma is associated with favorable outcomes, but the result of treatment can be less favorable in eyes with secondary uveal lymphoma, depending on the type of lymphoma and the extent and severity of ocular involvement.

2 Historical Perspective

In 1920, Triebenstein published the first report on lymphomatous infiltration of the uveal tract in a 63-year-old man and used the term *uveal lymphosarcoma* to refer to this condition [8]. Additional reports on isolated cases of *uveal sarcoma* were published by other investigators over the following several decades [9, 10].

In 1967, Crookes and Mullaney published a case report on a 44-year-old man who underwent enucleation of his right eye for management of a large intraocular mass. Histopathologic examination showed densely packed mature lymphocytic cells with numerous plasma cells at the periphery of the mass. Based on these features and the uneventful clinical course of the patient following enucleation, the authors concluded that the lymphoid mass was inflammatory and not neoplastic and they used the term *lymphoid hyperplasia of the uveal tract* in their publication [11]. In the same year, Gass described lymphoid infiltration of the choroid and ciliary body in a 55-year-old woman with retinal detachment and angle closure glaucoma. Evaluation of the enucleated eye showed thickening and dense infiltration of the choroid with predominantly immature lymphocytes with scattered plasma cells. Based on the presence of certain histopathologic features including cellular polymorphism, presence of foci of reticulum cell hyperplasia, metaplasia of the retinal pigment epithelium, and hyalinization of the choroid, he concluded that the infiltration represented reactive lymphoid hyperplasia secondary to an unknown stimulus and used the term *inflammatory pseudotumor of the uveal tract* to refer to this condition [12]. A few years later, Ryan and colleagues published a case report on a 51-year-old man with bilateral *inflammatory pseudotumor of the ciliary body* [13]. In 1972, Ryan and Zimmerman reviewed 19 enucleated eyes with massive infiltration of the uvea by lymphoid cells and used the term *reactive lymphoid hyperplasia* to describe the benign-appearing infiltrating lymphocytes [14].

Over the next several decades, a number of investigators started to cast doubt on the benign reactive nature of uveal lymphoid infiltrates and suggested that these infiltrates were in fact neoplastic in nature. In 1982, Mauriello and coworkers claimed that based on morphologic and immunohistologic features, the majority of cases of benign reactive lymphoid hyperplasia of the uveal tract in the Registry of Ophthalmic Pathology of the Armed Forces Institute of Pathology represented malignant lymphomas [15]. In 1987, Jakobiec suggested that the term reactive lymphoid hyperplasia be replaced with *uveal lymphoid infiltration* or *lym-*

A. Mashayekhi (✉)
Ophthalmology Department, Mayo Clinic Florida, Jacksonville, FL, USA
e-mail: Mashayekhi.Arman@mayo.edu

B. V. Chawla, M. E. Aronow (eds.), *Global Perspectives in Ocular Oncology*, https://doi.org/10.1007/978-3-031-08250-4_17

phoid tumor and in 1997 Ciulla and co-workers introduced the term *uveal lymphoid neoplasia* [16, 17]. Cockerham and co-workers used immunohistochemistry and polymerase chain reaction and, in a report published in 2000, were able to show that the majority of the 10 cases diagnosed as reactive lymphoid hyperplasia at the Armed Forces Institute of Pathology were low-grade uveal lymphoid neoplasias [18]. In a report published in 2002, Coupland and co-workers were able to show that the immunohistochemistry and polymerase chain reaction findings in all 13 cases with uveal lymphoproliferative lesions they studied were consistent with extranodal marginal zone B-cell lymphoma [19].

3 Clinical Features

3.1 Primary Choroidal Lymphoma

Primary choroidal lymphoma is a disease of the middle-aged to elderly with median age of diagnosis in the 60s although it can also develop in patients in their 30s and 40s [20–21]. This disease affects men more often than women [20–21]. Presenting symptoms included blurred or distorted vision although many patients with mild disease are asymptomatic. In the paper by Mashayekhi and co-workers 69% of patients had blurred vision and 17% were asymptomatic. Eye pain and redness are uncommon and were reported by only 5% and 7% of the patients, respectively [20]. Most cases are unilateral, but bilateral involvement is common and can be seen in 25% or more of patients [20–21].

Early in the course of the disease, funduscopy shows diffusely scattered, variably sized discrete multifocal creamy-yellow choroidal infiltrates (Fig. 1). With disease progression the thickness of the choroidal infiltrates increases, and the discrete patchy involvement becomes more confluent in appearance [16]. The progressive cellular infiltration leads to obscuration of choroidal vessels [20–22]. The range of tumor thickness on B-scan ultrasonography is wide and in one study varied between 0.9 and 8.9 mm with a mean of 3.0 mm [20].

Shallow serous retinal detachment has been reported in about half of eyes with choroidal lymphoma and is a common cause of decreased vision in such eyes [12, 20, 23, 24]. The retinal detachment is usually not extensive and in one study was limited to 1 quadrant or less in 60% of the involved eyes [20].

Another commonly seen feature noted in 41% of eyes with choroidal lymphoma in one study [20] is the presence of chorioretinal folds. This feature, usually visible on funduscopy and color fundus imaging, is more easily discernible on autofluorescence imaging or angiography [25]. Optic disc swelling, reported in only 6% of eyes, is caused by optic disc compression by circumpapillary choroidal lymphoma [20].

In some cases, uveal lymphoma involving the choroid or ciliary body extends through the sclera and manifests as one or more areas of epibulbar mass just outside the sclera. These areas of epibulbar extension, when located anteriorly, are visible as raised orange-pink (salmon-colored) masses under the bulbar or forniceal conjunctiva (Fig. 2) [25–27]. In contrast to conjunctival lymphoma that is mobile, epibulbar extension of uveal lymphoma is adherent to the sclera and is therefore not mobile. In one study, anterior epibulbar extension was present in 34% and posterior epibulbar extension in 47% of eyes with choroidal lymphoma [20]. In another study, 27% of eyes with uveal lymphoma were found to have con-

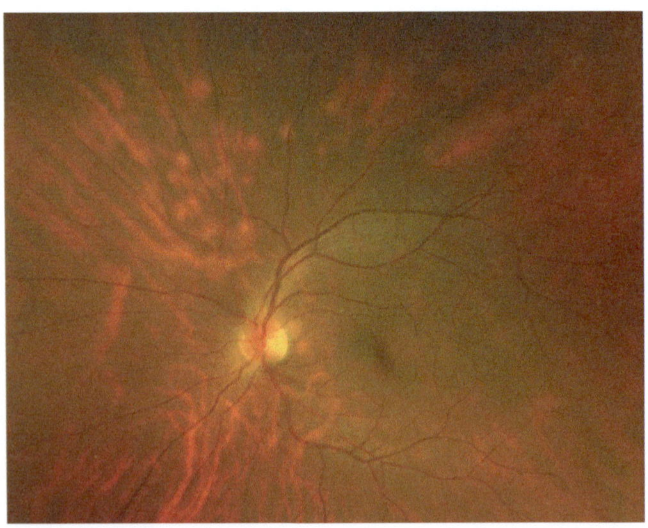

Fig. 1 Fundus photograph of the left eye in a 62-year-old male showing multi-focal yellow to white, creamy infiltrates in the choroid, predominantly in the superonasal quadrant

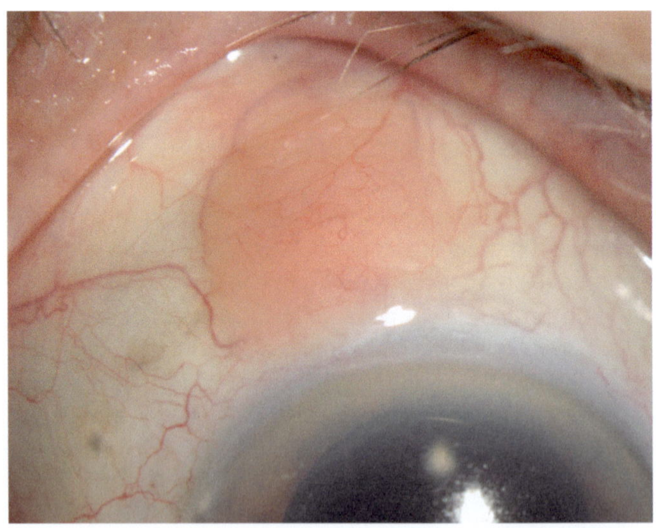

Fig. 2 Epibulbar "salmon patch" near the superior limbus in a 90-year-old female

junctival involvement [21]. Posterior epibulbar extension is visible on B-scan ultrasonography as one or more focal areas of echolucency just at the external surface of the sclera, usually in a macular or peripapillary location. Presence of anterior or posterior epibulbar extension not only greatly aids in making a clinical diagnosis of uveal lymphoma, but also provides a good source of material for tissue biopsy [21, 25, 27].

3.2 Secondary Choroidal Lymphoma

In one study on 59 patients with choroidal lymphoma, 18 (31%) were associated with systemic lymphoma [20]. In another study, out of 22 patients with uveal lymphoma, one had a known history of systemic lymphoma but staging studies performed at the time of initial diagnosis revealed extraocular systemic disease in a total of 5 patients (23%) [21].

In contrast to primary choroidal lymphoma, which is indolent and low-grade, most cases of secondary choroidal lymphoma originate from more aggressive forms of systemic lymphoma and are composed of higher-grade lymphoma cells [7, 20, 28]. Among the 18 patients with secondary choroidal lymphoma in one study, the associated systemic lymphomas included diffuse large B-cell lymphoma, (5 patients), chronic lymphocytic leukemia/small lymphocytic lymphoma, (4 patients), multiple myeloma (2 patients), Waldenstrom's macroglobulinemia (2 patients), extranodal marginal zone lymphoma (2 patients), plasmablastic lymphoma (1 patient), and non-Hodgkin lymphoma not otherwise specified (2 patients) [20]. Compared to primary choroidal lymphoma, secondary choroidal lymphoma is generally associated with worse visual acuity at presentation, is more likely to be bilateral, has higher rate of iris or ciliary body involvement, and is more likely to have associated vitreous cellular reaction [20, 28]. In a report on 28 patients with large B-cell lymphoma of the uvea, 11 were diagnosed at autopsy and 10 after enucleation. Life prognosis was poor with a median survival of only 14 months [7].

3.3 Iris Lymphoma

The majority of cases of uveal lymphoma affect the choroid, sometimes with concomitant ciliary body involvement, and clinically detectable involvement of the iris is quite rare [29, 30]. Similar to choroidal lymphoma, iris lymphoma can be primary (not associated with systemic lymphoma) or secondary (associated with systemic lymphoma) [7, 28–30].

The most common symptoms of iris lymphoma include blurred vision, eye redness, and eye pain. Examination shows diffuse iris thickening with or without areas of nodular iris elevation. Other associated findings include increased intraocular pressure, congestion of conjunctival/episcleral blood vessels, conjunctival/anterior epibulbar lymphoma (salmon patch lesions), corneal edema, keratic precipitates, variable degrees of anterior chamber reaction, pseudohypopyon, hyphema, abnormal iris vessels, and posterior synechiae. Concomitant ciliary body or choroidal involvement are common [7, 28, 29, 31, 32].

Increased intraocular pressure in eyes with iris or ciliary body lymphoma is common and was reported in 31% of eyes with iris involvement in one study [29]. Possible mechanisms of increased intraocular pressure include blockage of trabecular meshwork by lymphoma and inflammatory cells (secondary open angle) or closure of anterior chamber angle by the thickened iris and ciliary body (secondary angle closure) [12, 26, 28].

In contrast to choroidal lymphoma that is indolent and low-grade, iris lymphoma is generally high-grade on pathologic evaluation [7, 28, 29, 31–35] Most patients with iris lymphoma have known systemic lymphoma on presentation. Systemic lymphomas associated with iris lymphoma are aggressive with diffuse large B-cell lymphoma reported as the most common type in one study [28, 29, 33].

Involvement of the iris with anterior chamber reaction, keratic precipitates, and iris nodules has been reported in pediatric patients with posttransplant lymphoproliferative disorder and should be considered in the differential diagnosis of uveitis after organ transplant, especially in children [36]. Ocular involvement can be seen in the absence of systemic disease and may respond to reduction of immunosuppressive therapy or to intravenous rituximab [36, 37].

Signs and symptoms of iris lymphoma overlap with those of inflammatory anterior uveitis and many of these patients are initially treated with topical, peribulbar, or oral steroids before the correct diagnosis of iris lymphoma is considered. Other differential diagnoses for iris lymphoma include juvenile xanthogranuloma, amelanotic iris nevus, amelanotic iris melanoma, iris metastasis, or rare tumors such as leiomyoma, rhabdomyosarcoma, or iris hamartoma [32]. Some of features that point to a diagnosis of iris lymphoma include history of previous high-grade systemic lymphoma, presence of salmon-colored subconjunctival infiltrates, iris or ciliary body thickening on clinical examination or UBM, presence of abnormal iris vessels, and hyphema [29]. Definite diagnosis can be established with iris biopsy or analysis of aqueous fluid [29, 34].

4 Diagnostic Testing

4.1 Biopsy

Many cases of low-grade choroidal lymphoma can be diagnosed with high certainty based on the presence of typical clinical and imaging findings. In atypical cases when the diagnosis is not certain, a tissue biopsy can be helpful. Biopsy of an area of extrascleral extension of lymphoma, when present and especially when located anteriorly, is easier and less risky and should be attempted first [21, 25].

In experienced hands, fine needle aspiration biopsy (FNAB) is a reliable technique with low risk of complications [38, 39]. Transvitreal FNAB of intraocular tumors is generally more informative if the tumor is more than 2 mm in thickness [40]. Another technique is transretinal choroidal biopsy with vitrectomy probe [41, 42]. Kam and co-workers have reported successful biopsy of choroidal lymphoma using a 27-gauge vitrectomy cutter. They used a cut rate of 500 per minute with suction of 600 mm Hg and raised the intraocular pressure to 60 mm Hg at the time of biopsy to minimize the risk of hemorrhage [42]. Eye wall biopsy can also provide adequate tissue for diagnosis, but it is a riskier procedure and should be attempted only in atypical cases when other less risky biopsy techniques are not possible or are uninformative. Dirani and co-workers diagnosed a patient with choroidal lymphoma by full-thickness retinochoroidal biopsy [43]. Their technique consisted of pars plana vitrectomy followed by retinochoroidal biopsy (1.5 × 1.5 mm) using 23-gauge vertical scissors, endolaser, and silicone oil injection [43].

4.2 Ultrasonography

B-scan ultrasonography shows variable diffuse thickening of the choroid with low echogenicity [44]. Extrascleral extension is common, especially in the macular area and around the optic disc, and is seen as one or more focal areas of echolucency just outside the sclera (Fig. 3) [25]. Although this combination of ultrasonographic findings is typical for choroidal lymphoma, it can also be seen in some eyes with diffuse choroidal melanoma with concomitant extraocular extension. Ultrasound biomicroscopy is useful for evaluation of ciliary body or iris involvement.

4.3 Optical Coherence Tomography

Enhanced depth imaging optical coherence tomography (EDI-OCT) is extremely valuable in confirming the presence of choroidal thickening, especially in eyes with thin choroidal lymphoma not easily detectable on B-scan ultrasonography. The choroidal vessels are generally obscured by the infiltrate and are not visible on EDI-OCT. Another useful feature on EDI-OCT is the presence of a rippled or undulating surface that is very suggestive but not diagnostic of choroidal lymphoma [45].

4.4 Angiography

Both fluorescein angiography and indocyanine green angiography (Fig. 4) show tumor staining and hyperfluorescence in mid- to late frames. These features are not specific to choroidal lymphoma but are useful for determining the extent of choroidal involvement and will highlight the choroidal folds [6, 25].

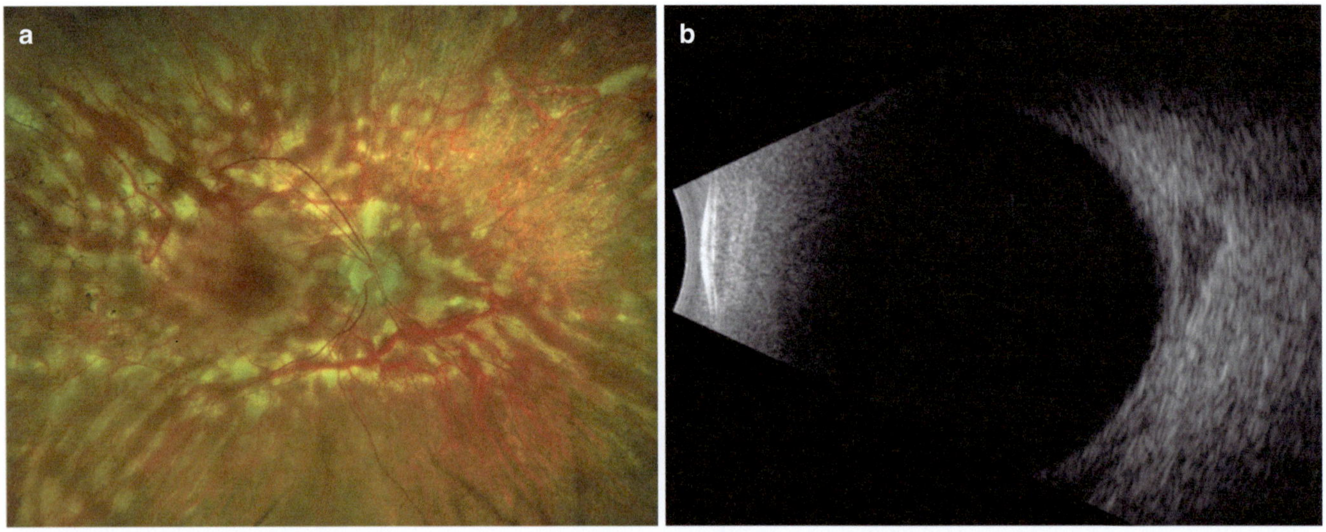

Fig. 3 (**a**)Multifocal choroidal infiltrates in a 60-year-old male with a blonde fundus. (**b**) B-scan ultrasonography highlights occult extrascleral extension which appears as a low-reflective orbital lesion near the optic nerve

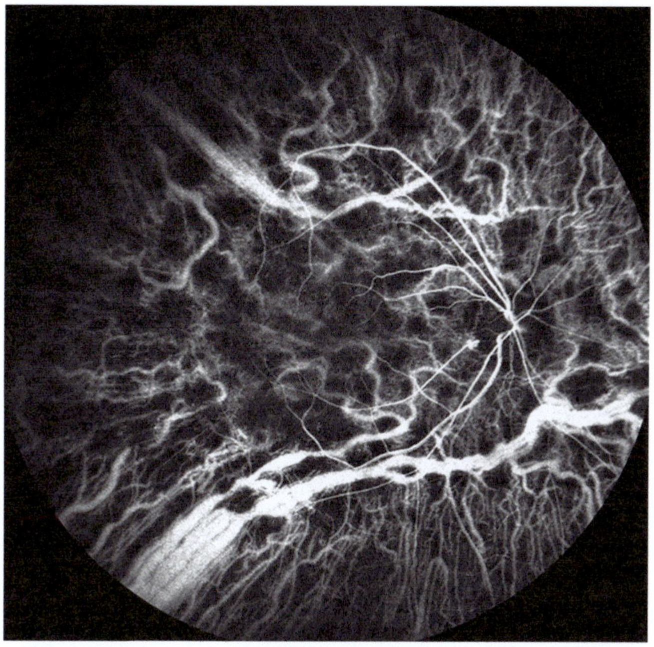

Fig. 4 Indocyanine green angiography highlights multi-focal, round choroidal infiltrates duc to the space occupying nature of lymphoma

5 Differential Diagnosis

The differential diagnosis of choroidal lymphoma is extensive and includes inflammatory (sarcoidosis, bird-shot chorioretinopathy, multifocal choroiditis, serpiginous choroidopathy [3], scleritis [24, 46, 47]), neoplastic (choroidal metastasis, amelanotic choroidal melanoma [23], choroidal hemangioma, vitreoretinal lymphoma, choroidal osteoma), and miscellaneous conditions (uveal effusion syndrome [48], fundus flavimaculatus [22]). The initial diagnoses in the 22 patients reported by Aronow and co-workers included scleritis, metastasis, central serous chorioretinopathy, sarcoidosis, birdshot chorioretinopathy, uveal effusion syndrome, and vitreoretinal lymphoma [21].

A thorough history and clinical examination, B-scan ultrasonography, EDI-OCT, and angiography is enough to make the correct diagnosis of uveal lymphoma in the majority of cases. In atypical cases, tissue biopsy can be helpful in establishing the correct diagnosis.

In a study on uveitis masquerade syndromes by Rothova and co-workers, out of 828 patients with presumed uveitis, 19 (2.3%) were found to have an intraocular malignancy [34]. Two of these eyes had iris involvement by lymphoma, one with diffuse large B-cell lymphoma and the other with transformed peripheral T-cell lymphoma [34].

6 Pathology

Cytopathological evaluation is the mainstay for diagnosis of uveal lymphoma. Primary uveal lymphoma represents a low-grade B cell non-Hodgkin lymphoma of the extranodal marginal zone B-cell lymphoma (EMZL) type comprised of a monomorphous population of small lymphocytes with scant cytoplasm and small indistinct nucleoli [19, 24, 26, 43]. A commonly seen histopathologic feature of uveal lymphomas is the presence of cells that morphologically resemble plasma cells and may contain immunoglobulin in their cytoplasm, a finding referred to as plasma cell (plasmacellular) differentiation [19]. Rare cases of uveal T-cell lymphoma have been reported [34, 35, 49]. A report on the histopathologic findings of the epibulbar (conjunctival and episcleral) biopsy specimens from four patients with uveal lymphoid infiltration has shown dense infiltration of the conjunctival stroma with lymphocytes with high nuclear-to-cytoplasmic ratios and scattered plasma cells. Some cells contained immunoglobulin (Russell bodies) and free immunoglobulin [27].

Pathologic findings of secondary uveal lymphoma can be variable depending on the origin of lymphomatous cells. There are multiple reports in the literature describing uveal involvement by B-cell lymphocytic leukemia [4], multiple myeloma [50, 51], small lymphocytic lymphoma [5], diffuse B-cell lymphoma [7], intravascular (angiotropic) large cell lymphoma [2, 7], follicle center non-Hodgkin lymphoma [3], plasmablastic lymphoma [7], natural killer cell lymphoma [28], and peripheral T-cell lymphoma [34, 35].

B-cell and T-cell lymphocytes express different markers on their surfaces. Identification of these surface markers by immunohistochemical techniques is very helpful for diagnosis and classification of lymphoma. On immunohistochemistry, the lymphoma cells are predominantly CD20-positive B cells with monotypic light chain restriction [52, 53].

Flow cytometry is another useful technique for diagnosis and classification of lymphoma and can be performed even in cases with scant material. Similar to immunohistochemistry, flow cytometry is based on the use of antibodies against different markers (antigens) present on the surface of viable B-cells and T-cells. Flow cytometry is also capable of detecting κ and λ light chains and can therefore help in determining B-cell monoclonality. Whereas in a reactive population of lymphocytes, the ratio of κ to λ light chains is approximately 2:1, in B-cell lymphoma there will be an even more pronounced predominance of one light chain [53].

Molecular testing, using polymerase chain reaction (PCR), is another technique used for diagnosis of lymphoma. The most commonly performed test for detection of B-cell clonality is looking for clonal rearrangements of the heavy chain of the immunoglobulin gene (IgH) [54, 55]. T-cell clonality is confirmed by demonstrating clonal rearrangements of the γ-chain of the T-cell receptor [53].

7 Treatment

7.1 Primary Uveal Lymphoma

All patients with primary uveal lymphoma should undergo thorough systemic evaluation to exclude systemic lymphoma soon after initial diagnosis. In a study on 59 patients with choroidal lymphoma, 14 had known systemic lymphoma at presentation and 4 were diagnosed with systemic lymphoma shortly after presentation. Of the 33 patients with primary choroidal lymphoma that had subsequent follow-up, none developed systemic lymphoma during a mean follow-up of 50 months [20]. Nevertheless, continued systemic evaluation on a regular basis, even in patients who are found to have negative initial work-up, is recommended.

Many cases of primary choroidal lymphoma, especially in their early stages, are asymptomatic and are discovered incidentally during routine eye examination. In light of the generally prolonged, indolent course of primary choroidal lymphoma, such asymptomatic cases can be safely monitored without treatment. Of 72 eyes with choroidal lymphoma in one study, 29% were initially observed without treatment. [44]

Although peribulbar or oral steroids were commonly used in the past for treatment of uveal lymphoma [16, 21, 27], this treatment has currently fallen out of favor as studies have shown it to be either totally ineffective or have only partial or temporary benefit [24, 55]. Of the 24 patients with choroidal lymphoma successfully treated with external beam radiation at the Oncology Service, Wills Eye Hospital, 10 had previously received periocular or oral steroids without adequate response [56].

Multiple studies have shown external beam radiation to be effective for treatment of uveal lymphoma and this treatment is currently the mainstay of treatment for symptomatic cases of this condition [39, 57]. In a report, 25 eyes of 24 patients with choroidal lymphoma were treated with external beam radiation using a mean total radiation dose of 2867 cGy (median, 3000; range, 1200–3600 cGy). After a mean follow-up period of 58 months, all eyes showed complete (18 eyes, 72%) or partial (7 eyes, 28%) regression of uveal lymphoma with complete resolution of subretinal or intraretinal fluid in all the treated eyes. One eye (4%) recurred after an initial partial response and only two eyes (8%) showed signs of mild radiation retinopathy [56]. In a study by Aronow and co-workers on 22 patients with uveal lymphoma, 16 (73%) were treated with external beam radiation using a median dose of 3060 cGy (range, 2340–3600 cGy) with complete remission in all treated eyes after a median follow-up of 29 months [21]. The authors recommended a dose of 2800–3600 cGy for low-grade indolent lymphomas and a higher dose of 3000–4000 cGy for higher grade lymphomas [21].

Recently, ultra-low dose radiation has become increasingly popular for treatment of ocular adnexal and choroidal lymphoma with good results [58, 59]. In 2019, Yang and co-workers published the results of ultra-low dose radiation (4 Gy delivered in two fractions) for management of 3 cases of primary choroidal lymphoma. After a mean follow-up of 14 months, there was evidence of tumor regression in all 3 cases with improvement in visual acuity and no radiation complications [58].

Systemic rituximab has been used by some ocular oncologists for treatment of uveal lymphoma [20, 21, 60]. Aronow and co-workers have recommended systemic administration of single-agent rituximab for patients with systemic lymphoma or with bilateral, multifocal ocular-only disease (involving the uvea and extensive orbital involvement). In their report, 5 out of 22 patients were treated with rituximab (median of 4 cycles) with stable disease in one patient and partial regression in two others [21]. Tiu Teo and co-workers have reported successful treatment of two patients with uveal lymphoma using systemic rituximab monotherapy. There were no systemic adverse events and no ocular tumor recurrence at 29 and 39 months after treatment [60]. In another study on 95 patients with ocular adnexal and uveal lymphoma, out of 11 patients with bilateral involvement 7 (64%) showed signs of disease progression after single-agent rituximab [57].

7.2 Secondary Uveal Lymphoma

The treatment of secondary uveal lymphoma is based on the status of systemic disease. Patients with active systemic lymphoma are generally treated with some form of immunotherapy or chemotherapy [21]. Treatment of secondary uveal lymphoma when the systemic disease is in remission is usually with some form of localized ocular therapy as described above. The outcome of treatment depends on the severity and extent of ocular involvement and may not be as favorable as in patients with primary uveal lymphoma [29].

References

1. Chambers JD, Mosher ML Jr. Intraocular involvement in systemic lymphoma. Surv Ophthalmol. 1966;11(5):562–4.
2. al-Hazzaa SA, Green WR, Mann RB. Uveal involvement in systemic angiotropic large cell lymphoma. Microscopic and immunohistochemical studies. Ophthalmology. 1993;100(6):961–5.

3. Rattray KM, Cole MD, Smith SR. Systemic non-Hodgkin's lymphoma presenting as a serpiginous choroidopathy: report of a case and review of the literature. Eye (Lond). 2000;14(Pt 5):706–10.
4. Coupland SE, Foss HD, Bechrakis NE, Hummel M, Stein H. Secondary ocular involvement in systemic "memory" B-cell lymphocytic leukemia. Ophthalmology. 2001;108(7):1289–95.
5. Ozcan AA, Paydas S, Soylu M, Yavuz S. Bilateral choroidal infiltration from indolent non-Hodgkin's lymphoma: a rapid course with poor prognosis. Leuk Lymphoma. 2005;46(4):615–7.
6. Saatci AO, Arikan G, Ozcan MA, Ozkal S, Kargi A, Undar B. Indocyanine green angiographic features of systemic non-Hodgkin's lymphoma and bilateral choroidal involvement. Ophthalmic Surg Lasers Imaging. 2006;37(3):236–9.
7. Valenzuela J, Yeaney GA, Hsi ED, Azzato EM, Peereboom DM, Singh AD. Large B-cell lymphoma of the uvea: histopathologic variants and clinicopathologic correlation. Surv Ophthalmol. 2020;65(3):361–70.
8. Triebenstein O. Ein Beitrag zur Frage der aleukamischen Augenveranderungen. Klin Monatsbl Augenheilkd. 1920;64:825–36.
9. Cook C. Uveal lymphosarcoma. Br J Ophthalmol. 1954;38:182–5.
10. Beasley H. Lymphosarcoma of the choroid. Am J Ophthalmol. 1961;51:1294–6.
11. Crookes GP, Mullaney J. Lymphoid hyperplasia of the uveal tract simulating malignant lymphoma. Am J Ophthalmol. 1967;63:962–7.
12. Gass JD. Retinal detachment and narrow-angle glaucoma secondary to inflammatory pseudotumor of the uveal tract. Am J Ophthalmol. 1967;64(Suppl 3):612–21.
13. Ryan SJ Jr, Frank RN, Green WR. Bilateral inflammatory pseudotumors of the ciliary body. Am J Ophthalmol. 1971;72(3):586–91.
14. Ryan SJ, Zimmerman LE, King FM. Reactive lymphoid hyperplasia. An unusual form of intraocular pseudotumor. Trans Am Acad Ophthalmol Otolaryngol. 1972;76(3):652–71.
15. Mauriello JA, Langloss JM, Weiner JM, Zimmerman LE. A clinicopathologic and immunohis- tologic study of lymphoproliferative lesions of the uveal tract. Invest Ophthalmol Vis Sci. 1982;22(ARVO Suppl):171.
16. Jakobiec FA, Sacks E, Kronish JW, et al. Multifocal static creamy choroidal infiltrates. An early sign of lymphoid neoplasia. Ophthalmology. 1987;94:397–406.
17. Ciulla TA, Bains RA, Jakobiec FA, et al. Uveal lymphoid neoplasia: a clinical-pathologic correlation and review of the early form. Surv Ophthalmol. 1997;41:467–76.
18. Cockerham GC, Hidayat AA, Bijwaard KE, Sheng ZM. Re- evaluation of "reactive lymphoid hyperplasia of the uvea": an immunohistochemical and molecular analysis of 10 cases. Ophthalmology. 2000;107:151–8.
19. Coupland SE, Foss H-D, Hidayat AA, et al. Extranodal marginal zone B cell lymphomas of the uvea: an analysis of 13 cases. J Pathol. 2002;197:333–40.
20. Mashayekhi A, Shukla SY, Shields JA, Shields CL. Choroidal lymphoma: clinical features and association with systemic lymphoma. Ophthalmology. 2014;121(1):342–51.
21. Aronow ME, Portell CA, Sweetenham JW, Singh AD. Uveal lymphoma: clinical features, diagnostic studies, treatment selection, and outcomes. Ophthalmology. 2014;121:334–41.
22. Gass JD, Weleber RG, Johnson DR. Non-Hodgkin's lymphoma causing fundus picture simulating fundus flavimaculatus. Retina. 1987;7(4):209–14.
23. Ben-Ezra D, Sahel JA, Harris NL, Hemo I, Albert DM. Uveal lymphoid infiltrates: immunohistochemical evidence for a lymphoid neoplasia. Br J Ophthalmol. 1989;73(10):846–51.
24. Gao X, Li B, You Q, Peng X. Primary extranodal marginal zone B-cell lymphoma with diffuse uveal involvement and focal infiltration of the trabecular meshwork: a case report and review of literature. BMC Ophthalmol. 2015;15:48.
25. Jusufbegovic D, Kim V, Char DH. Primary uveal lymphoma with epibulbar extension masquerading as an intraocular inflammation. Can J Ophthalmol. 2015;50(1):e24–6.
26. Rasić DM, Stanković Z, Terzić T, Kovacević D, Koturović Z, Marković V. Primary extranodal marginal zone lymphoma of the uvea associated with massive diffuse epibulbar extension and focal infiltration of the optic nerve and meninges, clinically presented as uveitis masquerade syndrome: a case report. Med Oncol. 2010;27(3):1010–6.
27. Grossniklaus HE, Martin DF, Avery R, Shields JA, Shields CL, Kuo IC, Green RL, Rao NA. Uveal lymphoid infiltration. Report of four cases and clinicopathologic review. Ophthalmology. 1998;105(7):1265–73.
28. Qian Y, Shen J, Che X, Yuan Y, Wang Z. Bilateral iris mass as the first manifestation of NK cell lymphoma: a case report. Eur J Ophthalmol. 2021:11206721211029136. https://doi.org/10.1177/11206721211029136. Epub ahead of print
29. Mashayekhi A, Shields CL, Shields JA. Iris involvement by lymphoma: a review of 13 cases. Clin Exp Ophthalmol. 2013;41:19–26.
30. Economou MA, Kopp ED, All-Ericsson C, Seregard S. Mantle cell lymphoma of the iris. Acta Ophthalmol Scand. 2007;85:341–3.
31. Coutinho AB, Muccioli C, Martins MC, Belfort R Jr, Sant'Anna AE, Burnier MN Jr. Extranodal B-cell lymphoma of the uvea: a case report. Can J Ophthalmol. 2005;40(5):623–6.
32. Kakkassery V, Coupland SE, Heindl LM. Iris lymphoma-a systematic guide for diagnosis and treatment. Surv Ophthalmol. 2021;66(1):41–53.
33. Vogel MH, Font RL, Zimmerman LE, Levine RA. Reticulum cell sarcoma of the retina and uvea. Report of six cases and review of the literature. Am J Ophthalmol. 1968;66(2):205–15.
34. Rothova A, Ooijman F, Kerkhoff F, Van Der Lelij A, Lokhorst HM. Uveitis masquerade syndromes. Ophthalmology. 2001;108(2):386–99.
35. Saga T, Ohno S, Matsuda H, Ogasawara M, Kikuchi K. Ocular involvement by a peripheral T-cell lymphoma. Arch Ophthalmol. 1984;102(3):399–402.
36. Cho AS, Holland GN, Glasgow BJ, Isenberg SJ, George BL, McDiarmid SV. Ocular involvement in patients with post-transplant lymphoproliferative disorder. Arch Ophthalmol. 2001;119(2):183–9.
37. Iu LP, Yeung JC, Loong F, Chiang AK. Successful treatment of intraocular post-transplant lymphoproliferative disorder with intravenous rituximab. Pediatr Blood Cancer. 2015;62(1):169–72.
38. Shields JA, Shields CL, Ehya H, Eagle RC Jr, De Potter P. Fine-needle aspiration biopsy of suspected intraocular tumors. The 1992 Urwick lecture. Ophthalmology. 1993;100(11):1677–84. https://doi.org/10.1016/s0161-6420(93)31418-1.
39. Fuller ML, Sweetenham J, Schoenfield L, Singh AD. Uveal lymphoma: a variant of ocular adnexal lymphoma. Leuk Lymphoma. 2008;49(12):2393–7.
40. Cohen VM, Dinakaran S, Parsons MA, Rennie IG. Transvitreal fine needle aspiration biopsy: the influence of intraocular lesion size on diagnostic biopsy result. Eye (Lond). 2001;15(Pt 2):143–7. https://doi.org/10.1038/eye.2001.48.
41. Sen J, Groenewald C, Hiscott PS, Smith PA, Damato BE. Transretinal choroidal tumor biopsy with a 25-gauge vitrector. Ophthalmology. 2006;113(6):1028–31.
42. Kam AW, Galvin J, Cherepanoff S, Miller AA, Fung AT. Primary choroidal lymphoma diagnosed with 27-gauge pars plana vitrectomy choroidal biopsy. Case Rep Ophthalmol. 2019;10(2):213–20.
43. Dirani A, Allaire G, Callejo S, Belair ML, Biernacki K, Corriveau C, Hammamji K. Choroidal extranodal marginal zone lymphoma diagnosed by full-thickness retinochoroidal biopsy: case report and review of the literature. Int Med Case Rep J. 2017;10:153–8.

44. Theophanous C, Pekmezci M, Damato BE, Kao AA, Bloomer MM, Stewart JM, Afshar AR. Choroidal lymphoma discovered on ultrasound in a patient with suspected corneal tumor. Ocul Oncol Pathol. 2018;4(5):318–21.
45. Shields CL, Arepalli S, Pellegrini M, Mashayekhi A, Shields JA. Choroidal lymphoma shows calm, rippled, or undulating topography on enhanced depth imaging optical coherence tomography in 14 eyes. Retina. 2014;34:1347–53.
46. Hoang-Xuan T, Bodaghi B, Toublanc M, Delmer A, Schwartz L, D'Hermies F. Scleritis and mucosal-associated lymphoid tissue lymphoma: a new masquerade syndrome. Ophthalmology. 1996;103(4):631–5.
47. Gaucher D, Bodaghi B, Charlotte F, Schneider C, Cassoux N, Lemaitre C, Leblond V, Rao N, LeHoang P. Lymphome oculaire de type MALT simulant une sclérite ou une uvéite postérieure [MALT-type B-cell lymphoma masquerading as scleritis or posterior uveitis]. J Fr Ophtalmol. 2005;28(1):31–8.
48. Holz FG, Boehmer HV, Mechtersheimer G, Ott G, Völcker HE. Uveal non-Hodgkin's lymphoma with epibulbar extension simulating choroidal effusion syndrome. Retina. 1999;19(4):343–6.
49. Lobo A, Larkin G, Clark BJ, et al. Pseudo-hypopyon as the presenting feature in B-cell and T-cell intraocular lymphoma. Clin Exp Ophthalmol. 2003;31:155–8.
50. Bronstein M. Ocular involvement in multiple myeloma. AMA Arch Ophthalmol. 1956;55(2):188–92.
51. Knapp AJ, Gartner S, Henkind P. Multiple myeloma and its ocular manifestations. Surv Ophthalmol. 1987;31(5):343–51.
52. Coupland SE, Joussen A, Anastassiou G, Stein H. Diagnosis of a primary uveal extranodal marginal zone B-cell lymphoma by chorioretinal biopsy: case report. Graefes Arch Clin Exp Ophthalmol. 2005;243:482–6.
53. Chute DJ. Uveal lymphoma. Monogr Clin Cytol. 2011:1–14.
54. Baehring JM, Androudi S, Longtine JJ, Betensky RA, Sklar J, Foster CS, Hochberg FH. Analysis of clonal immunoglobulin heavy chain rearrangements in ocular lymphoma. Cancer. 2005;104(3):591–7.
55. Hernández-Pons A, Gómez-Beltrán E, Fernández-Zarzoso M, Albert-Fort M, Martínez-Costa L. Choroidal lymphoma diagnosed by polymerase chain reaction-based clonality assessment. Eur J Ophthalmol. 2021;31(2):NP97–NP101.
56. Mashayekhi A, Hasanreisoglu M, Shields CL, Shields JA. External beam radiation for choroidal lymphoma: efficacy and complications. Retina (Philadelphia, Pa). 2016;36:2006–12.
57. Portell CA, Aronow ME, Rybicki LA, et al. Clinical characteristics of 95 patients with ocular adnexal and uveal lymphoma: treatment outcomes in extranodal marginal zone subtype. Clin Lymphoma Myeloma Leuk. 2014;14:203–10.
58. Yang X, Dalvin LA, Lim L-AS, et al. Ultra-low-dose (boom-boom) radiotherapy for choroidal lymphoma in three consecutive cases. Eur J Ophthalmol. 2019;1120672119888985
59. Pinnix CC, Dabaja BS, Milgrom SA, et al. Ultra-low- dose radiotherapy for definitive management of ocular adnexal B-cell lymphoma. Head Neck. 2017;39:1095–100.
60. Tiu Teo HM, Çiftçi S, Elner VM, Demirci H. Systemic anti-CD20 (rituximab) as primary treatment for symptomatic primary uveal lymphoma. Am J Ophthalmol Case Rep. 2019;15:100484.

Topical Chemotherapy for Ocular Surface Squamous Neoplasia

Osmel P. Alvarez, Ghada AlBayyat, Anat Galor, and Carol L. Karp

1 Introduction

Ocular surface squamous neoplasia (OSSN) is the most common non-pigmented malignancy of the ocular surface and comprises a spectrum of corneal and conjunctival lesions including dysplasia and squamous cell carcinoma [1, 2]. Historically, the primary treatment for OSSN was surgical excision with a no-touch technique; however, surgical treatment is associated with sequelae such as conjunctival hyperemia, conjunctival scarring, symblepharon formation, and limbal stem cell deficiency [1–4]. Recently, the tide has turned toward medical treatments in the form of topical chemotherapy [5–7]. Topical chemotherapies offer the unique advantage of treating the entire ocular surface, thereby addressing subclinical or microscopic disease. If treated surgically with resultant positive margins, such disease can lead to up to 56% recurrence rates [8]. Topical chemotherapies for OSSN include primarily interferon α-2b, 5-fluorouracil, and mitomycin C, as well as retinoids, cidofovir, anti-vascular endothelial growth factor agents, and aloe vera. Urea and dinitrochlorobenzene have also been studied as topical therapies for OSSN; however, they are not commonly used and have not been thoroughly studied for this use since the 1970s and 1980s [9–11].

2 Interferon α-2b

2.1 Description

Interferons are a family of naturally occurring, leukocyte-derived proteins released by several kinds of immune cells [12]. They are cytokines that help the immune system address threats to the body in a variety of ways [13]. Interferons have antiviral, antimicrobial, and antineoplastic qualities and can enhance phagocytic and cytotoxic mechanisms, inhibit biosynthetic enzymes, decrease blood vessel proliferation, induce apoptosis, and inactivate viral RNA [2, 14]. They have been used to treat hepatitis, cervical intraepithelial neoplasia, and cutaneous squamous cell carcinoma [15–17]. Interferon α has been used to treat hairy cell leukemia, follicular lymphoma, Kaposi's sarcoma, renal cell carcinoma, hepatitis C, chronic myeloid leukemia, melanoma, and more [18–22].

Interferon α-2b (IFNα2b) in particular is a glycoprotein with 166 amino acid residues that has anti-proliferative, immunomodulatory, and antiviral effects [23]. The first use of IFNα2b in the treatment of OSSN was in 1994 for a recurrent case of conjunctival intraepithelial neoplasia [1, 24]. Since then, a number of studies on IFNα2b have been published that demonstrate its usefulness as a topical chemotherapy agent for OSSN [25–38].

NIH Center Core Grant P30EY014801, RPB Unrestricted Award and Career Development Awards, Department of Veterans Affairs, Veterans Health Administration, Office of Research and Development, Clinical Sciences Research EPID-006-15S (Dr. Galor), R01EY026174 (Dr. Galor), The Dr. Ronald and Alicia Lepke Grant, The Lee and Claire Hager Grant, The H. Scott Huizenga Grant, The Grant and Diana Stanton-Thornbrough, The Robert Baer Family Grant, The Emilyn Page and Mark Feldberg Grant, The Robert Farr Family Grant, The Jose Ferreira de Melo Grant, Richard and Kathy Lesser Grant, The Michele and Ted Kaplan Grant and the Richard Azar Family Grant(institutional grants).

O. P. Alvarez · G. AlBayyat · C. L. Karp (✉)
Department of Ophthalmology, Bascom Palmer Eye Institute, University of Miami, Miami, FL, USA
e-mail: oalvare1@alumni.jh.edu; ckarp@med.miami.edu

A. Galor
Department of Ophthalmology, Bascom Palmer Eye Institute, University of Miami, Miami, FL, USA

Department of Ophthalmology, Miami Veterans Administration Medical Center, Miami, FL, USA
e-mail: agalor@med.miami.edu

B. V. Chawla, M. E. Aronow (eds.), *Global Perspectives in Ocular Oncology*, https://doi.org/10.1007/978-3-031-08250-4_18

2.2 Usage and Efficacy

IFNα2b has been used successfully as topical eye drops and as subconjunctival perilesional injections. Studies using topical IFNα2b eye drops as a sole treatment for OSSN have reported complete tumor resolution rates of 81%, 83%, 89%, 92%, and 100% [29, 32, 35, 38, 39] (Fig. 1). Studies combining IFNα2b injections and topical eye drops have also demonstrated similar resolution rates of 87–100% [30, 37] but with faster time to resolution. Another study found that IFNα2b drops and/or injections as primary treatment led to complete resolution in 70–100% of cases, while a combination of surgical excision and IFNα2b drops and/or injections led to 100% resolution [36]. IFNα2b drops and injections have low recurrence rates, with some studies reporting 0%, 4%, and 5% [32, 33, 36]. However, one study comparing IFNα2b (eye drops and/or injections) response in smokers and nonsmokers found that patients with history of smoking may have a higher recurrence rate than nonsmokers (23% vs. 13%, $p = 0.04$) [39].

IFNα2b has been used to treat both large and small tumors, and as primary treatment or as chemoreduction prior to surgical excision. It has been effective in eliminating tumors involving less than six clock hours and has been shown to eliminate and reduce tumors of greater involvement, including giant OSSN and tumors of 360-degree involvement [27, 31, 34].

2.3 Dosage and Administration

Topical IFNα2b is typically used with a one million IU/mL (MIU) dose and administered four times a day until tumor resolution and then at least 1–3 months [2, 36]. In terms of drug concentration, one study found no significant difference in outcomes when comparing 1 MIU/mL and 3 MIU/mL dosages [25]. Topical IFNα2b eye drops require compounding and refrigeration, and they may be labeled as stable for 15–30 days, depending on the pharmacy [1, 30].

For injections of IFNα2b, dosages may vary, with some studies specifying 3 MIU in 0.5 mL per injection given once weekly or up to thrice weekly for a mean total dosage of 15–18 MIU, and another study using 3–10 MIU injected monthly [30, 36, 37].

2.4 Adverse Effects

IFNα2b eye drops are notable for being very well-tolerated and generally have no side effects [2, 29, 32]. Patients receiving injections of IFNα2b may experience mild flu-like symptoms for about 48 h after a dose, but IFNα2b injections are still overall well-tolerated [2, 31].

2.5 Cost

Topical IFNα2b eye drops are relatively expensive. At our institution, they cost about $800 out of pocket for a month of treatment. However, the price may vary at other locations and may be significantly less in other countries [2]. In India, for example, interferon is very inexpensive. On the other hand, an advantage of the subconjunctival injections of IFNα2b is that they are commercially available and do not require compounding, and so are normally covered by health insurance [2].

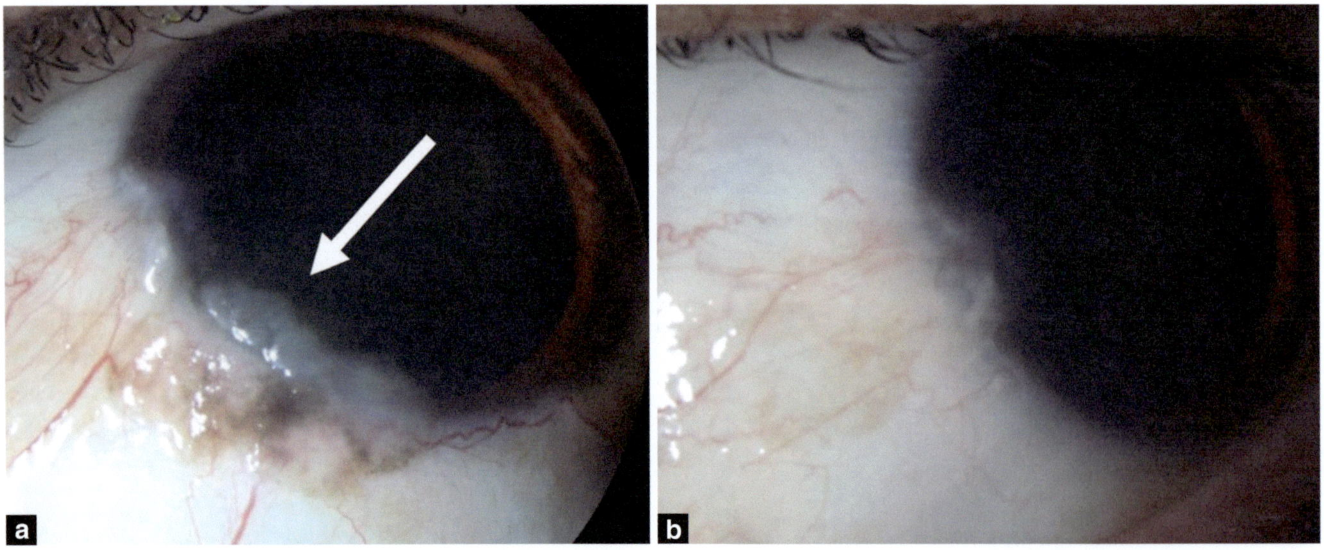

Fig. 1 (**a**) A 56-year-old Hispanic female with ocular surface squamous neoplasia on the left eye (arrow). Note gelatinous lesion on inferior nasal limbus and cornea. (**b**) Patient after 8 months of interferon α2b 1 MIU/mL eye drops four times daily. Note dramatic resolution of the tumor and the underlying nasal pterygium now visible more clearly

3 5-Fluorouracil

3.1 Description

5-Fluorouracil (5FU) is a fluoropyrimidine that blocks thymidylate synthase, thereby disrupting DNA replication and cell growth [40]. It is an antimetabolite used as an anticancer drug and has been used to treat colorectal, breast, and other cancers [40, 41]. 5FU has cytotoxic properties that are useful in ophthalmology, and it has been used in glaucoma surgery, pterygium surgery, vitreoretinal surgery, and more [41]. It was first used to treat OSSN in 1986 by de Keizer et al. [42].

3.2 Usage and Efficacy

5FU is primarily used as topical eye drops. In topical form, it has shown generally high-resolution rates, with studies reporting 82% and 100% [43, 44]. One study comparing IFN and 5FU reported 96% resolution with 5FU, compared to 81% for IFN [38] (Fig. 2). Recurrence rates for topical 5FU are low, with studies reporting 10%, 11.5%, and 14% recurrence [38, 43, 44].

Currently, evidence supporting the use of 5FU injections is limited. One study of six patients using subconjunctival perilesional injections reported that five lesions resolved entirely without recurrence, while one lesion recurred at the end of the study [45].

3.3 Dosage and Administration

Topical 5FU eye drops are compounded as 1% solutions and are stable at room temperature, so they may not require refrigeration [2, 43]. We now, however, do recommend refrigeration, and have done so for the last few years.

Several treatment regimens for topical 5FU have been studied. The most common regimen is in 4-week cycles: administration of 5FU eye drops four times per day for 1 week followed by 3 weeks of no treatment [38, 43]. Another study administered 5FU four times per day for 4 weeks followed by 3 months of no treatment until the next cycle [44]. In both methods, treatment cycles are repeated until tumor resolution.

One study using 5FU injections used 5 mg from a 25 mg/mL 5FU solution twice a week for four to 6 weeks, and then a total of 7.5 mg 5FU per week for 2–4 weeks [45].

3.4 Adverse Effects

Generally, topical 5FU is well-tolerated: in one study on 44 patients, 61% of patients reported at least one side effect, but only one patient discontinued 5FU treatment due to intolerance [43]. Topical 5FU drops may cause adverse effects including pain, tearing, redness, eyelid edema, photophobia, and keratopathy [38, 43]. Nonetheless, 5FU is considered a safe form of chemotherapy and has been shown to have no long-term complications and a low rate of sight-threatening effects [38, 41, 44].

3.5 Cost

5FU is relatively inexpensive when compared to other treatments, costing approximately $50 per cycle at our institution and less in other countries.

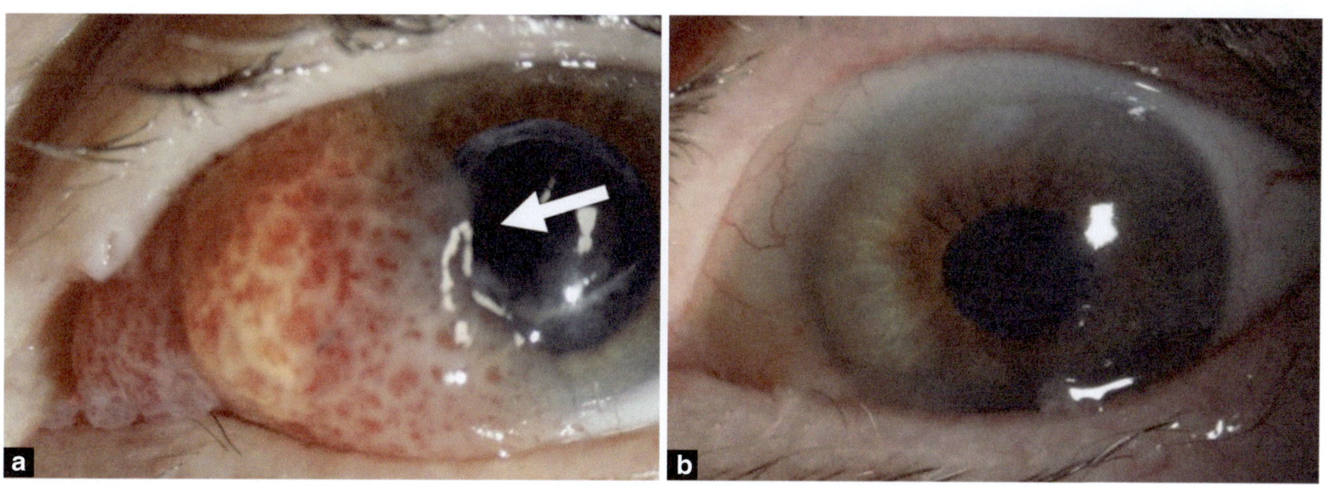

Fig. 2 (**a**) An 80-year-old white male with ocular surface squamous neoplasia on left eye (arrow). Note large papillomatous lesion on nasal conjunctiva and caruncle. (**b**) Patient after 3 cycles of 1 week of topical 5 fluorouracil 1% eye drops four times daily followed by 3 weeks off. Note dramatic resolution of lesion

4 Mitomycin C

4.1 Description

Mitomycin C (MMC) is an antimetabolite isolated from *Streptomyces caespitosus* [46]. It is an alkylating agent with antineoplastic and antibiotic properties that binds to DNA and inhibits DNA synthesis [47]. MMC has been used to treat other cancers, including bladder, colorectal, and pancreatic cancers [48–50]. In ophthalmology, MMC has also been used as an adjunct therapy in pterygium, glaucoma, and OSSN excision surgeries [1, 2, 26, 51, 52]. MMC was first used as a topical treatment for OSSN in 1994 and is now commonly used as a primary therapy [1, 53].

4.2 Usage and Efficacy

MMC is used as a topical chemotherapy in the form of eye drops [1, 2, 52]. MMC has generally high-resolution rates, with studies reporting 76%, 87%, and 100% [33, 54–57]. A randomized control trial showed 92% resolution in the MMC group and 0% resolution in the placebo group [58] (Fig. 3). Additionally, MMC can lead to relatively fast resolution times: one study comparing IFNα2b to MMC had mean times of resolution of 3.2 months for IFNα2b and 1.5 months for MMC [33]. Studies report relatively low recurrence rates of 0% and 4.3%, although one study reported 20% [33, 52, 54, 56, 57].

4.3 Dosage and Administration

MMC eye drops are unstable in solution and require refrigeration [1, 2]. They are typically labeled as stable for 15 days, depending on the pharmacy [1]. MMC is used most commonly in dosages of 0.02–0.04% [1]. Some studies report no significant difference in time to resolution or recurrence rates between patients receiving 0.02% and 0.04% dosages [52].

The most common treatment regimen is cycles of 1 week of 0.04% MMC topical eye drops four times per day followed by a few weeks off; these cycles are repeated until the lesion is resolved [33, 57, 59, 60]. However, many other treatment regimens have been reported in the literature. These include 0.04% MMC drops four times per day for 3 weeks, followed by 3 weeks of no treatment and then another 3 weeks of eye drops [61]; 0.02–0.04% MMC drops four times per day for 1 week, then 1–3 weeks off until the next cycle [2]; 0.04% MMC drops four times per day for 3 weeks [58]; 0.02% MMC drops four times per day for 4 weeks followed by 0.02% or 0.04% MMC drops four times per day for 2 weeks if recurrence was observed until tumor resolution [55]; 0.002% MMC drops four times per day continuously for 2–14 weeks [56]; and 0.02% MMC drops four times per day for 14–28 consecutive days [54].

In order to reduce the risk of punctal stenosis, MMC is commonly used in conjunction with punctal plugs, or patients may be instructed to manually occlude punctum while applying MMC eye drops [57, 58]. Additionally, patients should be instructed to use steroids and lubrication during the course of treatment to help ameliorate surface toxicity [33, 61].

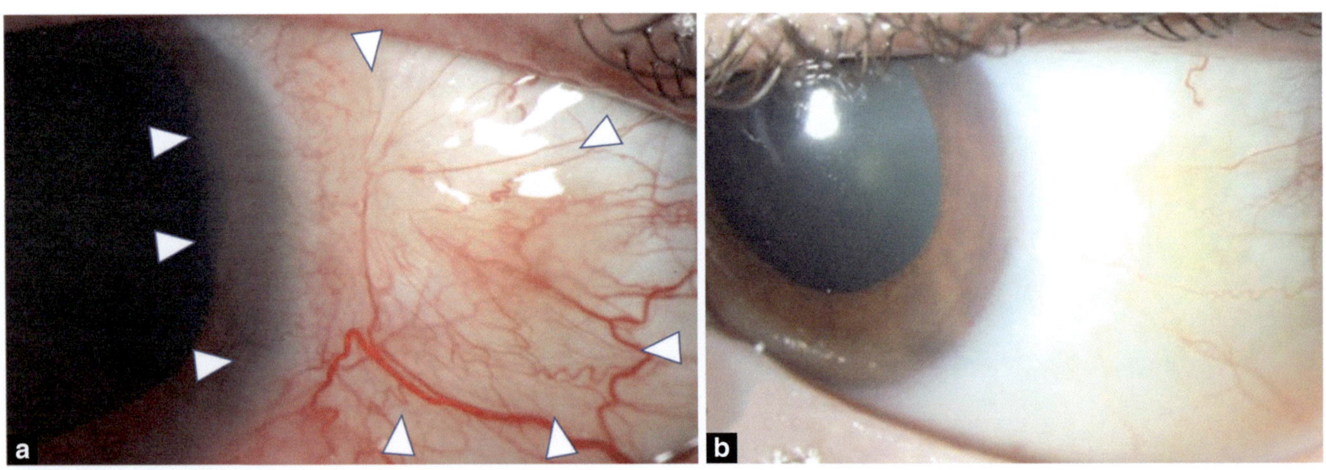

Fig. 3 (**a**) A 54-year-old Hispanic male with ocular surface squamous neoplasia temporally on the left eye (arrowheads). Note opalescent lesion on temporal cornea, and gelatinous lesion on the conjunctiva. (**b**) Patient after 3 1-week cycles of mitomycin C 0.04% eye drops four times daily with 2 weeks off between each cycle

4.4 Adverse Effects

Compared to IFNα2b and 5FU, MMC has more adverse effects [2]. These may include redness, pain, itching, tearing, conjunctival hyperemia, epithelial and lid toxicity, corneal erosion, hyperemia with burning sensation, punctate staining of cornea, and punctal stenosis [33, 52, 54–58, 61]. Patients may experience severe pain if MMC is used for more than 14 consecutive days [55]. The most feared consequence is limbal stem cell deficiency, which can rarely occur [62]. However, studies have found no long-term effects after discontinuation of treatment [52, 58].

4.5 Cost

Treatment with MMC is approximately six times cheaper than treatment with IFNα2b [33]. One cycle of MMC treatment costs approximately $100–190 in the United States, and is less expensive elsewhere [2].

5 Retinoic Acid

5.1 Description

Retinoic acid is a vitamin A compound that is important for cell processes such as growth, differentiation, and apoptosis [63]. Animal and in vitro studies have shown retinoids to be effective in combatting neoplastic cells [64, 65]. Evidence for usage of retinoic acid alone is limited to approximately five cases [65–68]. However, there exists significant evidence (over 100 documented cases) supporting the efficacy of retinoic acid in combination with IFNα2b. Therefore, further studies are needed to establish the effectiveness of retinoic acid alone for treating OSSN.

5.2 Usage and Efficacy

Thus far, only a few case reports describe the exclusive use of retinoic acid eye drops and ointments, and these have shown poor results [65, 68]. However, while the data on retinoic acid alone for OSSN is limited, two studies on over 80 eyes each showed favorable results when using IFNα2b in combination with retinoic acid to treat OSSN. These studies had high tumor resolution rates of 97.75% and 96.3% and low recurrence rates of 2.2% and 3.7% [66, 67]. One case report used this same combination treatment regimen in a patient whose OSSN did not respond to IFNα2b eye drops, injections, or retinoic acid eye drops individually [68].

5.3 Dosage and Administration

Retinoic acid has been used in the topical treatment of OSSN in the form of eye drops and ointments in various dosages on a limited basis. One case study documented the use of retinoic acid ointment with two patients [65]. In this case study, patients used 0.05% retinoic acid ointment three or two times per day and 0.01% retinoic acid ointment three times per day. The retinoic acid ointment was used for 10 weeks in one case and as continuous treatment for at least 8 months in the other. Because retinoic acid has not been thoroughly studied in the treatment of OSSN, an ideal treatment regimen has not yet been established.

In the combination studies of IFNα2b and retinoic acid, patients were given 1 MIU/mL IFNα2b topical eye drops four times per day and 0.01% retinoic acid eye drops once every other day [66, 67].

5.4 Adverse Effects

Retinoic acid has been shown to be a safe treatment with no long-term complications [67, 68]. It may have side effects such as mild allergic papillary conjunctivitis and lid irritation, but these are generally tolerable [26, 67]. There have been few cases of epithelial microcysts and marginal keratitis resulting from retinoic acid treatment in combination with IFNα2b [67].

5.5 Cost

Treatment with retinoic acid is relatively inexpensive, costing about $75 for 5 mL of 0.01% retinoic acid.

6 Anti-Vascular Endothelial Growth Factor Agents

6.1 Description

Anti-vascular endothelial growth factor agents (anti-VEGF agents) are monoclonal antibodies that bind to VEGF [69]. They have been used to treat a wide range of cancers and have also been used intravitreally to treat wet age-related macular degeneration, retinal vein occlusions, pachychoroid neovasculopathy, and as an adjuvant in pterygium excisions [1, 70–73].

6.2 Usage and Efficacy

The anti-VEGF agents, bevacizumab and ranibizumab, have been used as subconjunctival injections and eye drops. As injections, they have been more effective at reducing tumor size than complete elimination, while some tumors have not responded at all [74–77].

One case report on six patients using bevacizumab eye drops showed complete resolution in only two patients, and the rest eventually required surgical excision [78].

6.3 Dosage and Administration

Several studies have injected 0.5 gm of ranibizumab or bevacizumab once or twice per month [74, 75, 77]. Bevacizumab has been administered as eye drops in a 5 mg/mL dosage four times a day for 8 weeks [78].

6.4 Adverse Effects

No side effects have been reported for bevacizumab eye drops or bevacizumab and ranibizumab injections [74, 75, 77, 78].

6.5 Cost

Anti-VEGF agent therapies are expensive. Injections of ranibizumab and bevacizumab cost approximately $1500 and $600 each, respectively [79]. Bevacizumab eye drops are formulated from commercially available injection solutions, and thus may also be expensive [78].

7 Aloe Vera

7.1 Description

Aloe is a genus of plants that have long been used for medicinal purposes [80]. *Aloe vera* is the most well-known and most studied species of the genus, with over 4000 studies on it to date [80]. Aloe plants exhibit anticancer and antineoplastic properties and have antiproliferative, immunostimulatory, and antioxidant effects [2, 80]. However, evidence for the effectiveness of *Aloe vera* in treating OSSN is limited to one case report.

7.2 Usage and Efficacy

In a case report on one patient, *Aloe vera* oil drops were used to treat OSSN [81]. The lesion resolved completely and the patient had no recurrence for at least 6 years.

7.3 Dosage and Administration

The patient used commercially available *Aloe vera* oil drops four times per day for 3 months [81].

7.4 Adverse Effects

In this case report, the patient reported no side effects [81].

7.5 Cost

One bottle of *Aloe vera* oil costs approximately $25 [2].

8 Cidofovir

8.1 Description

Cidofovir is a nucleoside analog of deoxycytidine monophosphate that has broad spectrum antiviral activity toward DNA viruses like herpesviruses, papillomaviruses, and poxviruses [82, 83]. It is approved for intravenous use for the treatment of cytomegalovirus retinitis in patients with AIDS and has also been used intravitreally for this purpose [83, 84]. Evidence for the effectiveness of cidofovir in the treatment of OSSN is limited.

8.2 Usage and Efficacy

One study on six patients used cidofovir to successfully resolve OSSN in five patients with no reported recurrences after a mean follow-up period of 14 months [85]. Another case report on one patient used cidofovir to reduce OSSN before a surgical excision with no recurrence [86].

8.3 Dosage and Administration

Cidofovir has been used as topical eye drops with a 2.5 mg/mL concentration applied three, four, or more times per day for at least 4 weeks [85, 86].

8.4 Adverse Effects

One study using cidofovir to treat OSSN reported instances of conjunctivitis and punctal stenosis, both of which resolved after treatment and punctal plugs [85]. Another case report observed cicatrization of the inferior punctum 6 months after treatment, but the connection to cidofovir is uncertain [86]. Further studies are needed to establish the safety and efficacy of topical cidofovir.

8.5 Cost

Cidofovir is relatively expensive, costing about $300–400 for one vial of 75 mg/mL [2].

9 Conclusion

Traditionally, surgical excision has been the gold standard of treatment for OSSN. However, research over the past several decades has produced several chemotherapeutic options that offer low recurrence rates and few undesirable sequelae. These therapies also possess the benefit of treating the entire ocular surface, thereby treating subclinical or undetected disease. Currently, the three primary chemotherapies for OSSN are interferon α-2b, 5-fluorouracil, and mitomycin C, which are all generally effective but can vary greatly in price and tolerability. Other described options include retinoic acid, anti-vascular endothelial growth agents, aloe vera, and cidofovir, with less conclusive data. Clinicians now have multiple options available to medically treat patients with OSSN and avoid the complications of surgical excisions.

References

1. Nanji AA, Sayyad FE, Karp CL. Topical chemotherapy for ocular surface squamous neoplasia. Curr Opin Ophthalmol. 2013;24(4):336–42.
2. Al Bayyat G, Arreaza-Kaufman D, Venkateswaran N, Galor A, Karp CL. Update on pharmacotherapy for ocular surface squamous neoplasia. Eye Vis (Lond). 2019;6:24.
3. Nanji AA, Moon CS, Galor A, Sein J, Oellers P, Karp CL. Surgical versus medical treatment of ocular surface squamous neoplasia: a comparison of recurrences and complications. Ophthalmology. 2014;121(5):994–1000.
4. Sayed-Ahmed IO, Palioura S, Galor A, Karp CL. Diagnosis and medical management of ocular surface squamous neoplasia. Expert Rev Ophthalmol. 2017;12(1):11–9.
5. Adler E, Turner JR, Stone DU. Ocular surface squamous neoplasia: a survey of changes in the standard of care from 2003 to 2012. Cornea. 2013;32(12):1558–61.
6. Stone DU, Butt AL, Chodosh J. Ocular surface squamous neoplasia: a standard of care survey. Cornea. 2005;24(3):297–300.
7. Shields JA, Shields CL, De Potter P. Surgical management of conjunctival tumors. The 1994 Lynn B. McMahan lecture. Arch Ophthalmol. 1997;115(6):808–15.
8. Tabin G, Levin S, Snibson G, Loughnan M, Taylor H. Late recurrences and the necessity for long-term follow-up in corneal and conjunctival intraepithelial neoplasia. Ophthalmology. 1997;104(3):485–92.
9. Danopoulos ED, Danopoulou IE, Liarikos SB, Merkuris KM. Effects of urea treatment in malignancies of the conjunctiva and cornea. Ophthalmologica. 1979;178(4):198–203.
10. Ferry AP, Meltzer MA, Taub RN. Immunotherapy with dinitrochlorobenzene (DNCB) for recurrent squamous cell tumor of conjunctiva. Trans Am Ophthalmol Soc. 1976;74:154–71.
11. Petrelli R, Cotlier E, Robins S, Stoessel K. Dinitrochlorobenzene immunotherapy of recurrent squamous papilloma of the conjunctiva. Ophthalmology. 1981;88(12):1221–5.
12. De Andrea M, Ravera R, Gioia D, Gariglio M, Landolfo S. The interferon system: an overview. Eur J Paediatr Neurol. 2002;6(Suppl A):A41–6; discussion A55-8
13. Pestka S. The interferons: 50 years after their discovery, there is much more to learn. J Biol Chem. 2007;282(28):20047–51.
14. Baron S, Tyring SK, Fleischmann WR, Coppenhaver DH, Niesel DW, Klimpel GR, et al. The interferons. Mechanisms of action and clinical applications. JAMA. 1991;266(10):1375–83.
15. Edwards L, Berman B, Rapini RP, Whiting DA, Tyring S, Greenway HT, et al. Treatment of cutaneous squamous cell carcinomas by intralesional interferon alfa-2b therapy. Arch Dermatol. 1992;128(11):1486–9.
16. Chevaliez S, Pawlotsky JM. Interferon-based therapy of hepatitis C. Adv Drug Deliv Rev. 2007;59(12):1222–41.
17. Chakalova G, Ganchev G. Local administration of interferon-alpha in cases of cervical intraepithelial neoplasia associated with human papillomavirus infection. J BUON. 2004;9(4):399–402.
18. Decatris M, Santhanam S, O'Byrne K. Potential of interferon-alpha in solid tumours: part 1. BioDrugs. 2002;16(4):261–81.
19. Santhanam S, Decatris M, O'Byrne K. Potential of interferon-alpha in solid tumours: part 2. BioDrugs. 2002;16(5):349–72.
20. Talpaz M, Mercer J, Hehlmann R. The interferon-alpha revival in CML. Ann Hematol. 2015;94(Suppl 2):S195–207.
21. Jansen PL, De Bruijne J. Controlled-release interferon alpha 2b, a new member of the interferon family for the treatment of chronic hepatitis C. Expert Opin Investig Drugs. 2012;21(1):111–8.
22. Ascierto PA, Chiarion-Sileni V, Muggiano A, Mandalà M, Pimpinelli N, Del Vecchio M, et al. Interferon alpha for the adjuvant treatment of melanoma: review of international literature and practical recommendations from an expert panel on the use of interferon. J Chemother. 2014;26(4):193–201.
23. Asmana NR. Human interferon alpha-2b: a therapeutic protein for cancer treatment. Scientifica (Cairo). 2014;2014:970315.
24. Maskin SL. Regression of limbal epithelial dysplasia with topical interferon. Arch Ophthalmol. 1994;112(9):1145–6.
25. Galor A, Karp CL, Chhabra S, Barnes S, Alfonso EC. Topical interferon alpha 2b eye-drops for treatment of ocular surface squamous neoplasia: a dose comparison study. Br J Ophthalmol. 2010;94(5):551–4.
26. Giaconi JA, Karp CL. Current treatment options for conjunctival and corneal intraepithelial neoplasia. Ocul Surf. 2003;1(2):66–73.
27. Kaliki S, Bejjanki KM, Desai A, Mohamed A. Interferon alfa 2b for ocular surface squamous neoplasia: factors influencing the treatment response. Semin Ophthalmol. 2019;34(7–8):465–72.
28. Kanaya R, Kase S, Ishijima K, Ishida S. Usefulness of topical interferon alpha-2b eye drop as an adjunctive therapy following surgical resection in ocular surface squamous neoplasia. In Vivo. 2019;33(6):2211–5.

29. Karp CL, Moore JK, Rosa RH. Treatment of conjunctival and corneal intraepithelial neoplasia with topical interferon alpha-2b. Ophthalmology. 2001;108(6):1093–8.
30. Karp CL, Galor A, Chhabra S, Barnes SD, Alfonso EC. Subconjunctival/perilesional recombinant interferon α2b for ocular surface squamous neoplasia: a 10-year review. Ophthalmology. 2010;117(12):2241–6.
31. Kim HJ, Shields CL, Shah SU, Kaliki S, Lally SE. Giant ocular surface squamous neoplasia managed with interferon alpha-2b as immunotherapy or immunoreduction. Ophthalmology. 2012;119(5):938–44.
32. Kusumesh R, Ambastha A, Sinha B, Kumar R. Topical interferon α-2b as a single therapy for primary ocular surface squamous neoplasia. Asia Pac J Ophthalmol (Phila). 2015;4(5):279–82.
33. Kusumesh R, Ambastha A, Kumar S, Sinha BP, Imam N. Retrospective comparative study of topical interferon α2b versus Mitomycin C for primary ocular surface squamous neoplasia. Cornea. 2017;36(3):327–31.
34. Patel H, Jeang LJ, Shah A, Espana EM, Margo CE. Widespread ocular surface squamous neoplasia treated with topical interferon alpha-2b. Ocul Oncol Pathol. 2018;4(5):298–303.
35. Shah SU, Kaliki S, Kim HJ, Lally SE, Shields JA, Shields CL. Topical interferon alfa-2b for management of ocular surface squamous neoplasia in 23 cases: outcomes based on American joint committee on cancer classification. Arch Ophthalmol. 2012;130(2):159–64.
36. Shields CL, Kaliki S, Kim HJ, Al-Dahmash S, Shah SU, Lally SE, et al. Interferon for ocular surface squamous neoplasia in 81 cases: outcomes based on the American joint committee on cancer classification. Cornea. 2013;32(3):248–56.
37. Vann RR, Karp CL. Perilesional and topical interferon alfa-2b for conjunctival and corneal neoplasia. Ophthalmology. 1999;106(1):91–7.
38. Venkateswaran N, Mercado C, Galor A, Karp CL. Comparison of topical 5-fluorouracil and interferon alfa-2b as primary treatment modalities for ocular surface squamous neoplasia. Am J Ophthalmol. 2019;199:216–22.
39. Shields CL, Paulose SA, Yaghy A, Dalvin LA, Constantinescu AB, Lally SE, et al. Ocular surface squamous neoplasia managed with primary interferon α2b: a comparative analysis of 212 tumors in smokers versus nonsmokers. Cornea. 2021;40(11):1387–94.
40. Longley DB, Harkin DP, Johnston PG. 5-fluorouracil: mechanisms of action and clinical strategies. Nat Rev Cancer. 2003;3(5):330–8.
41. Abraham LM, Selva D, Casson R, Leibovitch I. The clinical applications of fluorouracil in ophthalmic practice. Drugs. 2007;67(2):237–55.
42. de Keizer RJ, de Wolff-Rouendaal D, van Delft JL. Topical application of 5-fluorouracil in premalignant lesions of cornea, conjunctiva and eyelid. Doc Ophthalmol. 1986;64(1):31–42.
43. Joag MG, Sise A, Murillo JC, Sayed-Ahmed IO, Wong JR, Mercado C, et al. Topical 5-fluorouracil 1% as primary treatment for ocular surface squamous neoplasia. Ophthalmology. 2016;123(7):1442–8.
44. Parrozzani R, Frizziero L, Trainiti S, Testi I, Miglionico G, Pilotto E, et al. Topical 1% 5-fluoruracil as a sole treatment of corneoconjunctival ocular surface squamous neoplasia: long-term study. Br J Ophthalmol. 2017;101(8):1094–9.
45. Sun Y, Hua R. Ocular surface squamous neoplasia: angiographic characteristics and response to subconjunctival/perilesional 5-fluorouracil injections. Drug Des Devel Ther. 2019;13:1323–34.
46. Abraham LM, Selva D, Casson R, Leibovitch I. Mitomycin: clinical applications in ophthalmic practice. Drugs. 2006;66(3):321–40.
47. Verweij J, Pinedo HM. Mitomycin C: mechanism of action, usefulness and limitations. Anti-Cancer Drugs. 1990;1(1):5–13.
48. Gabizon AA, Tahover E, Golan T, Geva R, Perets R, Amitay Y, et al. Pharmacokinetics of mitomycin-c lipidic prodrug entrapped in liposomes and clinical correlations in metastatic colorectal cancer patients. Investig New Drugs. 2020;38(5):1411–20.
49. Maffezzini M, Campodonico F, Canepa G, Manuputty EE, Tamagno S, Puntoni M. Intravesical mitomycin C combined with local microwave hyperthermia in non-muscle-invasive bladder cancer with increased European Organization for Research and Treatment of Cancer (EORTC) score risk of recurrence and progression. Cancer Chemother Pharmacol. 2014;73(5):925–30.
50. Miranda MB, Hartmann JT, Al-Batran SE, Kripp M, Gencer D, Hochhaus A, et al. Mitomycin C and capecitabine in pretreated patients with metastatic gastric cancer: a multicenter phase II study. J Cancer Res Clin Oncol. 2014;140(5):829–37.
51. Blasi MA, Maceroni M, Sammarco MG, Pagliara MM. Mitomycin C or interferon as adjuvant therapy to surgery for ocular surface squamous neoplasia: comparative study. Eur J Ophthalmol. 2018;28(2):204–9.
52. Daniell M, Maini R, Tole D. Use of mitomycin C in the treatment of corneal conjunctival intraepithelial neoplasia. Clin Exp Ophthalmol. 2002;30(2):94–8.
53. Frucht-Pery J, Rozenman Y. Mitomycin C therapy for corneal intraepithelial neoplasia. Am J Ophthalmol. 1994;117(2):164–8.
54. Ballalai PL, Erwenne CM, Martins MC, Lowen MS, Barros JN. Long-term results of topical mitomycin C 0.02% for primary and recurrent conjunctival-corneal intraepithelial neoplasia. Ophthalmic. Plast Reconstr Surg. 2009;25(4):296–9.
55. Frucht-Pery J, Sugar J, Baum J, Sutphin JE, Pe'er J, Savir H, et al. Mitomycin C treatment for conjunctival-corneal intraepithelial neoplasia: a multicenter experience. Ophthalmology. 1997;104(12):2085–93.
56. Prabhasawat P, Tarinvorakup P, Tesavibul N, Uiprasertkul M, Kosrirukvongs P, Booranapong W, et al. Topical 0.002% mitomycin C for the treatment of conjunctival-corneal intraepithelial neoplasia and squamous cell carcinoma. Cornea. 2005;24(4):443–8.
57. Wilson MW, Hungerford JL, George SM, Madreperla SA. Topical mitomycin C for the treatment of conjunctival and corneal epithelial dysplasia and neoplasia. Am J Ophthalmol. 1997;124(3):303–11.
58. Hirst LW. Randomized controlled trial of topical mitomycin C for ocular surface squamous neoplasia: early resolution. Ophthalmology. 2007;114(5):976–82.
59. Cohen VML, O'Day RF. Management issues in conjunctival tumours: ocular surface squamous neoplasia. Ophthalmol Ther. 2020;9(1):181–90.
60. Khong JJ, Muecke J. Complications of mitomycin C therapy in 100 eyes with ocular surface neoplasia. Br J Ophthalmol. 2006;90(7):819–22.
61. Russell HC, Chadha V, Lockington D, Kemp EG. Topical mitomycin C chemotherapy in the management of ocular surface neoplasia: a 10-year review of treatment outcomes and complications. Br J Ophthalmol. 2010;94(10):1316–21.
62. Dudney BW, Malecha MA. Limbal stem cell deficiency following topical mitomycin C treatment of conjunctival-corneal intraepithelial neoplasia. Am J Ophthalmol. 2004;137(5):950–1.
63. Das BC, Thapa P, Karki R, Das S, Mahapatra S, Liu TC, et al. Retinoic acid signaling pathways in development and diseases. Bioorg Med Chem. 2014;22(2):673–83.
64. Lotan R. Effects of vitamin A and its analogs (retinoids) on normal and neoplastic cells. Biochim Biophys Acta. 1980;605(1):33–91.
65. Herbort CP, Zografos L, Zwingli M, Schoeneich M. Topical retinoic acid in dysplastic and metaplastic keratinization of corneoconjunctival epithelium. Graefes Arch Clin Exp Ophthalmol. 1988;226(1):22–6.
66. Ip MH, Tat L, Coroneo MT. The treatment of recurrent conjunctival and corneal intraepithelial neoplasia with interferon alfa-2b and retinoic acid: ~9 years' follow-up on tumor control. Ocul Surf. 2020;18(3):354–9.

67. Krilis M, Tsang H, Coroneo M. Treatment of conjunctival and corneal epithelial neoplasia with retinoic acid and topical interferon alfa-2b: long-term follow-up. Ophthalmology. 2012;119(10):1969–73.
68. Skippen B, Tsang HH, Assaad NN, Coroneo MT. Rapid response of refractory ocular surface dysplasia to combination treatment with topical all-trans retinoic acid and interferon alfa-2b. Arch Ophthalmol. 2010;128(10):1368–9.
69. Ferrara N, Adamis AP. Ten years of anti-vascular endothelial growth factor therapy. Nat Rev Drug Discov. 2016;15(6):385–403.
70. Cho HJ, Jung SH, Cho S, Han JO, Park S, Kim JW. Intravitreal anti-vascular endothelial growth factor treatment for pachychoroid neovasculopathy. J Ocul Pharmacol Ther. 2019;35(3):174–81.
71. Kim LA, D'Amore PA. A brief history of anti-VEGF for the treatment of ocular angiogenesis. Am J Pathol. 2012;181(2):376–9.
72. Mak RK, Chan TC, Marcet MM, Choy BN, Shum JW, Shih KC, et al. Use of anti-vascular endothelial growth factor in the management of pterygium. Acta Ophthalmol. 2017;95(1):20–7.
73. Cheung N, Lam DS, Wong TY. Anti-vascular endothelial growth factor treatment for eye diseases. BMJ. 2012;344:e2970.
74. Finger PT, Chin KJ. Refractory squamous cell carcinoma of the conjunctiva treated with subconjunctival ranibizumab (Lucentis): a two-year study. Ophthalmic Plast Reconstr Surg. 2012;28(2):85–9.
75. Faramarzi A, Feizi S. Subconjunctival bevacizumab injection for ocular surface squamous neoplasia. Cornea. 2013;32(7):998–1001.
76. Paul S, Stone DU. Intralesional bevacizumab use for invasive ocular surface squamous neoplasia. J Ocul Pharmacol Ther. 2012;28(6):647–9.
77. Teng CC, Chin KJ, Finger PT. Subconjunctival ranibizumab for squamous cell carcinoma of the conjunctiva with corneal extension. Br J Ophthalmol. 2009;93(6):837–8.
78. Asena L, Dursun AD. Topical bevacizumab for the treatment of ocular surface squamous neoplasia. J Ocul Pharmacol Ther. 2015;31(8):487–90.
79. Ranibizumab (Lucentis): Visual Impairment due to Choroidal Neovascularization Secondary to Pathologic Myopia. 2015.
80. Harlev E, Nevo E, Lansky EP, Ofir R, Bishayee A. Anticancer potential of aloes: antioxidant, antiproliferative, and immunostimulatory attributes. Planta Med. 2012;78(9):843–52.
81. Damani MR, Shah AR, Karp CL, Orlin SE. Treatment of ocular surface squamous neoplasia with topical Aloe vera drops. Cornea. 2015;34(1):87–9.
82. Zabawski EJ, Cockerell CJ. Topical and intralesional cidofovir: a review of pharmacology and therapeutic effects. J Am Acad Dermatol. 1998;39(5 Pt 1):741–5.
83. Cundy KC. Clinical pharmacokinetics of the antiviral nucleotide analogues cidofovir and adefovir. Clin Pharmacokinet. 1999;36(2):127–43.
84. Rahhal FM, Arevalo JF, Munguia D, Taskintuna I, Chavez de la Paz E, Azen SP, et al. Intravitreal cidofovir for the maintenance treatment of cytomegalovirus retinitis. Ophthalmology. 1996;103(7):1078–83.
85. Ip MH, Robert George CR, Naing Z, Perlman EM, Rawlinson W, Coroneo MT. Topical Cidofovir for treatment-refractory ocular surface squamous neoplasia. Ophthalmology. 2018;125(4):617–9.
86. Sherman MD, Feldman KA, Farahmand SM, Margolis TP. Treatment of conjunctival squamous cell carcinoma with topical cidofovir. Am J Ophthalmol. 2002;134(3):432–3.

Surgical Management of Ocular Surface Squamous Neoplasia

Umiya Harley and Sachin M. Salvi

1 Introduction

Ocular surface squamous neoplasia (OSSN) is a well-established term [1] used to describe a spectrum of disease, representing the most common non-pigmented malignancy of the ocular surface [2]. In simple terms, it is essentially an abnormal growth of squamous epithelial cells affecting the conjunctiva and/or cornea, ranging from mild epithelial dysplasia to invasive squamous carcinoma (SSC) [3].

In this chapter, we describe the Sheffield Ocular Oncology Service (SOOS) approach to the surgical management of conjunctival and corneal OSSN. We have included rare OSSN-related problems such as disease spill over to the eyelid and anterior orbital involvement.

2 Clinical Assessment

Our practice at SOOS is a step-by-step approach from recognition to resolution (Fig. 1). Firstly, a thorough clinical assessment is done by obtaining a detailed history, including identifying the important risk factors of OSSN.

The major risk factor in the development of OSSN is exposure to solar ultraviolet light [4, 5], and is predominately seen in countries close to the equator for that reason. Individuals carrying the greatest risk are thought to be those living within 30° of the equator; sun exposed with fair eye color and skin, susceptible to sunburn [4].

OSSN can however affect any race, with incidence figures ranging from 0.03–1.9 per 100,000/year [4, 6–8] in Caucasian populations and a significantly higher incidence of 3–3.4 per 100,000/year in African ethnicity populations [9, 10] and is thought to be increasing [11]. It occurs predominantly in adults, with a higher predilection to the male gender in the Caucasian populations [12]. Other risk factors include smoking, radiation or chemical exposure, chronic irritation or atopy, p53 gene mutation/deletion, and hereditary deficiency of DNA repair such as in xeroderma pigmentosum [13]. Human immunodeficiency virus (HIV) is associated with an increased risk of OSSN [14, 15] and more controversially, human papilloma virus (HPV) 16 and 18 [16] has been implicated as a possible risk factor. HIV-related OSSN can be more aggressive and often the first presenting sign of HIV [17], therefore, it should be excluded in younger patients of any gender.

The signs and symptoms the patient may experience is variable; aside from the presence of a growth on the ocular surface, there may be redness, watering, and irritation. If the lesion has encroached over the center of the cornea, the visual acuity may be affected. The duration of growth in most cases is over several months but maybe weeks to years in some cases. Advanced cases may have associated severe pain and visual loss due to necrotizing scleritis [18].

A detailed clinical examination, including imaging, is vital for treatment planning. This includes documenting the location, size in clock hours, vascularity, mobility, and depth of the lesion.

The typical presentation of OSSN is a unilateral vascularized non-pigmented lesion located in the interpalpebral limbal area [1]. However, it can be found in any part of the conjunctiva, including the tarsus, and cornea. Rarely, it may present bilaterally or with multifocal lesions [1]. OSSN lesions can be flat or elevated, varying from yellow-pink, gray, or white in color [19]. The appearance is classified into gelatinous with superficial vessels; papilliform with a papillary appearance; leukoplakic with a white keratin plaque covering the lesion; or as a nodular lesion (Fig. 2). There may be an overlap of these appearances and the lesion may extend onto the peripheral cornea. The presence of large feeder vessels with a large immobile lesion is usually a sign of an invasive SCC.

U. Harley (✉) · S. M. Salvi
Sheffield Ocular Oncology Service, Royal Hallamshire Hospital, Sheffield, UK
e-mail: umiya.harley@nhs.net; sachin.salvi@nhs.net

B. V. Chawla, M. E. Aronow (eds.), *Global Perspectives in Ocular Oncology*, https://doi.org/10.1007/978-3-031-08250-4_19

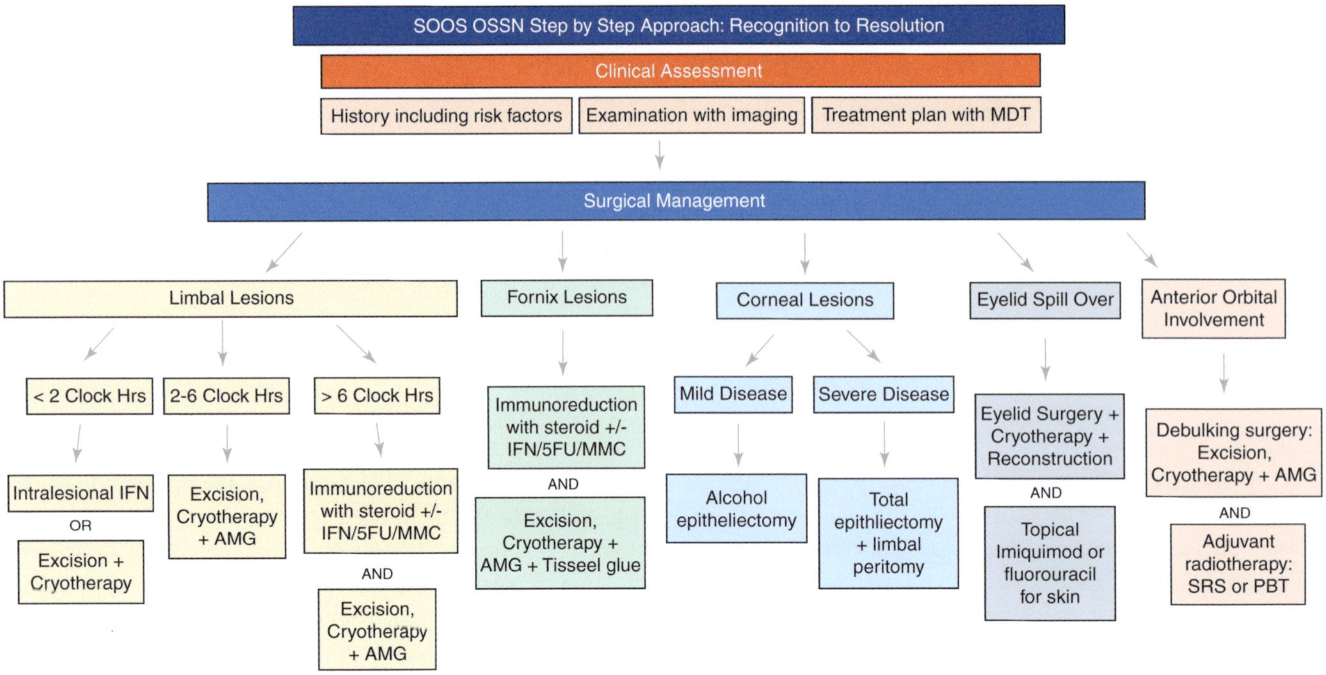

Fig. 1 Flow chart: SOOS OSSN management step-by-step approach from recognition to resolution

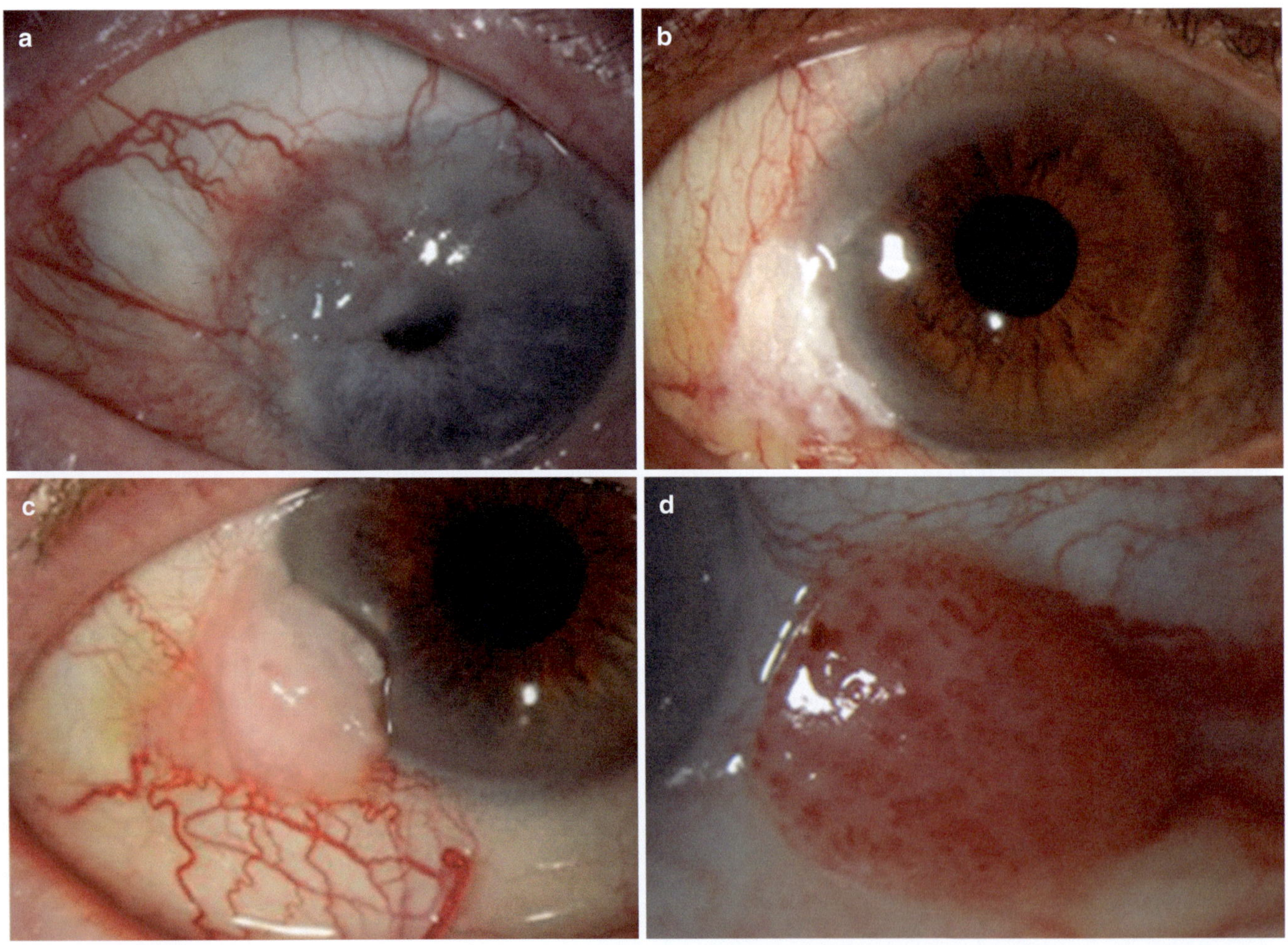

Fig. 2 Clinical appearance of OSSN: (**a**) gelatinous lesion at the limbus encroaching the cornea with feeder vessels, (**b**) flat leukoplakic plaque on the surface of the lesion, (**c**) raised leukoplakic lesion at the limbus with feeder vessels, (**d**) raised papilliferous lesion on the bulbar conjunctiva

OSSN may be associated with pigmentation in darker complexions, requiring differentiation from conjunctival melanoma (Fig. 3b). If HIV related, the lesions are often larger with feeder vessels and forniceal extension [11]. Differential diagnosis of OSSN includes pinguecula, pterygium, pannus, squamous papilloma, and granuloma.

OSSN is a clinical diagnosis, often not requiring a biopsy. However, the severity of the OSSN can be difficult to distinguish clinically without histopathological analysis, and thus histopathology remains the gold standard [20].

Histologically, OSSN presents as a spectrum of dysplastic changes of the ocular surface epithelium; mild, moderate,

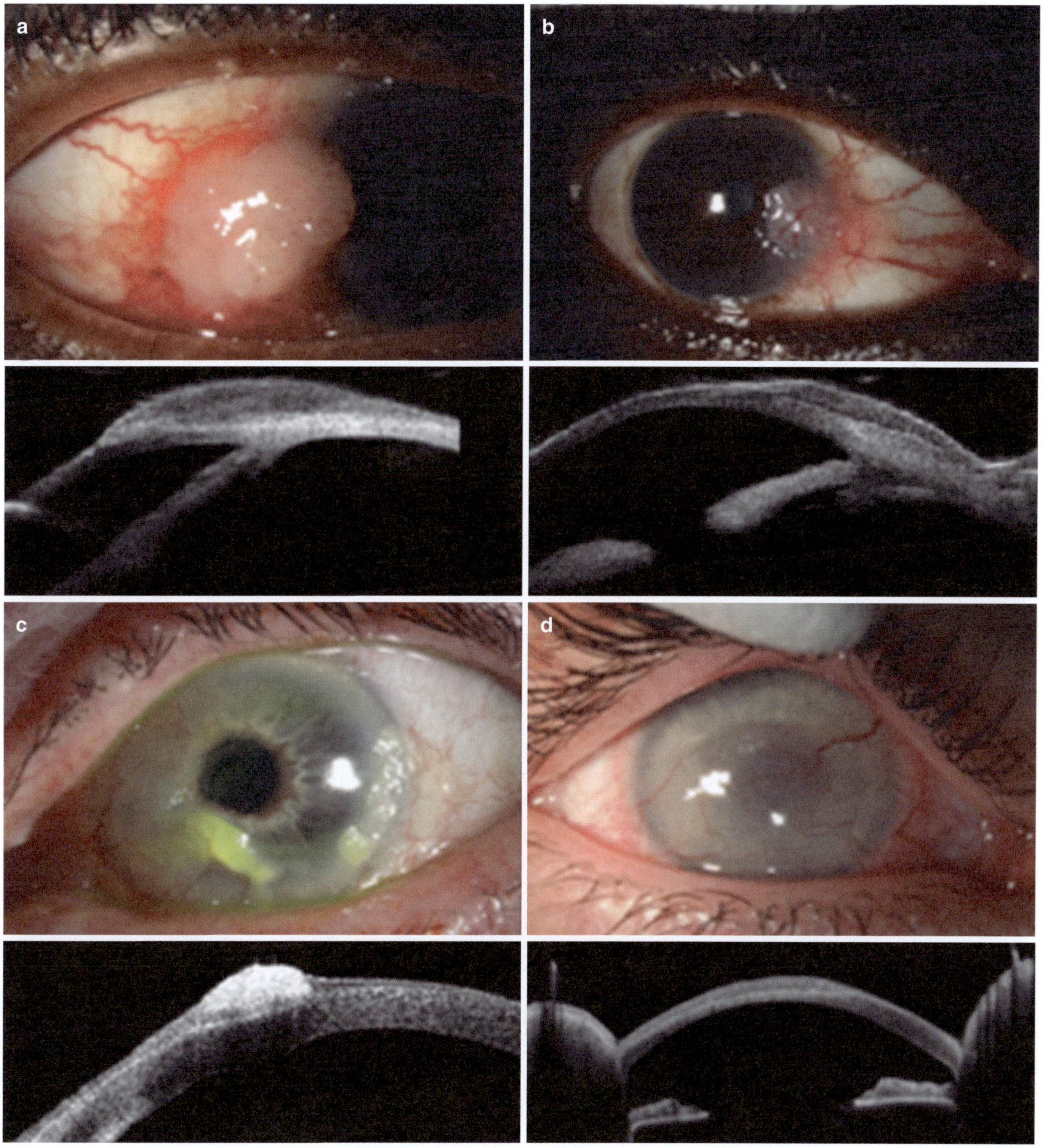

Fig. 3 Conjunctival limbal OSSN encroaching on the cornea: (**a** and **b**) UBM images showing thickened epithelium and depth of lesion. Corneal OSSN: (**c** and **d**) AS OCT showing the lesion disrupting the stromal layer

and severe cellular atypia, classified by the American Joint Committee on Cancer (AJCC) staging manual [21]. An intact basement membrane is characteristic of conjunctival intraepithelial neoplasia (CIN) of mild, moderate, or severe grade. Carcinoma in situ is the term used for severe atypia, respecting the basement membrane but involving the full thickness of the epithelium. Invasion of the basement membrane involving the stroma is characteristic of SCC; well, moderately, or poorly differentiated. A chronic inflammatory response and increased vascularity is often seen. Rare variants of invasive SCC such as mucoepidermoid carcinoma and spindle cell carcinoma demonstrate aggressive behavior with higher recurrence rates and intraocular spread and orbital invasion.

Non-invasive imaging modalities such as anterior segment optical coherence tomography (ASOCT) and ultrasound biomicroscopy (UBM) (Fig. 3) have become extremely useful aids to diagnosis and treatment planning, as they are able to identify the depth of lesions. There are other approaches to diagnosis such as impression cytology and confocal microscopy that have been explored [22].

Our practice at SOOS involves taking the patient's eye condition, general health, severity and extent of disease, and clinical suspicion into consideration before making a treatment plan with discussion at our multidisciplinary team (MDT) meeting.

3 Surgical Management of OSSN

Surgical management of OSSN still remains to be the gold standard for OSSN treatment [13], despite more conservative approaches to management which are increasing in popularity due to high recurrence rates and to avoid potential surgical complications [23]. The conservative medical treatments are not in the scope of this chapter and has been beautifully discussed in another chapter in this book. This section describes our surgical approach to managing conjunctival and corneal OSSN and the rarer situations of eyelid spill over and anterior orbital involvement.

3.1 Conjunctival OSSN

The main goal of managing a conjunctival lesion is to excise the tumor with clear margins and to make residual cells nonviable. Traditionally, surgery involved excision alone with "no touch" technique [24]; however, the recurrence rates were reported as high as 56% and up to 33% even with clear margins [23]. Adjuvant therapies such as cryotherapy, topical chemotherapeutic agents: interferon-a2b or -a2a (IFN), mitomycin C (MMC), and 5-fluorouracil (5FU), in addition to excision, have been shown to reduce the rates of recurrence [25–27].

We often commence patients on topical steroids prior to treatment as in our experience we find this reduces the inflammatory response to the tumor and helps demarcate tumor margins. Our preferred regime is preservative free dexamethasone eyedrops used four times a day until surgery (usually performed within 2 weeks).

For well-defined small limbal lesions, less than 2 clock hours, excision with 2 mm margin, double freeze thaw cryotherapy is the preferred surgical treatment with direct closure, generally under local anesthetic (LA). Direct closure in small lesions does not tend to cause surgical complications. Alternatively, immunoreduction with topical or intralesional chemotherapy agents such as IFN can be used to treat small lesions if the patient does not wish to undergo surgery. The authors do advocate the use of intralesional IFN, initially for immunoreduction of the lesion; however, if there is an incomplete response, surgical intervention is required (Fig. 4).

For larger limbal lesions, greater than 2 clock hours but less than 6 clock hours, our preference is to excise the lesion with a 2 mm margin, double freeze thaw cryotherapy and amniotic membrane graft (AMG). We have a low threshold to use AMG especially in medial lesions with our experience, due to its healing and anti-angiogenic properties which prevent chronic inflammation, granulation tissue formation, and scarring [28]. We prefer this to be done under general anesthetic (GA), although LA with sedation is also an option. Most lesions are in the limbal area; therefore, corneal involvement is common. Absolute alcohol epitheliectomy to the cornea is often required to remove the overlying lesion with the epithelium.

For limbal lesions greater than 6 clock hours, we prefer to immunoreduce the lesion with topical immunotherapy and chemotherapy agents such as IFN or 5FU or use intralesional IFN with topical steroids prior to surgical removal. This has the additional effect of reducing the inflammatory effect and reduces potential limbal cell damage from surgical removal. Again, we prefer surgical removal under GA for the excision with 2 mm margin, double freeze thaw cryotherapy and AMG.

Surgical excision of fornix lesions is often more challenging due to the increased risk of surgical complications including scarring, symblepharon, and restriction of eye movements due to the location. We again advocate the use of topical steroids and topical or intralesional chemotherapy agents pre-operatively to immunoreduce the lesion where possible. We prefer excision with 2 mm margin, double freeze thaw cryotherapy and AMG under GA, with the addition of the senior author's novel technique of using a fibrin sealant, such as Tisseel glue, stuck in place with squint hooks to reform the fornix.

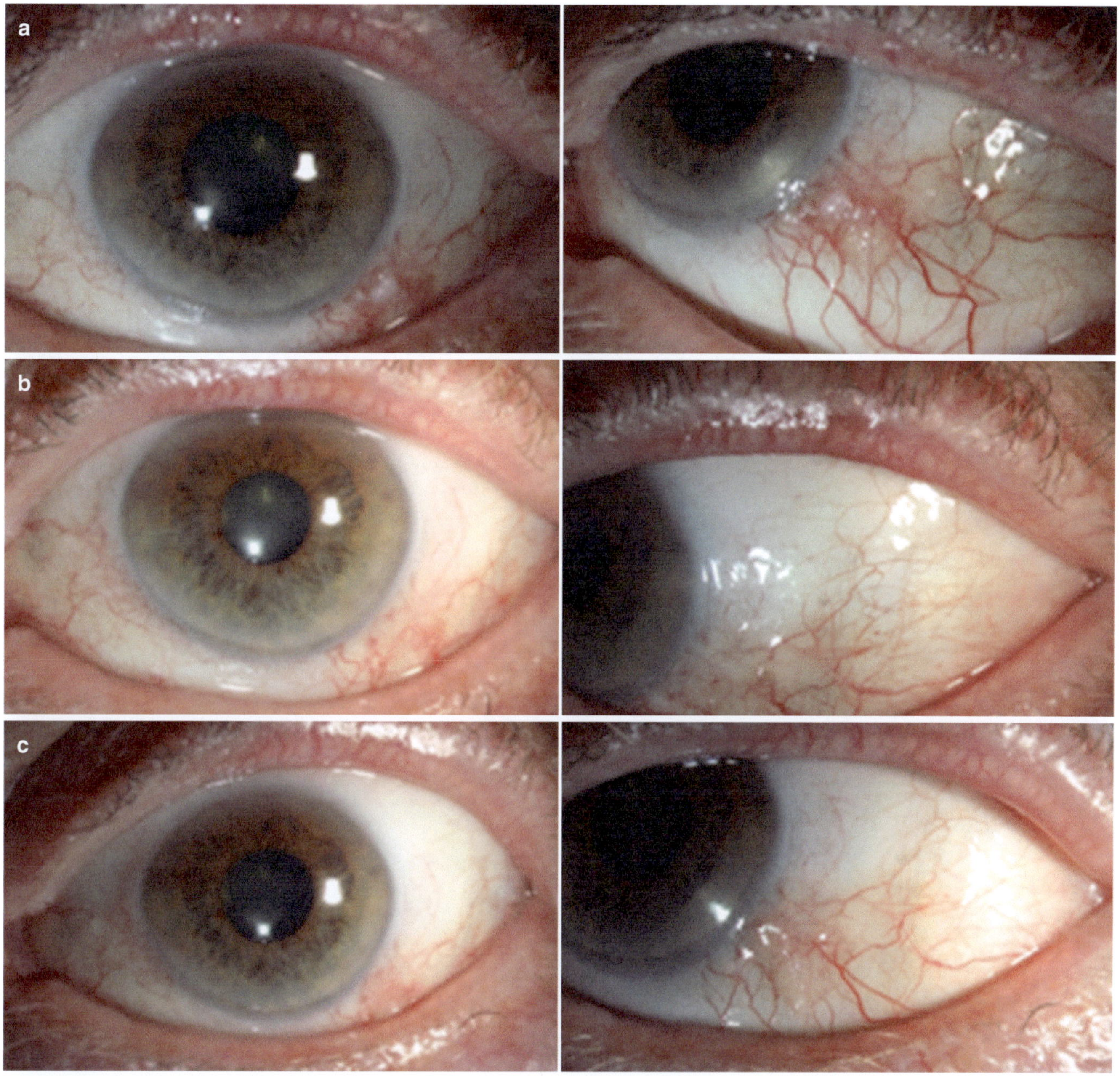

Fig. 4 Conjunctival limbal OSSN, (**a**) pre-treatment image, (**b**) regression of the lesion following IFN monthly intralesional injections for 3 months, (**c**) recurrence requiring excision, cryotherapy with map biopsies 4 months later

4 Surgical Technique for Conjunctival OSSN

4.1 Excision of Lesion

Our step-by-step approach to the surgical excision of conjunctival limbal lesion is as follows. Smaller lesions are undertaken under LA (Fig. 5), with topical anesthetic such a proxymetacaine or tetracaine. Larger lesions are preferred to be undertaken under GA (Fig. 6).

An important part of our surgical approach is planning the excision. Once the eye has been prepped and draped, the surgical field is dried using a cotton bud and the tumor is identified and marked with a marker pen. The lesion margins can be difficult to identify but the authors have observed that abnormal conjunctiva appears matte compared to normal

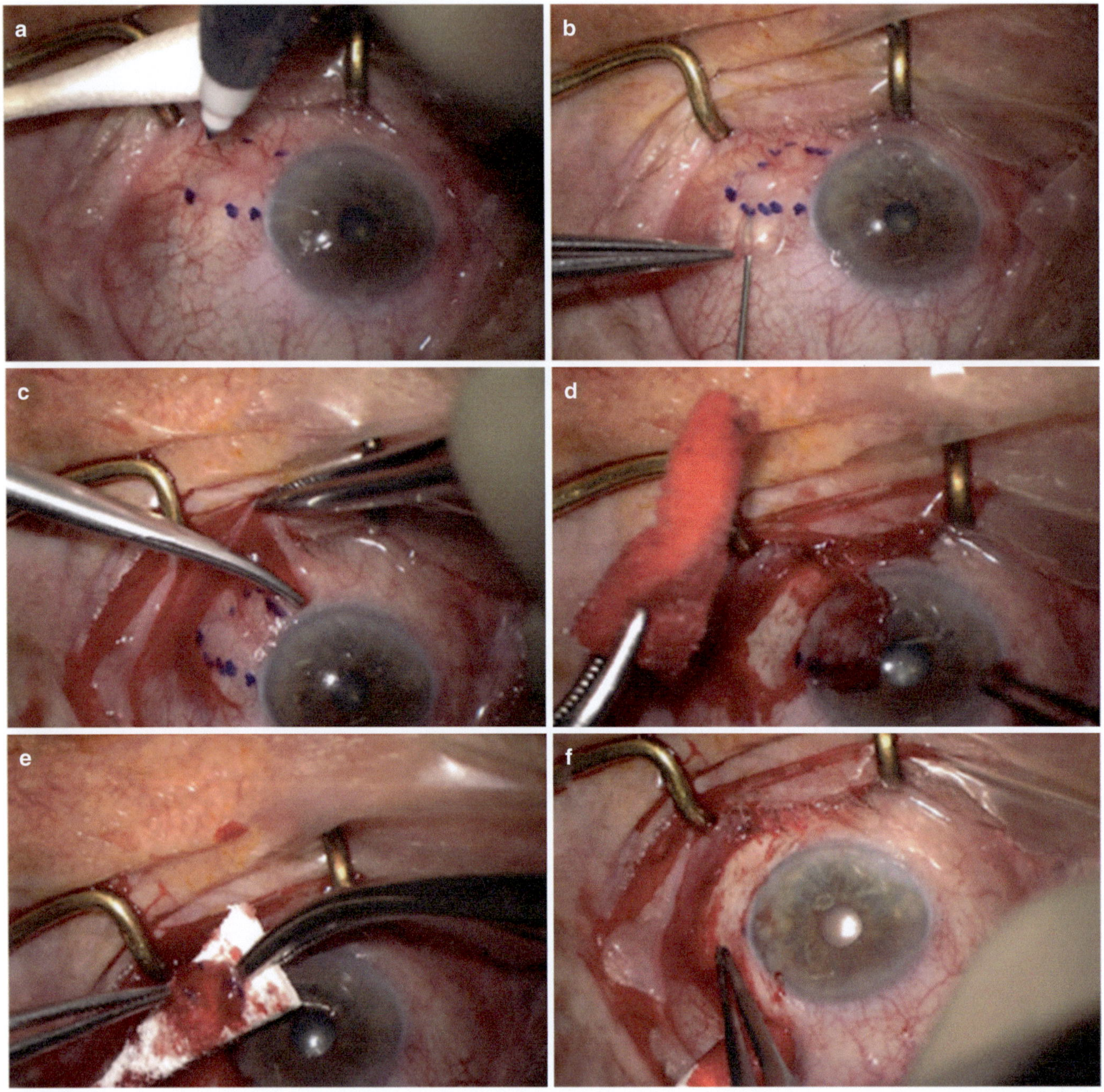

Fig. 5 Excision of small lesion (**a**) lesion marked, (**b**) subconjunctival local anesthetic injected, (**c**) no touch technique used to cut round the lesion starting at the limbus, (**d**) spear used to peel back the lesion off the sclera, (**e**) lesion cut at limbus and orientated on spear, (**f**) hemostasis achieved

conjunctiva. It is important to keep the surgical field dry throughout the surgery to reduce the risk of microscopic tumor cell spread. We use viscoelastic solution, such as Coatel, on the cornea to prevent it becoming dry and avoid the use of balance salt solution (BSS) irrigation.

The authors prefer to use sub-conjunctival Marcaine 0.5% with adrenaline injected from the non-involved conjunctiva to under the involved area and with gentle blunt diffusion with a cotton bud if required taking care not to touch the tumor area. We find this maneuver helps create a plane between the tenons and episclera, allowing preservation of deeper episcleral tissue during the surgery. It also allows us to identify if there is deeper scleral involvement prior to excision, suggested by adherence. This practice is not done in all centers as they fear this may cause seeding. We have not encountered this problem in our experience.

Moorfields forceps and Wescott scissors are used to excise the lesion with 2 mm margin, starting at the limbus using a “non-touch” technique. “Non-touch” technique is achieved by grasping the conjunctiva outside of the marked tumor ini-

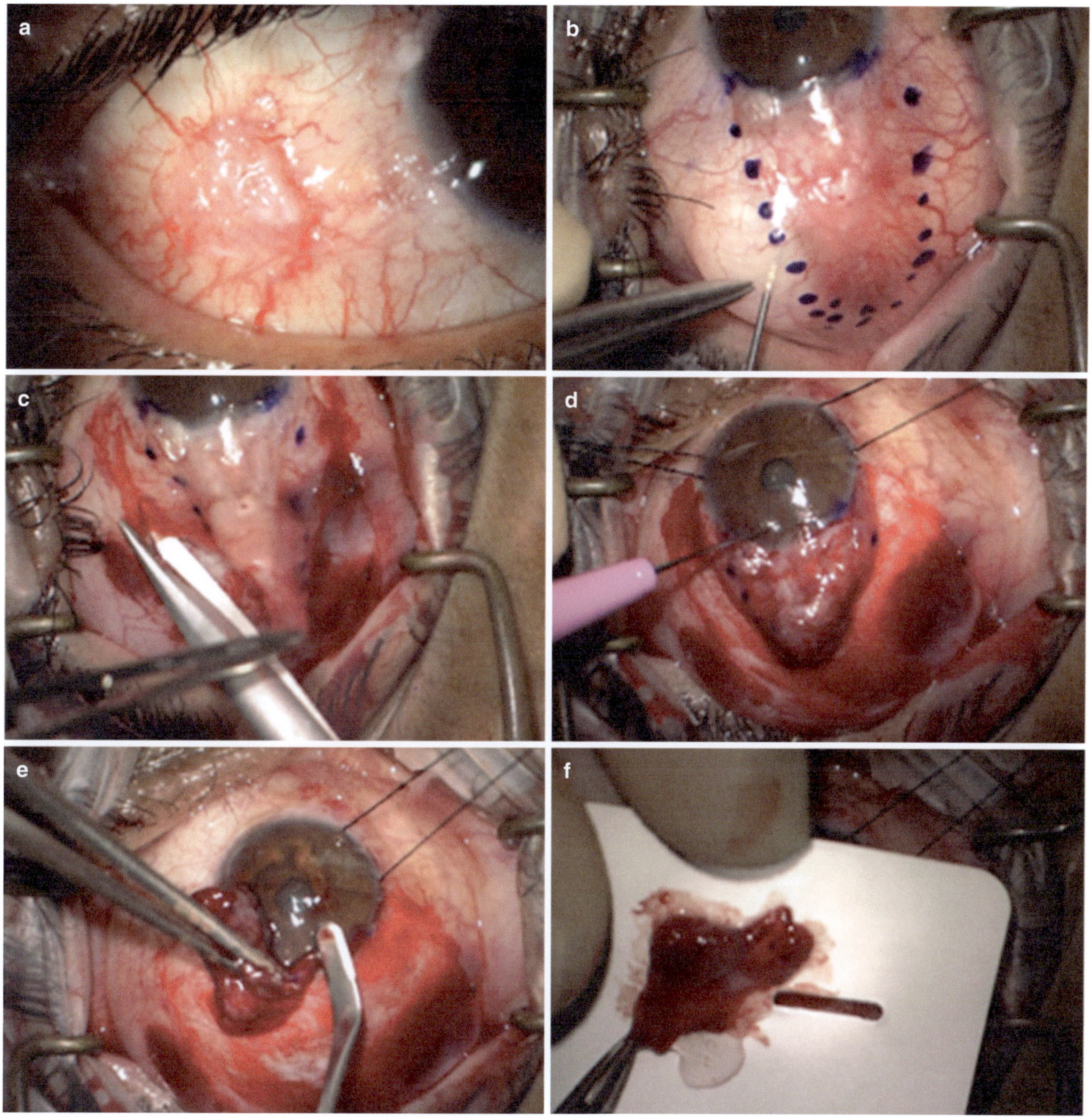

Fig. 6 Excision of large lesion with limbal and corneal involvement, (**a**) pre-operative image of temporal limbal lesion, (**b**) traction sutures used to ensure exposure, lesion marked and LA inserted, (**c**) no touch technique to excise lesion to limbus, (**d**) 15° blade used to mark corneal extent on epithelium, (**e**) crescent blade used to excise lesion from limbus, (**f**) orientated on paper to send for histology

tially and once the conjunctival portion has been excised from limbus to limbus, a disposable cotton bud or cellulose spear is used to peel the lesion from the underlying episclera up to the limbus. Cautery is used to achieve hemostasis. The tumor can now be grasped taking care not to crush the specimen, and using the Westcott scissor, the lesion can be cut from the limbus if there is no corneal involvement.

If there is a corneal extent of the lesion, a 15° blade is used to mark the advancing edge of the disease taking care to only mark the epithelium (Fig. 6d). A well is created using viscoelastic such as Coatel, which is applied to the unaffected cornea. Absolute alcohol is applied to the involved corneal area and limbus for 60 s and the desiccated corneal epithelium is gently scraped off the stroma from the line

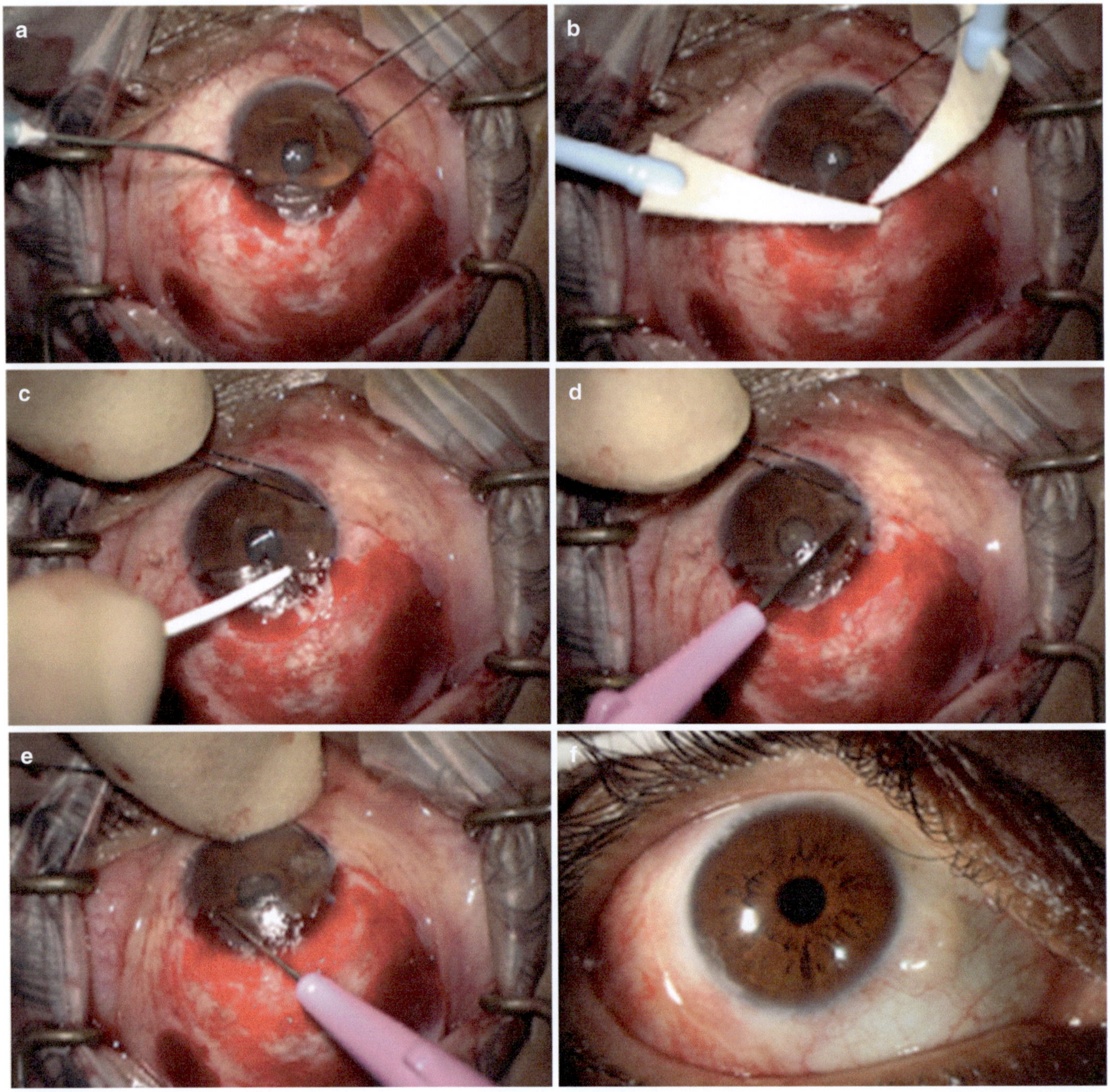

Fig. 7 Corneal involvement, (**a**) viscoelastic is used to create a well protecting the unaffected cornea, (**b**) absolute alcohol soaked in spears is applied for 60 s, (**c**) spear is used to scrape off the corneal epithelium, (**d** and **e**) blunt under surface of 15° blade used to scrape the epithelium, (**f**) 6 weeks post-operative image

marked with the 15° blade toward the limbus with the blunt end of a 15° blade, edge of crescent blade used vertically or cotton buds or spear (Fig. 7). Care is taken to avoid any unnecessary manipulation of the tumor.

If there is scleral involvement, we do not perform scleral bed dissection, as we feel this may cause complications such as scleral thinning and could lead to deeper spread of tumor following surgery. We instead prefer to treat scleral involvement 6 weeks later, to allow for post-operative healing, with adjuvant ruthenium plaque brachytherapy or proton beam therapy.

Once the lesion is excised it is placed on a spear or filter paper and orientated prior to being put into a formalin solution for histopathological analysis. Hemostasis is achieved with cautery if required.

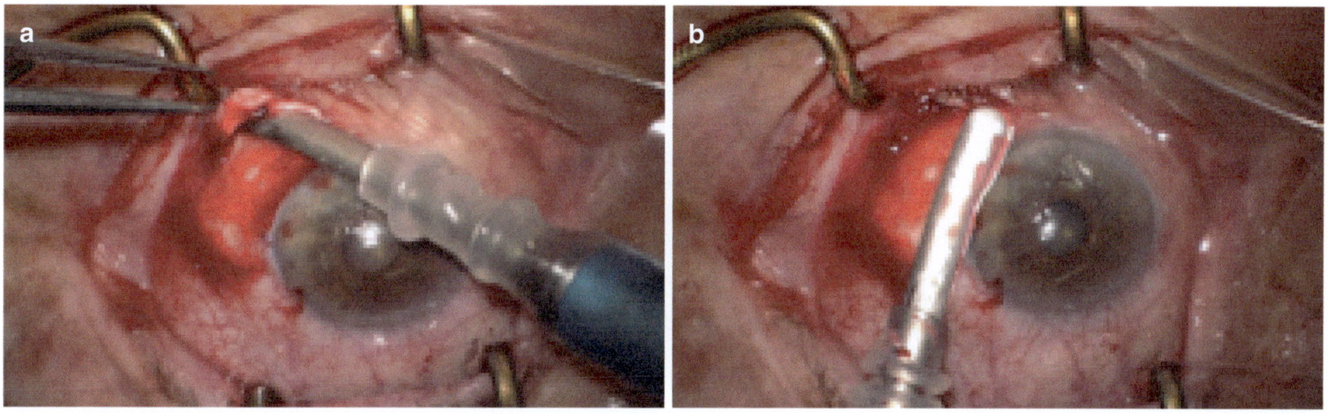

Fig. 8 Cryotherapy, double freeze thaw (**a**) conjunctival edge (**b**) limbus

4.2 Cryotherapy

Double freeze thaw cryotherapy is applied to the conjunctival edges, from an inside out approach, and to the limbus to treat any residual tumor cells and make them non-viable (Fig. 8). Maximal cell death is achieved by rapid freezing followed by a slow thawing. The authors prefer removing the sleeve or pushing back the sleeve of the disposable cryotherapy probe to allow a larger surface area to be treated. We avoid use of irrigation during this time. The episclera under the tumor is usually not treated. Once cryotherapy is completed, it is important that all the previously used instrument used for the excision are replaced with fresh set for the closure to prevent any seeding.

5 Closure of Conjunctival Defect

Direct closure of the conjunctiva for small lesions is achieved by undermining the conjunctiva and then suturing the edges with 8.0 Vicryl (Fig. 9).

For larger lesions, a wide excision is required, and closure is carried out using AMG to cover the exposed area (Fig. 10). The preserved human amniotic membrane is irrigated with BSS and carefully removed from its carrier sheet. The authors prefer to use two Moorfields forceps to grasp a corner each and then, with the help of an assistant who grasps and pulls away the paper on which the membrane lies, the AMG is placed on the eye stromal side down with ease. Cardinal sutures with 8.0 Vicryl are applied to suture the AMG starting at the limbus. A combination of 8.0 Vicryl interrupted sutures and a continuous 10.0 Vicryl is preferred. However, a fibrin sealant such as Tisseel glue is also an option, instead of the 10.0 Vicryl, and is smoothed out using a spear.

For fornix lesions, we prefer to use a fibrin sealant such as Tisseel glue to recreate the fornix. Once the cardinal sutures are applied, Tisseel glue is inserted into the area of the fornix and two squint hooks are placed for 2 min to allow the Tisseel to get stuck to the underlying bed and graft in its new position thus recreating the forniceal space (Fig. 11).

Map biopsies are undertaken during the initial excision only if multifocal disease is present or during the monitoring phase if there is a suspicion of a recurrence. The surgical approach (Fig. 12) is to again use LA to create a surgical plane and a small sample is taken from any suspicious areas in the bulbar, limbal, or tarsal conjunctiva. Simple non-tooth forceps such as Moorfields forceps are used to gently grasp and lift the conjunctiva and Wescott's scissors are used to take the 1–2 mm spindle shaped sample preferably in a single motion. Care is taken to ensure the full thickness of conjunctiva is biopsied as a superficial biopsy will not help distinguish between in situ and invasive disease. The specimen is gently unfolded on a spear or paper and each specimen is sent in a separate formalin pot for histopathology along with a detailed diagram showing anatomical location.

5.1 Corneal OSSN

Corneal OSSN in isolation without any limbal involvement is rare and can be exceedingly difficult to diagnose and manage. It is unclear whether the origin of the OSSN is from the limbus or corneal epithelium; however, histologically, it is like the conjunctiva and limbus, with an intact Bowman's layer [29]. Corneal OSSN lesions are usually opalescent with a mottled ground glass appearance, often with white dots and usually avascular (Fig. 13). However, they can develop in severe ocular surface disease with a vascularized appearance, making diagnosis challenging. Surgical removal

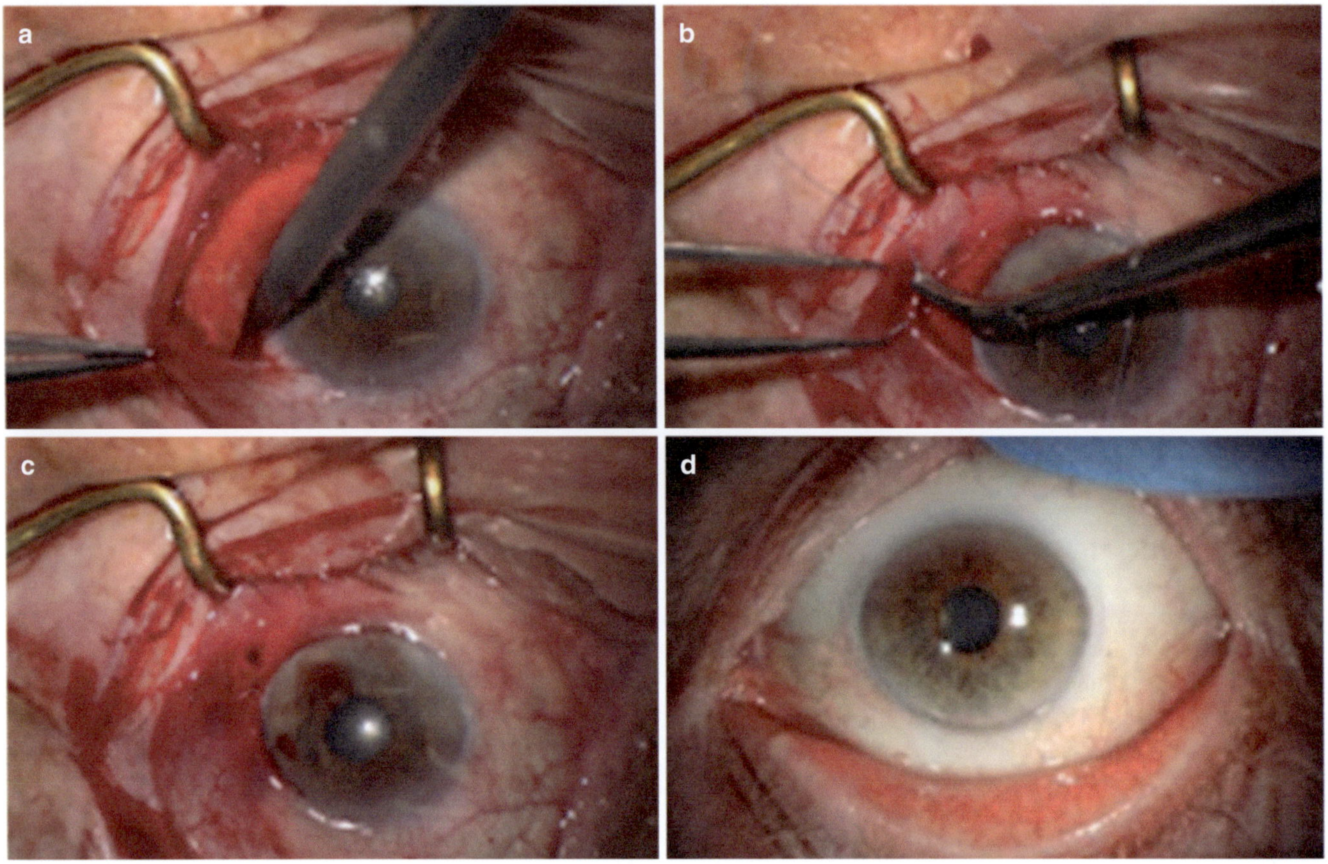

Fig. 9 Direct closure of conjunctival defect, (**a**) undermine the conjunctiva, (**b**) suture with 8.0 Vicryl, (**c**) closure of defect, (**d**) 6-month post-surgery

of the corneal epithelium is useful to aid diagnosis of OSSN and combined with topical chemotherapy agents can help control the disease [30].

6 Surgical Technique for Corneal OSSN

For mild epithelial superficial disease, absolute alcohol is used to remove the epithelium. This can be done under LA or GA. We prefer to use viscoelastic such as Coatel, which is applied 360° around the cornea to create a well. The absolute alcohol is applied to the cornea for 60 s, and the epithelium is scraped off with a spear cellulose sponge and sent off for histopathological analysis. Corneal punch biopsy can also be performed to aid diagnosis in patients with stromal involvement; though we often avoid this to prevent a dellen formation.

For more extensive corneal disease, a total epitheliectomy with a limbal peritomy is the preferred technique.

The blunt end of a 15° blade is used initially without alcohol to scrape any thickened corneal and limbal keratinization, which can often be peeled off or excised. Absolute alcohol is then applied and a spear cellulose sponge is used, as described in previous paragraph, to complete the total corneal epitheliectomy.

A 360 limbal peritomy is then completed and any feeder vessels are quaterized. A 1–2 frill of conjunctiva is also cut to remove any residual limbal disease. Limbal peritomy is recessed back by 1–2 mm and a bandage contact lens is inserted. Post-operative MMC, 5FU or IFN is used once the healing is completed, at least 6 weeks later, to prevent regrowth back onto the cornea (Fig. 14).

6.1 Eyelid and Anterior Orbital Involvement

OSSN spilling over to the eyelid and involving the orbital is extremely rare, often involving rare, aggressive variants of invasive SCC, such as poorly differentiated or mucoepidermoid carcinoma.

Eyelid spill over can be treated with double freeze thaw cryotherapy with additional eyelid surgery to excise the involving areas followed by reconstruction. Any suspicious areas away from the lid margin can be treated with topical treatment such as imiquimod or fluorouracil (Fig. 15).

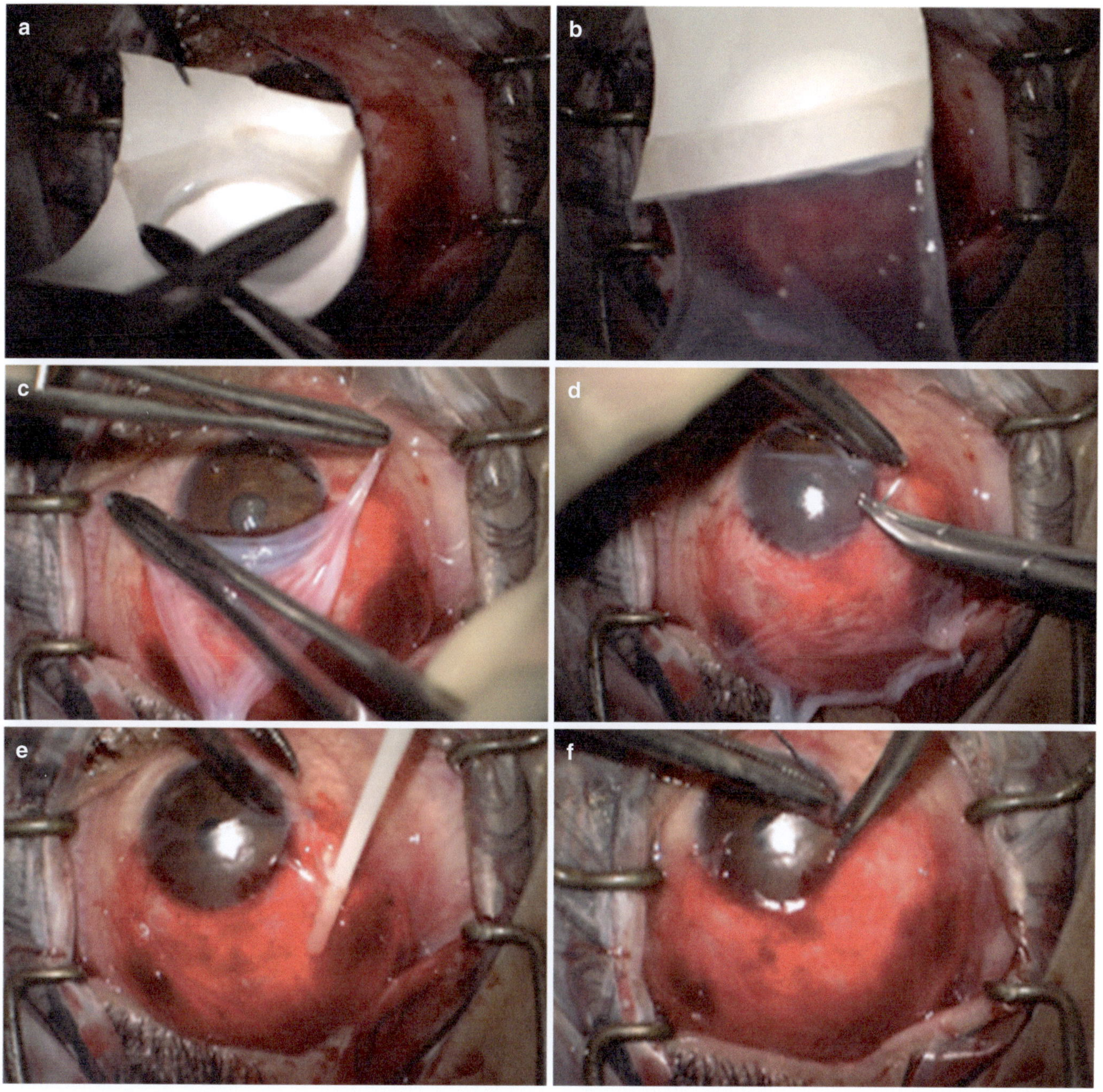

Fig. 10 Reconstruction with AMG: (**a**) two Moorfields forceps used to grasp the corners of the AMG and assistant using forceps to grasp the paper, (**b**) the AMG is pulled away from the paper, (**c**) placed stromal down, (**d**) cardinal sutures placed with 8.0 Vicryl, (**e**) fibrin sealant (Tisseel glue) is inserted and smoothed out using a spear, (**f**) excess AMG is cut at the limbus

For anterior orbital involvement, lesions can be surgically debulked using the surgical technique of excision, cryotherapy, and AMG (Fig. 16). However, further adjuvant radiotherapy such as stereotactic radiosurgery (SRS) or proton beam therapy (PBT) is often required to treat deeper involvement (of critical structures) and the residual microscopic disease. In some cases, radiation therapy such as SRS or PBT may be considered as the initial treatment when complete resection is not possible or as a salvage treatment to avoid exenteration [31, 32] (Fig. 17). In cases where more than two quadrants of the orbit are involved; poorly differentiated tumors or deeper orbital recurrence, exenteration surgery is the only treatment option [33] (Fig. 18).

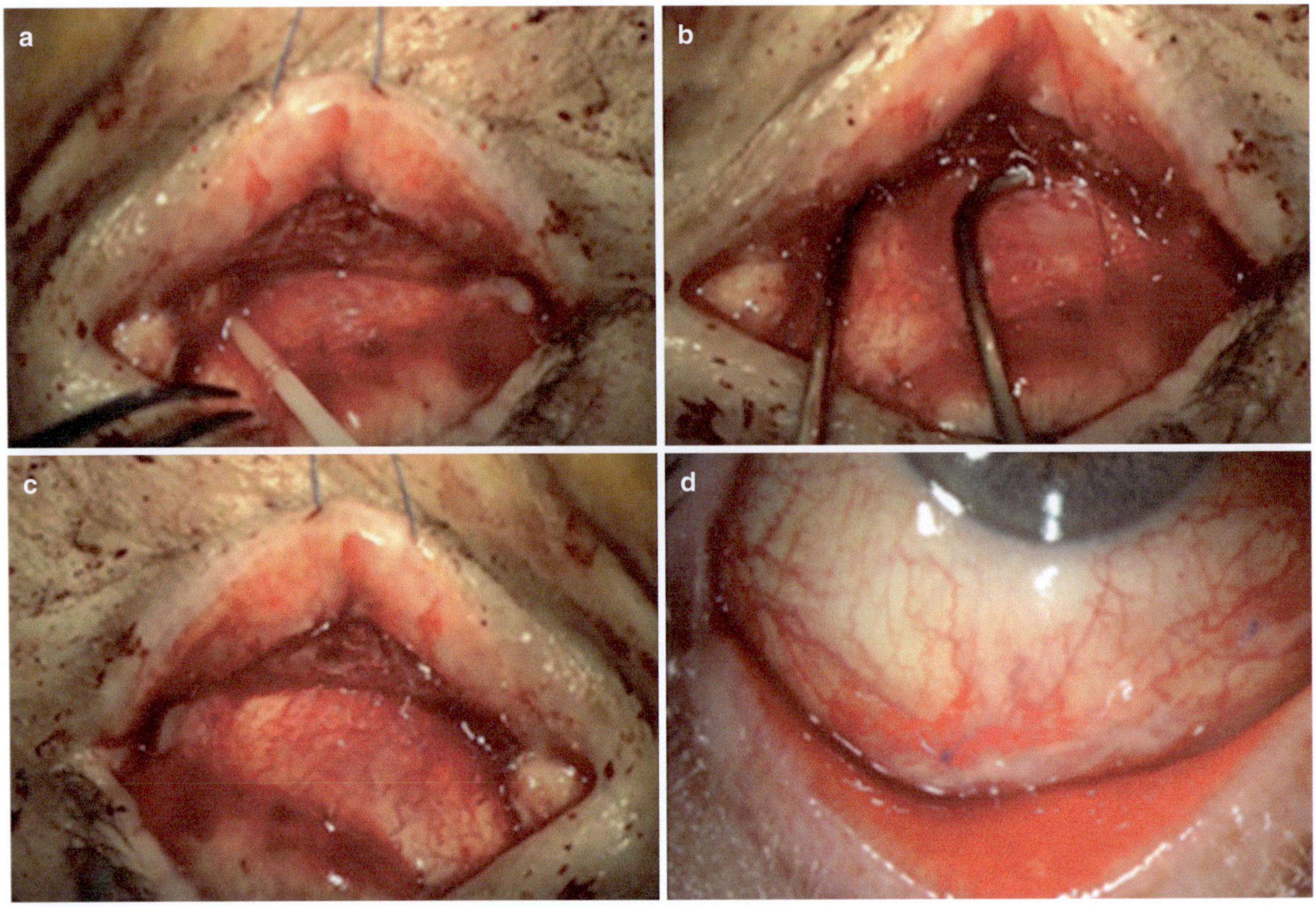

Fig. 11 Reconstruction of the inferior fornix: (**a**) fibrin sealant (Tisseel glue) is inserted once the cardinal sutures have been placed, (**b**) two squint hooks placed into the inferior fornix, (**c**) fornix recreated, (**d**) 2-week post-operative photo

7 Post-Operative Management

The post-operative management is largely dependent on the histopathological analysis and involvement of the margins. Despite a clear surgical margin, up to one-third of eyes may have a recurrence within 10 years, with a higher recurrence rate in cases with positive surgical margins, approximately 50% [34]. In addition, recurrent OSSN can grow more rapidly and become more invasive requiring more aggressive treatment with associated local invasion.

Thus, if the lesion has been completely excised and is not invasive; these patients are still monitored for recurrence; however, no further adjuvant therapy is required. Patients are usually followed up 3 monthly in year 1, 4 monthly in year 2, then 6 monthly for 3 years, as minimum follow up.

In our experience, the use of topical lubricants and ointments containing vitamin A provides a protective role and decrease the rate of recurrence. In addition, protective sunglasses, and the prompt treatment of any underlying inflammatory or allergic eye disease can reduce the risk of recurrence, including avoiding eye rubbing.

Any residual disease or incomplete margins identified from the histology requires further adjuvant therapy. For leukoplakic areas, we prefer to use topical 5FU treatment, 1 week on and 3 weeks off for at least 3 cycles. For moderate to severe dysplasia, topical IFN is used four times a day for 3–6 months. For in situ disease, 4 cycles of topical MMC 0.02%, 2 weeks on, 2 weeks off is considered 6 weeks post-surgery.

For residual invasive disease, we consider adjuvant ruthenium plaque brachytherapy (Fig. 19) or proton beam

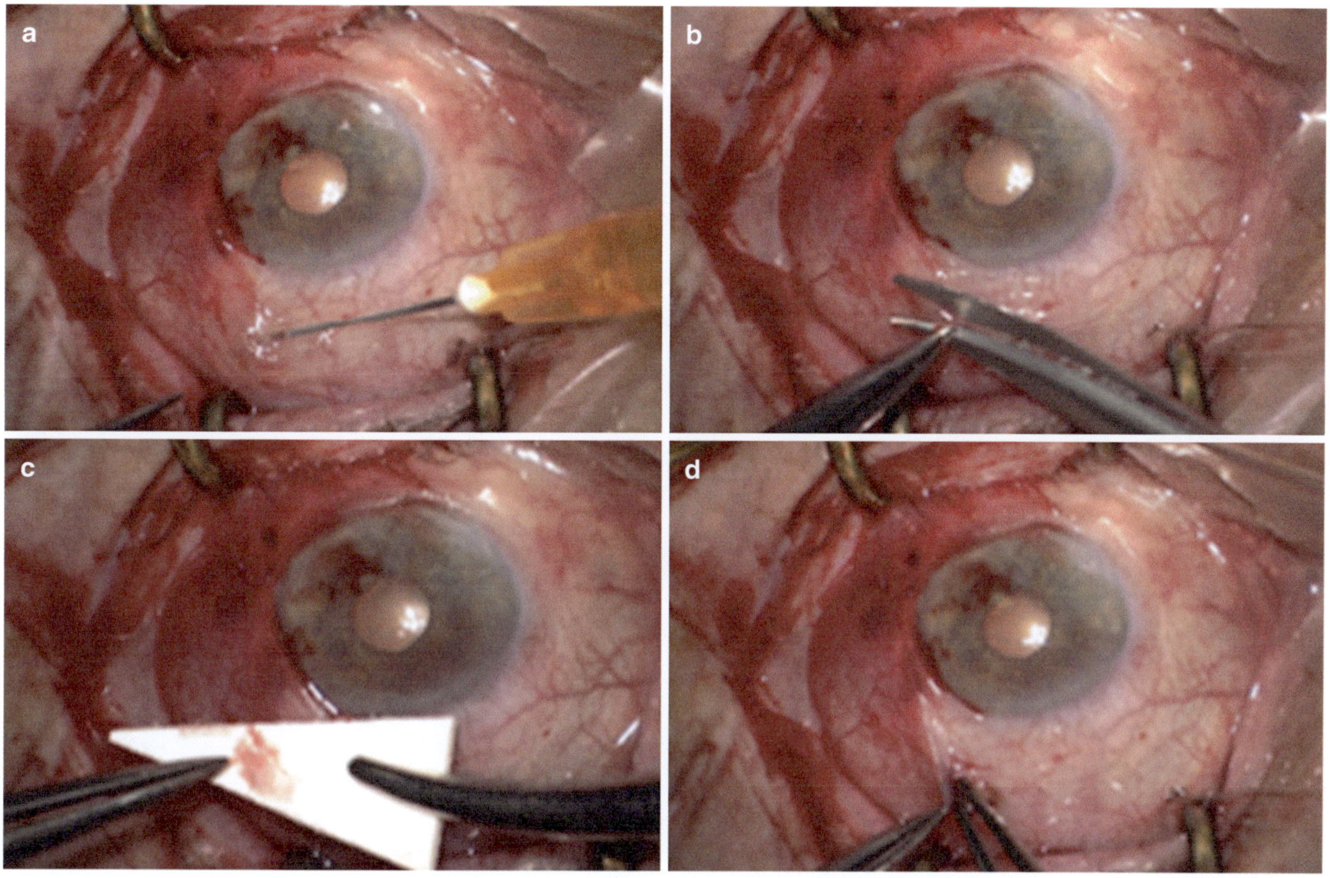

Fig. 12 Surgical approach to map biopsies (**a**) local anesthetic to area to be biopsied, (**b**) grasp conjunctiva with forceps and use Wescott scissors to cut biopsy in 2 snips, (**c**) place on spear for histological analysis into a formalin pot, (**d**) cautery to biopsy site

therapy, usually 6 weeks post-surgery to allow for healing. Baseline staging is undertaken only in patients with invasive disease which includes MRI neck/head/orbit and CT chest, abdomen, and pelvis. Surveillance is done with 6 monthly ultrasound neck for 5 years to look for local spread, then yearly thereafter, if the patient wishes to be monitored.

OSSN overall has a good prognosis, as the metastatic potential for conjunctival SCC is low ranging from 0% to 16%, with a higher risk of metastasis with orbital involvement [35–37]. Invasion through the sclera or cornea with intraocular spread is uncommon, but typically it can occur at the site of previous surgery or if there is immunosuppression. If there is spread, sites include the lymph nodes in the neck which often precedes the development of distant metastasis. If there is any suspicion of lymph node involvement or systemic spread, then appropriate medical professionals are involved via our multidisciplinary team. Our practice is to biopsy any enlarged lymph node found either clinically or by ultrasound and if this is positive, a radical neck dissection is undertaken. We do not routinely undertake sentinel lymph node biopsies as this is an investigational process and the therapeutic value is controversial [38].

We find that the above stepwise approach gives us excellent results in managing patients with OSSN at our National Sheffield Ocular Oncology Service in UK.

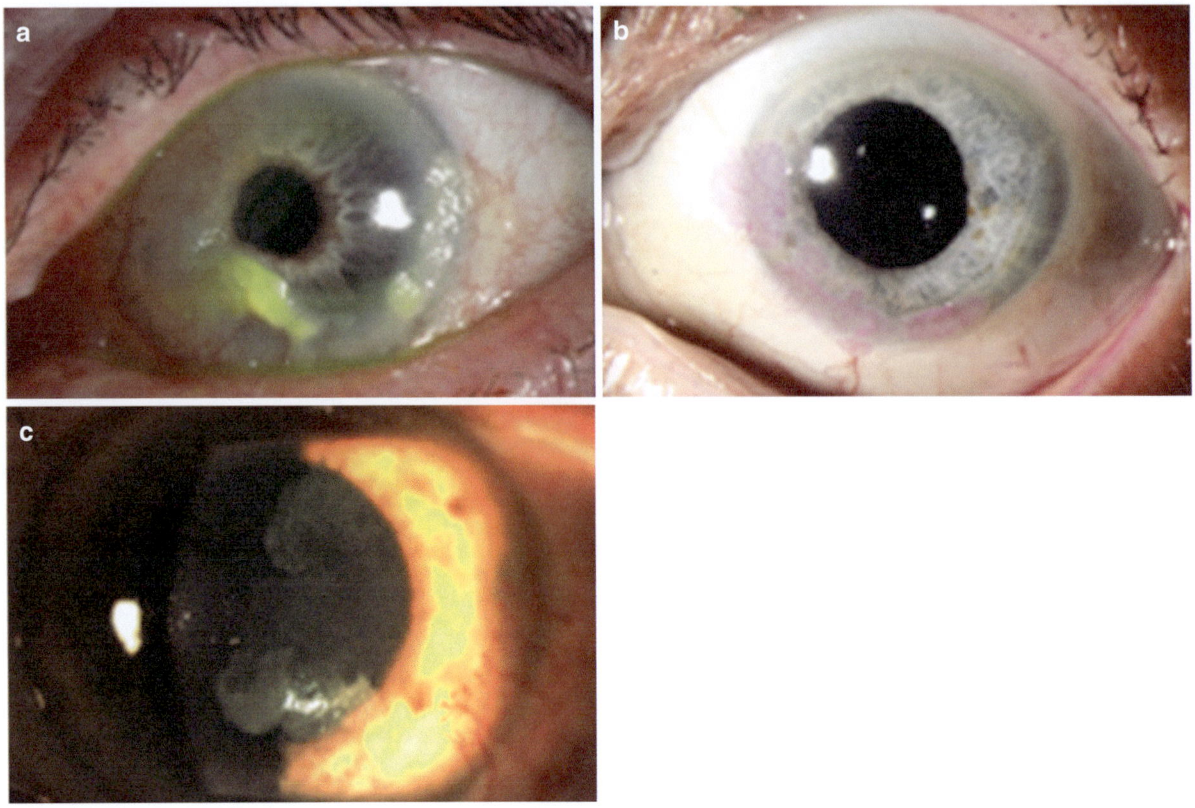

Fig. 13 Corneal OSSN (**a**) opalescent lesions on the cornea with vascularization staining with fluorescein, (**b**) mottled lesions on the cornea staining with Rose Bengal stain, (**c**) hazy appearance over the mottling at the limbus

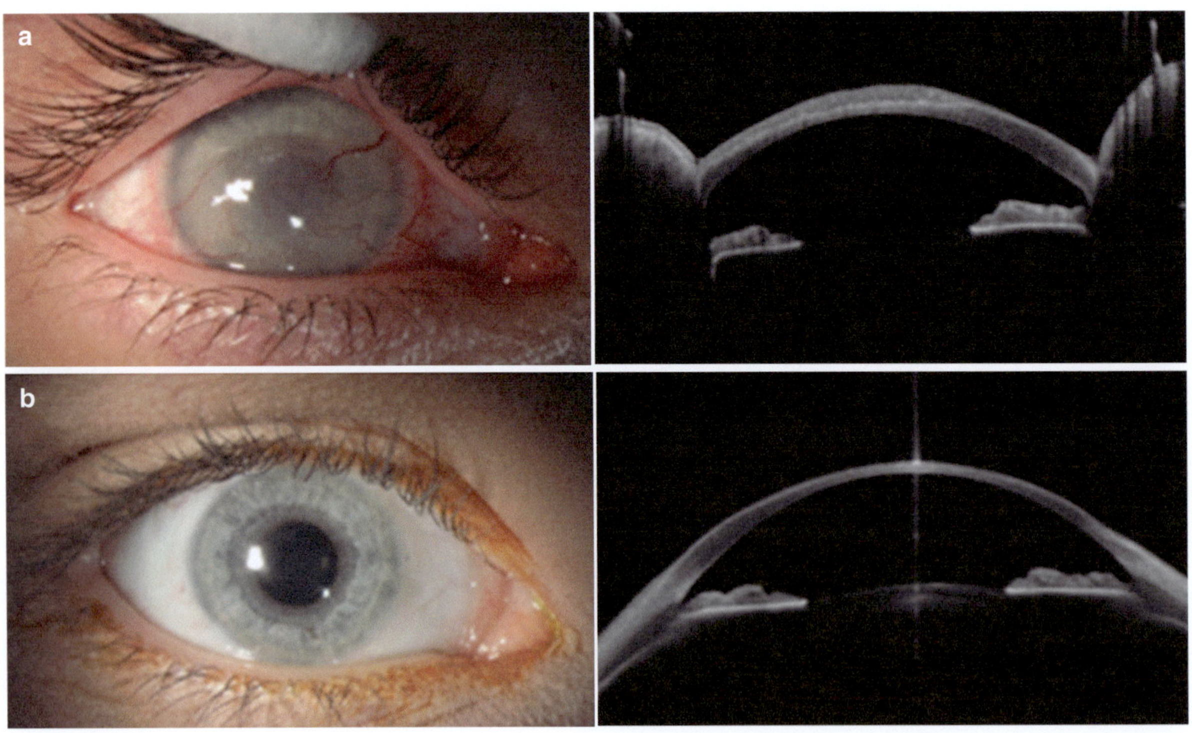

Fig. 14 Severe dysplasia with in situ SCC, (**a**) pre-operative images with AS OCT, (**b**) 6-month post-operative image following surgical management with total epitheliectomy and limbal peritomy

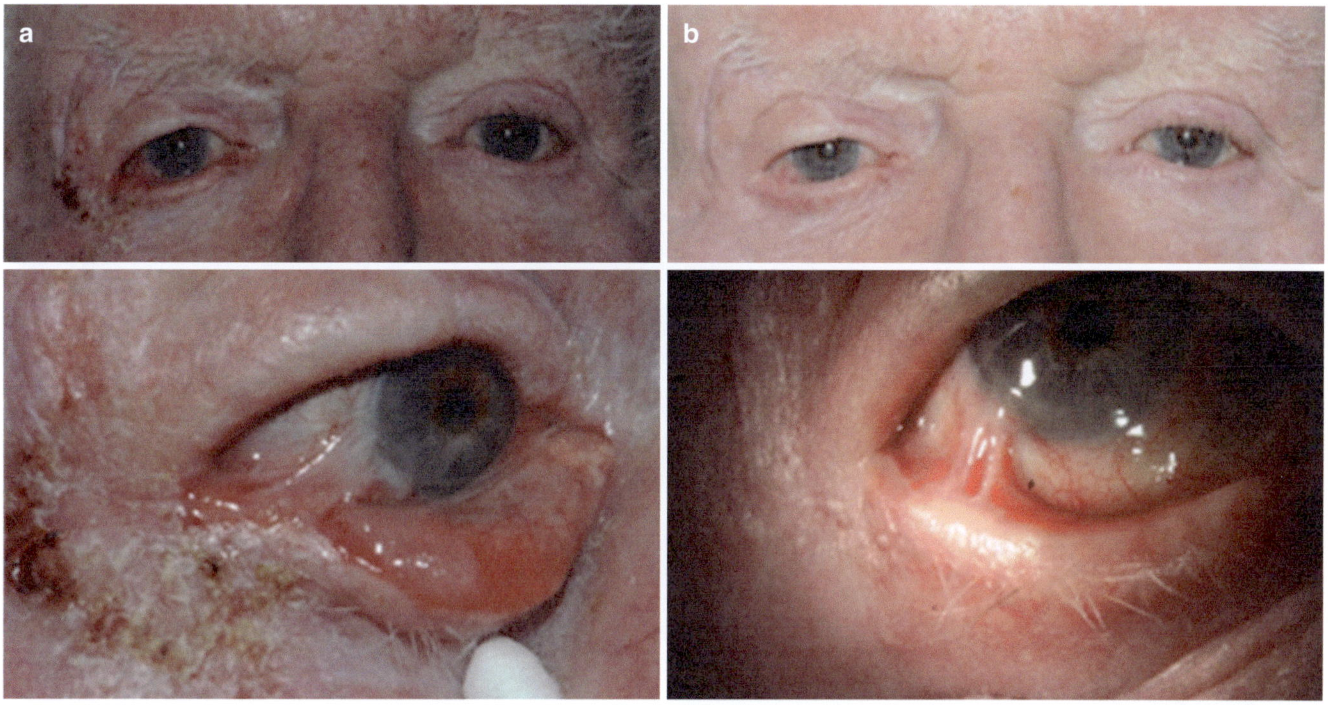

Fig. 15 Eyelid spillover of SCC: (**a**) Pre-treatment image of skin and conjunctival SCC, (**b**) Following treatment with topical 5% Imiquimod to skin (5 days a week × 6 weeks) and MMC 0.04% eye drops 6-month post-treatment

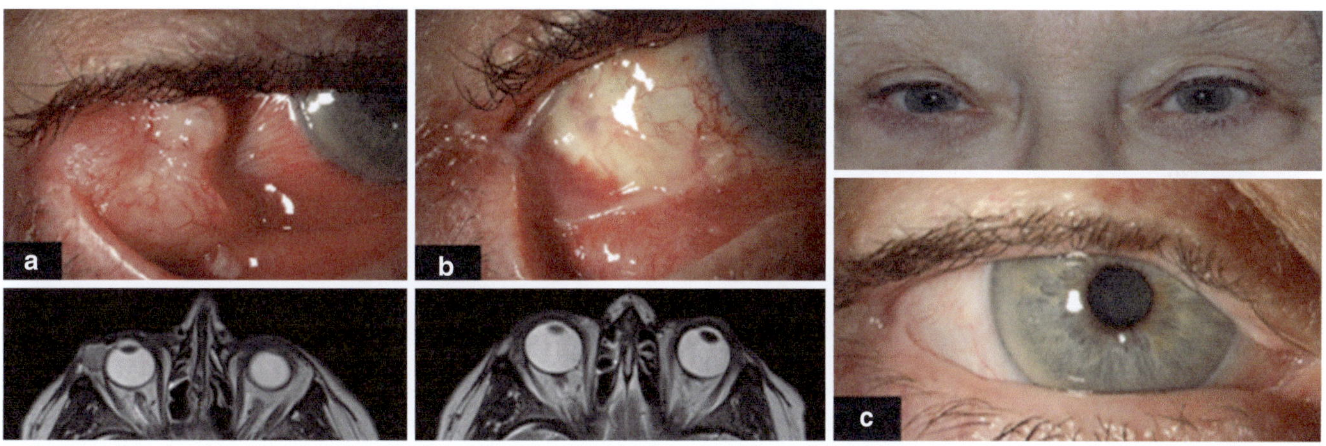

Fig. 16 Extensive SCC with anterior orbital involvement, (**a**) pre-treatment image with MRI orbit showing orbital extension, (**b**) Post-debulking surgery with excision, cryotherapy, and AMG with residual disease shown on MRI orbit treated with stereotactic radiosurgery (18–20 Gray), (**c**) 5 years post-treatment with no recurrence

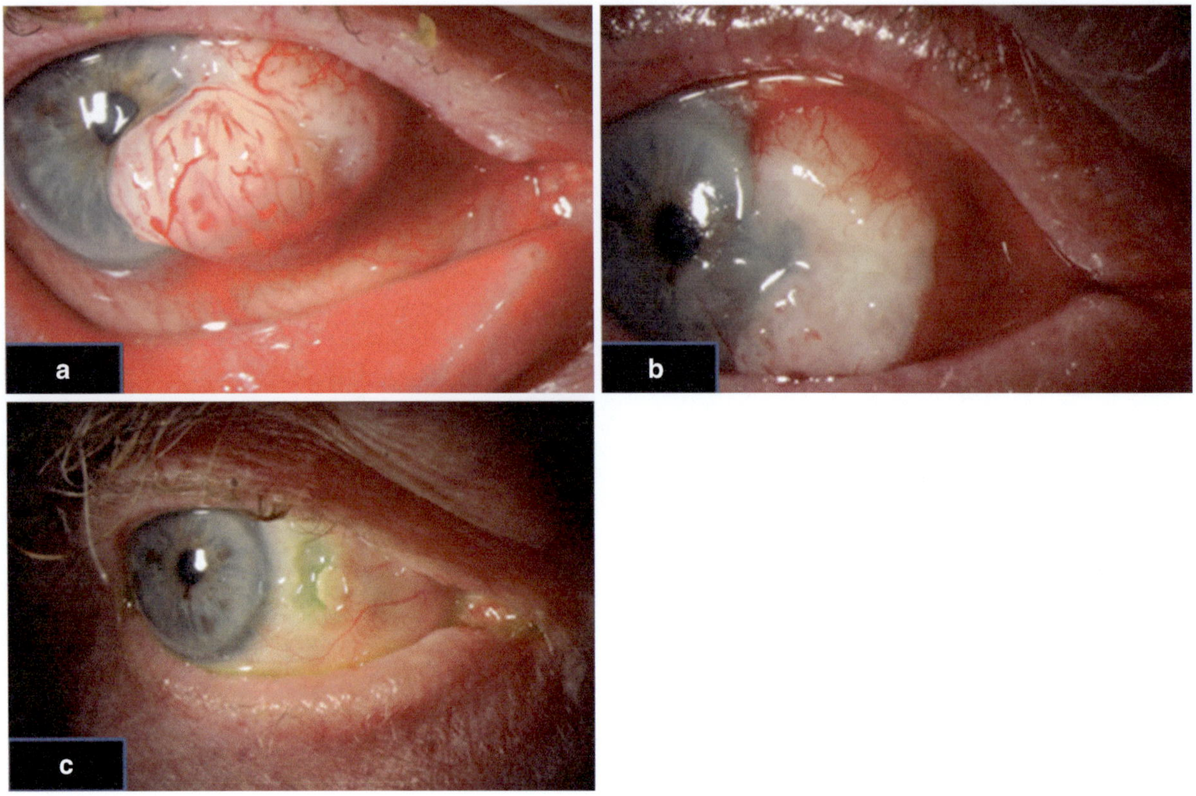

Fig. 17 Invasive SCC medially treated with PBT, (**a**) pre-treatment image, (**b**) 2 months post-PBT, (**c**) 7-month post-PBT showing completely regressed lesion

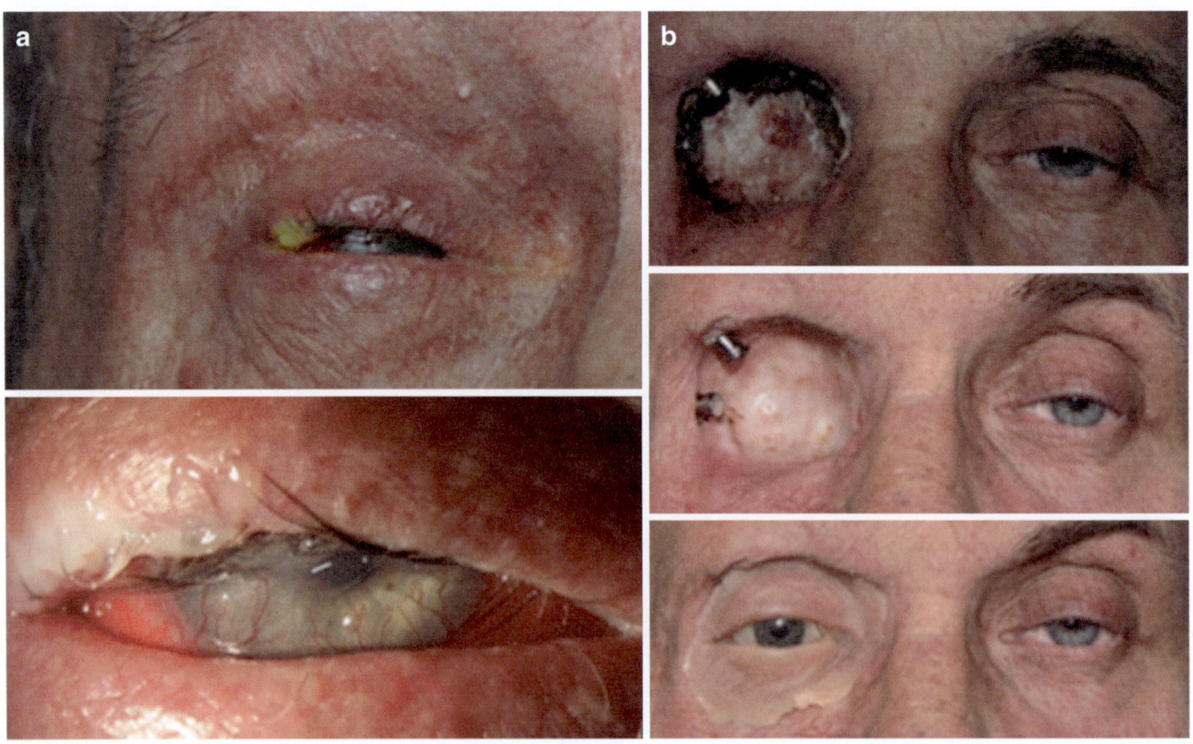

Fig. 18 Extensive SCC of cornea, eyelid and skin, (**a**) pre-operative image, (**b**) post-operative images following exenteration surgery, healing over 10-month period with excellent cosmesis

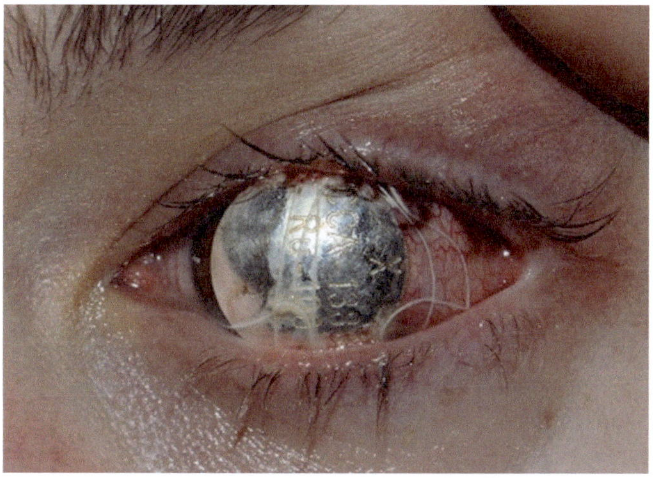

Fig. 19 Adjuvant treatment with Ruthenium plaque brachytherapy following excision of conjunctival OSSN, usually applied for 24 h

References

1. Lee GA, Hirst LW. Ocular surface squamous neoplasia. Surv Ophthalmol. 1995;39(6):429–50.
2. Shields CL, Demirci H, Karatza E, Shields JA. Clinical survey of 1643 melanocytic and nonmelanocytic conjunctival tumors. Ophthalmology. 2004;111(9):1747–54.
3. Shields CL, Chien JL, Surakiatchanukul T, Sioufi K, Lally SE, Shields JA. Conjunctival tumors: review of clinical features, risks, biomarkers, and outcomes— the 2017. J Donald M Gass Lecture Asia Pac J Ophthalmol (Phila). 2017;6(2):109–20.
4. Lee GA, Hirst LW. Incidence of ocular surface epithelial dysplasia in metropolitan Brisbane. A 10-year survey. Arch Ophthalmol. 1992;110(4):525–7.
5. Waddell K, Kwehangana J, Johnston WT, et al. A case-control study of ocular surface squamous neoplasia (OSSN) in Uganda. Int J Cancer. 2010;127:427–32.
6. Sun EC, Fears TR, Goedert JJ. Epidemiology of squamous cell conjunctival cancer. Cancer Epidemiol Biomark Prev. 1997;6(2):73–7.
7. Furahini G, Lewallen S. Epidemiology and management of ocular surface squamous neoplasia in Tanzania. Ophthalmic Epidemiol. 2010;17(3):171–6.
8. Emmanuel B, Ruder E, Lin SW, Abnet C, Hollenbeck A, Mbulaiteye S. Incidence of squamous-cell carcinoma of the conjunctiva and other eye cancers in the NIH-AARP diet and health study. Ecancermedicalscience. 2012;6:254.
9. Ateenyi-Agaba C. Conjunctival squamous-cell carcinoma associated with HIV infection in Kampala. Uganda Lancet. 1995;345(8951):695–6.
10. Gichuhi S, Sagoo MS, Weiss HA, Burton MJ. Epidemiology of ocular surface squamous neoplasia in Africa. Tropical Med Int Health. 2013;18(12):1424–43.
11. Makupa II, Swai B, Makupa WU, White VA, Lewallen S. Clinical factors associated with malignancy and HIV status in patients with ocular surface squamous neoplasia at Kilimanjaro Christian Medical Centre. Tanzania Br J Ophthalmol. 2012;96(4):482–4.
12. Dalvin LA, Salomão DR, Patel SV. Population-based incidence of conjunctival tumours in Olmsted County, Minnesota. Br J Ophthalmol. 2018;102:1728–34.
13. Cicinelli MV, Marchese A, Bandello F, Modorati G. Clinical management of ocular surface squamous neoplasia: a review of the current evidence. Ophthalmol Ther. 2018;7(2):247–62.
14. Guech-Ongey M, Engels EA, Goedert JJ, et al. Elevated risk for squamous cell carcinoma of the conjunctiva among adults with AIDS in the United States. Int J Cancer. 2008;122:2590–3.
15. Nagaiah G, Stotler C, Orem J, et al. Ocular surface squamous neoplasia in patients with HIV infection in sub-Saharan Africa. Curr Opin Oncol. 2010;22:437–42.
16. Scott IU, Karp CL, Nuovo GJ. Human papillomavirus 16 and 18 expression in conjunctival intraepithelial neoplasia. Ophthalmology. 2002;109:542–7.
17. Rathi SG, Ganguly Kapoor A, Kaliki S. Ocular surface squamous neoplasia in HIV-infected patients: current perspectives. HIV AIDS (Auckl). 2018;10:33–45.
18. Kim RY, Seiff SR, Howes EL Jr, O'Donnell JJ. Necrotizing scleritis secondary to conjunctival squamous cell carcinoma in acquired immunodeficiency syndrome. Am J Ophthalmol. 1990;109(2):231–3.
19. Kiire CA, Srinivasan S, Karp CL. Ocular surface squamous neoplasia. Int Ophthalmol Clin. 2010;50:35–46.
20. Kao AA, Galor A, Karp CL, Abdelaziz A, Feuer WJ, Dubovy SR. Clinicopathologic correlation of ocular surface squamous neoplasms at Bascom palmer eye institute: 2001 to 2010. Ophthalmology. 2012;119(9):1773–6.
21. Conway RM, Gf G, Pelayes D. Conjunctival carcinoma. AJCC cancer staging manual. 8th ed. Switzerland: Springer; 2017. p. 787–93.
22. Thomas BJ, Galor A, Nanji AA, et al. Ultra high-resolution anterior segment optical coherence tomography in the diagnosis and management of ocular surface squamous neoplasia. Ocul Surf. 2014;12:46–58.
23. Tabin G, Levin S, Snibson G, et al. Late recurrences and the necessity for long-term follow-up in corneal and conjunctival intraepithelial neoplasia. Ophthalmology. 1997;104:485–92.
24. Shields JA, Shields CL, De Potter P. Surgical management of conjunctival tumors. The 1994 Lynn B. McMahan Lecture. Arch Ophthalmol. 1997, 115:808–15.
25. Peksayar G, Altan-Yaycioglu R, Onal S. Excision and cryosurgery in the treatment of conjunctival malignant epithelial tumours. Eye (Lond). 2003;17:228–32.
26. Siganos CS, Kozobolis VP, Christodoulakis EV. The intraoperative use of mitomycin-C in excision of ocular surface neoplasia with or without limbal autograft transplantation. Cornea. 2002;21:12–6.
27. Midena E, Angeli CD, Valenti M, et al. Treatment of conjunctival squamous cell carcinoma with topical 5-fluorouracil. Br J Ophthalmol. 2000;84:268–72.
28. Agraval U, Rundle P, Rennie IG, Salvi S. Fresh frozen amniotic membrane for conjunctival reconstruction after excision of neoplastic and presumed neoplastic conjunctival lesions. Eye. 2017;31(6):884–9.
29. Waring GO III, Roth AM, Ekins MB. Clinical and pathologic description of 17 cases of corneal intraepithelial neoplasia. Am J Ophthalmol. 1984;97:547–59.
30. Fruct-Pery J, Sugar J, Baum J, et al. Mitomycin C treatment for conjunctival-corneal intraepithelial neoplasia: a multicenter experience. Ophthalmology. 1997;104:2085–93.
31. Graue GF, Tena LB, Finger PT. Electron beam radiation for conjunctival squamous carcinoma. Ophthal Plast Reconstr Surg. 2011;27:277–81.
32. Arepalli S, Kaliki S, Shields CL, Emirch J, Komarnicky L, Shields JA. Plaque radiotherapy in the management of scleral-invasive conjunctival squamous cell carcinoma: an analysis of 15 eyes. JAMA Ophthalmol. 2014;132:691–6.

33. Bata BM, Radatz MWR, Salvi SM. Gamma knife stereotactic radiosurgery for conjunctival squamous cell carcinoma invading the anterior orbit: a case series. Ocul Oncol Pathol. 2021 Jun;7(3):206–14.
34. Nanji AA, Moon CS, Galor A, Sein J, Oellers P, Karp CL. Surgical versus medical treatment of ocular surface squamous neoplasia: a comparison of recurrences and complications. Ophthalmology. 2014;121(5):994–1000.
35. Tunc M, Char DH, Crawford B, Miller T. Intraepithelial and invasive squamous cell carcinoma of the conjunctiva: analysis of 60 cases. Br J Ophthalmol. 1999 Jan;83(1):98–103.
36. Iliff WJ, Marback R, Green WR. Invasive squamous cell carcinoma of the conjunctiva. Arch Ophthalmol. 1975 Feb;93(2):119–22.
37. McKelvie PA, Daniell M, McNab A, Loughnan M, Santamaria JD. Squamous cell carcinoma of the conjunctiva: a series of 26 cases. Br J Ophthalmol. 2002 Feb;86(2):168–73.
38. Mendoza PR, Grossniklaus HE. Sentinel lymph node biopsy for eyelid and conjunctival tumours: what is the evidence? Int Ophthalmol Clin. 2015;55:123–36.

Part IV

Tools, Technology, and Innovations

Genomics: Past, Present, and Future

Stephanie N. Kletke and Brenda L. Gallie

1 Retinoblastoma: The Prototypic Genetic Cancer

In the early 1970s, research in cancer genetics was felt to be a fruitless endeavor. One co-author's motivation to pursue fellowship training in retinoblastoma was challenged by a pervasive attitude of dismissal: "Why would you want to study retinoblastoma, when no other cancer is related to genetics?." Fifty years later, advancements in cancer genomics continue to transform the practice of oncology and improve outcomes. Notably, no other cancer has contributed more to our understanding of the genetic basis underlying cancer development than retinoblastoma.

1.1 The Retinoblastoma Tumor Suppressor

Knudson proposed his landmark **"two-hit" hypothesis** for retinoblastoma development in 1971, based on comparison of the younger age at presentation in bilateral versus unilateral cases [1]. He proposed that heritable retinoblastoma (most commonly bilateral) results from a predisposing germline mutation followed by a second rate-limiting somatic mutation, while the non-heritable form (always unilateral) arises from two rate-limiting somatic mutations in the same retinal cell. In 1973, Comings identified that these two distinct mutational events inactivate both alleles of the same gene [2]. Chromosome 13q14 was subsequently identified as the predisposing-locus for retinoblastoma [3–11]. Restriction fragment length polymorphism (RFLP) studies comparing constitutional and tumor genetics identified loss of heterozygosity (LOH), the loss of the normal *RB1* allele with duplication of the mutant allele, as an important event in retinoblastoma tumorigenesis [12, 13]. This provided further evidence that the two mutational events affect both alleles at the same genetic locus. In the 1980s, this work led to the discovery of the *RB1* gene, the first tumor-suppressor to be identified [14–19]. Our genetic understanding of retinoblastoma continues to evolve, with broad implications for cancer genomics.

While retinoblastoma predisposition is dominantly inherited, the *RB1* mutation behaves recessively at the cellular level. Biallelic mutations in the *RB1* gene ($RB1^{-/-}$) are necessary to initiate both heritable and non-heritable retinoblastoma. In heritable (or germline) retinoblastoma, which accounts for nearly half of cases, a heterozygous constitutional *RB1* mutation (M1) is present in all, or a subset, of cells. A second somatic mutation (M2) inactivates the other allele in one or more retinal precursor cells. This often gives rise to bilateral, multifocal tumors (from independent M2 events) and confers lifelong risk for second primary cancers [20, 21]. All bilateral cases and approximately 15% of unilateral cases are heritable [22, 23], with a 50% risk that future offspring will inherit the *RB1* pathogenic variant. While 10% of individuals with heritable retinoblastoma have a known family history, the majority are sporadic (no family history) and result from a new germline mutation in the proband. This de novo mutation may arise pre-conception in a parental germ cell, most commonly in the mitotically active paternal germ cell [24–26], predisposing all cells of the child. If, however, the *RB1* mutation occurs post-conception in an early embryonic cell, only a subset of the child's cells carries the mutation, a concept termed mosaicism.

Non-heritable retinoblastoma is initiated by somatic loss of both *RB1* alleles (M1 and M2) in the same retinal cell. Rarely, a distinct non-heritable retinoblastoma genotype arises from high-level amplification of an oncogene, *MYCN*, despite normal *RB1* alleles [27]. Children with $MYCN^{A}$ $RB1^{+/+}$ retinoblastoma present with distinct, early-onset, aggressive disease. Both mechanisms lead to unilateral, unifocal tumors, with no risk of second cancers or transmission to future generations.

S. N. Kletke (✉) · B. L. Gallie
Department of Ophthalmology and Vision Sciences, The Hospital for Sick Children, University of Toronto, Toronto, ON, Canada
e-mail: stephanie.kletke@sickkids.ca; brenda.gallie@sickkids.ca

B. V. Chawla, M. E. Aronow (eds.), *Global Perspectives in Ocular Oncology*, https://doi.org/10.1007/978-3-031-08250-4_20

1.2 Genotype-Phenotype Correlations

The human *RB1* gene (OMIM #614041) spans 180 kilobases of genomic DNA and contains 27 coding exons [28, 29]. The complete sequencing was described in 1993 [30]. Transcription is initiated at multiple sites [28], producing a 4.7 kb mRNA transcript [15]. Retinoblastoma gene mutations are heterogenous, often unique to the affected family. Small deletions and insertions, frameshift, and nonsense point mutations spanning critical areas over the entire gene are common M1 events [31–35]. The resultant splicing errors and/or premature stop codons lead to reduced mRNA through nonsense mediated decay [36], with loss of tumor suppressor function. Large deletions of the long arm of chromosome 13, containing *RB1* and adjacent genes, result in retinoblastoma and variable craniofacial and systemic features, motor, and speech delays [37]. Promoter methylation, a potentially epigenetic mechanism preventing *RB1* transcription, frequently accounts for somatic M1 and M2 events [38–42]. Tumor formation is initiated following duplication of the mutant allele (LOH) in approximately half of tumors, occurring more frequently with M1 promoter methylation [38].

1.2.1 Penetrance and Expressivity

High penetrance and expressivity are seen in most hereditary retinoblastoma pedigrees. However, some families have low-penetrance phenotypes, with clinically unaffected *RB1* mutation carriers (**reduced penetrance**) and frequent unilateral, unifocal tumors (**reduced expressivity**) [43]. Low-penetrance phenotypes are associated with older age at first tumor detection [44]. These families may also have lower incidence of second primary cancers [45]. Penetrance may be quantified by the diseased-eye-ratio (DER), which reflects the proportion of eyes with a predisposing germline mutation that actually develop tumors [46]. For example, a pedigree consisting of two *RB1* mutation carriers, a proband with heritable unilateral retinoblastoma and an unaffected monozygotic twin, would have a DER of 0.25 (1 out of 4 at-risk eyes developed tumor). Low penetrance is defined as a DER ≤ 1, and high penetrance as a DER ≥ 1.5.

Elucidating the mechanisms underlying low penetrance has improved our understanding of genotype-phenotype correlations and informed genetic counseling. Such phenotypes arise from specific predisposing M1 mutations, in which some residual tumor suppressor function is retained [46–49]. Low-penetrance M1 events include missense [33, 35], in-frame [38, 50, 51], promoter [35, 47], some splice site [43, 52], and intronic variant mutations [53]. In contrast, null mutations that eliminate all tumor suppressor function are associated with high penetrance [38].

Large or complete deletions of 13q14, as seen in 13q deletion syndrome, are also counterintuitively associated with low penetrance [50]. Cells cannot survive without the protein product of *MED4*, which is located adjacent to *RB1* and may be included in deletions of the long arm of chromosome 13 [54]. Since loss of the normal allele is the most common M2 event, this would result in cell death due to co-deletion and complete loss of *MED4* [38]. Thus, large deletions often result in low-penetrance phenotypes, as tumors only form in the setting of an independent null M2 event, isolated to *RB1*.

Some low-penetrance pedigrees are explained by a **parent-of-origin** effect, in which the gender of the transmitting parent influences the retinoblastoma phenotype. This was first identified in pedigrees segregating the low-penetrance missense mutation c.1981C>T (p.Arg661Trp), in which individuals who inherit the mutation from their father are more likely to develop tumors [55]. The *RB1* gene is imprinted, such that hypermethylation of a CpG85 island on intron 2 of the maternal allele favors its transcriptional expression [55]. Since this missense mutation retains some tumor suppressor function, overexpression in the setting of a maternally inherited mutation is protective, as the cell retains sufficient retinoblastoma protein to prevent tumor formation. Other low-penetrance genotypes are also mechanistically explained by the parent-of-origin effect [56].

1.2.2 Mosaicism

Sporadic unilateral or bilateral retinoblastoma may arise from mutational mosaicism [57]. Mosaicism may be isolated somatic, isolated germline (mutation affects a dividing germ cell), or mixed somatic and germline (mutation occurs before the formation of germ cells in embryogenesis). The degree and distribution of tissue involvement depend on the timing of the mutational event following conception. Antecedent relatives to a mosaic proband do not require genetic testing, as mosaicism cannot be inherited. However, a mosaic proband's germline *RB1* variant may be transmitted to future offspring and level of risk may reflect the proportion of germline involvement. Though somatic mosaicism in the parent of a retinoblastoma proband is rare, parental mosaicism informs the risk for future pregnancies [58]. Mosaicism is detected in over 10% of cases, either in the proband or a parent [59, 60]. The introduction of highly sensitive allele-specific PCR (AS-PCR) and next-generation sequencing (NGS) technologies have further improved detection of low-level mosaicism [58, 60, 61]. This has important implications for genetic counseling of newly diagnosed families.

1.3 Cell Cycle Regulation by the Retinoblastoma Protein

The *RB1* gene encodes the 928 amino acid retinoblastoma tumor suppressor protein (pRB) [18], a critical cell-cycle regulator that prevents uncontrolled cellular proliferation. The cell-cycle contains two major regulatory checkpoints: the first occurs at the transition from G1 (gap phase) to S phase (DNA replication) and the second at the G2 (gap phase) to M phase (mitosis and cytokinesis) transition. The retinoblastoma protein regulates the G1 restriction checkpoint, preventing uncontrolled progression into S phase [62]. The function of pRB is dependent on its phosphorylation status, with higher levels of phosphorylation inactivating pRB and favoring cell proliferation [18, 63, 64]. In quiescent (G0) and early G1 cells, pRB is hypophosphorylated and active, becoming functionally inactivated by hyperphosphorylation in late G1, S, and G2 [65]. Dephosphorylation occurs in late mitosis [66]. The cyclic nature of pRB phosphorylation is regulated by different cyclin/cyclin-dependent kinase (CDK) complexes and cyclin kinase inhibitors (CKI), in response to growth-related signaling. Normally, this mediates phosphorylation of pRB only when the cell has adequate support to progress through the cell cycle.

A key molecular interaction occurs between pRB and the E2F family of transcription factors [67, 68]. E2F is functionally inactivated by its protein-protein complex with hypophosphorylated pRB in G1 cells [69]. Phosphorylation of pRB releases free E2F, which promotes the transcription of genes necessary for progression past the G1-S checkpoint. S-phase proteins and regulatory proteins are notable E2F targets [70].The interaction between pRB and E2F prevents cell-cycle progression by multiple pathways. First, pRB physically binds free E2F. Second, the pRB-E2F complex binds DNA and directly represses transcription of proteins involved in DNA replication, DNA repair, mitosis, transcription/chromatin structure [71] and even may modulate efficacy of chemotherapy [72, 73]. Thus, loss of pRB leads to uncontrolled cell cycle progression, central to the pathogenesis of retinoblastoma and many other human cancers.

1.4 Tumorigenesis: M1, M2, M3, and Beyond

Though the retinoblastoma tumor suppressor is widely expressed, its function is highly tissue specific. The cone photoreceptor precursor cell, present in the developing retina, is particularly sensitive to pRB loss [74, 75]. This reflects cell-specific mechanisms to evade apoptosis, the normal response to cellular dysregulation [75, 76]. The loss of both *RB1* alleles (M1 and M2) in the susceptible cone precursor is insufficient to induce retinoblastoma. Rather, it initiates the formation of a retinoma, the benign retinoblastoma precursor [77]. Retinoma may be incidentally noted or clinically diagnosed in retinoblastoma patients or their family members (incidence, 1.8–10%) [78, 79]. It appears as a translucent retinal mass with variable calcification, surrounded by pigmentary changes [78]. Though benign, retinomas must be monitored by serial eye examination, given the lifelong risk of malignant transformation [80]. Studies of enucleated retinoblastoma eyes with contiguous retinoma suggest this transformation results from accumulation of genomic instability, following biallelic *RB1* loss [77].

A human *RB1*$^{-/-}$ cell progresses to retinoblastoma only after additional genomic changes arise. These events have been termed M3 to Mn [75], and have been reviewed elsewhere [81, 82]. A unique genomic signature, consisting of recurrent somatic chromosomal copy number alterations (SCNA) that occur independent of M1/M2 events, is noted in most retinoblastoma tumors post-enucleation [83]. In contrast, recurrent somatic gene mutations are rare [84]. Gain of 6p, the most notable SCNA in retinoblastoma, was first identified in 60% of enucleated retinoblastoma tumors in the early 1980s [85, 86]. The other common chromosomal changes, including gains of 1q and 2p and loss of 16q, have been extensively evaluated [83, 87–93]. Gains of 1q and 6p are most frequently noted, often in the same tumor [83]. Knowledge of SCNA led to the identification of important candidate cancer genes: oncogenes represented by gains and tumor suppressors by losses. These include *MDM4* and *KIF14* at 1q32.1 [94, 95], *MYCN* at 2p24.3 [96], *DEK* and *E2F3* at 6p22.3 [97], *SYK* at 9q22 [98], and *CDH11* at 16q21 [99]. Though not yet clinically validated, these genomic changes may hold promise as biomarkers for prognostication of tumor response or as targets for therapeutic intervention.

In contrast to most cancers, the critical p53 tumor suppressor is rarely mutated in retinoblastoma [100]. However, evidence suggests the p53 pathway contributes to genomic instability after *RB1* loss, through the important regulators MDM2 and MDM4 (MDMX). While MDM2 downregulates p53 [101], MDM4 functions to stabilize the interaction [102]. Interestingly, these proto-oncoproteins may be upregulated even in the absence of genomic amplification. Single nucleotide polymorphisms (SNPs) of both *MDM2* and *MDM4* increase protein levels and subsequent p53 inhibition [103–106]. This pathway highlights one mechanism by which *RB1*$^{-/-}$ cells may evade p53-mediated apoptosis, warranting further investigation [107].

2 Where Are We Now?

Emerging insights from the retinoblastoma genome translate to improved clinical care for children and their families. Retinoblastoma genetics is transforming the practice of ocular oncology and is the foundation for our gold-standard approach to staging, screening, diagnosis, counseling, and follow-up in 2021.

2.1 Retinoblastoma Staging: "H Status"

Hereditary predisposition to retinoblastoma confers an increased risk for additional tumors in both eyes and second primary cancers, as well as special considerations for the entire family. The importance of germline status to retinoblastoma outcomes was highlighted by the recent, unprecedented incorporation of "heritable trait" into the eighth edition American Joint Committee on Cancer tumor-node-metastasis (AJCC TNM) staging, now termed TNMH (only retinoblastoma has gained the "H" in cancer staging [108]). This gold-standard staging is evidence-based and most accurately predicts ocular and overall survival for the child. Cancer predisposition is denoted by "H" and reflects both clinical and/or genetic evidence of germline status:

- **HX:** Unknown genetic risk, including variants of unknown significance.
- **H0:** Absence of the familial *RB1* mutation in blood *OR* normal *RB1* alleles in blood and confirmed *MYCN*[A] in tumor.
- **H0*:** Normal *RB1* in blood with <1% risk for undetected mosaicism [109].
- **H1:** Bilateral *OR* trilateral retinoblastoma [110] *OR* family history *OR* confirmed germline *RB1* mutation.

2.2 Screening Based on Genetic Risk

Children at risk to carry the proband's pathogenic *RB1* variant require screening. While conventional surveillance involves an intensive clinical exam schedule, molecular genetic testing can accurately determine risk. First, the proband should have blood testing by a high-sensitivity lab to detect *RB1* mutations, informed by tumor genetics when possible [111]. At-risk relatives can then be offered testing for the familial germline mutation. Carriers (H1) require clinical surveillance for early tumor detection, to reduce the need for invasive therapies. Genetic testing is also important to promote awareness of second cancer risk in H1 adults. Children who test negative for the proband's allele (H0) are at population risk (0.007%) for retinoblastoma and do not require clinical screening. Molecular genetic testing is significantly more cost-effective for the healthcare system, as fewer family members require surveillance after post-test risk adjustment [38, 112]. If molecular testing is not feasible, pre-test risk is estimated based on the proband's disease laterality and relationship to the at-risk relative. Though genetic testing for relatives is not currently standard of care in the absence of a known familial mutation, cost-benefit analysis comparing clinical screening and molecular analysis in this setting may inform future recommendations.

The American Association of Ophthalmic Oncologists and Pathologists (AAOOP) recently published retinoblastoma screening guidelines for at-risk relatives [113]. Prior to genetic testing, it is recommended that screening follow a schedule determined by pre-test risk. Mutation carrier risk is stratified into 3 categories: (1) **high > 7.5%** (includes offspring of bilateral probands (50%) and known mutation carriers), (2) **intermediate, 1–7.5%** (includes siblings of bilateral (2.5%) and offspring of unilateral probands (7.5%)), and (3) **low < 1%** (includes siblings of unilateral probands (0.4%)) [113]. Risk estimation is informed by mutation carrier rates from known retinoblastoma pedigrees. Expert consensus recommends screening at-risk children from birth to age 7 years, more frequent for younger children and those at higher risk, with exam frequency decreasing as they become older. Though screening protocols are associated with earlier tumor detection, less severe tumor burden, and improved ocular salvage and vision outcome [114–116], genetic testing refines risk and eliminates clinical surveillance for children shown to NOT be at risk. Importantly, the AAOOP guideline applies only to asymptomatic children. When a tumor is identified, the child is managed with EUAs and follow-up as dictated by tumor response.

2.3 Prenatal Diagnosis for Familial Retinoblastoma

Conventional screening of at-risk neonates involves examination within the first week of life and post-natal familial *RB1* mutation test (ideally on cord blood). Some centers also perform fetal magnetic resonance imaging (MRI) and ultrasound. While large tumors have been detected on fetal ultrasound as early as 21 weeks' gestation [117], small tumors are missed by both imaging modalities [118].

The importance of early diagnosis when tumors are small, enabling timely intervention with focal therapies, is highlighted by the natural history of retinoblastoma. Early tumors threaten vision in the macula, forming in the less visually significant peripheral retina as the child gets older [119–122]. Furthermore, tumor size doubles in only 2 weeks at this age [123, 124]. There is a critical window in which tumors may be amenable to focal therapy alone. Larger tumors require chemotherapy, imposing unique risks to neonates. Though intra-arterial chemotherapy (IAC) has been reported as early as 35 days post-natal [125], most centers do not consider IAC before 3 months due to immature and small circumference vasculature. Intravenous chemotherapy (IVC) in neonates requires reduced dosage and/or agents, risking later resistance to chemotherapy.

Given nearly 100% risk of developing tumors in both eyes, neonates detected prenatally to be H1 may be delivered safely at early-term to facilitate prompt dilated retinal exam [111]. This approach enables earlier detection of visually significant tumors, that can be treated when smaller, improving visual outcomes and ocular salvage, without adverse outcomes of early delivery [44]. Prenatal molecular analysis by amniocentesis (after 16 weeks' gestation) has a procedure-specific miscarriage risk of 0.1% [126]. Infants who are found to be H1 have the option of early-term delivery (36 weeks' gestation). These tiny neonates receive timely, vision salvaging therapy through effective collaboration between families, pediatric ophthalmology, high-risk obstetrics, neonatology, anesthesia, perioperative services, oncology, genetic counseling, nursing, ocular imaging, and social work.

Early delivery of H1 infants is standard of care at our center and offered to all families. H1 neonates are examined within 48 h after delivery, and if no tumors are detected, awake dilated retinal exam is repeated every few days. Follow-up is gradually extended to weekly in the first month, then every 2 weeks until 3 months of age (Fig. 1). Subsequent exams occur every 2–4 weeks under anesthesia. Once a tumor is identified, treatment is performed under EUA, repeated every 2–4 weeks based on tumor response. Screening for neonatal tumors includes wide-field retinal imaging and hand-held spectral domain optical coherence tomography (OCT) at every exam [127], to discover, treat, and evaluate response to therapy. OCT detects "invisible" tumors, too small to be detected visually [128, 129]. Screening OCT is continued until 9 months of age, when the likelihood of new macular tumors is low. Laser therapy (532 nm) for invisible tumors is accurately guided by OCT, by identifying tumor location relative to anatomic boundaries and confirming laser burn placement [130]. Subsequently, OCT detects subclinical recurrence over scars [127, 131].

Genetic counseling informs, and thus empowers, retinoblastoma families about their reproductive options. Parental decision-making is influenced by an understanding of associated risks [132, 133]. Prenatal molecular diagnosis optimizes early intervention for at-risk neonates or may inform parents who wish to terminate an affected pregnancy. Preimplantation genetic diagnosis (PGD) is also an option, involving in vitro fertilization, mutation testing of embryos, and selection of H0 embryos for implantation [134, 135]. Early genetic testing supports fully informed counseling for parents of the proband and retinoblastoma survivors of childbearing age. Effective counseling continues lifelong, informing families of novel diagnostic and therapeutic options and clarifying perceived risks.

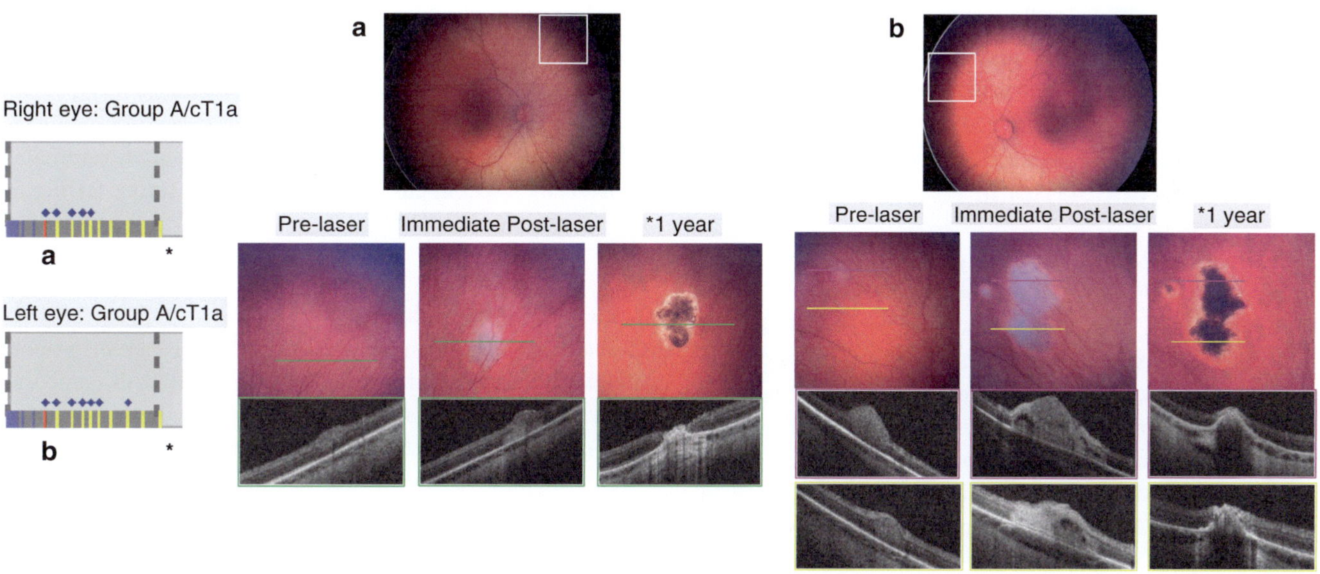

Fig. 1 Prompt screening following prenatal diagnosis of retinoblastoma and early-term delivery. The neonate was confirmed prenatally by amniocentesis to carry her father's pathogenic *RB1* variant (H1). He had a history of bilateral retinoblastoma and required enucleation of one eye. On day 1 after delivery at 36 weeks' gestation, the baby was examined in clinic and at frequent intervals for 3 months (purple bars, eCancerCare timeline), with no tumors detected. Screening was transitioned to EUAs, at which time the first tumor was detected in each eye (red bars). OCT detected a subclinical superonasal tumor in the right eye (**a**, green), which appeared as a homogenous inner nuclear layer mass. Two superonasal tumors were detected in the left eye (**b**), one apparent clinically (red) and one identified only by OCT (yellow). Fundus imaging confirmed retinal/tumor whitening post-laser photocoagulation and OCT confirmed tumor edema. eCancerCare timeline illustrates the events: staging EUA, red bar; EUAs, yellow bars; and focal therapy, blue diamonds. At 1 year of age (*), she has 2 flat, inactive scars (clinically and by OCT) in the right eye and 4 in the left eye. Visual prognosis is excellent

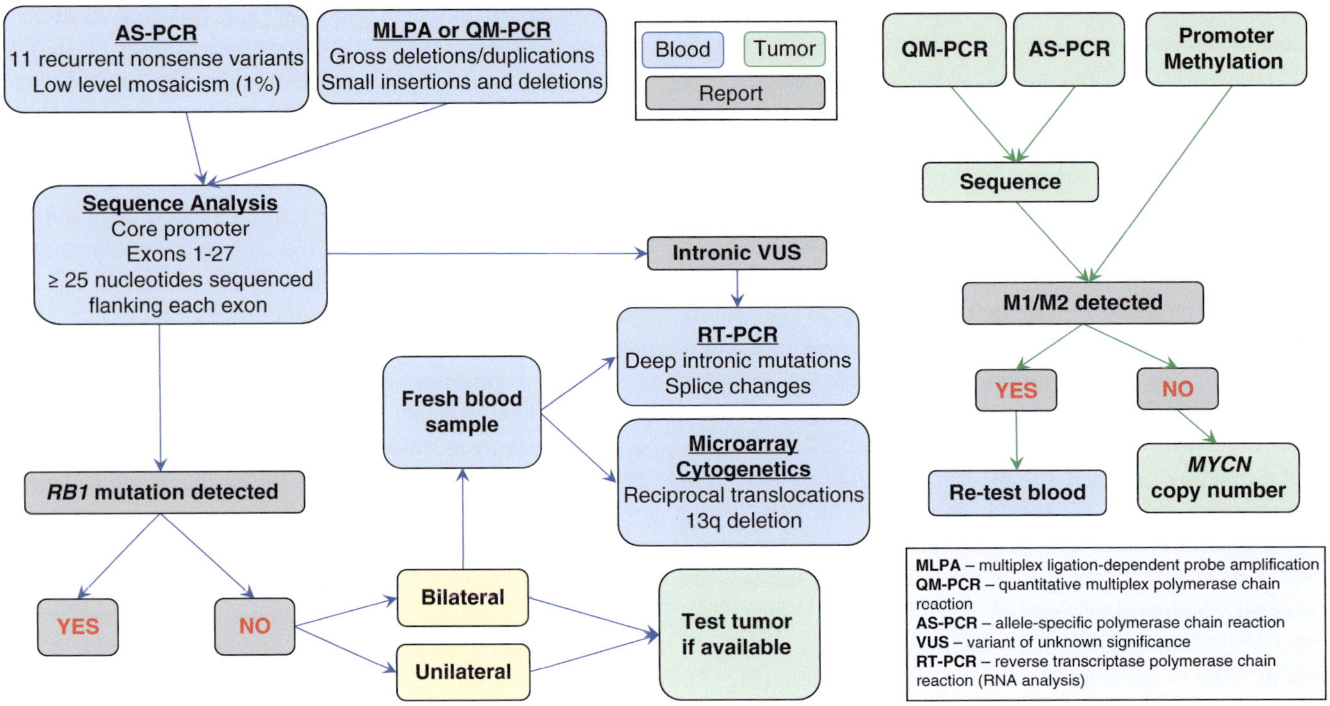

Fig. 2 *RB1* molecular testing strategy in 2021 (adapted from Impact Genetics). Tests of peripheral blood (blue) and available tumor (green) for a unilateral or bilateral proband include multiplex ligation-dependent probe amplification (MLPA) or quantitative multiplex polymerase chain reaction (QM-PCR) [38], sequence analysis and allele-specific polymerase chain reaction (AS-PCR) [38, 58] and for tumor, promoter methylation. Variants detected by AS-PCR are confirmed by sequencing. If no germline mutation is found for a bilateral (H1) proband, additional testing may be performed on a new blood sample, including reverse transcriptase polymerase chain reaction (RT-PCR) RNA studies and microarray/cytogenetic analysis (fluorescence in situ hybridization (FISH) or karyotyping). When testing does not identify a germline mutation, tumor (if available) is tested for M1 and M2. Blood is then specifically re-tested for the tumor mutations. Molecular tumor studies (green) also include identification of *RB1* promoter methylation [139] and microsatellite marker analysis for loss of heterozygosity (LOH). For unilateral tumors in which no *RB1* mutation is identified, QM-PCR assesses for *MYCN* amplification [27]

2.4 Molecular Testing Strategies for Retinoblastoma

Our current gold-standard strategy for *RB1* molecular analysis identifies over 96% of mutations (Impact Genetics' data). Both peripheral blood and tumor are tested, if available (Fig. 2). DNA extracted from fresh tumor samples (submitted in sterile tissue culture medium) is preferred to formalin-fixed or paraffin-embedded specimens [111]. Tumor has previously not been available if the eye was salvaged or enucleated remotely. Now the advantage of sampling cell-free DNA (cfDNA) from the aqueous humor can provide the tumor *RB1* pathogenic alleles [136–138].

Even high-sensitivity molecular analysis does not identify the germline mutation in 4% of bilateral (H1) probands, which may reflect low-level mosaicism or deep intron mutations altering splicing. A germline mutation is identified in 19% of sporadic unilateral (H1) probands (Impact Genetics' data). Sporadic unilateral probands without detectable germline mutation (H0*) comprise 2 groups: when M1/M2 tumor mutations are known, the residual germline mutation risk decreases to 0.3%, compared to 0.6% in the absence of tumor testing (Impact Genetics' data). If only one tumor mutation is identified, the residual risk for a germline mutation remains <1%. Tumor specimens can be banked for future testing as technologies evolve [111].

2.4.1 Global Partnerships

Globally, retinoblastoma centers of excellence are disproportionately concentrated in high-income areas with comparatively low disease burden [140]. Children in low national income countries present with more advanced disease [141, 142], leading to worse eye salvage and survival [142]. Lack of retinoblastoma screening and awareness campaigns, diagnostic delays and limited access to care contribute to these disparities. Though genetic testing and counseling are standard of care in high-income areas, access in low-and-middle-income countries (LMIC) is limited.

International collaboration supports building sustainable cancer care capacity in LMIC. The Kenyan National Retinoblastoma Strategy (KNRbS), established in 2008 through global partnership with Daisy's Eye Care Fund (DECF), is one such initiative [143]. Through multidisciplinary collaboration, the KNRbS developed comprehensive national guidelines to improve retinoblastoma care in 2014

[144]. Genetic testing and counseling were identified as high-needs areas, prompting the establishment of the KNRbS task force to develop a cancer genetics service [145]. Important challenges for implementation include accessibility, psychosocial and cultural factors, and lack of genetic counselors with specialized knowledge [146]. Furthermore, genetics education and counseling for retinoblastoma families is limited [147]. To address these needs, a cancer genetics educational program was developed for Kenyan clinicians to improve genetic counseling competencies [148]. Molecular testing is not yet routinely available in Kenya, so counseling focuses on risk assessment in the setting of unknown genetics (HX). However, capacity is within reach and will improve outcomes. Global partnerships can prioritize universally accessible genetic testing and counseling.

2.5 Molecular Markers of Metastasis

The presence of subclinical retinoblastoma cells in bone marrow (BM), cerebrospinal fluid (CSF) or other extraocular sites is termed minimal disseminated disease (MDD). GD2 synthase and CRX, both highly expressed in metastatic retinoblastoma cells, have been proposed as molecular markers to detect MDD. In children with high-risk retinoblastoma, detection of GD2 synthase mRNA in the CSF confers a higher risk for CNS retinoblastoma [149]. However, mRNA yield from CSF limits its reliability as a molecular marker [149]. The cone-rod homeobox (CRX) transcription factor has also been explored as a marker for metastatic surveillance, given its unique role in photoreceptor differentiation. It is expressed in BM metastasis and may be used to monitor response to therapy [150]. CRX mRNA is also detected in bone and soft tissue metastasis and may play a role when diagnosis is uncertain [151]. In the absence of overt extraocular disease, detection of CRX mRNA in BM and CSF is associated with worse disease-free survival [152], highlighting a potential application of biomarkers in prognostication at diagnosis.

Molecular genetic analysis is more definitive than other proposed tumor markers and is the current gold standard for diagnosis of metastasis. Following tumor analysis, M1 and M2 may serve as unique molecular markers in metastatic surveillance, including monitoring of treatment response and evaluating for recurrence. Unique AS-PCR primers can precisely identify the tumor mutations in BM, CSF, and other metastatic sites [83, 153]. Serial molecular monitoring is performed to assess therapeutic response (minimal residual disease, MRD) and confirm disease remission [153]. *RB1* mutation detection is also more sensitive than cytopathology in identifying systemic recurrence [153]. When pathology and cytology are inconclusive, molecular analysis can differentiate metastasis from a second primary cancer [154]. For individuals with non-heritable retinoblastoma, both M1 and M2 can be used for metastatic surveillance, while the M2 somatic event is informative in germline cases. If the tumor is homozygous for M1, the distinct tumor specific SCNAs (M3 to Mn) may serve instead as molecular markers [83, 154].

2.6 Aqueous Humor: A Liquid Biopsy

Recently, there has been widespread interest in cell-free DNA (cfDNA) as a genomic biomarker in oncology [155, 156]. First identified in plasma in the 1940s [157], cfDNA includes DNA fragments from various sources present in body fluids. Tumor cells release DNA during secretion, apoptosis and necrosis. This tumor-derived cfDNA is termed circulating tumor DNA (ctDNA) in plasma and cell-free tumor DNA (cftDNA) in other body fluids [158]. The potential clinical application to cancer diagnosis, prognostication, therapeutic monitoring, and surveillance is promising.

Since retinoblastoma biopsy risks extraocular spread, the search for biomarkers has focused on tumor and aqueous humor (AH) after enucleation. Several potential biomarkers, including lactate dehydrogenase (LDH), survivin, proteins and cytokines, have been identified in AH and were previously reviewed [159]. However, studies limited to enucleated eyes offer little prognostic insight. Anterior chamber paracentesis is now routinely performed to lower intraocular pressure before intravitreal chemotherapy injection, with very low risk of extraocular dissemination [160–162]. Even in eyes harboring active tumor, a small volume (0.1–0.15 mL) of AH is aspirated through clear cornea anterior to peripheral iris with minimal risk of complications or tumor dissemination. Berry et al. have confirmed that AH collected in vivo contains cftDNA for genetic analysis, an exciting application of **"liquid biopsy"** to retinoblastoma [136].

Further studies confirmed that the genetic profile of AH cftDNA resembles tumor tissue and remains stable over time [136, 163]. Specifically, the SCNAs identified in cftDNA, most commonly 6p gain, correspond to the retinoblastoma genomic signature previously described (see above). In heritable cases with multifocal tumors, the aqueous profile therefore reflects the heterogenous M3 to Mn changes accumulated by all tumors in the eye [163]. In addition to genomic changes, both M1 and M2 can be detected [137]. Despite small volumes collected, current technologies can determine both *RB1* mutations and the SCNA profile from a single sample [138].

Further studies suggest that SCNA may have prognostic biomarker potential [163]. Specifically, gain of 6p, the copy number change in 60% of enucleated retinoblastoma, identified first in 1984 [83, 85, 86], was associated with ten-fold increased odds of failed attempted eye salvage [164]. While promising, causality cannot be inferred from small retrospective studies with few samples collected at diagnosis. An important parameter is tumor fraction (TFx), the proportion of cfDNA in the sample derived from tumor [138]. Currently, TFx is estimated from aqueous SCNA. Relative increases in both TFx and SCNA amplitudes correlate with worse disease burden [165]. Thus, these biomarkers are proposed predictors of therapeutic response. However, estimation of TFx can only be assumed when SCNA are detected and understanding the half-life of cftDNA in the aqueous is important to clarify the role of biomarkers in therapeutic monitoring.

Although plasma is an important source of ctDNA for other solid tumors, only recently has its potential emerged for retinoblastoma. Retinoblastoma cfDNA is more concentrated in AH than plasma [166]. The fraction of plasma cfDNA that is ctDNA taken at the time of enucleation for advanced disease has been confirmed to match the tumor genomic *RB1* pathogenic allele [167]. As technologies evolve, plasma ctDNA may contribute to non-invasive systemic surveillance in retinoblastoma (see below).

3 The Future of Retinoblastoma Genomics

3.1 Expanding the Role of Aqueous Cell-Free DNA

3.1.1 Diagnosis

Though not yet clinically available, routine *RB1* mutation testing of AH cftDNA will play an important role when tumor tissue is unavailable. Clinically meaningful testing strategies will have high sensitivity and rapid turn-around time. In the future, retinoblastoma will benefit from robust multicenter clinical trials that provide strong evidence supporting novel therapies. As eye salvage improves, aqueous will replace tumor DNA to inform blood testing, especially in unilateral cases and those bilateral cases without a detectable germline mutation. It will also facilitate earlier diagnosis of aggressive *RB1*$^{+/+}$ *MYCN*^{A} tumors [168]. As discussed, genetic testing refines risk and improves counseling for the proband and entire family.

A minimally invasive test of AH cftDNA will aid in diagnostic uncertainty, complementing clinical exam and imaging. Detection of *RB1* mutations may confirm retinoblastoma when media opacity (e.g., cataract, vitreous hemorrhage) prevents fundus view and distinguish retinoblastoma from mimickers (e.g., uveitis, Coats disease). Serial tests may detect early recurrence when standard clinical monitoring is challenging, such as inactive seed remnants in anterior diffuse disease and regressed calcified tumors that mask recurrence within or under calcium.

In the future, cfDNA analysis may be used for metastatic surveillance in high-risk children. Serial non-invasive tests of plasma ctDNA could detect changes in *RB1* mutation fractions (M1/M2 in non-heritable or M2 in germline cases) indicative of systemic disease. The sensitivity to quantify tumor activity by variant allele fraction (VAF) requires prospective validation.

3.1.2 Prognosis

The role of 6p gain at diagnosis by cfDNA to predict failure of ocular salvage requires further prospective evaluation. Will high-sensitivity assays detect cftDNA in cT1a eyes? Is lack of detectable SCNA reflective of the tumor genomic profile or simply low tumor cfDNA content in the aqueous? Do salvaged eyes have lower TFx at baseline, thus predicting better outcomes, or is TFx reduced during treatment as tumor burden improves? Does relative change in TFx reliably predict therapeutic response in a clinically meaningful way? Will specific biomarkers predict high-risk histopathology? We need global collaborative prospective research with long-term follow-up to answer remaining questions. Research standard operating procedures and a centralized laboratory for cfDNA analysis will be beneficial [155]. This may one day lead to a standardized cftDNA protocol to sample AH at presentation, develop an individualized treatment plan based on prognostic factors, and serially sample AH during and after treatment to monitor response. Analysis of cfDNA will require fast turn-around to impact clinical decision-making in real time. Ultimately, cfDNA may complement, though not replace, clinical judgement in retinoblastoma.

3.2 Non-Invasive Prenatal Diagnosis

Cell-free fetal DNA (cffDNA) was first detected in maternal plasma in 1997 [169] and Non-invasive Prenatal Testing (NIPT) [158] is now established. The fraction of cffDNA (**fetal fraction**) increases during pregnancy, sufficiently to allow molecular diagnostics [170]. Non-invasive prenatal diagnosis (NIPD) involves testing of cffDNA for sex determination, chromosomal aneuploidies such as Trisomy 21, and more recently monogenic diseases [171]. Since cffDNA is obtained from non-invasive samples of maternal plasma, the potential risks of chorionic villus sampling or amniocentesis are avoided. When applied to single-gene disorders, NIPD successfully detects mutations inherited from the father. However, detection of maternally inherited mutations is more complex, as maternal cfDNA exceeds the fetal fraction in plasma. A technique known as relative haplotype dosage (RHDO) circumvents this issue [172]. This involves determining whether the fetus inherited a particular haplotype from mother or father [173]. NIPD as early as 8 weeks gestation has been successfully applied to familial retinoblastoma [174]. Amplicon-based massively parallel sequencing (MPS) was used to detect paternal variants and capture-based targeted MPS with RHDO for maternal alleles. This is an exciting non-invasive alternative to previous prenatal H1 diagnosis by amniocentesis to improve care for retinoblastoma families when combined with early-term delivery of H1 infants.

3.3 Targeted Therapies

An important priority for future research is the identification of targetable biomarkers in retinoblastoma. While certain SCNA may provide prognostic information, ideal biomarkers will have corresponding molecular therapies targeting specific tumorigenic pathways. For instance, preclinical studies demonstrate early evidence that small molecular inhibitors of MDM2/MDM4 can restore p53-mediated apoptosis in retinoblastoma [175–177]. The development of novel small molecular therapies, combined with innovative local drug delivery systems such as episcleral devices [178] in clinical trial [179] may promote precision care. These exciting ideas must be evaluated through high-quality preclinical and clinical trials to confirm efficacy and safety. In the future, sampling of AH cftDNA at diagnosis may identify biomarkers eligible for treatment with specific molecular therapies, and care will be individualized to the child based on tumor genomic signatures.

3.4 Molecular Surveillance for Second Cancers

Though the lifetime risk of second cancers among germline *RB1* mutation carriers (H1) exceeds the recommended threshold for surveillance [180], a comprehensive, universal screening guideline is lacking. This places significant burden on patients, who must attempt to navigate their own care and follow-up in a system lacking knowledge of their unique risks. Some centers recommend annual whole-body MRI (WB-MRI) screening, but there is no consensus [181]. The feasibility of annual WB-MRI surveillance for asymptomatic H1 survivors was demonstrated by a small retrospective pilot study [182]. However, sensitivity (67%) for detecting second cancers was limited at longer follow-up [183]. Currently, consensus does not support surveillance of H1 survivors with WB-MRI, given lack of robust evidence and psychosocial implications of false-positive results [184].

We propose that future second cancer surveillance for H1 individuals with a constitutional M1 *RB1* pathogenic allele will be a routine, non-invasive test of plasma cfDNA. Detection of an M2 *RB1* variant allele will be followed longitudinally and suggest the presence of an emerging second cancer. Genomic profiling of the ctDNA fraction may identify signatures characteristic of common second cancers. Focused imaging studies will then localize the second cancer. Similar to OCT detection of invisible retinal tumors, molecular surveillance will detect subclinical second cancers and improve survival. This is an immediate priority for further research, as recently identified by a group of Canadian retinoblastoma survivors, researchers, and health professionals [185].

4 Uveal Melanoma: A Genetic Comparison

The genetics of uveal melanoma (UM), the most common primary eye cancer in adults, provides complementary insight into cancer genomics. Retinoblastoma is initiated following loss of both alleles of the same gene and M1 is germline in approximately half of cases. In contrast, uveal melanoma nearly always results from somatic mutations in several genes. Though the sequence of progressive genomic changes has yet to be elucidated, *GNAQ* and other G-protein signaling genes play a role early in tumorigenesis [186]. However, they are not associated with outcomes. While retinoblastoma survival outcomes are excellent when diagnosis is timely, they are relatively poor in UM. Thus, genetic studies have focused on metastatic prognostication.

Uveal melanoma micrometastasis likely start within a 5-year window prior to treatment of the primary ocular tumor [187]. The liver is the most common site, though widespread dissemination also occurs [188]. Unfortunately, no treatment options have proven efficacious, and most patients die within a year of metastasis diagnosis [189]. Early studies focused on the prognostic potential of somatic chromosomal alterations in UM. The most important predictor of poor prognosis from metastatic disease is monosomy 3 [190], followed by gain of the long arm of chromosome 8 [191]. In contrast, 6p alterations are associated with improved outcomes [192]. Though a candidate tumor suppressor gene was subsequently identified at 3p21.1 (*BAP1*) [193], the significance of these chromosomal changes has yet to be fully elucidated.

Two distinct genetic testing strategies have been developed for prognostication in routine clinical care. Since UM is often treated conservatively, sufficient tissue for genetic analysis can be retrieved by fine needle aspiration biopsy [194]. The RNA-based test found that UM is divided into two transcriptomic groups: class 1 (low metastatic risk) and class 2 (high metastatic risk) [195, 196]. These gene expression profiles (GEP) correlate with other prognostic features. A 15 gene GEP was prospectively validated and found to predict prognosis better than chromosomal and clinicopathologic markers [197, 198]. Subsequently, *PRAME* (preferentially expressed antigen in melanoma) was identified as a poor prognostic biomarker in class 1

UM [199]. When added to GEP, *PRAME* status demonstrated better prognostic potential than the clinical AJCC TNM eighth edition staging [200]. More recently, the Cancer Genome Atlas (TCGA) expanded this genetic classification to four molecular subtypes, with two poor prognostic groups (monosomy 3) and 2 higher prognostic groups (disomy 3) [201]. These groups, termed A through D [202], consider specific genomic characteristics, with *BAP1* being more common in the setting of monosomy 3. The TCGA classification also better predicts metastasis compared to the AJCC TNM [203].

Metastatic prognostication for UM analyzes recurrent somatic chromosomal changes identified by MLPA and predicts metastasis when combined with clinical and histopathologic predictors [204, 205]. Tumor clinical features, including basal diameter and thickness, ciliary body involvement, and extraocular extension, are incorporated into the AJCC TNM staging [206]. Unlike retinoblastoma, the UM AJCC does not currently include genetic status. However, an online algorithm (the Liverpool Uveal Melanoma Prognosticator Online, LUMPO) was developed to provide a unique estimate of all-cause mortality for the patient, incorporating DNA-based genetic testing, clinical and histologic features [207]. The utility of this algorithm was validated by several international centers [208].

Though the series of genetic changes leading to UM has yet to be confirmed, genetic information plays an important role in survival prognosis. With further insight, genetic-based algorithms will evolve, and novel targeted molecular therapies will improve outcomes. Knowledge of an individual's unique genomic profile will inform criteria for clinical trials and enable patient-centered surveillance and counseling.

References

1. Knudson AG. Mutation and cancer: statistical study of retinoblastoma. Proc Natl Acad Sci U S A. 1971;68(4):820–3.
2. Comings DE. A general theory of carcinogenesis. Proc Natl Acad Sci U S A. 1973;70(12):3324–8.
3. Yunis JJ, Ramsay N. Retinoblastoma and subband deletion of chromosome 13. Am J Dis Child. 1978;132(2):161–3.
4. Connolly MJ, Payne RH, Johnson G, Gallie BL, Allderdice PW, Marshall WH, et al. Familial, EsD-linked, retinoblastoma with reduced penetrance and variable expressivity. Hum Genet. 1983;65(2):122–4.
5. Godbout R, Dryja TP, Squire J, Gallie BL, Phillips RA. Somatic inactivation of genes on chromosome 13 is a common event in retinoblastoma. Nature. 1983;304(5925):451–3.
6. Halloran SL, Boughman JA, Dryja TP, Mukai S, Long D, Roberts DF, et al. Accuracy of detection of the retinoblastoma gene by esterase D linkage. Arch Ophthalmol. 1985;103(9):1329–31.
7. Sparkes RS, Murphree AL, Lingua RW, Sparkes MC, Field LL, Funderburk SJ, et al. Gene for hereditary retinoblastoma assigned to human chromosome 13 by linkage to Esterase D. Science. 1983;219:971–2.
8. Wilson MG, Ebbin AJ, Towner JW, Spencer WH. Chromosomal anomalies in patients with retinoblastoma. Clin Genet. 1977;12(1):1–8.
9. Knight LA, Gardner HA, Gallie BL. Segregation of chromosome 13 in retinoblastoma. Lancet. 1978;1(8071):989.
10. Sparkes RS, Muller H, Klisak I. Retinoblastoma with 13q- chromosomal deletion associated with maternal paracentric inversion of 13q. Science. 1979;203(4384):1027–9.
11. Sparkes RS, Sparkes MC, Wilson MG, Towner JW, Benedict W, Murphree AL, et al. Regional assignment of genes for human esterase D and retinoblastoma to chromosome band 13q14. Science. 1980;208(4447):1042–4.
12. Cavenee WK, Dryja TP, Phillips RA, Benedict WF, Godbout R, Gallie BL, et al. Expression of recessive alleles by chromosomal mechanisms in retinoblastoma. Nature. 1983;305(5937):779–84.
13. Dryja TP, Cavenee W, White R, Rapaport JM, Petersen R, Albert DM, et al. Homozygosity of chromosome 13 in retinoblastoma. N Engl J Med. 1984;310(9):550–3.
14. Dryja TP, Rapaport JM, Joyce JM, Petersen RA. Molecular detection of deletions involving band q14 of chromosome 13 in retinoblastomas. Proc Natl Acad Sci U S A. 1986;83(19):7391–4.
15. Friend SH, Bernards R, Rogelj S, Weinberg RA, Rapaport JM, Albert DM, et al. A human DNA segment with properties of the gene that predisposes to retinoblastoma and osteosarcoma. Nature. 1986;323(6089):643–6.
16. Dryja TP, Friend S, Weinberg RA. Genetic sequences that predispose to retinoblastoma and osteosarcoma. Symp Fundam Cancer Res. 1986;39:115–9.
17. Lee WH, Bookstein R, Hong F, Young LJ, Shew JY, Lee EY. Human retinoblastoma susceptibility gene: cloning, identification, and sequence. Science. 1987;235(4794):1394–9.
18. Lee WH, Shew JY, Hong FD, Sery TW, Donoso LA, Young LJ, et al. The retinoblastoma susceptibility gene encodes a nuclear phosphoprotein associated with DNA binding activity. Nature. 1987;329(6140):642–5.
19. Fung YK, Murphree AL, T'Ang A, Qian J, Hinrichs SH, Benedict WF. Structural evidence for the authenticity of the human retinoblastoma gene. Science. 1987;236(4809):1657–61.
20. Temming P, Viehmann A, Arendt M, Eisele L, Spix C, Bornfeld N, et al. Pediatric second primary malignancies after retinoblastoma treatment. Pediatr Blood Cancer. 2015;62(10):1799–804.
21. MacCarthy A, Bayne AM, Draper GJ, Eatock EM, Kroll ME, Stiller CA, et al. Non-ocular tumours following retinoblastoma in Great Britain 1951 to 2004. Br J Ophthalmol. 2009;93(9):1159–62.
22. Vogel F. Genetics of retinoblastoma. Hum Genet. 1979;52(1):1–54.
23. Lohmann DR, Gerick M, Brandt B, Oelschlager U, Lorenz B, Passarge E, et al. Constitutional RB1-gene mutations in patients with isolated unilateral retinoblastoma. Am J Hum Genet. 1997;61(2):282–94.
24. Dryja TP, Morrow JF, Rapaport JM. Quantification of the paternal allele bias for new germline mutations in the retinoblastoma gene. Hum Genet. 1997;100(3–4):446–9.
25. Dryja TP, Mukai S, Petersen R, Rapaport JM, Walton D, Yandell DW. Parental origin of mutations of the retinoblastoma gene. Nature. 1989;339:556–8.
26. Zhu XP, Dunn JM, Phillips RA, Goddard AD, Paton KE, Becker A, et al. Preferential germline mutation of the paternal allele in retinoblastoma. Nature. 1989;340(6231):312–3.
27. Rushlow DE, Mol BM, Kennett JY, Yee S, Pajovic S, Theriault BL, et al. Characterisation of retinoblastomas without RB1 mutations: genomic, gene expression, and clinical studies. Lancet Oncol. 2013;14(4):327–34.

28. Hong FD, Huang H-JS, To H, Young LJ, Oro A, Bookstein R, et al. Structure of the human retinoblastoma gene. Proc Natl Acad Sci U S A. 1989;86:5502–6.
29. McGee TL, Yandell DW, Dryja TP. Structure and partial genomic sequence of the human retinoblastoma susceptibility gene. Gene. 1989;80:119–28.
30. Toguchida J, McGee TL, Paterson JC, Eagle JR, Tucker S, Yandell DW, et al. Complete genomic sequence of the human retinoblastoma susceptibility gene. Genomics. 1993;17(3):535–43.
31. Lohmann DR, Brandt B, Hopping W, Passarge E, Horsthemke B. The spectrum of RB1 germ-line mutations in hereditary retinoblastoma. Am J Hum Genet. 1996;58(5):940–9.
32. Lohmann DR. RB1 gene mutations in retinoblastoma. Hum Mutat. 1999;14(4):283–8.
33. Valverde JR, Alonso J, Palacios I, Pestana A. RB1 gene mutation up-date, a meta-analysis based on 932 reported mutations available in a searchable database. BMC Genet. 2005;6:53.
34. Dommering CJ, Mol BM, Moll AC, Burton M, Cloos J, Dorsman JC, et al. RB1 mutation spectrum in a comprehensive nationwide cohort of retinoblastoma patients. J Med Genet. 2014;51(6):366–74.
35. Taylor M, Dehainault C, Desjardins L, Doz F, Levy C, Sastre X, et al. Genotype-phenotype correlations in hereditary familial retinoblastoma. Hum Mutat. 2007;28(3):284–93.
36. Holbrook JA, Neu-Yilik G, Hentze MW, Kulozik AE. Nonsense-mediated decay approaches the clinic. Nat Genet. 2004;36(8):801–8.
37. Mitter D, Ullmann R, Muradyan A, Klein-Hitpass L, Kanber D, Ounap K, et al. Genotype-phenotype correlations in patients with retinoblastoma and interstitial 13q deletions. Eur J Hum Genet. 2011;19(9):947–58.
38. Richter S, Vandezande K, Chen N, Zhang K, Sutherland J, Anderson J, et al. Sensitive and efficient detection of RB1 gene mutations enhances care for families with retinoblastoma. Am J Hum Genet. 2003;72(2):253–69.
39. Greger V, Passarge E, Hopping W, Messmer E, Horsthemke B. Epigenetic changes may contribute to the formation and spontaneous regression of retinoblastoma. Hum Genet. 1989;83(2):155–8.
40. Ohtani-Fujita N, Dryja TP, Rapaport JM, Fujita T, Matsumura S, Ozasa K, et al. Hypermethylation in the retinoblastoma gene is associated with unilateral, sporadic retinoblastoma. Cancer Genet Cytogenet. 1997;98(1):43–9.
41. Greger V, Debus N, Lohmann D, Hopping W, Passarge E, Horsthemke B. Frequency and parental origin of hypermethylated RB1 alleles in retinoblastoma. Hum Genet. 1994;94(5):491–6.
42. Raizis AM, Racher HM, Foucal A, Dimaras H, Gallie BL, George PM. DNA hypermethylation/boundary control loss identified in retinoblastomas associated with genetic and epigenetic inactivation of the RB1 gene promoter. Epigenetics. 2021;16(9):940–54.
43. Zhang K, Nowak I, Rushlow D, Gallie BL, Lohmann DR. Patterns of missplicing caused by RB1 gene mutations in patients with retinoblastoma and association with phenotypic expression. Hum Mutat. 2008;29(4):475–84.
44. Soliman SE, Dimaras H, Khetan V, Gardiner JA, Chan HS, Heon E, et al. Prenatal versus postnatal screening for familial retinoblastoma. Ophthalmology. 2016;123(12):2610–7.
45. Dommering CJ, Marees T, van der Hout AH, Imhof SM, Meijers-Heijboer H, Ringens PJ, et al. RB1 mutations and second primary malignancies after hereditary retinoblastoma. Fam Cancer. 2012;11(2):225–33.
46. Lohmann DR, Brandt B, Hopping W, Passarge E, Horsthemke B. Distinct RB1 gene mutations with low penetrance in hereditary retinoblastoma. Hum Genet. 1994;94:349–54.
47. Otterson GA, Chen W, Coxon AB, Khleif SN, Kaye FJ. Incomplete penetrance of familial retinoblastoma linked to germ-line mutations that result in partial loss of RB function. Proc Natl Acad Sci U S A. 1997;94(22):12036–40.
48. Kratzke RA, Otterson GA, Hogg A, Coxon AB, Geradts J, Cowell JK, et al. Partial inactivation of the RB product in a family with incomplete penetrance of familial retinoblastoma and benign retinal tumors. Oncogene. 1994;9(5):1321–6.
49. Harbour JW. Molecular basis of low-penetrance retinoblastoma. Arch Ophthalmol. 2001;119(11):1699–704.
50. Albrecht P, Ansperger-Rescher B, Schuler A, Zeschnigk M, Gallie B, Lohmann DR. Spectrum of gross deletions and insertions in the RB1 gene in patients with retinoblastoma and association with phenotypic expression. Hum Mutat. 2005;26(5):437–45.
51. Bremner R, Du DC, Connolly-Wilson MJ, Bridge P, Ahmad KF, Mostachfi H, et al. Deletion of RB exons 24 and 25 causes low-penetrance retinoblastoma. Am J Hum Genet. 1997;61(3):556–70.
52. Schubert EL, Strong LC, Hansen MF. A splicing mutation in RB1 in low penetrance retinoblastoma. Hum Genet. 1997;100(5–6):557–63.
53. Soliman SE, Racher H, Lambourne M, Matevski D, MacDonald H, Gallie B. A novel deep intronic low penetrance RB1 variant in a retinoblastoma family. Ophthalmic Genet. 2018;39(2):288–90.
54. Dehainault C, Garancher A, Castera L, Cassoux N, Aerts I, Doz F, et al. The survival gene MED4 explains low penetrance retinoblastoma in patients with large RB1 deletion. Hum Mol Genet. 2014;23(19):5243–50.
55. Eloy P, Dehainault C, Sefta M, Aerts I, Doz F, Cassoux N, et al. A parent-of-origin effect impacts the phenotype in low penetrance retinoblastoma families segregating the c.1981C>T/p.Arg661Trp mutation of RB1. PLoS Genet. 2016;12(2):e1005888.
56. Imperatore V, Pinto AM, Gelli E, Trevisson E, Morbidoni V, Frullanti E, et al. Parent-of-origin effect of hypomorphic pathogenic variants and somatic mosaicism impact on phenotypic expression of retinoblastoma. Eur J Hum Genet. 2018;26(7):1026–37.
57. Carlson EA, Desnick RJ. Mutational mosaicism and genetic counseling in retinoblastoma. Am J Med Genet. 1979;4(4):365–81.
58. Rushlow D, Piovesan B, Zhang K, Prigoda-Lee NL, Marchong MN, Clark RD, et al. Detection of mosaic RB1 mutations in families with retinoblastoma. Hum Mutat. 2009;30(5):842–51.
59. Sippel KC, Fraioli RE, Smith GD, Schalkoff ME, Sutherland J, Gallie BL, et al. Frequency of somatic and germ-line mosaicism in retinoblastoma: implications for genetic counseling. Am J Hum Genet. 1998;62(3):610–9.
60. Amitrano S, Marozza A, Somma S, Imperatore V, Hadjistilianou T, De Francesco S, et al. Next generation sequencing in sporadic retinoblastoma patients reveals somatic mosaicism. Eur J Hum Genet. 2015;23(11):1523–30.
61. Chen Z, Moran K, Richards-Yutz J, Toorens E, Gerhart D, Ganguly T, et al. Enhanced sensitivity for detection of low-level germline mosaic RB1 mutations in sporadic retinoblastoma cases using deep semiconductor sequencing. Hum Mutat. 2014;35(3):384–91.
62. Goodrich DW, Wang NP, Qian Y-W, Lee EY-HP, Lee W-H. The retinoblastoma gene product regulates progression through the G_1 phase of the cell cycle. Cell. 1991;67:293–302.
63. Chen PL, Scully P, Shew JY, Wang JY, Lee WH. Phosphorylation of the retinoblastoma gene product is modulated during the cell cycle and cellular differentiation. Cell. 1989;58(6):1193–8.
64. Brown VD, Phillips RA, Gallie BL. Cumulative effect of phosphorylation of pRB on regulation of E2F activity. Mol Cell Biol. 1999;19(5):3246–56.
65. Hamel PA, Gallie BL, Phillips RA. The retinoblastoma protein and cell cycle regulation. Trends Genet. 1992;8:180–5.
66. Ludlow JW, Shon J, Pipas JM, Livingston DM, DeCaprio JA. The retinoblastoma susceptibility gene product undergoes cell cycle-dependent dephosphorylation and binding to and release from SV40 large T. Cell. 1990;60(3):387–96.

67. Chellappan SP, Hiebert S, Mudryl M, Horowitz JM, Nevins JR. The E2F transcription factor is a cellular target for the RB protein. Cell. 1991;65:1053–61.
68. Lees JA, Saito M, Vidal M, Valentine M, Look T, Harlow E, et al. The retinoblastoma protein binds to a family of E2F transcription factors. Mol Cell Biol. 1993;13(12):7813–25.
69. Helin K, Harlow E, Fattaey A. Inhibition of E2F-1 transactivation by direct binding of the retinoblastoma protein. Mol Cell Biol. 1993;13(10):6501–8.
70. Polager S, Kalma Y, Berkovich E, Ginsberg D. E2Fs up-regulate expression of genes involved in DNA replication, DNA repair and mitosis. Oncogene. 2002;21(3):437–46.
71. Markey MP, Angus SP, Strobeck MW, Williams SL, Gunawardena RW, Aronow BJ, et al. Unbiased analysis of RB-mediated transcriptional repression identifies novel targets and distinctions from E2F action. Cancer Res. 2002;62(22):6587–97.
72. Guarducci C, Bonechi M, Benelli M, Biagioni C, Boccalini G, Romagnoli D, et al. Cyclin E1 and Rb modulation as common events at time of resistance to palbociclib in hormone receptor-positive breast cancer. NPJ Breast Cancer. 2018;4:38.
73. de Leeuw R, McNair C, Schiewer MJ, Neupane NP, Brand LJ, Augello MA, et al. MAPK reliance via acquired CDK4/6 inhibitor resistance in cancer. Clin Cancer Res. 2018;24(17):4201–14.
74. Xu XL, Singh HP, Wang L, Qi DL, Poulos BK, Abramson DH, et al. Rb suppresses human cone-precursor-derived retinoblastoma tumours. Nature. 2014;514(7522):385–8.
75. Gallie BL, Campbell C, Devlin H, Duckett A, Squire JA. Developmental basis of retinal-specific induction of cancer by RB mutation. Cancer Res. 1999;59(7 Suppl):1731s–5s.
76. Xu XL, Fang Y, Lee TC, Forrest D, Gregory-Evans C, Almeida D, et al. Retinoblastoma has properties of a cone precursor tumor and depends upon cone-specific MDM2 signaling. Cell. 2009;137(6):1018–31.
77. Dimaras H, Khetan V, Halliday W, Orlic M, Prigoda NL, Piovesan B, et al. Loss of RB1 induces non-proliferative retinoma: increasing genomic instability correlates with progression to retinoblastoma. Hum Mol Genet. 2008;17(10):1363–72.
78. Gallie BL, Ellsworth RM, Abramson DH, Phillips RA. Retinoma: spontaneous regression of retinoblastoma or benign manifestation of the mutation? Br J Cancer. 1982;45(4):513–21.
79. Balmer A, Munier F, Gailloud C. Retinoma. Case studies. Ophthalmic Paediatr Gen. 1991;12(3):131–7.
80. Eagle RC Jr, Shields JA, Donoso L, Milner RS. Malignant transformation of spontaneously regressed retinoblastoma, retinoma/retinocytoma variant. Ophthalmology. 1989;96(9):1389–95.
81. Corson TW, Gallie BL. One hit, two hits, three hits, more? Genomic changes in the development of retinoblastoma. Genes Chromosomes Cancer. 2007;46(7):617–34.
82. Theriault BL, Dimaras H, Gallie BL, Corson TW. The genomic landscape of retinoblastoma: a review. Clin Experiment Ophthalmol. 2014;42(1):33–52.
83. Bowles E, Corson TW, Bayani J, Squire JA, Wong N, Lai PB, et al. Profiling genomic copy number changes in retinoblastoma beyond loss of RB1. Genes Chromosomes Cancer. 2007;46(2):118–29.
84. Kooi IE, Mol BM, Massink MP, Ameziane N, Meijers-Heijboer H, Dommering CJ, et al. Somatic genomic alterations in retinoblastoma beyond RB1 are rare and limited to copy number changes. Sci Rep. 2016;6:25264.
85. Squire J, Phillips RA, Boyce S, Godbout R, Rogers B, Gallie BL. Isochromosome 6p, a unique chromosomal abnormality in retinoblastoma: verification by standard staining techniques, new densitometric methods, and somatic cell hybridization. Hum Genet. 1984;66(1):46–53.
86. Squire J, Gallie BL, Phillips RA. A detailed analysis of chromosomal changes in heritable and non-heritable retinoblastoma. Hum Genet. 1985;70(4):291–301.
87. Mairal A, Pinglier E, Gilbert E, Peter M, Validire P, Desjardins L, et al. Detection of chromosome imbalances in retinoblastoma by parallel karyotype and CGH analyses. Genes Chromosomes Cancer. 2000;28(4):370–9.
88. Chen D, Gallie BL, Squire JA. Minimal regions of chromosomal imbalance in retinoblastoma detected by comparative genomic hybridization. Cancer Genet Cytogenet. 2001;129(1):57–63.
89. Herzog S, Lohmann DR, Buiting K, Schuler A, Horsthemke B, Rehder H, et al. Marked differences in unilateral isolated retinoblastomas from young and older children studied by comparative genomic hybridization. Hum Genet. 2001;108(2):98–104.
90. Lillington DM, Kingston JE, Coen PG, Price E, Hungerford J, Domizio P, et al. Comparative genomic hybridization of 49 primary retinoblastoma tumors identifies chromosomal regions associated with histopathology, progression, and patient outcome. Genes Chromosomes Cancer. 2003;36(2):121–8.
91. van der Wal JE, Hermsen MA, Gille HJ, Schouten-Van Meeteren NY, Moll AC, Imhof SM, et al. Comparative genomic hybridisation divides retinoblastomas into a high and a low level chromosomal instability group. J Clin Pathol. 2003;56(1):26–30.
92. Potluri VR, Helson L, Ellsworth RM, Reid T, Gilbert F. Chromosomal abnormalities in human retinoblastoma. A review. Cancer. 1986;58(3):663–71.
93. Kooi IE, Mol BM, Massink MP, de Jong MC, de Graaf P, van der Valk P, et al. A meta-analysis of retinoblastoma copy numbers refines the list of possible driver genes involved in tumor progression. PLoS One. 2016;11(4):e0153323.
94. Corson TW, Huang A, Tsao MS, Gallie BL. KIF14 is a candidate oncogene in the 1q minimal region of genomic gain in multiple cancers. Oncogene. 2005;24(30):4741–53.
95. Gratias S, Schuler A, Hitpass LK, Stephan H, Rieder H, Schneider S, et al. Genomic gains on chromosome 1q in retinoblastoma: consequences on gene expression and association with clinical manifestation. Int J Cancer. 2005;116(4):555–63.
96. Lee WH, Murphree AL, Benedict WF. Expression and amplification of the N-myc gene in primary retinoblastoma. Nature. 1984;309(5967):458–60.
97. Orlic M, Spencer CE, Wang L, Gallie BL. Expression analysis of 6p22 genomic gain in retinoblastoma. Genes Chromosomes Cancer. 2006;45(1):72–82.
98. Zhang J, Benavente CA, McEvoy J, Flores-Otero J, Ding L, Chen X, et al. A novel retinoblastoma therapy from genomic and epigenetic analyses. Nature. 2012;481(7381):329–34.
99. Marchong MN, Chen D, Corson TW, Lee C, Harmandayan M, Bowles E, et al. Minimal 16q genomic loss implicates cadherin-11 in retinoblastoma. Mol Cancer Res. 2004;2(9):495–503.
100. Kato MV, Shimizu T, Ishizaki K, Kaneko A, Yandell DW, Toguchida J, et al. Loss of heterozygosity on chromosome 17 and mutation of the p53 gene in retinoblastoma. Cancer Lett. 1996;106(1):75–82.
101. Oliner JD, Kinzler KW, Meltzer PS, George DL, Vogelstein B. Amplification of a gene encoding a p53-associated protein in human sarcomas. Nature. 1992;358:80–3.
102. Medina-Medina I, Martinez-Sanchez M, Hernandez-Monge J, Fahraeus R, Muller P, Olivares-Illana V. p53 promotes its own polyubiquitination by enhancing the HDM2 and HDMX interaction. Protein Sci. 2018;27(5):976–86.
103. McEvoy J, Ulyanov A, Brennan R, Wu G, Pounds S, Zhang J, et al. Analysis of MDM2 and MDM4 single nucleotide polymorphisms, mRNA splicing and protein expression in retinoblastoma. PLoS One. 2012;7(8):e42739.
104. Bond GL, Hu W, Bond EE, Robins H, Lutzker SG, Arva NC, et al. A single nucleotide polymorphism in the MDM2 promoter attenuates the p53 tumor suppressor pathway and accelerates tumor formation in humans. Cell. 2004;119(5):591–602.

105. Castera L, Sabbagh A, Dehainault C, Michaux D, Mansuet-Lupo A, Patillon B, et al. MDM2 as a modifier gene in retinoblastoma. J Natl Cancer Inst. 2010;102(23):1805–8.
106. de Oliveira Reis AH, de Carvalho IN, de Sousa Damasceno PB, Ferman SE, Lucena E, Lopez-Camelo JS, et al. Influence of MDM2 and MDM4 on development and survival in hereditary retinoblastoma. Pediatr Blood Cancer. 2012;59(1):39–43.
107. Pritchard EM, Dyer MA, Guy RK. Progress in small molecule therapeutics for the treatment of retinoblastoma. Mini Rev Med Chem. 2016;16(6):430–54.
108. Mallipatna A, Gallie BL, Chévez-Barrios P, Lumbroso-Le Rouic L, Chantada GL, Doz F, et al. Retinoblastoma. In: Amin MB, Edge SB, Greene FL, editors. AJCC cancer staging manual. 8th ed. New York, NY: Springer; 2017. p. 819–31.
109. Soliman SE, Racher H, Zhang C, MacDonald H, Gallie BL. Genetics and molecular diagnostics in retinoblastoma—an update. Asia Pac J Ophthalmol (Phila). 2017;6(2):197–207.
110. de Jong MC, Kors WA, de Graaf P, Castelijns JA, Kivela T, Moll AC. Trilateral retinoblastoma: a systematic review and meta-analysis. Lancet Oncol. 2014;15(10):1157–67.
111. Canadian Retinoblastoma Society. National Retinoblastoma Strategy Canadian Guidelines for Care: Stratégie thérapeutique du rétinoblastome guide clinique canadien. Can J Ophthalmol. 2009;44(Supp 2):S1–88.
112. Noorani HZ, Khan HN, Gallie BL, Detsky AS. Cost comparison of molecular versus conventional screening of relatives at risk for retinoblastoma. Am J Hum Genet. 1996;59(2):301–7.
113. Skalet AH, Gombos DS, Gallie BL, Kim JW, Shields CL, Marr BP, et al. Screening children at risk for retinoblastoma: consensus report from the American association of ophthalmic oncologists and pathologists. Ophthalmology. 2018;125(3):453–8.
114. Yousef YA, Alkhoms A, AlJabari R, AlJboor M, Mohammad M, Lahlouh M, et al. Programmed screening for retinoblastoma enhances early diagnosis and improves management outcome for high-risk children. Ophthalmic Genet. 2020;41(4):308–14.
115. Soliman SE, ElManhaly M, Dimaras H. Knowledge of genetics in familial retinoblastoma. Ophthalmic Genet. 2017;38(3):226–32.
116. Rothschild PR, Levy D, Savignoni A, Lumbroso-Le Rouic L, Aerts I, Gauthier-Villars M, et al. Familial retinoblastoma: fundus screening schedule impact and guideline proposal. A retrospective study. Eye (Lond). 2011;25(12):1555–61.
117. Maat-Kievit JA, Oepkes D, Hartwig NG, Vermeij-Keers C, van Kamp IL, van de Kamp JJ. A large retinoblastoma detected in a fetus at 21 weeks of gestation. Prenat Diagn. 1993;13(5):377–84.
118. Paquette LB, Miller D, Jackson HA, Lee T, Randolph L, Murphree AL, et al. In utero detection of retinoblastoma with fetal magnetic resonance and ultrasound: initial experience. AJP Rep. 2012;2(1):55–62.
119. Abramson DH, Gombos DS. The topography of bilateral retinoblastoma lesions. Retina. 1996;16(3):232–9.
120. Abramson DH, Mendelsohn ME, Servodidio CA, Tretter T, Gombos DS. Familial retinoblastoma: where and when? Acta Ophthalmol Scand. 1998;76(3):334–8.
121. Brinkert AW, Moll AC, Jager MJ, Den Otter W, Koten JW, Faber JA, et al. Distribution of tumors in the retina in hereditary retinoblastoma patients. Ophthalmic Genet. 1998;19(2):63–7.
122. King BA, Parra C, Li Y, Helton KJ, Qaddoumi I, Wilson MW, et al. Spatiotemporal patterns of tumor occurrence in children with intraocular retinoblastoma. PLoS One. 2015;10(7):e0132932.
123. Shah PK, Narendran V, Kalpana N. In vivo growth of retinoblastoma in a newborn infant. Indian J Ophthalmol. 2010;58(5):421–3.
124. Abramson DH, Schefler AC, Beaverson KL, Rollins IS, Ruddat MS, Kelly CJ. Rapid growth of retinoblastoma in a premature twin. Arch Ophthalmol. 2002;120(9):1232–3.
125. Manjandavida FP, Xia J, Zhang J, Tang XY, Yi HR. In-utero ultrasonography detection of fetal retinoblastoma and neonatal selective ophthalmic artery chemotherapy. Indian J Ophthalmol. 2019;67(6):958–60.
126. Akolekar R, Beta J, Picciarelli G, Ogilvie C, D'Antonio F. Procedure-related risk of miscarriage following amniocentesis and chorionic villus sampling: a systematic review and meta-analysis. Ultrasound Obstet Gynecol. 2015;45(1):16–26.
127. Soliman SE, VandenHoven C, MacKeen LD, Heon E, Gallie BL. Optical coherence tomography-guided decisions in retinoblastoma management. Ophthalmology. 2017;124(6):859–72.
128. Saktanasate J, Vongkulsiri S, Khoo CT. Invisible retinoblastoma. JAMA Ophthalmol. 2015;133(7):e151123.
129. Berry JL, Cobrinik D, Kim JW. Detection and intraretinal localization of an 'invisible' retinoblastoma using optical coherence tomography. Ocul Oncol Pathol. 2016;2(3):148–52.
130. Soliman SE, VandenHoven C, MacKeen LD, Gallie BL. Secondary prevention of retinoblastoma revisited: laser photocoagulation of invisible new retinoblastoma. Ophthalmology. 2020;127(1):122–7.
131. Gaillard MC, Houghton S, Stathopoulos C, Munier FL. OCT-guided management of subclinical recurrent retinoblastoma. Ophthalmic Genet. 2018;39(3):338–43.
132. Dommering CJ, van den Heuvel MR, Moll AC, Imhof SM, Meijers-Heijboer H, Henneman L. Reproductive decision-making: a qualitative study among couples at increased risk of having a child with retinoblastoma. Clin Genet. 2010;78(4):334–41.
133. Foster A, Boyes L, Burgess L, Carless S, Bowyer V, Jenkinson H, et al. Patient understanding of genetic information influences reproductive decision making in retinoblastoma. Clin Genet. 2017;92(6):587–93.
134. Yahalom C, Macarov M, Lazer-Derbeko G, Altarescu G, Imbar T, Hyman JH, et al. Preimplantation genetic diagnosis as a strategy to prevent having a child born with an heritable eye disease. Ophthalmic Genet. 2018;39(4):450–6.
135. Dhanjal S, Kakourou G, Mamas T, Saleh N, Doshi A, Gotts S, et al. Preimplantation genetic diagnosis for retinoblastoma predisposition. Br J Ophthalmol. 2007;91(8):1090–1.
136. Berry JL, Xu L, Murphree AL, Krishnan S, Stachelek K, Zolfaghari E, et al. Potential of aqueous humor as a surrogate tumor biopsy for retinoblastoma. JAMA Ophthalmol. 2017;135(11):1221–30.
137. Gerrish A, Stone E, Clokie S, Ainsworth JR, Jenkinson H, McCalla M, et al. Non-invasive diagnosis of retinoblastoma using cell-free DNA from aqueous humour. Br J Ophthalmol. 2019;103(5):721–4.
138. Xu L, Shen L, Polski A, Prabakar RK, Shah R, Jubran R, et al. Simultaneous identification of clinically relevant RB1 mutations and copy number alterations in aqueous humor of retinoblastoma eyes. Ophthalmic Genet. 2020;41(6):526–32.
139. Zeschnigk M, Lohmann D, Horsthemke B. A PCR test for the detection of hypermethylated alleles at the retinoblastoma locus. J Med Genet. 1999;36(10):793–4.
140. Dimaras H, Corson TW, Cobrinik D, White A, Zhao J, Munier FL, et al. Retinoblastoma. Nat Rev Dis Primers. 2015;1:15021.
141. Group GRS. Global retinoblastoma presentation and analysis by national income level. JAMA Oncol. 2020;6(5):685–95.
142. Tomar AS, Finger PT, Gallie B, Kivela TT, Mallipatna A, Zhang C, et al. Global retinoblastoma treatment outcomes: association with national income level. Ophthalmology. 2021;128(5):740–53.
143. Hill JA, Kimani K, White A, Barasa F, Livingstone M, Gallie BL, et al. Achieving optimal cancer outcomes in East Africa through multidisciplinary partnership: a case study of the Kenyan National Retinoblastoma Strategy group. Global Health. 2016;12(1):23.
144. Health KMo. Kenya national retinoblastoma strategy: Best Practice guidelines; 2014.
145. He LQ, Njambi L, Nyamori JM, Nyenze EM, Kimani K, Matende I, et al. Developing clinical cancer genetics services in resource-

limited countries: the case of retinoblastoma in Kenya. Public Health Genomics. 2014;17(4):221–7.
146. Zhong A, Darren B, Loiseau B, He LQB, Chang T, Hill J, et al. Ethical, social, and cultural issues related to clinical genetic testing and counseling in low- and middle-income countries: a systematic review. Genet Med. 2018.
147. Gedleh A, Lee S, Hill JA, Umukunda Y, Qaiser S, Kabiru J, et al. "Where does it come from?" Experiences among survivors and parents of children with retinoblastoma in Kenya. J Genet Couns. 2018;27(3):574–88.
148. Hill J, Lee M, Njambi L, Corson T, Dimaras H. Cancer genetics education in a low- to middle-income country: evaluation of an interactive workshop for clinicians in Kenya. Ann Glob Health. 2015;81(1):152–3.
149. Laurent VE, Sampor C, Solernou V, Rossi J, Gabri M, Eandi-Eberle S, et al. Detection of minimally disseminated disease in the cerebrospinal fluid of children with high-risk retinoblastoma by reverse transcriptase-polymerase chain reaction for GD2 synthase mRNA. Eur J Cancer. 2013;49(13):2892–9.
150. Torbidoni AV, Laurent VE, Sampor C, Ottaviani D, Vazquez V, Gabri MR, et al. Association of cone-rod homeobox transcription factor messenger RNA with pediatric metastatic retinoblastoma. JAMA Ophthalmol. 2015;133(7):805–12.
151. Meredith DM, Charville GW, Fletcher CDM, Hornick JL. Distantly metastatic retinoblastoma to soft tissue and bone: a challenging diagnosis highlighting the utility of CRX. Am J Surg Pathol. 2021;45(6):820–4.
152. Laurent VE, Torbidoni AV, Sampor C, Ottaviani D, Vazquez V, Gabri MR, et al. Minimal disseminated disease in nonmetastatic retinoblastoma with high-risk pathologic features and association with disease-free survival. JAMA Ophthalmol. 2016;134(12):1374–9.
153. Dimaras H, Rushlow D, Halliday W, Doyle JJ, Babyn P, Abella EM, et al. Using RB1 mutations to assess minimal residual disease in metastatic retinoblastoma. Transl Res. 2010;156(2):91–7.
154. Racher H, Soliman S, Argiropoulos B, Chan HS, Gallie BL, Perrier R, et al. Molecular analysis distinguishes metastatic disease from second cancers in patients with retinoblastoma. Cancer Genet. 2016;209(7–8):359–63.
155. Andersson D, Fagman H, Dalin MG, Stahlberg A. Circulating cell-free tumor DNA analysis in pediatric cancers. Mol Aspects Med. 2020;72:100819.
156. Stewart CM, Tsui DWY. Circulating cell-free DNA for non-invasive cancer management. Cancer Genet. 2018;228–229:169–79.
157. Mandel P, Metais P. Nuclear acids in human blood plasma. C R Seances Soc Biol Fil. 1948;142(3–4):241–3.
158. Bronkhorst AJ, Ungerer V, Diehl F, Anker P, Dor Y, Fleischhacker M, et al. Towards systematic nomenclature for cell-free DNA. Hum Genet. 2021;140(4):565–78.
159. Ghiam BK, Xu L, Berry JL. Aqueous humor markers in retinoblastoma, a review. Transl Vis Sci Technol. 2019;8(2):13.
160. Munier FL, Gaillard MC, Balmer A, Soliman S, Podilsky G, Moulin AP, et al. Intravitreal chemotherapy for vitreous disease in retinoblastoma revisited: from prohibition to conditional indications. Br J Ophthalmol. 2012;96(8):1078–83.
161. Munier FL, Soliman S, Moulin AP, Gaillard MC, Balmer A, Beck-Popovic M. Profiling safety of intravitreal injections for retinoblastoma using an anti-reflux procedure and sterilisation of the needle track. Br J Ophthalmol. 2012;96(8):1084–7.
162. Francis JH, Abramson DH, Ji X, Shields CL, Teixeira LF, Schefler AC, et al. Risk of extraocular extension in eyes with retinoblastoma receiving intravitreous chemotherapy. JAMA Ophthalmol. 2017;135(12):1426–9.
163. Berry JL, Xu L, Kooi I, Murphree AL, Prabakar RK, Reid M, et al. Genomic cfDNA analysis of aqueous humor in retinoblastoma predicts eye salvage: the surrogate tumor biopsy for retinoblastoma. Mol Cancer Res. 2018;16(11):1701–12.
164. Xu L, Polski A, Prabakar RK, Reid MW, Chevez-Barrios P, Jubran R, et al. Chromosome 6p amplification in aqueous humor cell-free DNA is a prognostic biomarker for retinoblastoma ocular survival. Mol Cancer Res. 2020;18(8):1166–75.
165. Polski A, Xu L, Prabakar RK, Kim JW, Shah R, Jubran R, et al. Cell-free DNA tumor fraction in the aqueous humor is associated with therapeutic response in retinoblastoma patients. Transl Vis Sci Technol. 2020;9(10):30.
166. Berry JL, Xu L, Polski A, Jubran R, Kuhn P, Kim JW, et al. Aqueous humor is superior to blood as a liquid biopsy for retinoblastoma. Ophthalmology. 2019;127(4):552–4.
167. Kothari P, Marass F, Yang JL, Stewart CM, Stephens D, Patel J, et al. Cell-free DNA profiling in retinoblastoma patients with advanced intraocular disease: An MSKCC experience. Cancer Med. 2020;9(17):6093–101.
168. Berry JL, Cobrinik D, Hicks J. Potential of aqueous humor as a surrogate tumor biopsy for retinoblastoma-reply. JAMA Ophthalmol. 2018;136(5):598.
169. Lo YM, Corbetta N, Chamberlain PF, Rai V, Sargent IL, Redman CW, et al. Presence of fetal DNA in maternal plasma and serum. Lancet. 1997;350(9076):485–7.
170. Lo YM, Tein MS, Lau TK, Haines CJ, Leung TN, Poon PM, et al. Quantitative analysis of fetal DNA in maternal plasma and serum: implications for noninvasive prenatal diagnosis. Am J Hum Genet. 1998;62(4):768–75.
171. Saito H, Sekizawa A, Morimoto T, Suzuki M, Yanaihara T. Prenatal DNA diagnosis of a single-gene disorder from maternal plasma. Lancet. 2000;356(9236):1170.
172. Lo YM, Chan KC, Sun H, Chen EZ, Jiang P, Lun FM, et al. Maternal plasma DNA sequencing reveals the genome-wide genetic and mutational profile of the fetus. Sci Transl Med. 2010;2(61):61ra91.
173. Young E, Bowns B, Gerrish A, Parks M, Court S, Clokie S, et al. Clinical service delivery of noninvasive prenatal diagnosis by relative haplotype dosage for single-gene disorders. J Mol Diagn. 2020;22(9):1151–61.
174. Gerrish A, Bowns B, Mashayamombe-Wolfgarten C, Young E, Court S, Bott J, et al. Non-invasive prenatal diagnosis of retinoblastoma inheritance by combined targeted sequencing strategies. J Clin Med. 2020;9(11):3517.
175. Brennan RC, Federico S, Bradley C, Zhang J, Flores-Otero J, Wilson M, et al. Targeting the p53 pathway in retinoblastoma with subconjunctival nutlin-3a. Cancer Res. 2011;71(12):4205–13.
176. Grace CR, Ban D, Min J, Mayasundari A, Min L, Finch KE, et al. Monitoring ligand-induced protein ordering in drug discovery. J Mol Biol. 2016;428(6):1290–303.
177. Togashi K, Okada M, Suzuki S, Sanomachi T, Seino S, Yamamoto M, et al. Inhibition of retinoblastoma cell growth by CEP1347 through activation of the P53 pathway. Anticancer Res. 2020;40(9):4961–8.
178. Pontes de Carvalho RA, Krausse ML, Murphree AL, Schmitt EE, Campochiaro PA, Maumenee IH. Delivery from episcleral exoplants. Invest Ophthalmol Vis Sci. 2006;47(10):4532–9.
179. Phase I. Sustained-Release Topotecan Episcleral Plaque (Chemoplaque) for Retinoblastoma [Internet]; 2020. https://clinicaltrials.gov/ct2/show/NCT04428879.
180. Brodeur GM, Nichols KE, Plon SE, Schiffman JD, Malkin D. Pediatric cancer predisposition and surveillance: an overview, and a tribute to Alfred G. Knudson Jr. Clin Cancer Res. 2017;23(11):e1–5.
181. Kamihara J, Bourdeaut F, Foulkes WD, Molenaar JJ, Mosse YP, Nakagawara A, et al. Retinoblastoma and neuroblastoma predisposition and surveillance. Clin Cancer Res. 2017;23(13):e98–e106.

182. Friedman DN, Lis E, Sklar CA, Oeffinger KC, Reppucci M, Fleischut MH, et al. Whole-body magnetic resonance imaging (WB-MRI) as surveillance for subsequent malignancies in survivors of hereditary retinoblastoma: a pilot study. Pediatr Blood Cancer. 2014;61(8):1440–4.
183. Friedman DN, Hsu M, Moskowitz CS, Francis JH, Lis E, Fleischut MH, et al. Whole-body magnetic resonance imaging as surveillance for subsequent malignancies in preadolescent, adolescent, and young adult survivors of germline retinoblastoma: an update. Pediatr Blood Cancer. 2020;67(7):e28389.
184. Tonorezos ES, Friedman DN, Barnea D, Bosscha MI, Chantada G, Dommering CJ, et al. Recommendations for long-term follow-up of adults with heritable retinoblastoma. Ophthalmology. 2020;127(11):1549–57.
185. Flegg K, Gelkopf MJ, Johnson SA, Dimaras H. Canadian retinoblastoma research advisory board priority setting steering C. The top 10 retinoblastoma research priorities in Canada as determined by patients, clinicians and researchers: a patient-oriented priority-setting partnership. CMAJ Open. 2020;8(2):E420–E8.
186. Onken MD, Worley LA, Long MD, Duan S, Council ML, Bowcock AM, et al. Oncogenic mutations in GNAQ occur early in uveal melanoma. Invest Ophthalmol Vis Sci. 2008;49(12):5230–4.
187. Eskelin S, Pyrhonen S, Summanen P, Hahka-Kemppinen M, Kivela T. Tumor doubling times in metastatic malignant melanoma of the uvea: tumor progression before and after treatment. Ophthalmology. 2000;107(8):1443–9.
188. Collaborative Ocular Melanoma Study G. Assessment of metastatic disease status at death in 435 patients with large choroidal melanoma in the Collaborative Ocular Melanoma Study (COMS): COMS report no. 15. Arch Ophthalmol. 2001;119(5):670–6.
189. Diener-West M, Reynolds SM, Agugliaro DJ, Caldwell R, Cumming K, Earle JD, et al. Development of metastatic disease after enrollment in the COMS trials for treatment of choroidal melanoma: Collaborative Ocular Melanoma Study Group Report No. 26. Arch Ophthalmol. 2005;123(12):1639–43.
190. Prescher G, Bornfeld N, Hirche H, Horsthemke B, Jockel KH, Becher R. Prognostic implications of monosomy 3 in uveal melanoma. Lancet. 1996;347(9010):1222–5.
191. Sisley K, Rennie IG, Parsons MA, Jacques R, Hammond DW, Bell SM, et al. Abnormalities of chromosomes 3 and 8 in posterior uveal melanoma correlate with prognosis. Genes Chromosomes Cancer. 1997;19(1):22–8.
192. White VA, Chambers JD, Courtright PD, Chang WY, Horsman DE. Correlation of cytogenetic abnormalities with the outcome of patients with uveal melanoma. Cancer. 1998;83(2):354–9.
193. Harbour JW, Onken MD, Roberson ED, Duan S, Cao L, Worley LA, et al. Frequent mutation of BAP1 in metastasizing uveal melanomas. Science. 2010;330(6009):1410–3.
194. Onken MD, Worley LA, Davila RM, Char DH, Harbour JW. Prognostic testing in uveal melanoma by transcriptomic profiling of fine needle biopsy specimens. J Mol Diagn. 2006;8(5):567–73.
195. Onken MD, Worley LA, Ehlers JP, Harbour JW. Gene expression profiling in uveal melanoma reveals two molecular classes and predicts metastatic death. Cancer Res. 2004;64(20):7205–9.
196. Tschentscher F, Husing J, Holter T, Kruse E, Dresen IG, Jockel KH, et al. Tumor classification based on gene expression profiling shows that uveal melanomas with and without monosomy 3 represent two distinct entities. Cancer Res. 2003;63(10):2578–84.
197. Worley LA, Onken MD, Person E, Robirds D, Branson J, Char DH, et al. Transcriptomic versus chromosomal prognostic markers and clinical outcome in uveal melanoma. Clin Cancer Res. 2007;13(5):1466–71.
198. Onken MD, Worley LA, Char DH, Augsburger JJ, Correa ZM, Nudleman E, et al. Collaborative Ocular Oncology Group report number 1: prospective validation of a multi-gene prognostic assay in uveal melanoma. Ophthalmology. 2012;119(8):1596–603.
199. Field MG, Decatur CL, Kurtenbach S, Gezgin G, van der Velden PA, Jager MJ, et al. PRAME as an independent biomarker for metastasis in uveal melanoma. Clin Cancer Res. 2016;22(5):1234–42.
200. Cai L, Paez-Escamilla M, Walter SD, Tarlan B, Decatur CL, Perez BM, et al. Gene expression profiling and PRAME status versus tumor-node-metastasis staging for prognostication in uveal melanoma. Am J Ophthalmol. 2018;195:154–60.
201. Robertson AG, Shih J, Yau C, Gibb EA, Oba J, Mungall KL, et al. Integrative analysis identifies four molecular and clinical subsets in uveal melanoma. Cancer Cell. 2017;32(2):204–20 e15.
202. Jager MJ, Brouwer NJ, Esmaeli B. The cancer genome atlas project: an integrated molecular view of uveal melanoma. Ophthalmology. 2018;125(8):1139–42.
203. Mazloumi M, Vichitvejpaisal P, Dalvin LA, Yaghy A, Ewens KG, Ganguly A, et al. Accuracy of the cancer genome atlas classification vs american joint committee on cancer classification for prediction of metastasis in patients with uveal melanoma. JAMA Ophthalmol. 2020;138(3):260–7.
204. Damato B, Dopierala J, Klaasen A, van Dijk M, Sibbring J, Coupland SE. Multiplex ligation-dependent probe amplification of uveal melanoma: correlation with metastatic death. Invest Ophthalmol Vis Sci. 2009;50(7):3048–55.
205. Damato B, Dopierala JA, Coupland SE. Genotypic profiling of 452 choroidal melanomas with multiplex ligation-dependent probe amplification. Clin Cancer Res. 2010;16(24):6083–92.
206. Kujala E, Damato B, Coupland SE, Desjardins L, Bechrakis NE, Grange JD, et al. Staging of ciliary body and choroidal melanomas based on anatomic extent. J Clin Oncol. 2013;31(22):2825–31.
207. Damato B, Eleuteri A, Taktak AF, Coupland SE. Estimating prognosis for survival after treatment of choroidal melanoma. Prog Retin Eye Res. 2011;30(5):285–95.
208. Cunha Rola A, Taktak A, Eleuteri A, Kalirai H, Heimann H, Hussain R, et al. Multicenter external validation of the Liverpool uveal melanoma prognosticator online: an OOG collaborative study. Cancers (Basel). 2020;12(2):477.

Application of Deep Learning Models in the Evaluation of Histopathology of Uveal Melanoma

Sarah E. Coupland, Hongrun Zhang, Hayley Jones, and Yalin Zheng

1 Introduction

It is no longer adequate for the diagnostic histopathologist to classify cancer types based on morphology alone. Instead, there is an expectation that the pathologist integrates cancer morphology with immunohistology and any available genomic data ('tissue phenome') [1], in order to produce an integrated report using updated tumour classification and staging systems, e.g. those of the World Health Organization (WHO) and the American Joint Committee on Cancer/Tumor, Node, Metastasis (AJCC/TNM) systems, respectively. Furthermore, where possible, all other patient and available meta-data should be incorporated, potentially through the setting of a multidisciplinary tumour board meeting and subsequent follow-up visits. This current paradigm is based on the notion that 'complete knowledge' of disease-related information allows for educated decisions on the exact prognosis for individual patients, and thereby enables the selection of the best available treatment. Furthermore, it allows for the 'organised collation' of knowledge that will allow for improved therapies in the future [2–4]. Today, free or commercially available software solutions allow pathologists not only to collate available information, but also obtain more actionable knowledge and relevant insights when applying machine or deep learning solutions.

This above-mentioned paradigm also exists within ophthalmic pathology and oncology, as evidenced by the updated '4th WHO Volume of Eye Tumours' [5] and the eighth AJCC/TNM staging manual of ocular tumours [6]. Feeding into these important references are multi-collaborative studies, such as The Cancer Genome Atlas (TCGA) [7], which provided detailed information about uveal melanoma (UM). Of note, the UM-TCGA project, which examined 80 primary tumours, revealed valuable genomic data, linked not only to the clinical outcome but also to the digitalized images of the tumour specimens. This extensive library of information continues to be 'mined' by researchers, in order to better understand the biology of the disease but also to improve prognostication algorithms.

The main focus of this chapter will be the application of digital pathology (DP) and artificial intelligence (AI) in UM, and how these new technologies can aid histopathologists, serving as adjunctive tools. The basic principles applied to UM also can be utilized in other eye cancers, and indeed are already being done [8, 9].

2 Uveal Melanoma

Uveal melanoma is the most common primary intraocular malignancy in adults, with an incidence of between 5 and 8 individuals per million persons per year [10]. Although treatments for the ocular tumour have high rates of success in local control [11], approximately 50% of patients develop metastatic disease to the liver. Disseminated UM is currently incurable, although promising therapies are on the horizon [12]. Various parameters are well known for determining UM patient prognosis, and this enables their stratification into metastatic risk groups for surveillance of the liver [13]. Should the metastases be detected earlier, patients can either

S. E. Coupland (✉)
George Holt Chair of Pathology, Liverpool, UK
e-mail: s.e.coupland@liverpool.ac.uk

H. Zhang
Institute of Life Course and Medical Sciences/Institute of Systems, Molecular and Integrative Biology, University of Liverpool, Liverpool, UK
e-mail: Hongrun.Zhang@liverpool.ac.uk

H. Jones
Institute of Risk Management/Institute of Systems, Molecular and Integrative Biology, University of Liverpool, Liverpool, UK
e-mail: Hayley.Jones2@liverpool.ac.uk

Y. Zheng
Healthcare Eye and Vision Science, Institute of Life Course and Medical Sciences, University of Liverpool, Liverpool, UK
e-mail: yzheng@liverpool.ac.uk

B. V. Chawla, M. E. Aronow (eds.), *Global Perspectives in Ocular Oncology*, https://doi.org/10.1007/978-3-031-08250-4_21

Table 1 Published digital image analyses of UM (in chronological sequence)

Authors	Sample type	Parameter assessed	Methods used
Arnljots et al. [19]	Enucleation	Tumour volume	Pappus' second centroid theorem
Stålhammar et al. [25]	Enucleation	Nuclear BAP1 positivity based on IHC stains	QuPathBioimage analysis v.0.1.2
Stålhammar et al. [24]	Enucleation	PAS+ patterns and relationship to other metastasis-related risk parameters	QuPathBioimage analysis v.0.1.2
Sun et al. [26]	Enucleation	Nuclear BAP1 positivity based on IHC stains	DenseNet-121 based network and ImageNet
Herrspiegel et al. [20]	Enucleation	Tumour cell morphometry and relationship to other metastasis-related risk parameters	QuPathBioimage analysis v.0.1.2
Zhang et al. [27]	Enucleation	Nuclear BAP1 positivity based on H&E stains	Deep convolutional neural networks (Resnet18 pre-trained on ImageNet) and auto-encoder-decoders (U-net)
Slater et al. [22]	Tissue microarrays	Cytoplasmic protein expression	Visiopharm integrator system and Oncotopix (v.4.2.2.0)
Liu et al. [21]	FNAB	Gene expression profile on basis of H&E sections	Deep convolutional neural networks (Resnet-152)
Stålhammar et al. [23]	Enucleation	Heterogeneity of nuclear BAP1 positivity based on IHC stains	QuPathBioimage analysis v.0.2.3
Zhang et al. [28]	Enucleation	Nuclear BAP1 positivity based on H&E stains	Deep convolutional neural networks (ResNet-18, ResNet-50, DenseNet-121, AlexNet, and VGG-16); all pre-trained on ImageNet

undergo liver surgery for removal of metastatic UM nodules, or be registered into clinical trials [14].

Prognostic parameters for primary UM include clinical features (age and gender of the patient; intraocular tumour location; size and extent of tumour growth), and both histomorphological and genetic features of the tumour. Histomorphological features include the presence/absence of epithelioid cells, connective tissue loops, necrosis and extraocular melanoma growth. Further, the number of mitoses per 40 high power fields (HPF) in UM is associated with prognosis, with a cut-off of greater than 5/40 HPF being relevant [15].

With respect to the genetic features, one of the strongest parameters is the status of chromosome 3 in the UM cells: loss of one copy of chromosome 3 (i.e. monosomy 3) is associated with a poor prognosis [15]. Located on chromosome 3 (3p21.1) is the gene *BAP1* (BRCA1 associated protein-1), which encodes for the deubiquitinating enzyme, ubiquitin carboxy-terminal hydrolase. Somatic inactivating *BAP1* mutations have been reported in 18–48% of all UM, and in around 84% of UM with monosomy 3; this is strongly associated with metastasis and poor patient prognosis [16]. The bi-allelic inactivation of *BAP1* frequently leads to a loss of nuclear *BAP1* protein expression (nBAP1) on immunohistochemistry (IHC)—as such, it can be used as a surrogate marker since its nuclear expression corresponds to a high degree with both *BAP1* mutational and chromosome 3 status [17, 18].

Digital image analysis (DIA) of UM samples has been undertaken to improve the assessment of some of the above-mentioned parameters in histological sections and cytological spins [19–28]. The studies undertaken to date are summarized in Table 1. As can be observed from this table, the application of DIA with associated AI is at its infancy in UM, and remains at the moment in the domain of 'research-use only' applications.

3 Artificial Intelligence

Before progressing, it is important to provide some definitions of terms that appear in DP and AI written texts. The term AI dates back to more than 60 years ago when the availability of high-power hardware was limited [2]. Since then, the development of AI has in part been shaped by the field of neuroscience and other non-medical applications. By understanding the human brain, scientists have attempted to build new intelligent machines capable of performing complex tasks. While the development and application of AI algorithms has been fast paced, including in histopathology [1, 29–31], their actual use in clinical practice is still markedly below its potential. This is partly because for any new algorithm to be incorporated into existing or future laboratory workflows, it has to stand the test of thorough scientific validation and robust clinical utility without causing any harm or confusing the human factor [32–35]. Consequently, there is

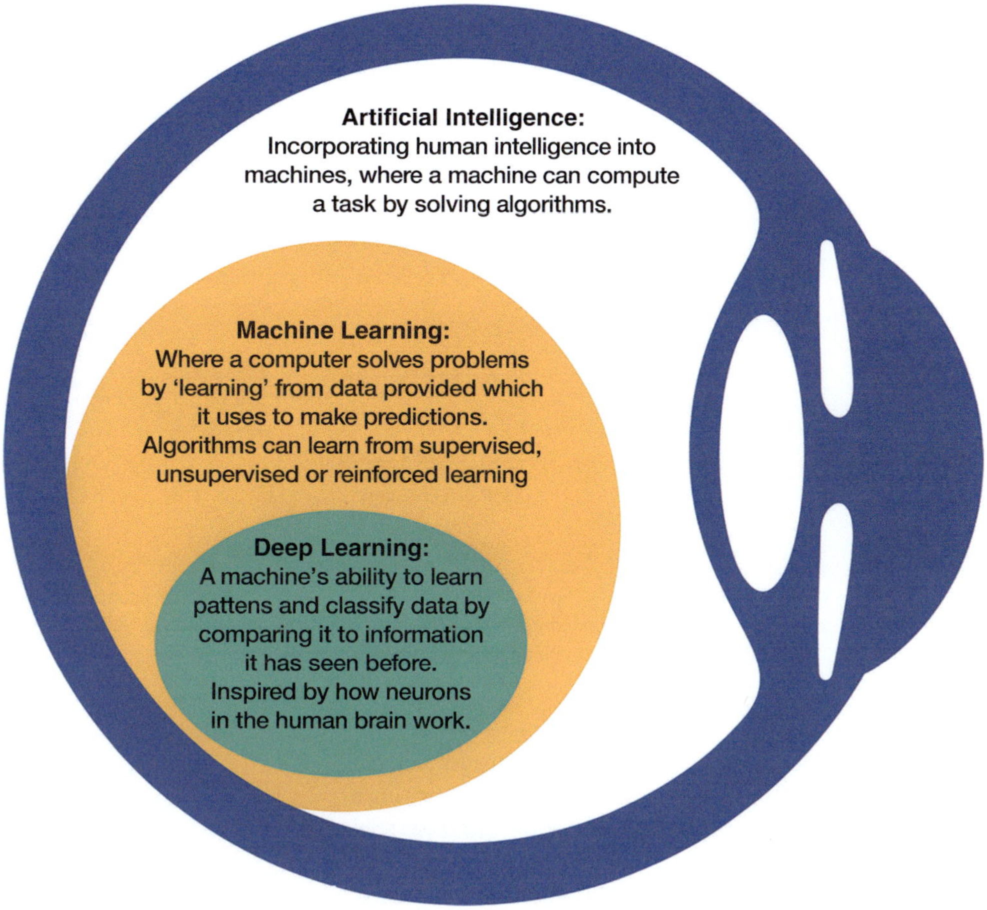

Fig. 1 Schematic representation explaining the relationship between artificial intelligence, machine learning and deep learning

much to be gained by combining AI and the human intelligence of experienced pathologists.

AI is a general concept that incorporates various specific subfields (Fig. 1), one of which is machine learning (ML), a computer science that can perform various tasks by learning from images and data without requiring the user to define explicit rules. ML has made tremendous progress in the last decades, especially in the fields of image analysis, natural language processing and pattern recognition. This development has been fostered by the availability of large data sets for training these systems as well as reasonably priced computing power, especially graphics processing units (GPU). With respect to pathology, this has led to the application of ML algorithms to recognize histopathological images captured usually using whole slide images (WSI) [34, 36–38].

Figure 2 shows typical steps for histopathological image analysis using machine learning. Prior to the application of ML algorithms, some pre-processing is usually performed. For example, when cancer regions of interest (ROI) are detected in WSI, local mini patches are sampled from the ROI in a large WSI [27, 39, 40]. These patches then go through the staining normalization procedure to eliminate the stain variances in each WSI [41]. In sequence, 'feature extraction' is made to extract useful information from mini patches that will be compatible to the subsequent ML algorithms. The feature extraction is often guided by expert knowledge to extract explicit features, such as size, shape and colour. Following feature extraction, classification by ML algorithms for target prediction is imposed on: (1) features of mini patches for individual patch prediction, or (2) slide representation features aggregated from the mini patch features for slide-level prediction. Typically, feature extraction and ML decision-making are separate process in traditional ML paradigm.

Within the family of ML methods is 'deep learning' (DL) (Fig. 1), which is based on 'deep' artificial neural networks with representation learning [34, 36–38]. DL algorithms, such as convolutional neural networks, start the analysis from 'feature extraction' and can generate novel insights depending on the quantity and quality of available data. Often referred to as 'end-to-end' approach, features and classifiers are simultaneously optimized in DL, which is the main difference between DL and traditional ML [42]. The features learned in DL often outperform other traditional

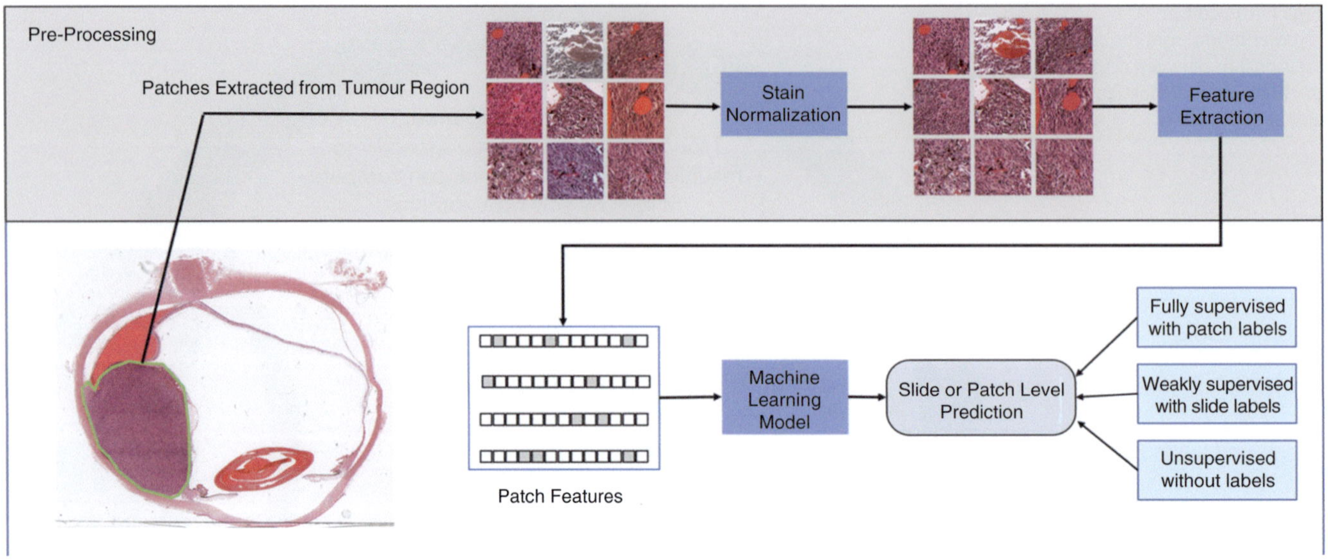

Fig. 2 Diagram illustrating the various steps involved in the interpretation of whole slide images of haematoxylin-and-eosin stained slides of uveal melanoma, with subsequent stain normalization, feature extraction, analysis of patch features, and then application of the machine learning, prior to a validation study using supervised and unsupervised patches

hand-crafted features in histopathological image analysis. Learning can be 'supervised,' 'semi-supervised' or 'unsupervised,' with each of these methods having differing goals and hence results.

In 2012, the ImageNet image classification by AlexNet [43] led to revolutionary successes in DL architecture and to the exponential growth in convolutional network methodologies, architectures and applications. This growth is fuelled by ever-increasing computational power (e.g. in the field of GPU development and deployment), the availability of freely available open-source packages (such as Caffe [44] or Tensorflow [45]) and the availability of robust big data.

These DL neural networks can perform wonderful feats thanks to their extremely large and complicated web of parameters. But their complexity could also be considered their curse: the inner workings of neural networks are often perceived as a mystery—i.e. a 'black box,' which has aroused some distrust. But the question remains whether the practising pathologist really needs to fully understand how any software comes to a certain conclusion coming from text, data or images, and how to trust the conclusion that comes from such a 'black box'. Ultimately, it is still the responsibility of the human factor (i.e. the pathologist) to validate and assess any software-based solutions regarding diagnostic plausibility and clinical utility, based on personal expert knowledge or empirical experience. What is certainly clear is that histopathologists have to try to keep up with this fast pace of innovation and development, and there are various teaching programmes across the globe trying to enable this.

4 Possible Solutions Through Software in Uveal Melanoma Diagnostics

The future is exciting for the application of digital pathology, artificial intelligence, deep and machine learning in uveal melanoma diagnostics and prognostication. Areas that can be explored in the future include:

A. *Tumour cell-related:*
   - Proportion of epithelioid cells within uveal melanoma sections, and thereby aiding the cellular subtyping of these tumours.
   - Mitosis counting per tumour area on histological sections.
   - Chromosome 3 status: on the basis of either histological sections or cytology.
   - Mutation status: on the basis of either histological sections or cytology.
   - Gene expression profiling prediction: on the basis of either histological sections or cytology.

B. *Non-tumour cell-related, considered to be of prognostic relevance:*
   - Inflammatory cell component and type (e.g. macrophages versus lymphocytes).
   - Extracellular matrix density.
   - Vascular patterns.

Challenges for real-world clinical use include the small datasets used in the existing research testing and validation studies in UM, and the relative lack of internal and external validation. These limitations could be overcome by multicentre collaborative studies, with investment in high-quality whole slide scanners and the involvement of multidisciplinary teams.

5 Conclusion

Digital pathology has already proven to be a reliable tool in the education and training of histopathologists and critical in translational research. Although still in its infancy, digital pathology in general and especially software-assisted decision support systems are here to stay and wait at the front door to enter routine histopathology given all the challenges ahead of pathologists. While there are still regulatory barriers, there are multiple reasons for the clinical adoption of this technology, including technical advances in the digital technology and the availability of cognitive computing. The question remains when to enter the routine use of clinical software support. Other clinical disciplines—e.g. radiology—have already embraced this 'disruptive technology' as the digital interface with the global community of domain experts, and to allow the real-time accessibility of all available data and best solution for comprehensive patient profiling and optimal therapy matching.

References

1. Huss R, Coupland SE. Software-assisted decision support in digital histopathology. J Pathol. 2020;250(5):685–92.
2. Howard J. Artificial intelligence: implications for the future of work. Am J Ind Med. 2019;62(11):917–26.
3. Pablo RJ, Roberto DP, Victor SU, Isabel GR, Paul C, Elizabeth OR. Big data in the healthcare system: a synergy with artificial intelligence and blockchain technology. J Integr Bioinform. 2021;19(1):20200035.
4. Yu KH, Beam AL, Kohane IS. Artificial intelligence in healthcare. Nat Biomed Eng. 2018;2(10):719–31.
5. Grossniklaus HE, Eberhart CG, Kivela TT. WHO classification of the tumours of the eye. Lyon: IARC; 2018.
6. Finger PT, Coupland SE. AJCC cancer staging manual. New York: Springer; 2017.
7. Robertson AG, Shih J, Yau C, Gibb EA, Oba J, Mungall KL, Hess JM, Uzunangelov V, Walter V, Danilova L, Lichtenberg TM, Kucherlapati M, Kimes PK, Tang M, Penson A, Babur O, Akbani R, Bristow CA, Hoadley KA, Iype L, Chang MT, Network TR, Cherniack AD, Benz C, Mills GB, Verhaak RGW, Griewank KG, Felau I, Zenklusen JC, Gershenwald JE, Schoenfield L, Lazar AJ, Abdel-Rahman MH, Roman-Roman S, Stern MH, Cebulla CM, Williams MD, Jager MJ, Coupland SE, Esmaeli B, Kandoth C, Woodman SE. Integrative analysis identifies four molecular and clinical subsets in uveal melanoma. Cancer Cell. 2018;33(1):151.
8. Strijbis VIJ, de Bloeme CM, Jansen RW, Kebiri H, Nguyen HG, de Jong MC, Moll AC, Bach-Cuadra M, de Graaf P, Steenwijk MD. Multi-view convolutional neural networks for automated ocular structure and tumor segmentation in retinoblastoma. Sci Rep. 2021;11(1):14590.
9. Wang L, Ding L, Liu Z, Sun L, Chen L, Jia R, Dai X, Cao J, Ye J. Automated identification of malignancy in whole-slide pathological images: identification of eyelid malignant melanoma in gigapixel pathological slides using deep learning. Br J Ophthalmol. 2020;104(3):318–23.
10. Jager MJ, Shields CL, Cebulla CM, Abdel-Rahman MH, Grossniklaus HE, Stern MH, Carvajal RD, Belfort RN, Jia R, Shields JA, Damato BE. Uveal melanoma. Nat Rev Dis Primers. 2020;6(1):24.
11. Damato B, Heimann H. Personalized treatment of uveal melanoma. Eye (Lond). 2013;27(2):172–9.
12. Nathan P, Hassel JC, Rutkowski P, Baurain JF, Butler MO, Schlaak M, Sullivan RJ, Ochsenreither S, Dummer R, Kirkwood JM, Joshua AM, Sacco JJ, Shoushtari AN, Orloff M, Piulats JM, Milhem M, Salama AKS, Curti B, Demidov L, Gastaud L, Mauch C, Yushak M, Carvajal RD, Hamid O, Abdullah SE, Holland C, Goodall H, Piperno-Neumann S, IMCgp100-202 Investigators. Overall survival benefit with Tebentafusp in metastatic uveal melanoma. N Engl J Med. 2021;385(13):1196–206.
13. Cunha Rola A, Taktak A, Eleuteri A, Kalirai H, Heimann H, Hussain R, Bonnett LJ, Hill CJ, Traynor M, Jager MJ, Marinkovic M, Luyten GPM, Dogrusoz M, Kilic E, de Klein A, Smit K, van Poppelen NM, Damato BE, Afshar A, Guthoff RF, Scheef BO, Kakkassery V, Saakyan S, Tsygankov A, Mosci C, Ligorio P, Viaggi S, Le Guin CHD, Bornfeld N, Bechrakis NE, Coupland SE. Multicenter external validation of the Liverpool uveal melanoma prognosticator online: an OOG collaborative study. Cancers (Basel). 2020;12(2):477.
14. Sacco JJ, Kalirai H, Kenyani J, Figueiredo CR, Coulson JM, Coupland SE. Recent breakthroughs in metastatic uveal melanoma: a cause for optimism? Future Oncol. 2018;14(14):1335–8.
15. Damato B, Duke C, Coupland SE, Hiscott P, Smith PA, Campbell I, Douglas A, Howard P. Cytogenetics of uveal melanoma: a 7-year clinical experience. Ophthalmology. 2007;114(10):1925–31.
16. Harbour JW, Onken MD, Roberson ED, Duan S, Cao L, Worley LA, M. L. Council, Matatall KA, Helms C, Bowcock AM. Frequent mutation of BAP1 in metastasizing uveal melanomas. Science. 2010;330(6009):1410–3.
17. Farquhar N, Thornton S, Coupland SE, Coulson JM, Sacco JJ, Krishna Y, Heimann H, Taktak A, Cebulla CM, Abdel-Rahman MH, Kalirai H. Patterns of BAP1 protein expression provide insights into prognostic significance and the biology of uveal melanoma. J Pathol Clin Res. 2018;4(1):26–38.
18. Kalirai H, Dodson A, Faqir S, Damato BE, Coupland SE. Lack of BAP1 protein expression in uveal melanoma is associated with increased metastatic risk and has utility in routine prognostic testing. Br J Cancer. 2014;111(7):1373–80.
19. Arnljots TS, Al-Sharbaty Z, Lardner E, All-Eriksson C, Seregard S, Stålhammar G. Tumour thickness, diameter, area or volume? The prognostic significance of conventional versus digital image analysis-based size estimation methods in uveal melanoma. Acta Ophthalmol. 2018;96(5):510–8.
20. Herrspiegel C, See TRO, Mendoza PR, Grossniklaus HE, Stålhammar G. Digital morphometry of tumor nuclei correlates to BAP-1 status, monosomy 3, gene expression class and survival in uveal melanoma. Exp Eye Res. 2020;193:107987.
21. Liu TA, Zhu H, Chen H, Arevalo JF, Hui FK, Paul HY, Wei J, Unberath M, Correa ZM. Gene expression profile prediction in uveal melanoma using deep learning: a pilot study for the development of an alternative survival prediction tool. Ophthalmol Retina. 2020;4(12):1213–5.
22. Slater K, Heeran AB, Garcia-Mulero S, Kalirai H, Sanz-Pamplona R, Rahman A, Al-Attar N, Helmi M, O'Connell F, Bosch R, Portela A, Villanueva A, Gallagher WM, Jensen LD, Piulats JM, Coupland SE, O'Sullivan J, Kennedy BN. High cysteinyl leukotriene receptor 1 expression correlates with poor survival of uveal melanoma

patients and cognate antagonist drugs modulate the growth, cancer secretome, and metabolism of uveal melanoma cells. Cancers. 2020;12(10):2950.
23. Stålhammar G, Grossniklaus HE. Intratumor heterogeneity in uveal melanoma BAP-1 expression. Cancers. 2021;13(5):1143.
24. Stålhammar G, See TRO, Phillips S, Seregard S, Grossniklaus HE. Digital image analysis of BAP-1 accurately predicts uveal melanoma metastasis. Transl Vis Sci Technol. 2019;8(3):11.
25. Stålhammar G, See TRO, Phillips SS, Grossniklaus HE. Density of PAS positive patterns in uveal melanoma: correlation with vasculogenic mimicry, gene expression class, BAP-1 expression, macrophage infiltration, and risk for metastasis. Mol Vis. 2019;25:502–16.
26. Sun M, Zhou W, Qi X, Zhang G, Girnita L, Seregard S, Grossniklaus HE, Yao Z, Zhou X, Stålhammar G. Prediction of BAP1 expression in uveal melanoma using densely-connected deep classification networks. Cancers (Basel). 2019;11(10):1579.
27. Zhang H, Kalirai H, Acha-Sagredo A, Yang X, Zheng Y, Coupland SE. Piloting a deep learning model for predicting nuclear BAP1 immunohistochemical expression of uveal melanoma from hematoxylin-and-eosin sections. Transl Vis Sci Technol. 2020;9(2):50.
28. Zhang H, Meng Y, Qian X, Yang X, Coupland SE, Zheng Y. A regularization term for slide correlation reduction in whole slide image analysis with deep learning. Proceedings of Machine Learning Research (Medical Imaging with Deep Learning (MIDL)); 2021:1–13.
29. Howard FM, Dolezal J, Kochanny S, Schulte J, Chen H, Heij L, Huo D, Nanda R, Olopade OI, Kather JN, Cipriani N, Grossman RL, Pearson AT. The impact of site-specific digital histology signatures on deep learning model accuracy and bias. Nat Commun. 2021;12(1):4423.
30. Krause J, Grabsch HI, Kloor M, Jendrusch M, Echle A, Buelow RD, Boor P, Luedde T, Brinker TJ, Trautwein C, Pearson AT, Quirke P, Jenniskens J, Offermans K, van den Brandt PA, Kather JN. Deep learning detects genetic alterations in cancer histology generated by adversarial networks. J Pathol. 2021;254(1):70–9.
31. Schneider L, Laiouar-Pedari S, Kuntz S, Krieghoff-Henning E, Hekler A, Kather JN, Gaiser T, Frohling S, Brinker TJ. Integration of deep learning-based image analysis and genomic data in cancer pathology: a systematic review. Eur J Cancer. 2021;160:80–91.
32. Bengtsson E, Danielsen H, Treanor D, Gurcan MN, MacAulay C, Molnar B. Computer-aided diagnostics in digital pathology. Cytometry A. 2017;91(6):551–4.
33. Colling R, Pitman H, Oien K, Rajpoot N, Macklin P, CM-Path AI in Histopathology Working Group, Snead D, Sackville T, Verrill C. Artificial intelligence in digital pathology: a roadmap to routine use in clinical practice. J Pathol. 2019;249(2):143–50.
34. van der Laak J, Litjens G, Ciompi F. Deep learning in histopathology: the path to the clinic. Nat Med. 2021;27(5):775–84.
35. Williams BJ, Treanor D. Practical guide to training and validation for primary diagnosis with digital pathology. J Clin Pathol. 2020;73(7):418–22.
36. Ehteshami Bejnordi B, Veta M, Johannes van Diest P, van Ginneken B, Karssemeijer N, Litjens G, van der Laak J, Hermsen M, Manson QF, Balkenhol M, Geessink O, Stathonikos N, van Dijk MC, Bult P, Beca F, Beck AH, Wang D, Khosla A, Gargeya R, Irshad H, Zhong A, Dou Q, Li Q, Chen H, Lin HJ, Heng PA, Haß C, Bruni E, Wong Q, Halici U, Öner M, Cetin-Atalay R, Berseth M, Khvatkov V, Vylegzhanin A, Kraus O, Shaban M, Rajpoot N, Awan R, Sirinukunwattana K, Qaiser T, Tsang YW, Tellez D, Annuscheit J, Hufnagl P, Valkonen M, Kartasalo K, Latonen L, Ruusuvuori P, Liimatainen K, Albarqouni S, Mungal B, George A, Demirci S, Navab N, Watanabe S, Seno S, Takenaka Y, Matsuda H, Ahmady Phoulady H, Kovalev V, Kalinovsky A, Liauchuk V, Bueno G, Fernandez-Carrobles MM, Serrano I, Deniz O, Racoceanu D, Venâncio R. Diagnostic assessment of deep learning algorithms for detection of lymph node metastases in women with breast cancer. JAMA. 2017;318(22):2199–210.
37. Litjens G, Kooi T, Bejnordi BE, Setio AAA, Ciompi F, Ghafoorian M, van der Laak J, van Ginneken B, Sanchez CI. A survey on deep learning in medical image analysis. Med Image Anal. 2017;42:60–88.
38. Litjens G, Sánchez CI, Timofeeva N, Hermsen M, Nagtegaal I, Kovacs I, Hulsbergen-van de Kaa C, Bult P, van Ginneken B, van der Laak J. Deep learning as a tool for increased accuracy and efficiency of histopathological diagnosis. Sci Rep. 2016;6:26286.
39. Hou L, Samaras D, Kurc TM, Gao Y, Davis JE, Saltz JH. Patch-based convolutional neural network for whole slide tissue image classification. Proc IEEE Comput Soc Conf Comput Vis Pattern Recognit. 2016;2016:2424–33.
40. Kosaraju SC, Hao J, Koh HM, Kang M. Deep-Hipo: multi-scale receptive field deep learning for histopathological image analysis. Methods. 2020;179:3–13.
41. Macenko M, Niethammer M, Marron JS, Borland D, Woosley JT, Guan X, C. Schmitt and N. E. Thomas A method for normalizing histology slides for quantitative analysis. 2009 IEEE International Symposium on Biomedical Imaging: From Nano to Macro, IEEE; 2009.
42. Echle A, Rindtorff NT, Brinker TJ, Luedde T, Pearson AT, Kather JN. Deep learning in cancer pathology: a new generation of clinical biomarkers. Br J Cancer. 2021;124(4):686–96.
43. Krizhevsky A, Sutskever I, Hinton GE. ImageNet Classification with Deep Convolutional Neural Networks; 2012
44. Jia, Y., E. Shelhamer, J. Donahue, S. Karayev, J. Long, R. Girshick, S. Guadarrama and T. Darrell (2015). Caffe: convolutional architecture for fast feature embedding.
45. Abadi M, Agarwal A, Barham P, Brevdo E, Chen Z, Citro C, Corrado GS, Davis A, Dean J, Devin M, Ghemawat S, Goodfellow I, Harp A, Irving G, Isard M, Jia Y, Jozefowicz R, Kaiser L, Kudlur M, Levenberg J, Mane D, Monga R, Moore S, Murray D, Olah C, Schuster M, Shlens J, Steiner B, Sutskever I, Talwar K, Tucker P, Vanhoucke V, Vasudevan V, Viegas F, Vinyals O, Warden P, Wattenberg M, Wicke M, Yu Y, Zheng X. TensorFlow: large-scale machine learning on heterogeneous distributed systems. arXiv preprint arXiv. 2016:1603.04467.

Developing Prognostic Tools for Estimating Risk of Metastatic Death and Non-Metastatic Death in Individuals with Choroidal Melanoma

Bertil E. Damato, Antonio Eleuteri, Azzam F. G. Taktak, Heinrich Heimann, and Sarah E. Coupland

1 Introduction

Choroidal melanoma is fatal in approximately 50% of all patients, usually as a result of hematogenous metastatic spread to the liver [1]. Metastatic disease usually develops after ocular treatment, months or years after apparent good health. Studies based on tumor-doubling times suggest that lethal uveal melanomas start to metastasize years before treatment of the primary tumor [2, 3].

It is useful to determine not only whether a patient with choroidal melanoma will die of metastatic disease but also to estimate when death is likely to happen. If convincing, a low risk of metastatic death should enhance patients' well-being, while also minimizing expenditure on long-term systemic surveillance. This would benefit both patients and over-stretched healthcare services. Conversely, a high risk of metastatic death would enable counseling, systemic surveillance, and possibly systemic adjuvant therapy to be targeted at patients in greatest need of such care. A prognostic tool would also indicate change in risk of metastatic death over time in each affected patient, so that frequency of liver imaging could be adjusted accordingly.

An accurate prognostic tool also enhances opportunities for evaluating the impact of ocular and systemic therapies on survival. For example, with sufficient data, risk of metastatic death after endoresection could be compared to that after enucleation or radiotherapy, with stratification according to known predictive factors.

The standard tool for predicting metastatic mortality after treatment of choroidal melanoma is the Tumor, Node, Metastasis (TNM) staging system of the American Joint Committee on Cancer (AJCC) [4]. This estimates survival probability according to largest basal tumor diameter, tumor thickness, ciliary body involvement, and extraocular spread. The prognostic accuracy of this tool is limited by its reliance on anatomic predictors without exploiting highly informative histologic and genetic data and by failing to account for the effects of deaths from other causes, hence providing biased estimates of metastatic mortality. TNM staging is therefore relevant only to large groups of patients (as in clinical trials) and not individual patients.

In 2007, we developed a prognostic index to provide Kaplan–Meier estimates of risk of metastatic death according to chromosome-3 loss, largest basal tumor diameter, and presence of epithelioid cells (Fig. 1) [5]. This model had several weaknesses, such as (1) over-predicting metastatic mortality because of bias caused by censoring non-metastatic deaths; (2) bias caused by missing data; (3) inability to estimate risk in patients with rare combinations of metastasis predictors; and (4) inaccuracy caused by non-linear associations between continuous variables (e.g., basal tumor diameter) and metastatic death.

B. E. Damato (✉)
Nuffield Laboratory of Ophthalmology, University of Oxford, Oxford, UK

Ocular Oncology Service, Moorfields Eye Hospital, London, UK

Department of Ocular Oncology, Royal Liverpool University Hospital, Liverpool, UK

Department of Molecular and Clinical Cancer Medicine, Institute of Systems, Molecular and Integrative Biology, University of Liverpool, Liverpool, UK
e-mail: Bertil.Damato@NHS.net

A. Eleuteri · A. F. G. Taktak
Department of Medical Physics and Clinical Engineering, Liverpool University Hospitals NHS Foundation Trust, University of Liverpool, Liverpool, UK

Department of Physics, University of Liverpool, Liverpool, UK
e-mail: antonio.eleuteri@liverpool.ac.uk; afgt@liverpool.ac.uk

H. Heimann
Department of Ocular Oncology, Royal Liverpool University Hospital, Liverpool, UK
e-mail: heinrich.heimann@rlbuht.nhs.uk

S. E. Coupland
Department of Molecular and Clinical Cancer Medicine, Institute of Systems, Molecular and Integrative Biology, University of Liverpool, Liverpool, UK
e-mail: s.e.coupland@liverpool.ac.uk

B. V. Chawla, M. E. Aronow (eds.), *Global Perspectives in Ocular Oncology*, https://doi.org/10.1007/978-3-031-08250-4_22

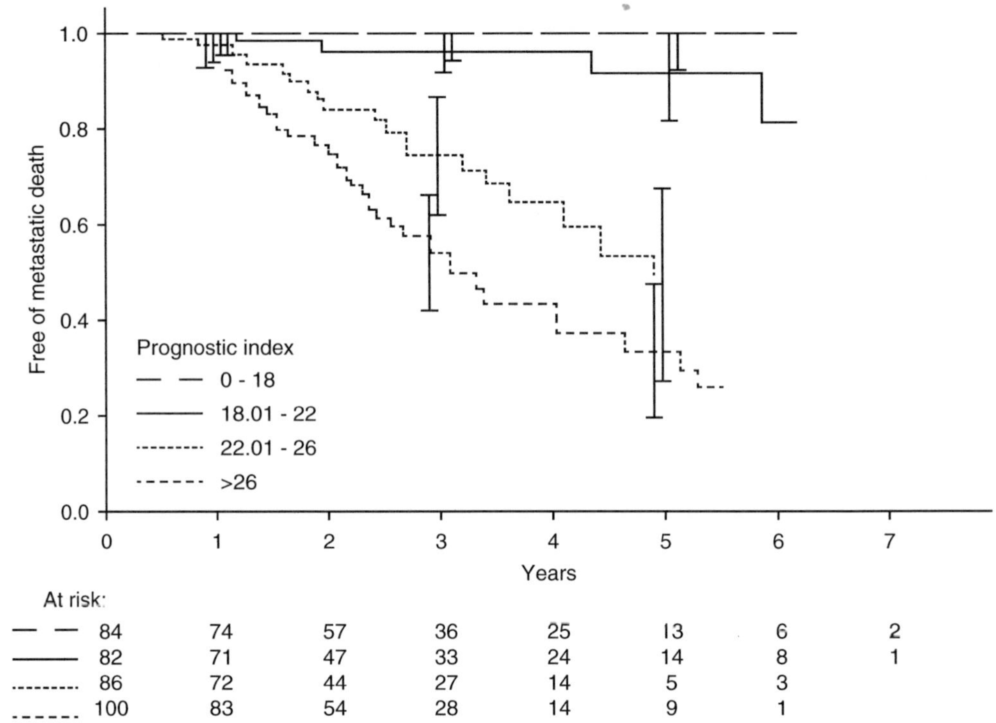

Fig. 1 Kaplan–Meier survival curves showing disease-specific mortality according to prognostic index, which was computed from largest basal tumor diameter in millimeters, plus 5 (if monosomy 3 was present), and plus 6 (if epithelioid cells were present). (Damato, B. et al. Cytogenetics of Uveal Melanoma: A 7-Year Clinical Experience. Ophthalmology. 114, (10), 2007, 1925–1931)

These shortcomings were addressed by developing the Liverpool Uveal Melanoma Prognosticator Online (LUMPO) [6]. The earliest version used artificial neural networks to model metastatic mortality, censoring deaths from other causes, and inferring risk of metastatic death by comparing model predictions of mortality of patients with choroidal melanoma with that of the general population, matched by age and sex (Fig. 2). An enhanced version of the model, LUMPO II, was published a few years later, which did not use an artificial neural network model, but an accelerated failure time model, which also implemented multiple imputation of missing data, thus improving the quality of model predictions [7]. This version of the tool was validated externally in a study comparing data from 390 patients treated at the University of California, San Francisco, with 1175 patients treated at the Liverpool Ocular Oncology Centre [8]. In both groups of patients, no statistical differences were found between predicted and observed survival, with respect to all-cause mortality and metastatic mortality.

In 2018, LUMPO II was superseded by LUMPO III, which predicts metastatic death specifically instead of inferring risk according to all-cause mortality [9]. This chapter describes LUMPO III and discusses its strengths as well as problems with its deployment in centers around the world.

2 LUMPO III

2.1 Access

The LUMPO III program, version 10.1, is easily reached by searching online for "LUMPO" (https://mpcetoolsforhealth.liverpool.ac.uk/LUMPONet/LUMPONet.html, accessed on October 8, 2021).

2.2 Data Input

The online form allows the following data to be entered: (1) demographics (date, patient's name and medical record number, practitioner's name and position, age (range, 40–79 years) and sex); (2) anatomic tumor features (diameter and thickness (rounded to whole numbers), ciliary body involvement, and extraocular spread (absent, <=5 mm, >5 mm)); (3) histologic features (melanoma cell type (epithelioid cells present or absent), presence of closed loops and mitotic count per 40 high-power fields (0–1,2-3,4–7,>7)); (4) genetic type (chromosome 3 loss and 8q gain (no, yes, not available)); and, for the purpose of computing TNM stage, metastatic status (i.e., disease in regional lymph nodes and distant organs) (Fig. 3). For patients undergoing systemic surveillance, the program also indicates when the next liver scan should be performed,

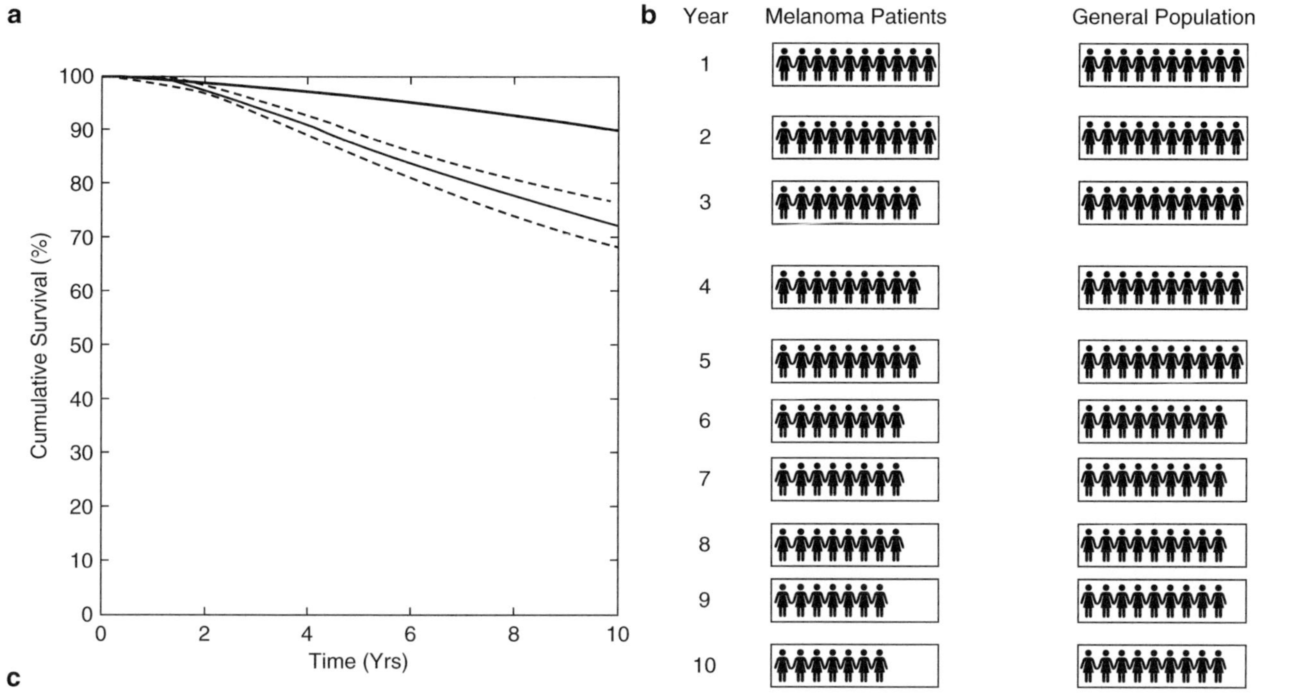

c

Year	0	1	2	3	4	5	6	7	8	9	10
Number of close matches in database*	102	95	86	78	61	53	50	44	39	35	26
Survival in General population	100	99.32	98.59	97.79	96.91	95.94	94.88	93.74	92.50	91.14	89.69
Predicted Survival	100	99.15	97.31	94.43	90.90	87.19	83.63	80.36	77.39	74.69	72.22
Relative Survival§	100	99.82	98.70	96.56	93.81	90.88	88.14	85.72	83.67	81.96	80.52

**Close matches are determined by grouping age to the nearest decade and largest tumour diameter into < 10, 10-15 and > 15 mm categories*

§Calculated as (Predicted from patient population)/(Observed from general population)

Fig. 2 (**a**) Curves showing 10-year all-cause survival of a 60-year-old woman with a low-grade 13-mm choroidal melanoma (thin solid line) as compared with survival of the age-matched female population in Britain (thick solid line). Dashed lines define the 95% credibility interval. (**b**) Pictogram showing survival of patients with choroidal melanoma and of the matched British population. (**c**) Number of close matches in database, survival in general population, survival in melanoma patients, and relative survival. (Damato et al. Artificial Neural Networks Estimating Survival Probability after Treatment of Choroidal Melanoma. Ophthalmology. 115(9), 2008, 1598–1607)

according to the date of the latest scan, the estimated survival time after detection of metastasis, and the number of negative scans that would be acceptable for each positive scan.

2.3 Output

LUMPO III gives the following outputs: (1) all-cause survival probability, (2) probability of death from metastasis, and (3) probability of death from other causes. These are estimated for each post-treatment year up to a maximum of 10 years. Prognostications are provided as text as well as in a table, graph, boxplot, and, to aid communication with patients, a pictogram. The program also computes the TNM size category and stage.

2.4 Data Collection

The model was developed with data from 4161 patients treated at the Liverpool Ocular Oncology Centre, UK, for uveal melanoma involving choroid and if they resided in England, Scotland, or Wales. The patients comprised 2142 males and 2019 females, with a median age of 62.5 years.

Diagnosis was based on clinical findings on ophthalmoscopy and slit-lamp examination and, if these were inconclusive, on tumor biopsy. Largest basal tumor diameter and tumor thickness were measured by ultrasonography, which was also used to detect extraocular spread. Tumor dimensions were rounded to whole numbers, because of the limited accuracy of ultrasonography (i.e., +/− 0.5 mm). Choroidal tumors were categorized as involving ciliary body even if

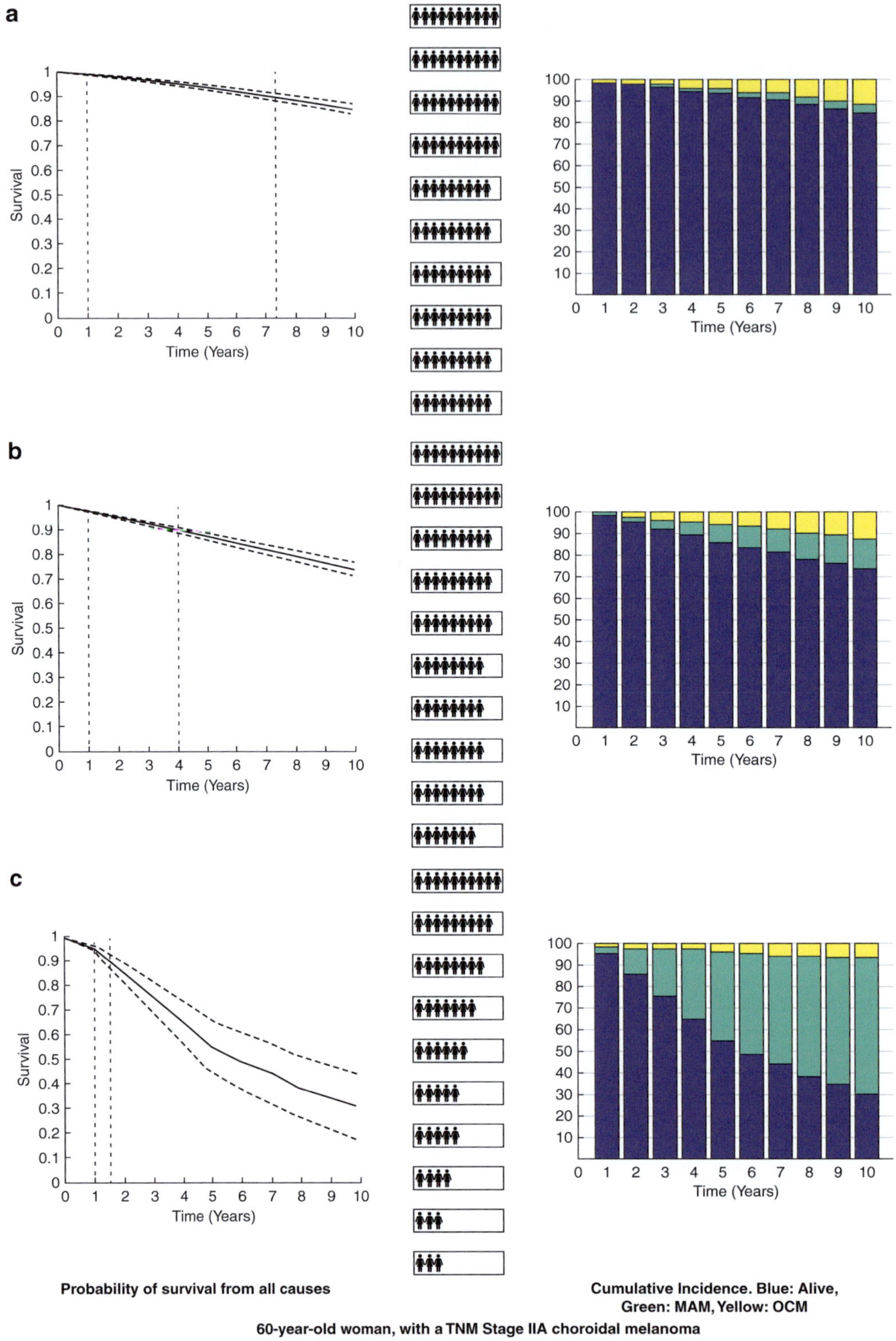

Fig. 3 LUMPO III outputs showing graphs indicating probability of survival from all causes on left, and bar charts indicating cumulative incidences of survival, melanoma-associated mortality (MAM) and mortality from other causes (OCM) for a 60-year-old woman with a choroidal melanoma having a basal diameter of 13 mm and a thickness of 6 mm, without ciliary body involvement or extraocular spread (TNM T size category, 2a; stage, IIA) (**a**) Low-grade histology and no lethal chromosomal abnormalities, indicating 10-year probabilities of survival, metastatic death and non-metastatic death of 0.85, 0.04, and 0.11, respectively. This model also suggests that after a normal scan 1 year after treatment the next scan should be performed 6 years and 4 months later for it to have a 1-in-10 chance of detecting metastases, assuming a 6-month survival time after detection of metastases. (**b**) Without histologic and genetic data, the 10-year probabilities of survival, metastatic death, and non-metastatic death are 0.74, 0.14, and 0.12, respectively, with the time to next scan estimated at 3 years, for a 1-in-10 chance of positivity. (**c**) High-grade pathology with chromosome-3 loss and 8q gain, indicating 0.31-, 0.63-, and 0.06–10-year probabilities of survival, metastatic death, and non-metastatic death, respectively, with time to next scan shortened to 6 months. According to the TNM staging system, the 10-year survival probability is 0.85

they extended only to pars plana. The tumors had a median basal diameter and median thickness of 12.4 mm and 5.0 mm respectively, with 26.5% involving ciliary body and 6.7% extending extraocularly.

Histologic grade of malignancy was determined by light microscopy, using hematoxylin and eosin stains for melanoma cytomorphology and PAS without counter stain for assessing extravascular matrix patterns. Epithelioid cells and closed loops were found in 58.1% of 2187 cases and 49.9% of 1198 cases with a mitotic count exceeding 7 per 40 high-power fields in 17.5% of 1762 cases.

Chromosome 3 loss, chromosome 8q gain and other genetic aberrations were identified by a succession of techniques as more sensitive methods became available over the years. These methods included: fluorescence in-situ hybridization (FISH), microsatellite analysis, multiplex ligation-dependent probe amplification (MLPA), and immunohistochemical assessment of nuclear BAP1 protein expression [5, 10, 11].

Most patients were treated by plaque brachytherapy, proton beam radiotherapy, local resection and laser therapy, or a combination of these modalities, resorting to enucleation when such methods were considered unlikely to succeed [12].

Patients considered to have a high-risk of metastatic disease were referred to an oncologist for long-term surveillance, which consisted of liver ultrasonography or, preferably, magnetic resonance imaging. Metastatic disease, which almost always involved the liver, was treated with various forms of chemotherapy or immunotherapy or, in rare cases, by partial hepatectomy.

At the time of diagnosis of the ocular tumor, demographic data on all patients were sent to the National Health Service (NHS) Cancer Registry, which automatically informed us of the date and certified cause of death of any patients who had died in the previous month. The median follow-up was 6.5 years (quartiles range, 3.19–11.61), exceeding 5 years in 2512 patients and 10 years in 1264. A total of 1665 deaths were recorded, 893 attributed to metastatic disease and 772 to other causes.

Clinical, pathologic, and cytogenetic data were collected contemporaneously, during clinical consultations, using synoptic paper forms that prevented free text, except for concurrent ocular and systemic disease. Within a few days, a data manager entered this information into a computerized registry, which was based on Advanced Revelation software (OpenInsight, Westwood, NJ, USA) and which was customized for our oncology service and maintained by a team of software engineers (Sprezzatura Ltd., London, UK).

2.5 LUMPO Model

LUMPO III was implemented as a Markov state-space model with semi-parametric Cox transition intensities, to predict (1) absolute risk of non-metastatic death, estimated according to age and sex, and (2) absolute risk of metastatic death, which also included the anatomic, histologic, and genetic predictors mentioned above. A detailed description of the mathematical methods is beyond the scope of this article, but described in a paper by Eleuteri et al. [9]

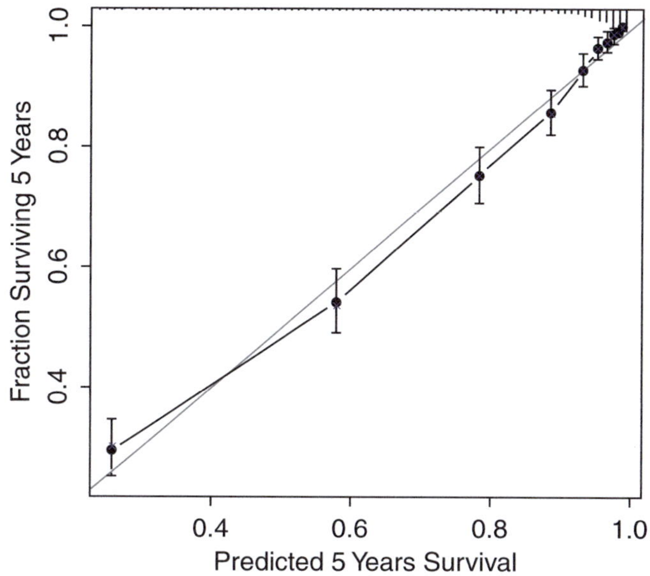

Fig. 4 Calibration performance, showing the model's predicted 5-year survival vs. observed fraction. The dots represent the estimated performance. The crosses represent the estimated performance corrected for optimism. The straight line represents the ideal prediction. The black vertical dashes at the top of the graph are a "rug plot" showing the distribution of predicted all-cause survival. (Eleuteri A. et al. Prognostication of metastatic death in uveal melanoma patients: A Markov multi-state model. Computers in Biology and Medicine. 102, 2018, 151–156)

2.6 Internal Validation

The ability of LUMPO III to rank outcomes as a function of predictive factors (i.e., discrimination) was expressed in terms of the C-index, which was 0.86 (95% confidence interval, 0.84–0.88) (Fig. 4). (C-indices over 0.7 and 0.8 indicate good and strong models respectively). Comparisons between predicted and actual metastatic mortality in different risk groups (i.e., calibration) showed that LUMPO III reliably provides personalized metastatic death prognostication [9].

2.7 External Validation

Cunha-Rola et al. evaluated LUMPO III with anonymized data of 1836 patients from seven ocular oncology centers around the world [13]. The C-index measuring discrimination was 0.72 (95% confidence interval, 0.68–0.75). Agreement between observed and predicted survival probabilities was generally good although all-cause survival probability was over-predicted in some centers and under-predicted in others. This is possibly because of inconsistent categorization of predictive factors such as tumor cell type, ciliary body involvement, and extravascular matrix patterns. For example, the prevalence of tumors with epithelioid cells varied between centers from 3% to 100%. Furthermore, the sensitivity with which chromosome 3 loss and 8q gain were detected varied according to the analytic methods that were used. Figure 3 shows how probability of metastatic death varies greatly according to whether or not predictors are detected. Apart from validating LUMPO III, Cunha-Rola's study highlights how important it is for all users to assess and categorize metastasis predictors in a standardized fashion, ideally also performing their own validations before deploying this tool in their practice.

3 Prognostic Tables

The author and associates have prepared a set of prognostic tables for situations where TNM staging and LUMPO III are not available (Table 1) [14].

Using a backward selection algorithm, we analyzed the predictive power of LUMPO III's predictors in 4174 patients who had been treated for choroidal melanoma, 889 of whom had known chromosome-3 status. A total of 1553 patients had died by the end of the study, with death attributed to metastatic disease in 956 patients, 816 of whom had a monosomy-3 melanoma. This analysis identified largest basal tumor diameter and chromosome-3 status as the factors most predictive of metastatic death and showed age to be the most important predictor of death from other causes.

The printed chart comprises three tables for patients having melanoma with disomy3, monosomy3 or unknown chromosome-3 status. Each table provides 2-, 5-, and 10-year metastatic-mortality absolute risks according to largest basal tumor diameter with separate sections for patients less than 81 years old and those older than 80 years, respectively.

Compared to the eighth edition of the TNM staging system, our predictive models had similar accuracy when chromosome-3 status was unknown and were superior when chromosome-3 status was known. For largest basal tumor diameter with or without known chromosome-3 status, the metastatic-death-specific concordance, C-indices at 2, 5, and 10 years were 0.85, 0.85, and 0.84 and 0.79, 0.77, and 0.74, respectively, as compared with 0.81, 0.79, and 0.76 for Kaplan–Meier prognostication using the eighth edition of the TNM staging system.

4 Clinical Impact of LUMPO

The accurate prognostication provided by LUMPO III increased the scope of genetic typing of uveal melanomas at our center. This, in turn, stimulated us to further develop tumor biopsy techniques and genetic analytic methods [15, 16]. These advances resulted in prognostic biopsy being offered to all our patients undergoing plaque or proton beam radiotherapy, including those with small tumors [17]. Conversely, the advances in genetic tumor typing stimulated further development of LUMPO III, which is ongoing.

Reliable prognostication made it possible for us to target systemic surveillance at patients with high risk of metastasis. This made it affordable for our hospital in Liverpool to offer patients liver imaging with magnetic resonance imaging instead of ultrasonography. A study by Marshall et al. showed that 90 (48%) of 188 patients developed detectable metastases a median of 18 months after ocular treatment [18]. The metastases were detected before symptoms in 83 (92%) of the 90 patients, with 49% of these having less than five hepatic lesions all measuring less than 2 cm in diameter. Of these 90 patients, 12 (14%) underwent hepatic resection, all surviving for at least a year afterward.

In 2009, Cook et al. reported that 97% of 298 eligible patients with uveal melanoma whom we treated by enucleation or local resection accepted an offer of cytogenetic prognostication [19]. None of these patients expressed any regret about having this test and there was no evidence of any harm. The main benefit perceived by patients was that they would have greater control and that screening for metastatic disease and early treatment might enhance chances of survival. This was despite counseling that prognostication, screening, and treatment were unlikely to prolong life and that the main purpose of cytogenetic studies was to allow life-planning. Since that study, scope for systemic surveillance has improved following the development of tebentafusp and other novel therapies showing encouraging results in clinical trials [20].

5 Conclusions

We have improved survival prognostication following treatment for choroidal melanoma so that absolute risk estimates of metastatic death are relevant to individual patients. This has been achieved by creating advanced mathematical models using anatomic, histologic, genetic, and mortality data that were collected prospectively from large numbers of patients over several decades. Prognostic accuracy depends greatly on the quality of genetic tumor analysis and on strict adherence to standardized protocols for assessing and categorizing the predictors of metastatic disease and death. These developments have enhanced our ability to target systemic surveillance and counseling at high-risk patients.

Table 1 Absolute risk of metastatic death (and a 95% bootstrapped confidence interval) according to choroidal melanoma basal tumor diameter and age if genetic analysis shows (A) disomy 3; (B) monosomy 3; or if (C) chromosome-3 status is unknown

a

DISOMY-3 MELANOMA							
Treatment age <81 yrs				Treatment age >80 yrs			
LBTD [mm]	Years after treatment			LBTD [mm]	Years after treatment		
	2	5	10		2	5	10
<10.1	0.1 [0, 0.5]	0.7 [0, 1.6]	2.1 [0.7, 4]	<10.1	0.1 [0, 0.5]	0.6 [0, 1.4]	1.4 [0.4, 2.6]
10.1-12.0	0.8 [0.2, 1.7]	1.7 [0.5, 3.4]	3.7 [1.5, 6.7]	10.1-12.0	0.7 [0.1, 1.6]	1.5 [0.5, 3]	2.7 [1.1, 4.8]
12.1-14.0	1.1 [0, 2.5]	3.3 [1, 6]	6.5 [2.7, 11]	12.1-14.0	1 [0, 2.4]	2.9 [0.9, 5.3]	4.9 [2, 8.3]
14.1-16.0	1.5 [0, 4]	5.3 [1.8, 9.6]	11 [4.9, 18]	14.1-16.0	1.5 [0, 3.8]	4.6 [1.6, 8.4]	8 [3.7, 13]
16.1-18.0	3.1 [0, 8.7]	12 [5.1, 21]	17 [8, 28]	16.1-18.0	2.9 [0, 8.3]	11 [4.5, 19]	14 [6.5, 22]
18.1-28.0	6 [0, 14]	12 [2.4, 25]	18 [6.2, 32]	18.1-28.0	5.7 [0, 14]	11 [2.3, 22]	15 [4.6, 26]

b

MONOSOMY-3 MELANOMA							
Treatment age <81 yrs				Treatment age >80 yrs			
LBTD [mm]	Years after treatment			LBTD [mm]	Years after treatment		
	2	5	10		2	5	10
<10.1	2.5 [0.6, 5.2]	13 [6.4, 21]	26 [13, 41]	<10.1	2.4 [0.5, 5]	11 [5.5, 18]	19 [9.6, 30]
10.1-12.0	5 [2.2, 8.4]	20 [12, 28]	37 [22, 51]	10.1-12.0	4.8 [2.1, 8.1]	18 [11, 25]	28 [17, 38]
12.1-14.0	8 [4.9, 12]	33 [24, 42]	53 [38, 65]	12.1-14.0	7.9 [4.7, 12]	29 [21, 37]	42 [30, 51]
14.1-16.0	13 [9.2, 18]	42 [35, 50]	66 [55, 75]	14.1-16.0	13 [8.8, 17]	37 [30, 44]	52 [43, 60]
16.1-18.0	21 [16, 27]	59 [51, 67]	77 [67, 85]	16.1-18.0	20 [15, 26]	53 [46, 61]	64 [56, 71]
18.1-28.0	32 [26, 38]	70 [63, 78]	80 [73, 87]	18.1-28.0	31 [25, 37]	64 [57, 71]	71 [64, 77]

c

UNKNOWN CHROMOSOME 3 STATUS							
Treatment age <81 yrs				Treatment age >80 yrs			
LBTD [mm]	Years after treatment			LBTD [mm]	Years after treatment		
	2	5	10		2	5	10
<10.1	0.6 [0.2, 1.1]	3.1 [2.1, 4.2]	6.6 [5, 8.3]	<10.1	0.6 [0.2, 1]	2.7 [1.8, 3.6]	4.7 [3.6, 6]
10.1-12.0	2 [1.2, 3]	7 [5.3, 8.9]	13 [10, 15]	10.1-12.0	1.9 [1.1, 2.9]	6.1 [4.6, 7.8]	9.7 [7.8, 12]
12.1-14.0	4 [2.6, 5.4]	15 [13, 18]	25 [21, 28]	12.1-14.0	3.8 [2.5, 5.1]	14 [11, 16]	19 [17, 22]
14.1-16.0	7.9 [5.7, 10]	25 [22, 30]	41 [36, 45]	14.1-16.0	7.6 [5.5, 9.8]	22 [19, 26]	32 [28, 36]
16.1-18.0	15 [11, 19]	43 [37, 48]	55 [50, 61]	16.1-18.0	14 [11, 18]	38 [33, 43]	46 [41, 51]
18.1-28.0	25 [21, 30]	56 [50, 62]	65 [59, 70]	18.1-28.0	24 [20, 29]	51 [45, 56]	56 [51, 62]

References

1. Kujala E, Makitie T, Kivelä T. Very long-term prognosis of patients with malignant uveal melanoma. Invest Ophthalmol Vis Sci. 2003;44(11):4651–9.
2. Eskelin SK, T. Uveal melanoma: implications of tumor doubling time (letter). Ophthalmology. 2001;108:830–1.
3. Singh AD. Uveal melanoma: implications of tumor doubling time. Ophthalmology. 2001;108(5):829–31.
4. Kujala E, Damato B, Coupland SE, Desjardins L, Bechrakis NE, Grange JD, Kivel ä T. Staging of ciliary body and choroidal melanomas based on anatomic extent. J Clin Oncol. 2013;31(22):2825–31.
5. Damato B, Duke C, Coupland SE, Hiscott P, Smith PA, Campbell I, Douglas A, Howard P. Cytogenetics of uveal melanoma: a 7-year clinical experience. Ophthalmology. 2007;114(10):1925–31.
6. Damato B, Eleuteri A, Fisher AC, Coupland SE, Taktak AF. Artificial neural networks estimating survival probability after treatment of choroidal melanoma. Ophthalmology. 2008;115(9):1598–607.
7. Eleuteri A, Damato B, Coupland SE, Taktak AFG. Enhancing survival prognostication in patients with choroidal melanoma by integrating pathologic, clinical and genetic predictors of metastasis. IJBET. 2012;8:18–35.
8. DeParis SW, Taktak A, Eleuteri A, Enanoria W, Heimann H, Coupland SE, Damato B. External validation of the Liverpool uveal melanoma prognosticator online. Invest Ophthalmol Vis Sci. 2016;57(14):6116–22.
9. Eleuteri A, Taktak AFG, Coupland SE, Heimann H, Kalirai H, Damato B. Prognostication of metastatic death in uveal melanoma patients: a Markov multi-state model. Comput Biol Med. 2018;102:151–6.
10. Damato B, Dopierala JA, Coupland SE. Genotypic profiling of 452 choroidal melanomas with multiplex ligation-dependent probe amplification. Clin Cancer Res. 2010;16(24):6083–92.
11. Kalirai H, Dodson A, Faqir S, Damato BE, Coupland SE. Lack of BAP1 protein expression in uveal melanoma is associated with increased metastatic risk and has utility in routine prognostic testing. Br J Cancer. 2014;111(7):1373–80.
12. Damato B, Heimann H. Personalized treatment of uveal melanoma. Eye. 2013;27(2):172–9.
13. Cunha Rola A, Taktak A, Eleuteri A, Kalirai H, Heimann H, Hussain R, Bonnett LJ, Hill CJ, Traynor M, Jager MJ, et al. Multicenter external validation of the Liverpool uveal melanoma prognosticator online: an OOG collaborative study. Cancers (Basel). 2020;12(2):477.
14. Damato B, Eleuteri A, Hussain R, Kalirai H, Thornton S, Taktak A, Heimann H, Coupland SE. Parsimonious models for predicting mortality from choroidal melanoma. Invest Ophthalmol Vis Sci. 2020;61(4):35.
15. Thornton S, Coupland SE, Olohan L, Sibbring JS, Kenny JG, Hertz-Fowler C, Liu X, Haldenby S, Heimann H, Hussain R, et al. Targeted next-generation sequencing of 117 routine clinical samples provides further insights into the molecular landscape of uveal melanoma. Cancers (Basel). 2020;12(4):1039.
16. Angi M, Kalirai H, Taktak A, Hussain R, Groenewald C, Damato BE, Heimann H, Coupland SE. Prognostic biopsy of choroidal melanoma: an optimised surgical and laboratory approach. Br J Ophthalmol. 2017;101(8):1143–6.
17. Hussain RN, Kalirai H, Groenewald C, Kacperek A, Errington RD, Coupland SE, Heimann H, Damato B. Prognostic biopsy of choroidal melanoma after proton beam radiation therapy. Ophthalmology. 2016;123(10):2264–5.
18. Marshall E, Romaniuk C, Ghaneh P, Wong H, McKay M, Chopra M, Coupland SE, Damato BE. MRI in the detection of hepatic metastases from high-risk uveal melanoma: a prospective study in 188 patients. Br J Ophthalmol. 2013;97(2):159–63.
19. Cook SA, Damato B, Marshall E, Salmon P. Psychological aspects of cytogenetic testing of uveal melanoma: preliminary findings and directions for future research. Eye. 2009;23(3):581–5.
20. Damato BE, Dukes J, Goodall H, Carvajal RD. Tebentafusp: T cell redirection for the treatment of metastatic uveal melanoma. Cancers (Basel). 2019;11(7):971.

Applications of Plaque Brachytherapy in Anterior Segment Ocular Tumors: A Clinical Review

Puneet Jain, Bhavna V. Chawla, and Paul T. Finger

1 Introduction

Epibulbar plaque brachytherapy (EPB) is evolving to increase its role in treatment of anterior segment tumors [1, 2]. At first, there was concern if the cornea would tolerate radiation. However, experience taught us that the epithelial cells repopulate and the relatively non-mitotic endothelial cells were relatively impervious [3]. Anterior segment EPB has contributed to improved globe-salvage and vision preservation [4].

While brachytherapy for choroidal tumors started in the late 1920s, the use of brachytherapy for anterior segment tumors started much later, in the 1970s [5, 6]. Then, over the last half a century, brachytherapy sources have evolved from high energy cobalt-60 (^{60}Co) and beta-emitting ruthenium-106 (^{106}Ru), strontium-90 (^{90}Sr),*to low energy seeded plaques (iodine-125, palladium-103) and most recently pure high-dose-rate yttrium-90 (^{90}Y) [1, 7–9]. Anterior segment applications of EPB has similarly evolved utilizing beta and low energy gamma plaques. Of interest, the most recent American Brachytherapy Society (ABS) consensus guidelines for uveal melanoma and retinoblastoma were written by 47 doctors from 9 countries. Therein, the ABS suggested that plaque brachytherapy should be performed at a qualified subspecialty center that provides coordinated patient care, comprised of an ocular oncology specialist, a radiation oncologist, and a medical physicist. It did not include guidance for treatment of anterior epibulbar, intrascleral, or invasive ocular surface malignancies [9].

*The strontium-90 in ophthalmic ^{90}Sr applicators emits two kinds of beta-irradiation. Note that ^{90}Sr is in secular equilibrium with its daughter product yttrium-90 (^{90}Y), with the latter more capable of deeper penetration.

Table 1 enumerates the anterior segment ocular tumors for which plaque brachytherapy is currently used.

Table 1 Indications for brachytherapy of anterior segment ocular tumors

Benign	Malignant
1. Pterygium	1. Conjunctival melanoma
	2. OSSN or conjunctival SCC
	3. Iris melanoma
	4. Ciliary body melanoma

OSSN ocular surface squamous neoplasia, *SCC* squamous cell carcinoma

2 Pterygium

Pterygium is a wing-like overgrowth of the bulbar conjunctiva onto the cornea. The condition itself is benign; however, high recurrence rates post-surgery pose a challenge [10].

The current gold standard treatment is surgical excision with use of adjuvant therapies like anti-mitotic drugs, conjunctival autografting, amniotic membrane grafting, or radiation therapy. The aim of these adjuvant modalities is to lower the recurrence rates and reduce scarring. High-dose-rate ^{90}Sr brachytherapy has been used in management of pterygium. The total radiation dose ranges from 10 to 60 Gy in 1 to 6 fractions [10, 11]. For it to be effective, the radiation therapy has to be started within 72 hours of pterygium excision [10]. Reported recurrence rates are under 15% in such a setting. Adverse effects of plaque brachytherapy

P. Jain
Oculoplasty and Ocular Oncology Department, Eye-Q Super-Specialty Eye Hospitals, Gurgaon, India
e-mail: pjain@eyecancer.com

B. V. Chawla
Ocular Oncology Service, Rajendra Prasad Centre for Ophthalmic Sciences, All India Institute of Medical Sciences, New Delhi, India
e-mail: bhavna2424@aiims.edu

P. T. Finger (✉)
The Department of Ocular Tumor, Orbital Disease and Ophthalmic Radiation Therapy, The New York Eye Cancer Center, New York, NY, USA
e-mail: pfinger@eyecancer.com

B. V. Chawla, M. E. Aronow (eds.), *Global Perspectives in Ocular Oncology*, https://doi.org/10.1007/978-3-031-08250-4_23

post-excision include scleral thinning, scleral ulceration, scleritis, and cataract [10].

3 Conjunctival Melanoma

Conjunctival melanoma (also known as malignant melanoma of the conjunctiva) is a rare ocular tumor comprising approximately 5% of ocular melanomas and much less than 1% of all melanomas [12, 13]. However, the incidence of conjunctival melanoma has been increasing, local treatment failure common leading to high tumor mortality [14]. Fortunately, phase-I clinical case series have found the diffuse multifocal and metastatic conjunctival melanoma responds to systemic immunotherapy [15, 16]. The American Joint Committee on Cancer (AJCC) Staging System (eighth edition) has been validated to predict both local treatment failure and mortality [12, 13].

Treatment generally follows tumor stage as well as local ophthalmiconcology center practices. When possible, primary treatment typically includes excision with margins, and/or adjuvant cryotherapy. Excision can also be coupled with adjuvant plaque radiation therapy or topical chemotherapy. Orbital exenteration has been employed with the tumor and is confined to the orbit, while coordination of care is needed for larger surgeries when the tumor extends into the sinus or brain. Systemic immunotherapy should be considered for locally unresectable and metastatic conjunctival melanoma [16].

At The New York Eye Cancer Center, local control is typically achieved after excision of the nodular components with subsequent topical mitomycin 0.02% and/or topical interferon alpha 2B [17–20]. Radiation therapy (e.g., plaque brachytherapy, proton beam therapy) is typically employed for intrascleral or intraocular invasion or when all other treatments fail [13]. Over the last two decades, eye cancer specialists have shifted toward the use of topical chemotherapy agents as primary or adjuvant therapy. That said, these topical agents have limited penetration and have not been found effective for invasive melanomas.

Plaque brachytherapy can be used alone or more commonly together with surgical excision, or after as an adjuvant procedure [5, 13, 21–26]. Brachytherapy sources used for conjunctival melanoma include: ^{60}Co, ^{90}Sr, ^{106}Ru, ^{125}I, and ^{103}Pd [5, 13, 21–28]. In general, melanomas are treated to a minimum dose of 50 Gy; however, published doses range from 150 to 500 Gy to a depth of 1 mm [27]. Fractionated ^{90}Sr doses have been delivered to a total dose of 50–60 Gy with a reported local control rate of 90% [23, 25].

Indications for plaque brachytherapy currently include: histopathologically proven tumor-positive resected-base margins, corneoscleral invasion, and recurrent tumors. Some investigators have used plaque brachytherapy for early-stage tumors as an adjuvant to surgery in order to reduce local recurrence [22]. Regardless of tumor stage, a combination of surgery and episcleral plaque brachytherapy has been shown to reduce local tumor recurrence and the need for secondary treatments (exenteration, immunotherapy) [21, 26]. Also, brachytherapy typically obviates the need for scleral dissection and can thereby preserve scleral integrity. Similarly, ^{125}I plaque brachytherapy has been used to avoid exenteration by treating residual or recurrent melanoma of the palpebral conjunctiva [28].

Plaque brachytherapy has been applied for 1–3 mm of intraocular penetration. Therefore, it offers an accountable radiation dose delivery to the tumor, with minimal radiation exposure to the radiosensitive lens, retina, and optic nerve. Generally, well-tolerated, adverse effects of plaque brachytherapy for conjunctival melanoma have been limited to the ocular surface (e.g., ocular irritation, episcleritis, corneal ulceration, keratopathy, and rarely scleral thinning). However, with time intraocular complications may include cataract, retinopathy, and secondary neovascular glaucoma [5, 26].

4 Ocular Surface Squamous Neoplasia

Malignant ocular surface squamous neoplasia (M-OSSN) is the most common ocular surface malignancy with an incidence of 0.03–3.4 per million [29, 30]. M-OSSN is a comprehensive clinical term comprising cases with mild epithelial dysplasia to eyes suffering from invasive squamous cell carcinoma. While the latter can exhibit intraocular and/or orbital invasion as well as regional lymph node spread, distant metastasis is rare [31]. At The New York Eye Cancer Center, we typically perform metastatic surveys (e.g., PET/CT imaging) for any high-risk squamous carcinomas, e.g., larger (in volume) than a typical lima-bean(1–3 cm), those who are immunocompromised and when the tumor locally extends into and beyond the orbit.

Morphological patterns include the papilliform, gelatinous, and leukoplakic forms, with some degree of overlap [29]. Histopathologically, there can be mild dysplasia, moderate dysplasia, severe dysplasia, carcinoma in-situ or invasive squamous cell carcinoma of which there can be of the spindle, epidermoid, clear, or mucoepidermoid cell-types. When possible, M-OSSN tumor staging should be performed according to the American Joint Committee on Cancer (AJCC) Staging System (eighth edition) [31, 32]. However, in that the AJCC system was based on histopathological diagnoses, it may not be as useful in patients managed with primary topical chemotherapy where tissue diagnosis is unavailable [33–35].

Though surgical excision has been a mainstay of treatment, the advent of topical chemotherapy (interferon alfa–

2b, 5-fluorouracil, and mitomycin C) has allowed outpatient cure [2, 30]. However, when the tumor invades the sclera or cornea topical chemotherapy has been considered inadequate, eye and vision-sparing plaque brachytherapy can be employed [35]. Lastly, orbital exenteration, sinusectomy, craniotomy and immunotherapy have been reserved for advanced cases when the tumor invades the orbital tissues and sinuses and/or brain [2, 29–31, 36–38]. Recent reports suggest that immunotherapy, specifically programmed cell death PD-1 inhibitor medication (e.g., cemiplimab), can be used for local tumors that cannot be treated by surgery or radiation and those with metastatic disease [39, 40].

4.1 Plaque Brachytherapy

Plaque brachytherapy for OSSN is mainly used as adjuvant therapy to positive deep margins, scleral or corneal infiltration, or minimal intraocular invasion [41]. Sometimes, these indications are discovered after excision (reported as base positivity on histopathological examination) and for clinically apparent recurrent tumors post-surgery [6, 36, 42–50]. At The New York Eye Cancer Center, the most common indications are failure to alternative local treatments and localized intraocular invasion. Brachytherapy sources that have been used for OSSN include radium seeds, ^{90}Sr, ^{106}Ru, ^{125}I, ^{103}Pd, and phosphorus-32 (^{32}P), of these ^{106}Ru and ^{125}I are most common [6, 30, 31, 36, 42]. Local tumor control rates of up to 100% have been reported with use of ^{125}I plaques, in cases of corneo-scleral invasion. Side effects of plaque brachytherapy in the treatment of OSSN include cataracts, transient epithelial defects, scleral thinning, conjunctival telangiectasia, glaucoma, and limbal stem cell deficiency [31, 36, 42, 44].

5 Iris Melanoma

Iris melanoma is the most common malignant tumor of the iris, but the least common type of uveal melanoma (<5% of uveal melanoma) [51]. Iris melanoma have been associated with a better prognosis and lower metastatic potential (11.7%) than a ciliary body or choroidal melanoma (50%) [3, 4, 52]. This finding has been attributed to the remote anatomical location, smaller tumor volumes, and lower biological activity [4]. It can be of 2 types—nodular and diffuse [53, 54].

Both diagnosis and treatment are aided by anterior segment ultrasonography biomicroscopy (UBM). Ultrasound typically reveals that malignant iris tumors do not respect the underlying pigment epithelium and may invade into the supraciliary space. Nodular tumors are easier to diagnose than the relatively rare diffuse variant. Tumor size, used for both surgical and radiation treatment planning, is best measured by UBM imaging. Staging should be performed according to AJCC (eighth edition) cancer staging system for uveal melanoma [52].

5.1 Iris Melanoma Primary Treatment

Treatment is guided by clinical features of the tumor (size, location, and tumor seeding) and any associated complications (secondary glaucoma) [3]. In general, superficial characteristics are best observed for change by comparing slit-lamp photographs over time. Treatment can either be surgical iridectomy or radiation therapy (plaque brachytherapy or proton beam irradiation). Surgical resection is an extensive intraocular procedure, risks anterior segment complications and creates a non-pupil-sparing large optical iridectomy [55].

In contrast, radiation therapy does not require intraocular surgery, obviates those complications, and preserves pupillary function. That said, there exist marked differences between radiation techniques. For example, the protons used in proton beam therapy are generated externally generated, collimated for ocular use and directed toward the eye. As the protons approach the eye, they sequentially interact with the eyelashes, eyelid, conjunctiva, cornea, iris tumor, ciliary body, and lens. These "entry-dose" interactions result in a high probability of eyelash loss, skin and conjunctival telangiectasia, limbal stem cell deficiency, cataract, and neovascular glaucoma. Further complicating treatment, eye movements within the proton field can displace the target volume during treatment. If the eye is closed, then Bell's phenomenon can also displace the target from the beam. In contrast, low-energy (^{125}I, ^{103}Pd) seeds are housed within high-Z gold plaque carriers. The gold has been shown to block >99.95% of the radiation, creating a virtually unidirectional source sewn onto the eye as to cover the tumor and free margin (ABS normal plaque position) [9]. Thus, the gold of the plaque shields the eyelids and eye lashes. The area of treatment is limited to that beneath the plaque and should the eye move, the attached plaque moves with it, never leaving the iris melanoma target. Though both cataract and dry eye are common after anterior segment plaque therapy, in my experience these complications are much less severe and thus more manageable than that seen after proton beam. In general, radiation has been shown to be a safe pupil-sparing, globe-salvaging, and vision-saving alternative to surgical resection [56, 57].

Plaque radionuclides used to treat iris melanoma include ^{125}I, ^{106}Ru, ^{90}Y, and ^{103}Pd [3, 55, 58, 59]. In a retrospective analysis of 50 patients over a mean 5.2 years follow-up, ^{103}Pd plaque brachytherapy was found to achieve 100% local tumor control rate [3, 57]. This very high local control rate was thought due (in part) to careful definition of tumor margins as determined by combining slit-lamp and goniophotography with high frequency ultrasound imaging (UBM) and iris fluorescein angiography, then adding 2–3 mm "tumor-free" radiation margins to create the treatment zone. A minimum tumor dose of 85 Gy was used for ^{125}I and ^{103}Pd plaques. Post-treatment features of tumor regression in iris melanoma with ^{103}Pd plaque brachytherapy were described [40]. These include increased tumor pigmentation and ultrasonographic tumor reflectivity, with a decrease in tumor height and vascularity.

The reported adverse effects include cataract (most common), secondary glaucoma, transient keratitis, corneal epitheliopathy, iris stromal atrophy, uveitis, and inflammation at the limbus [3, 55, 58, 59]. Corneal complications have been minimized by the use of Finger's amniotic membrane buffer technique [60]. No case of radiation retinopathy or scleromalacia has been found after epicorneal ^{103}Pd plaque brachytherapy [3, 61].

^{106}Ru plaque brachytherapy for iris melanoma has also been shown to achieve 100% local tumor control rate. The most common complications reported with its use are cataract, uveitis, dry eye, and thinning of the sclera [55].

Cases of diffuse multifocal iris melanoma have been treated by enucleation. However, Shields treated non-resectable tumors with ^{125}I plaques yielding a local tumor control rate of 92% [62]. Most recently, total-front-of-the-eye covering ^{103}Pd plaques buffered with amniotic membrane have been successfully used for management of multifocal iris melanomas with a 100% local tumor control rate [54, 56].

6 Epicorneal Plaque Surgery

Suturing a metal plaque to the corneal surface typically causes discomfort and pain. This is why in 2008, Finger introduced the use of the epicorneal amniotic membrane buffer technique (AMBT) to protect the corneal surface form the gold and ^{103}Pd seeds in gold eye plaques [60]. In AMBT a single layer amniotic membrane graft (approximately 0.1 mm in thickness) is placed between the plaque and the cornea with its sticky-side up on the cornea. There should be no folding of the membrane as it offsets the plaque away from the tumor. This procedure has been shown to reduce pain and improves patient comfort while the plaque stays in situ [60] (Fig. 1).

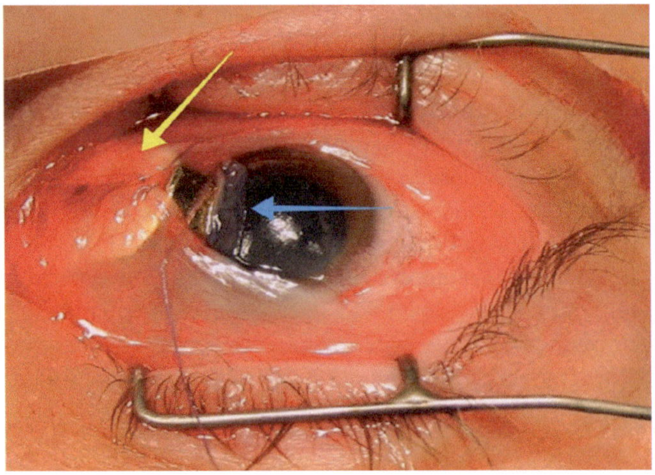

Fig. 1 Intra-operative picture showing plaque placement in a case of irido-ciliary melanoma (yellow arrow). Note the amniotic membrane sandwiched between the plaque and the cornea (blue arrow). After this photograph, the Gunderson flap is closed to provide a smooth surface for the eye lid to glide over the plaque for its duration

7 Ciliary Body Melanoma

Ciliary body melanoma comprises less than 10% of uveal melanomas, but this location has been shown to be a risk factor for metastasis [63]. This is likely due (in part) to their being hidden behind the iris, able to silently enlarge in height and width without visual symptoms prior to being detected. Ciliary body melanoma can grow anteriorly to involve the iris, posteriorly to involve the choroid, or outwardly through the sclera. However, one must always consider its relatively lethal, lateral spread along the ciliary body, termed the "ring melanoma." As ring melanomas spread, they ring themselves around the anterior segment. The worst variant, ring melanomas typically bear a very large basal diameter and thus a worse prognosis [64]. Tumor staging should be performed according to the eighth edition AJCC cancer staging system for uveal melanoma [65].

Local tumor control has been achieved with either surgical resection, radiation therapy, or enucleation depending on tumor-size, visual potential, available treatments, and patient preference. Surgical resection can be considered in small-sized melanoma but it is associated with complications like lens subluxation, vitreous hemorrhage, retinal detachment, and tumor dissemination in the operating field. Further, obtaining a tumor negative lateral and scleral margins of resection has been historically difficult. In general, failures of local resection have prompted the use of adjuvant plaque therapy to improve local control [66–68].

8 American Brachytherapy Society Consensus Guidelines

In 2014, 47 eye cancer specialists from 9 countries (The ABS Ophthalmic Oncology Task Force) developed consensus guidelines for plaque brachytherapy for choroidal melanoma

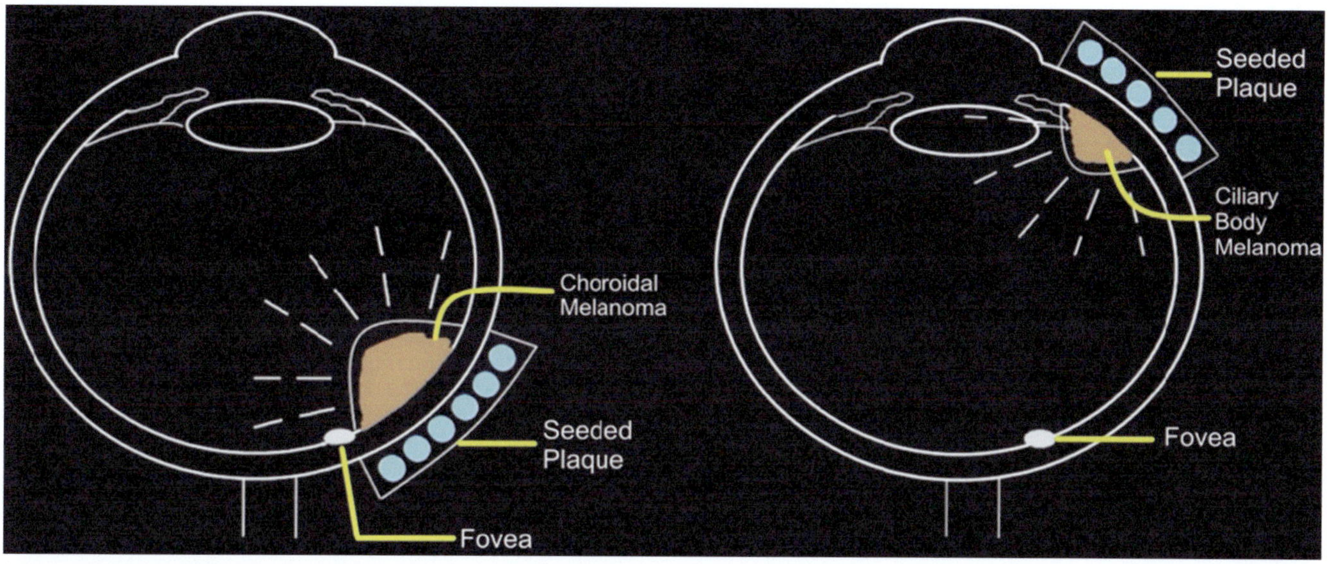

Fig. 2 Plaque placement in episcleral plaque brachytherapy for a choroidal melanoma (left side) and a ciliary body melanoma (right side). Note the distance of the plaque from the fovea in case of a ciliary body melanoma. This distance is the reason behind a very low radiation dose delivery to the macula [3, 61]

and retinoblastoma [9]. In these guidelines, treatment by enucleation was reserved for the few cases where globe salvage is not possible, eyes with poor or no visual potential, and when it is the patient's preference [9].

Broadly speaking, ciliary body melanomas measuring <16 mm in basal dimension with a tumor height <10 mm are amenable to low energy (^{125}I and ^{103}Pd) plaque brachytherapy [63]. Further, ciliary body melanoma with <3 mm clinically visible extrascleral extension has been managed with episcleral brachytherapy with good efficacy and a reasonable rate of globe preservation [67]. Radioisotopes reportedly used for this tumor include ^{60}Co, ^{106}Ru, ^{125}I, and ^{103}Pd. A tumor apex dose of 85–90 Gy has been used with the ^{125} I plaque [67, 68]. The reported local tumor control rates have been 98–100% with globe retention rates of 93–100% when plaque brachytherapy has been used for ciliary body melanoma without extrascleral extension [4, 66–68]. Complications include radiation-induced cataract, secondary glaucoma including neovascular glaucoma, vitreous hemorrhage, radiation retinopathy, and keratopathy. Of interest, Yousef and Chaugule observed no cases of radiation maculopathy or optic neuropathy utilizing ^{103}Pd-brachytherapy for anterior uveal melanomas [3, 61] (Fig. 2).

Though ciliary body melanoma location carries a significantly worse systemic prognosis than a similar-sized posterior uveal melanoma, the prognosis for local control and visual acuity preservation after plaque irradiation is superior [66]. Systemic surveillance should be performed for all iris, ciliary body, and choroidal melanoma patients [67–72].

9 Limitations of Plaque Brachytherapy

Episcleral plaque brachytherapy has a few limitations. Despite it being a type of radiation therapy, it does require 2 surgical procedures—insertion of the plaque and plaque removal. Both these surgeries need to be carried out in an operating room. The availability is limited and cost of therapy is greater than resection or enucleation. The ABS guidelines suggest that plaque brachytherapy be performed by subspecialty trained eye cancer specialist and at established ocular oncology centers. The details of setting up a plaque brachytherapy service are beyond the scope of this chapter but have been described [72]. Though it is an expensive treatment modality, anterior segment plaque brachytherapy is less expensive than proton beam and it provides excellent vision, globe, and life-preserving benefits.

10 Summary

In summary, plaque brachytherapy has been found useful in treatment of conjunctival melanoma, invasive squamous cell carcinoma, and uveal melanoma. For malignant OSSN, plaque brachytherapy is typically employed as an adjunct to surgical excision and not used as primary, sole therapy. For anterior uveal melanomas, plaque brachytherapy has been found to be a pupil-sparing, globe salvaging, life and vision preserving therapy, especially for diffuse and multifocal iris melanomas. Anterior segment plaque radiation therapy has provided excellent local cancer control, a few durable vision-limiting side-effects, and excellent cosmesis.

Disclosures Dr. Finger has a majority interest in LV Liberty Vision Corporation (https://www.libertyvision.com) providing a new radiation source for ophthalmology.

References

1. Finger PT. Radiation therapy for orbital tumors: concepts, current use, and ophthalmic radiation side effects. Surv Ophthalmol. 2009;54(5):545–68. https://doi.org/10.1016/j.survophthal.2009.06.004.
2. Jain P, Finger PT. Newer technologies in ocular oncology. In: Ichhpujani P, editor. Current advances in ophthalmic technology. Singapore: Springer; 2019. p. 101–12.
3. Chaugule SS, Finger PT. Regression patterns of iris melanoma after Palladium-103 (^{103}Pd) plaque brachytherapy. Ophthalmology. 2017;124(7):1023–30.
4. Finger PT. Plaque radiation therapy for malignant melanoma of the iris and ciliary body. Am J Ophthalmol. 2001;132(3):328–35.
5. Lederman M, Wybar K, Busby E. Malignant epibulbar melanoma: natural history and treatment by radiotherapy. Br J Ophthalmol. 1984;68(9):605–17.
6. Lommatzsch P. Beta-ray treatment of malignant epithelial tumors of the conjunctiva. Am J Ophthalmol. 1976;81(2):198–206. https://doi.org/10.1016/0002-9394(76)90731-5.
7. Finger PT. Plaque brachytherapy for choroidal melanoma: strategies and techniques to reduce risk and maximize outcomes. Expert Rev Ophthalmol. 2020;15(4):201–10. https://doi.org/10.1080/17469899.2020.1781618.
8. Finger PT, Rivard MJ, Chaugule SS, Shanmugam PM, Saakyan S, Krema H, et al. Ophthalmic radiotherapy: plaques and implants. In: Chaugule S, Honavar S, Finger P, editors. Surgical ophthalmic oncology: a collaborative open access reference. Switzerland: Springer Nature; 2019. p. 147–58.
9. Simpson ER, Gallie B, Laperrierre N, Beiki-Ardakani A, Kivelä T, Raivio V, et al. The American brachytherapy society consensus guidelines for plaque brachytherapy of uveal melanoma and retinoblastoma. Brachytherapy. 2014;13(1):1–14.
10. Ali AM, Thariat J, Bensadoun RJ, Thyss A, Rostom Y, El-Haddad S, Gérard JP. The role of radiotherapy in the treatment of pterygium: a review of the literature including more than 6000 treated lesions. Cancer Radiother. 2011;15:140–7. https://doi.org/10.1016/j.canrad.2010.03.020.
11. Shahraki T, Arabi A, Feizi S. Pterygium: an update on pathophysiology, clinical features, and management. Ther Adv Ophthalmol. 2021;13:251584142110201.
12. Jain P, Finger PT, Damato B, Coupland SE, Heimann H, Kenawy N, et al. Multicenter, international assessment of the eighth edition of the American joint committee on cancer cancer staging manual for conjunctival melanoma. JAMA Ophthalmol. 2019;137(8):905–11.
13. Jain P, Finger PT, Fili M, Damato B, Coupland SE, Heimann H, et al. Conjunctival melanoma treatment outcomes in 288 patients: a multicentre international data-sharing study. Br J Ophthalmol. 2021;105(10):1358–64. https://doi.org/10.1136/bjophthalmol-2020-316293.
14. Yu GP, Hu DN, McCormick S, Finger PT. Conjunctival melanoma: is it increasing in the United States? Am J Ophthalmol. 2003;135(6):800–6.
15. Sagiv O, Thakar SD, Kandl TJ, Ford J, Sniegowski MC, Hwu WJ, et al. Immunotherapy with programmed cell death 1 inhibitors for 5 patients with conjunctival melanoma. JAMA Ophthalmol. 2018;136(11):1236–41.
16. Finger PT, Pavlick AC. Checkpoint inhibition immunotherapy for advanced local and systemic conjunctival melanoma: a clinical case series. J Immunother Cancer. 2019;7(1):1–7.
17. Finger PT, Milner MS, McCormick SA. Topical chemotherapy for conjunctival melanoma. Br J Ophthalmol. 1993;77(11):751–3.
18. Finger PT, Czechonska G, Liarikos S. Topical mitomycin chemotherapy for conjunctival melanoma and PAM with atypia. Br J Ophthalmol. 1998;82(5):476–9.
19. Kurli M, Finger PT. Topical mitomycin chemotherapy for conjunctival malignant melanoma and primary acquired melanosis with atypia: 12 years' experience. Graefes Arch Clin Exp Ophthalmol. 2005;243(11):1108–14.
20. Chaugule SS, Park J, Finger PT. Topical chemotherapy for giant ocular surface squamous neoplasia of the conjunctiva and cornea: is surgery necessary? Indian J Ophthalmol. 2018;66(1):55–60.
21. Lommatzsch PK, Lommatzsch RE, Kirsch I, Fuhrmann P. Therapeutic outcome of patients suffering from malignant melanomas of the conjunctiva. Br J Ophthalmol. 1990;74(10):615–9.
22. Zografos L, Uffer S, Bercher L, Gailloud C. Combined surgical excision, cryotherapy and radiotherapy in malignant melanomas of the conjunctiva. Klin Monatsbl Augenheilkd. 1994;204(5):385–90.
23. Krause L, Ritter C, Wachtlin J, Kreusel KM, Höcht S, Foerster MH, et al. Rezidivhäufigkeit nach exzision von bindehautmelanomen und adjuvanter strontium-90-kontaktbestrahlung. Klin Monatsbl Augenheilkd. 2008;225(7):649–52.
24. Karim R, Conway RM. Conservative resection and adjuvant plaque brachytherapy for early-stage conjunctival melanoma. Clin Exp Ophthalmol. 2011;39(4):293–8.
25. Cohen VML, Papastefanou VP, Liu S, Stoker I, Hungerford JL. The use of strontium-90 beta radiotherapy as adjuvant treatment for conjunctival melanoma. J Oncol. 2013;22013:349162. https://doi.org/10.1155/2013/349162.
26. Damato B, Coupland SE. An audit of conjunctival melanoma treatment in Liverpool. Eye. 2009;23(4):801–9. https://doi.org/10.1038/eye.2008.154.
27. Zehetmayer M, Menapace RKW. Combined local excision and brachytherapy with Ru-106 in the treatment of epibulbar malignancies. Ophthalmologica. 1993;207:137–9.
28. Stannard CE, Sealy GRH, Hering ER, Pereira SB, Knowles R, Hill JC. Malignant melanoma of the eyelid and palpebral conjunctiva treated with iodine-125 brachytherapy. Ophthalmology. 2000;107(5):951–8.
29. Lee G, Hirst L. Ocular surface squamous neoplasia. Surv Ophthalmol. 1995;39(6):429–50.
30. Cicinelli MV, Marchese A, Bandello F, Modorati G. Clinical management of ocular surface squamous neoplasia: a review of the current evidence. Ophthalmol Ther. 2018;7(2):247–62. https://doi.org/10.1007/s40123-018-0140-z.
31. Yousef YA, Finger PT. Squamous carcinoma and dysplasia of the conjunctiva and cornea: an analysis of 101 cases. Ophthalmology. 2012;119(2):233–40. https://doi.org/10.1016/j.ophtha.2011.08.005.
32. Conway RM, Graue GF, Pelayes D, et al. Conjunctival carcinoma. In: Amin MB, Edge SB, Greene FL, et al., editors. AJCC cancer staging manual. 8th ed. Switzerland: Springer; 2017. p. 787–93.
33. Semenova EA, Milman T, Finger PT, Natesh S, Kurli M, Schneider S, et al. The diagnostic value of exfoliative cytology vs histopathology for ocular surface squamous neoplasia. Am J Ophthalmol. 2009;148(5):772–778.e1. https://doi.org/10.1016/j.ajo.2009.06.015.
34. Honavar S. Ocular surface squamous neoplasia: are we calling a spade a spade? Indian J Ophthalmol. 2017;65(10):907–9.
35. Semenova E, Finger PT, Choi W. Squamous cell carcinoma invading a transplanted cornea: eye-and vision-sparing palladium-103 plaque radiation therapy for a functionally monocular patient. Cornea. 2018;37(11):1468–70.
36. Arepalli S, Kaliki S, Shields CL, Emrich J, Komarnicky L, Shields JA. Plaque radiotherapy in the management of scleral-invasive con-

junctival squamous cell carcinoma: an analysis of 15 eyes. JAMA Ophthalmol. 2014;132(6):691–6.
37. Graue GF, Tena LB, Finger PT. Electron beam radiation for conjunctival squamous carcinoma. Ophthal Plast Reconstr Surg. 2011;27(4):277–81.
38. Finger PT, Tena LB, Semenova E, Aridgides P, Choi WH. Extrascleral extension of choroidal melanoma: post-enucleation high-dose-rate interstitial brachytherapy of the orbit. Brachytherapy. 2014;13(3):275–80. https://doi.org/10.1016/j.brachy.2013.09.002.
39. Migden MR, Rischin D, Schmults CD, Guminski A, Hauschild A, Lewis KD, et al. PD-1 blockade with cemiplimab in advanced cutaneous squamous-cell carcinoma. N Engl J Med. 2018;1–11
40. Wessely A, Steeb T, Leiter U, Garbe C, Berking C, Heppt MV. Immune checkpoint blockade in advanced cutaneous squamous cell carcinoma: what do we currently know in 2020? Int J Mol Sci. 2020;21(23):1–26.
41. Finger PT, Tran HV, Turbin RE, Perry HD, Abramson DH, Chin K, et al. High-frequency ultrasonographic evaluation of conjunctival intraepithelial neoplasia and squamous cell carcinoma. Arch Ophthalmol. 2003;121(2):168–72.
42. Walsh-Conway N, Conway RM. Plaque brachytherapy for the management of ocular surface malignancies with corneoscleral invasion. Clin Exp Ophthalmol. 2009;37(6):577–83.
43. Singh R, Lomi N, Chawla B. Expanded indications of plaque brachytherapy. Delhi J Ophthalmol. 2019;29(4):22–6.
44. Seale ER. Carcinoma of limbus: report of 19 cases treated with radium and effect of gamma radiation upon eye. AMA Arch Dermatol. 1953;68(3):286–95.
45. Goldberg JR, Becker SC, Rosenbaum HD. Gamma radiation. In the treatment of squamous-cell carcinoma of the limbus. Am J Ophthalmol. 1963;55(4):811–5.
46. Cerezo L, Otero J, Aragón G, Polo E, de la Torre A, Valcárcel F, et al. Conjunctival intraepithelial and invasive squamous cell carcinomas treated with strontium-90. Radiother Oncol. 1990;17(3):191–7.
47. Kearsley JH, Fitchew RSTR. Adjunctive radiotherapy with strontium-90 in the treatment of conjunctival squamous cell carcinoma. Int J Radiat Oncol Biol Phys. 1988;14(3):435–43. https://doi.org/10.1016/0360-3016(88)90257-x.
48. Häberle H, Pham DT, Scholman HJWJ. Ruthenium 106-applicator for radiation treatment of carcinoma in situ of the cornea and conjunctiva. Ophthalmologe. 1995;92(6):866–9.
49. Buc D, Pilon F, Donnarieix D, Kemeny JL, Bacin FRD. Treatment of conjunctival epithelial tumors: brachytherapy with ruthenium-106. J Fr Ophtalmol. 2003;26(9):929–39.
50. Marr BP, Abramson DH, Cohen GN, Williamson MJ, McCormick B, Barker CA. Intraoperative high-dose rate of radioactive phosphorus 32 brachytherapy for diffuse recalcitrant conjunctival neoplasms: a retrospective case series and report of toxicity. JAMA Ophthalmol. 2015;133(3):283–9.
51. Jain P, Aronow ME, Chawla B. Advances in clinical management of uveal melanoma. Adv Ophthalmol Optom. 2020;5:103–18. https://doi.org/10.1016/j.yaoo.2020.04.003.
52. Khan S, Finger PT, Yu GP, Razzaq L, Jager MJ, De Keizer RJW, et al. Clinical and pathologic characteristics of biopsy-proven iris melanoma: a multicenter international study. Arch Ophthalmol. 2012;130(1):57–64.
53. Finger PT, Milman T. Microincision, aspiration cutter-assisted multifocal iris biopsy for melanoma. Eur J Ophthalmol. 2017;27(1):62–6.
54. Finger PT, Tomar AS, Chin KJ. Palladium-103 plaque therapy for multifocal iris melanoma: radiation of the entire anterior segment of the eye. Eur J Ophthalmol. 2021;31(3):1375–83.
55. Agraval U, Sobti M, Russell HC, Lockington D, Ritchie D, Cauchi P, et al. Use of ruthenium-106 brachytherapy for iris melanoma: the Scottish experience. Br J Ophthalmol. 2018;102(1):74–8.
56. Petousis V, Finger PT, Milman T. Multifocal iris melanoma treated with total anterior segment palladium-103 plaque radiation therapy. Graefes Arch Clin Exp Ophthalmol. 2011;249(6):937–40.
57. Maheshwari A, Finger P, Malpani A, Jain P, Tomar A, Garg G. Doctor reported outcomes: real-world data from a tertiary eye cancer center. Indian J Ophthalmol. 2021;69(1):135–9.
58. Fernandes BF, Krema H, Fulda E, Pavlin CJ, Payne DG, McGowan HD, et al. Management of iris melanomas with ^{125}I plaque radiotherapy. Am J Ophthalmol. 2010;149(1):70–76.e2. https://doi.org/10.1016/j.ajo.2009.08.007.
59. Tsimpida M, Hungerford J, Arora A, Cohen V. Plaque radiotherapy treatment with ruthenium-106 for iris malignant melanoma. Eye. 2011;25(12):1607–11. https://doi.org/10.1038/eye.2011.222.
60. Finger PT. Finger's amniotic membrane buffer technique. Arch Ophthalmol. 2008;126(4):531.
61. Yousef YAFP. Lack of radiation maculopathy after palladium-103 plaque radiotherapy for iris melanoma. Int J Radiat Oncol Biol Phys. 2012;83(4):1107–12.
62. Shields CL, Naseripour M, Shields JA, Freire JCJ. Custom-designed plaque radiotherapy for nonresectable iris melanoma in 38 patients: tumor control and ocular complications. Am J Ophthalmol. 2003;135(5):648–56.
63. Simpson ER. Ciliary body melanoma: a special challenge. Can J Ophthalmol. 2004;39(4):365–71. https://doi.org/10.1016/S0008-4182(04)80007-3.
64. Demirci H, Shields CL, Shields JA, Honavar SG, Eagle RC. Ring melanoma of the ciliary body. Retina. 2002;22(6):698–706.
65. Kivelä T, Simpson RE, Grossniklaus HE, et al. Uveal melanoma. In: Amin MB, Edge SB, Greene FL, editors. The 8th edition AJCC cancer staging manual. New York: Springer International Publishing: American Joint Commission on Cancer; 2017. p. 805–17.
66. Krema H, Simpson ER, Pavlin CJ, Payne D, Vasquez LM, Mcgowan H. Management of ciliary body melanoma with iodine-125 plaque brachytherapy. Can J Ophthalmol. 2009;44(4):395–400. https://doi.org/10.3129/i09-097.
67. Gündüz K, Shields CL, Shields JA, Cater JBL. Plaque radiotherapy for management of ciliary body and choroidal melanoma with extraocular extension. Am J Ophthalmol. 2000;130:97–102.
68. Lumbroso-Le Rouic L, Charif Chefchaouni M, Levy C, Plancher C, Dendale R, Asselain B, Solignac S, Mazal A, Desjardins L. 125I plaque brachytherapy for anterior uveal melanomas. Eye (Lond). 2004 Sep;18(9):911–6. https://doi.org/10.1038/sj.eye.6701361.
69. Garg G, Finger PT, Kivelä TT, Simpson ER, Gallie BL, Saakyan S, et al. Patients presenting with metastases: stage IV uveal melanoma, an international study. Br J Ophthalmol. 2022;106(4):510–7.
70. Pavlick AC, Finger PT. In: Schachat AP, editor. Section 153: systemic evaluation and management of patients with metastatic uveal melanoma Ryan's retina. 6th ed. Elsevier Inc.; 2018. p. 2608–12.
71. Finger PT, Pavlick AC. In: DeVita Jr VT, Lawrence TS, Rosenberg SA, editors. Cancer: principles and practice of oncology. 11th ed. Philadelphia, PA: Wolters Kluwer, Lippincott, Williams and Wilkins; 2019. p. 1899–908.
72. Chaugule S, Honavar S, Finger P, editors. Surgical ophthalmic oncology: a collaborative open access reference. Switzerland: Springer International Publishing; 2019. p. 1–216.

The Role of Telemedicine in Ocular Oncology

Aluisio Rosa Gameiro Filho, Nakul Singh, and Rubens N. Belfort

1 Introduction

The constant evolution of technology is changing the way we live. With the advent of highly developed mobile devices and robust telecommunication networks, we can instantly communicate with others across the globe through high-definition video. These information and communication technologies (ICTs) also have great potential to play a significant role in providing cost-effective and high-quality health-care services.

"Tele" derives from the Greek word "distance." The term telemedicine was coined in the 1970s, and despite having more than 104 peer-reviewed definitions already in use [1], the World Health Organization defines it as "the delivery of health-care services, where distance is a critical factor, by all health-care professionals using information and communication technologies for the exchange of valid information for the diagnosis, treatment, and prevention of disease and injuries, research and evaluation" [2]. Telemedicine is an open and constantly evolving science, which incorporates new advances in technology, and has the capacity to easily adapt to the changes in health needs.

The first published account of telemedicine dates from the nineteenth century when electrocardiography data were transmitted over telephone wires [3]. In the 1960s, advances were made mostly due to military and space technology [4]. Since then, many advances in telecommunications and mobile devices have allowed for wide access of affordable Internet—according to the International Telecommunication Union (ITU), almost 85% of the world's population is covered by a 4G network [5]. The decreased cost of advanced mobile devices, with built-in audio and video capture, has permitted telemedicine to flourish. Telemedicine can increase convenience and patient access to health care. It is growing fast, with valuation growing over 20 billion in the next few years [6]. Moreover, telemedicine has the potential to help communities traditionally underserved by health services.

The global pandemic of coronavirus disease 2019 (COVID-19) has catalyzed rapid uptake of telemedicine, particularly in ophthalmology. In some places, in-person medical appointments with ophthalmologists dropped by 80% [7], with telemedicine appointments being the only way many clinicians were able to deliver health care during the pandemic due to social-distancing regulations [8–13]. These extremely unusual circumstances have prompted re-examination of many of the ways clinicians deploy telemedicine, in both resource-rich and resource-poor settings. In this chapter, we will review the types of telemedicine, outline the needs for telemedicine, discuss applications of telemedicine to ophthalmology (teleophthalmology), with a special focus on ocular oncology and our own experiences in Brazil. We will discuss further considerations in implementing telemedicine for ocular oncology, and conclude by imagining future directions of the field. We believe ocular oncology care is poised to benefit from the advances in telemedicine because telemedicine promises to extend the reach of a few number of ocular oncology care centers in the world, and that these benefits will be especially impactful in low-income countries.

A. R. G. Filho · R. N. Belfort (✉)
Department of Ophthalmology, Universidade Federal de São Paulo/Escola Paulista de Medicina (UNIFESP - EPM) and Instituto da Visão (IPEPO), São Paulo, SP, Brazil
e-mail: aluisio.gameiro@unifesp.br; rubens@belfort.med.br

N. Singh
Department of Ophthalmology, Massachusetts Eye and Ear, Boston, MA, USA
e-mail: nakul_singh@meei.harvard.edu

B. V. Chawla, M. E. Aronow (eds.), *Global Perspectives in Ocular Oncology*, https://doi.org/10.1007/978-3-031-08250-4_24

2 Definitions and Types of Telemedicine

Telemedicine is one part of a broader concept of "eHealth," which is defined by WHO as "the cost-effective and secure use of ICTs in support of health and health-related fields, including health-care services, health surveillance, health literature and health education, knowledge and research." eHealth is considered a key area of priority for WHO since 2005 [14]. A related concept to eHealth is mHealth, which is defined as health practices supported by mobile devices, such as mobile phones.

Telemedicine can be classified in several ways. One way to classify it depends on the time that the information is transmitted between the people involved: (1) asynchronous, also known as store-and-forward, in which the process involves the exchange of pre-recorded data, at different times or (2) synchronous or real-time, which requires immediate exchange of information between both involved individuals, such as video conferences.

Telemedicine can not only describe interactions between health professionals and patients but also interactions between health professionals and other health professionals. Activities that are also covered by the definition of telemedicine include virtual consultations, case discussions, or even lectures.

3 Telemedicine Can Alleviate Health-Care Access Disparities

The total number of ophthalmologists around the world was estimated at 204,909 in 2010 [15]; however, the distribution of these professionals is not uniform. Six countries (China, USA, Russia, Japan, Brazil, and India) account for roughly 50%, whereas 23 countries have less than 1 ophthalmologist per million inhabitants [15]. The WHO recommends a ratio of 1 ophthalmologist per 17,000 people [16]. Furthermore, although the population of ophthalmologists is growing, the average growth of the population aged 60+ years old (the population that in theory demands more for ocular attention) is growing more than twice as fast as the ophthalmologists [15].

In Brazil in particular, an upper-middle-income country, in 2019, there were an estimated 20,445 ophthalmologists for a population of 208,494,900 inhabitants, which is equivalent to a ratio of 1 ophthalmologist per 9224 inhabitants, However, 50% of these professionals are concentrated in only 14 cities [17]. While the most developed southeast region of the country has a rate of 1 professional per 7257 inhabitants, the poorest regions in the north have only 1 professional per 19,742 people, resulting in inaccessible eye care to many people.

This is not a problem limited to low-income and/or middle-income countries—even the richest countries face problems regarding geographic barriers to eye care, with severe disparities in health-care access. In rural areas especially, there is a shortage of specialists, and appointments can demand traveling long distances, with associated time and financial burdens. Canada, for example, has a ratio of 1 ophthalmologist per 29,851 people; although there are areas in the country wherein the ratio is only 1:112,360 [18]. In the United States, it takes an average of 20 days to secure a 20-min appointment with a physician, and attending that appointment can take 2 h, including transportation and wait times [19].

While there are significant disparities in in-person health-care access between urban and rural areas, there is less disparity in telecommunication coverage: virtually all urban areas of the world and 92% of rural areas are covered by a mobile broadband network [5], which in some low and middle-income countries surpass other infrastructure such as paved roads, running water, or even electricity [2].

By leveraging the well-developed telecommunication network and low-cost mobile devices, telemedicine can overcome geographic barriers to health care and increase access for populations for which it was otherwise unavailable. It can alleviate barriers to care for patients by avoiding long trips and reducing costs.

4 Teleophthalmology

Teleophthalmology refers to ophthalmology practiced as telemedicine. Teleophthalmology has been deployed to aid in screening populations, making diagnoses, or managing diseases [20]. Historically, most of Ophthalmology's experience in telemedicine is store-and-forward, which is already being used for several eye conditions.

Perhaps one of the most advanced teleophthalmology programs have been implemented in addressing diabetic retinopathy (DR), a leading cause of blindness among the working-age population [21]. Several telemedicine programs for DR have been implemented to increase the rate of diabetics screened for retinopathy [22–28]. In most programs, a health-care professional, in selected primary care centers, obtains images using non-mydriatic cameras, which are forwarded to a reading center. Images are evaluated and treatment recommendations are made. These telemedicine screening models demonstrated cost-effectiveness and efficacy, as well as good acceptance by its users [22]. Prospective studies showed that such telemedicine screening programs for DR have led to early diagnosis and referrals. These programs also reduce costs—near 29 USD per patient per referral [29]. Moreover, some automated, deep-learning screening technologies are already being tested, with encouraging results [6].

Retinopathy of prematurity (ROP) is another area of prior attention, with a few telemedicine programs already developed [6, 30–32]. One such program is the Stanford University Networks for Diagnosis of Retinopathy of Prematurity (SUNDROP), which showed a sensitivity of 100%, specificity of 99.8%, positive predictive value (PPV) of 95.5%, and negative predictive value (NPV) of 100%, compared to bedside indirect fundoscopy [33].

Initiatives for other conditions, such as age-related macular degeneration (AMD) and glaucoma [34], also have shown good and promising results.

5 Telemedicine and Ocular Oncology

A few institutions have implemented telemedicine in ocular oncology. In 2016, Balaskas et al. [35] tested how telemedicine may be applied to the management of 102 patients with choroidal melanocytic lesions at Moorfields Eye Hospital or Manchester Royal Eye Hospital. The patients underwent a full ophthalmic and medical history as well as imaging tests (wide-field color imaging, autofluorescence [AF], optical coherence tomography [OCT], and ultrasound [USG]). The authors compared the management decisions (discharge back to optometrists/follow-up or referral to a specialist in ocular oncology) by three groups: (1) expert ophthalmologists, based on the imaging tests and direct clinical assessment (gold-standard); (2) expert ophthalmologist based on the analysis of the images with a short patient history; or (3) decisions made by a reading center grading, also based on the images with a short patient history. The reading center was composed of optometrists working on a diabetic retinopathy telemedicine program, who underwent subsequent training. The short patient history noted the presence or absence of "retinal symptoms," such as blur, metamorphopsias, floaters, and flashes. There was considerable agreement in management between the expert ophthalmologists who performed the full clinical assessment and the reading center graders (96.1%). The agreement between the clinical and the masked ophthalmologists was 100%. The images were very sensitive for identifying known risk factors of high-risk lesions, with 94% sensitivity for orange pigment on AF and 100% sensitivity for subretinal fluid on OCT.

In 2018, Lapere and Weis [36] published a pilot study in which 71 patients with choroidal or iris nevus were offered the choice of in-person follow-up or teleophthalmology assessment by an ophthalmologist, where identical investigations (fundus photography; USG or ultrasound biomicroscopy [UBM]) and spectral-domain OCT (SD-OCT) were performed. They found a result of 100% sensitivity and 92% specificity of teleophthalmology as a tool in monitoring choroidal and iris nevus, with a positive predictive value of 57% and a negative predictive value of 100% to detect growth of a lesion.

In 2019, Roelofs and Weis [37] published a retrospective study with 99 eyes with either choroidal or iris nevi, after reviewing clinical records in chronological order. All patients underwent the same routine protocol, consisting of the standard fundus or slit-lamp photos; B-scan USG or UBM, depending on the location of the lesion; and OCT through the macula and over the choroidal lesion performed by specialized technicians. These images were then uploaded to a central software platform, and reviewed by a masked ophthalmologist specialized in ocular oncology. A 100% sensitivity and 100% negative predictive value were found for the detection of either axial and/or basal growth. Likewise, a specificity of 99% and a positive predictive value of 91% were detected. Moreover, when taking into consideration only the iris lesions, the sensitivity was 100% and specificity of 99%.

Together, the three aforementioned studies show encouraging results of teleophthalmology assessment of choroidal and iris nevi.

Telemedicine can also support transnational partnerships that encourage centers with more experience to support less experienced centers develop expertise and self-sufficiency for managing high-morbidity disease. Recently, Yousef [38] published the results of a telemedicine-based partnership between the King Hussein Cancer Center (KHCC) in Jordan, St Jude Children's Research Hospital, and Hamilton Eye Institute at the University of Tennessee Health Science Center in Memphis for treating retinoblastoma. Before the partnership was established in 2003, there was no centralized tertiary center to treat retinoblastoma in Jordan, the mortality rate of retinoblastoma was approximately 40% and the eye salvage rate was less than 5%. In the course of the partnership, all the new cases and major therapeutic decisions of KHCC were discussed with St Jude's. During the first 7 years of the partnership, 142 patients were treated, and the mortality rate was 6%. From 2015 to 2019, 157 patients were treated, and the mortality rate further dropped to only 5%. The eye salvage rate increased to 62% in the last 4 years of the study. The program showed that expertise was developed at KHCC: in the first 5 years of the program, 70% of consultations recommended changes in the management of the patient. This rate dropped to 7% in the last 7 years of the program. Over time, the need for telemedicine consultations decreased gradually: all cases of retinoblastoma required consultation during the first 4 years of the program, whereas after 6 years of the partnership, half of the cases were managed independently. Finally, after 12 years, most of the cases were managed without the need for consultations with St

Jude's experts. Moreover, this program promoted the development of other kinds of capacity at KHCC: at the beginning of the program only systemic chemotherapy, enucleation, and external-bean radiation were available for treating patients with retinoblastoma. With time, focal therapy (with laser or cryotherapy), other modalities of chemotherapy (intravitreal, intra-arterial, and sub-Tenon), as well as radioactive plaque therapy were implemented. Furthermore, since 2005, KHCC is the center where all retinoblastoma cases are treated in Jordan.

The aforementioned case study demonstrated the benefits of implementing a twinning telemedicine program to create a state-of-the-art multidisciplinary team specialized in retinoblastoma. The telemedicine program allowed KHCC to gain experience and know-how to manage patients with retinoblastoma with impressive results: Jordan's current rates of survival and eye salvage for patients with retinoblastoma are comparable to developed countries. Teleconsultations with more experienced colleagues can lead not only to better patient care, but also serve as a teaching tool for the medical team as well.

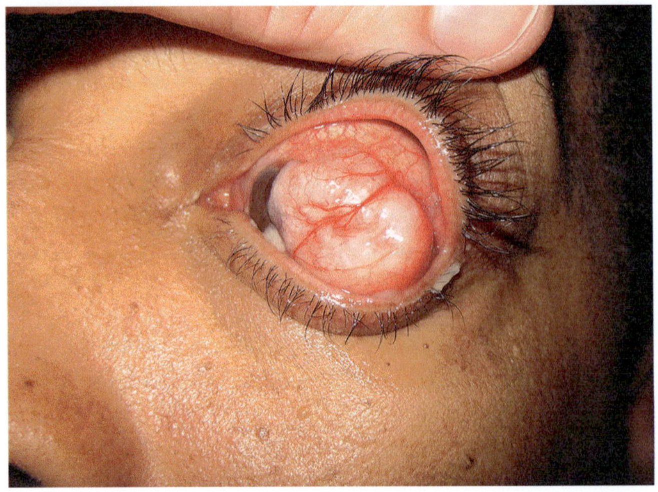

Fig. 1 Patient from Manaus with a squamous carcinoma of the conjunctiva on the left eye

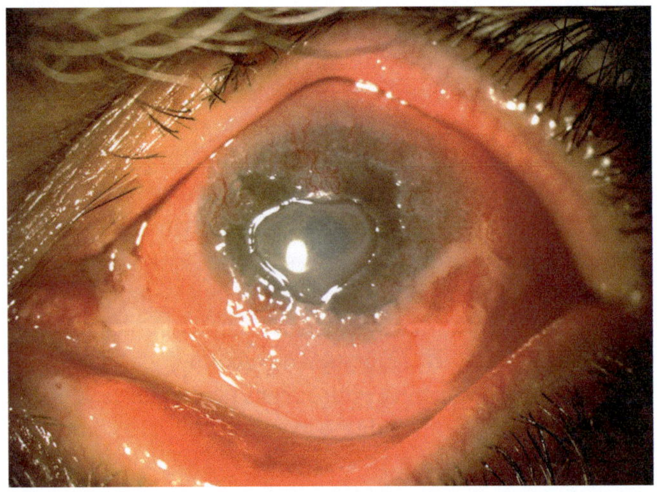

Fig. 2 Patient with SCC of the right eye who had to wait for 13 months since first symptoms to a consultation with an ocular oncologist

6 Telemedicine and Ocular Oncology: São Paulo Experience

In Brazil, there are a few ocular oncology centers, most of them in major cities. Our hospital is situated in São Paulo, the largest metropolitan area in Brazil with population of more than 21 million people. The design of the current public health system of Brazil mandates that patients with suspected eye cancer under the public health system are referred to an ocular oncologist by a general ophthalmologist through a bureaucratic process that can take months. Depending on their city of origin, some patients need to travel for many days because they live far from a major city. Given the nature of the pathology, like retinoblastoma and choroidal melanoma, establishing the correct diagnosis and treatment plan as quickly as possible is important for prognosis and patient survival. More advanced disease is associated with a higher disease burden on the patient, with higher mortality, cost, and suffering to the patient and their family. Examples of patients who have suffered from late diagnosis due to their remote locations are seen in Figs. 1, 2, 3, and 4.

It is our main objective to provide early diagnosis and treatment for every patient with eye cancer in Brazil. Since most of the ocular cancers are rare, it is our stance that it is inefficient to try to train all general ophthalmologists in Brazil to independently manage ocular malignancies. Rather, we can share our expertise with those general ophthalmologists to support them where they are. We aim to empower the general ophthalmologists to diagnose and treat less complex ocular malignancy cases, as well as guide the referral of the more complex ones, such as retinoblastoma and melanoma to ocular oncologists in tertiary centers. To this end, we provide free peer-to-peer consultation with our team of ocular oncologists, free educational videos for ophthalmologists and patients on common eye malignancies, and online educational courses to increase the awareness of ocular cancer. Our group has also leveraged social media to proactively seek out specific groups of patients for complex care-management.

The primary way our team supports ocular oncology care in Brazil is through "Oncophone" [39], which is our service to provide free consultation to general ophthalmologists who can send case details, clinical pictures, and ancillary exams of patients with suspicion of ocular malignancies over the

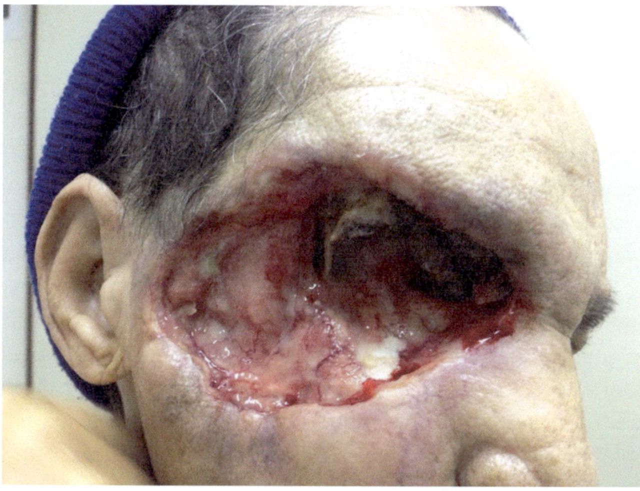

Fig. 3 Patient from an underserved state in Brazil presented with this very advanced squamous carcinoma of the skin to our service in São Paulo

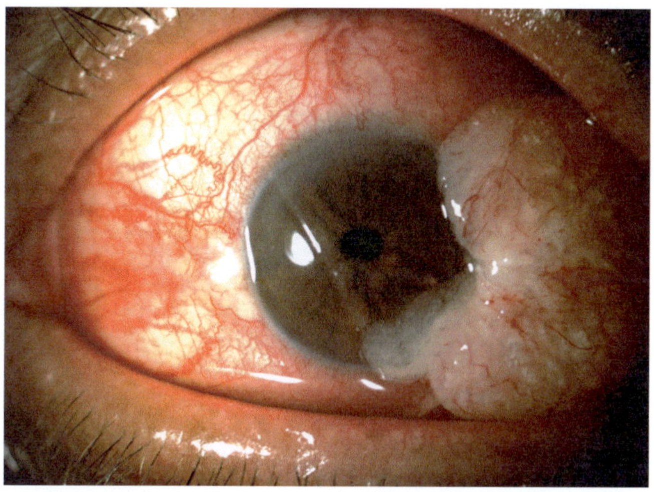

Fig. 4 Patient with a squamous carcinoma of the ocular surface had to travel 12 h by boat and 5 h by airplane to be seen by an ocular oncologist

messaging service WhatsApp®. We provide fast response from our group of specialists, helping early diagnosis and treatment for patients. Oncophone has been widely accepted by our colleagues, and we serve hundreds of consultations every year to Brazil and other Latin American countries. We favor WhatsApp as a telemedicine tool for several reasons: WhatsApp is the main software for instant communications in Brazil—it is free, quick, reliable, user-friendly, and encrypted. WhatsApp allows the transfer of text, images, videos, and documents in high quality. Most importantly, it is already widely used—there are an estimated 2 billion users in 2020 [40]. Several studies have shown the utility of WhatsApp for communication between physicians [40–43]. By creating Oncophone, we have leveraged a widely available and flexible telecommunication technology to extend our ocular oncology center reach to assist our colleagues in ophthalmology, wherever they may be.

In order to promote early diagnosis and treatment for every patient with eye cancer in Brazil, we believe there must be a high level of awareness for ocular cancer among the eye care providers. To this end, we have published videos on YouTube (www.cancerocular.com.br/videos) with information for general ophthalmologists to treat the most common eye cancers. For each topic, we have two videos, one with information for doctors and health professionals, and another for the lay audience of patients and families. The channel has over 157,000 views and has been added by the American Academy of Ophthalmology as part of the "One Network," an online portal with ophthalmic news and education. We also have an Instagram account (@centro_oncologia_ocular) with more than 6800 followers who share ocular oncology case histories and photos weekly. Before the social distancing policies of the pandemic, we hosted local free 1 day ocular oncology courses in partnership with ophthalmology residency programs. During the pandemic, we have moved our educational activities to a virtual setting. One such series was "OncoSunday," where we hosted weekly online teleconference meetings on Sundays. The courses were presented in Portuguese, with instant translation to English, and we hosted specialists in ocular oncology from Brazil and all over the world. We had a wide reach, and we estimate to have hosted between 500 and 750 ophthalmologists in each Sunday meeting.

Finally, in order to reach special patient populations who may suffer a higher burden of ocular malignancy, we have also used social media to recruit patients with very rare diseases like phacomatoses or xeroderma pigmentosum (XP). As an example, we had only 7 XP patients being followed up in our ambulatory service, and we noticed that these patients did not have access to ocular oncologists before coming to our institution. For that reason, we have decided to make an active search for patients with XP with posts in social media, such as Facebook® and Instagram®, with excellent responses. Nowadays, we follow 47 patients with this disease on our service.

7 Barriers to Overcome for Teleophthalmology

While teleophthalmology has a lot to offer patients and providers, it is not the panacea for health delivery and still has several barriers to overcome, including technological, cultural, financial, and regulatory.

For teleophthalmology consults from providers to patients, the main technological barrier that needs to be overcome is a high quality, remote ophthalmologic exam.

Presently, the video eye exam can only provide very basic information, like patient symptoms, and the equivalent of a penlight exam of the external and anterior segment. But basic steps of the eye exam, like measuring visual acuity, intraocular pressure, pupil response, refraction, or fundus exam, are currently not supported with widely available technology like smartphones. These constitute the foundations of an ophthalmic evaluation, and as such, severely limit the diagnostic capability of virtual ophthalmologists. In the future, there might be home-based technology that allows IOP measurement and even posterior segment exams that will allow follow-up of patients without the need frequent for office visits [44].

There are also cultural barriers to adoption of teleophthalmology. Many patients tend to resist the concept of seeing their doctors over the computer [45]. A systematic review analyzing the effectiveness of video consultations in clinical oncology showed that despite the overall positive results, patients reported reluctance to communicate with providers using video-based systems, and a feeling of emotional distance between the patient and providers was also observed. Moreover, the ideal group for telemedicine is composed of patients who mostly live far from big medical centers, many in rural areas. These individuals, especially the elderly, tend to have less familiarity with ICT, or in extreme cases, are ICT illiterate [45]. There needs to be creative and careful solutions to addressing these issues, most likely by augmenting the capacity of local resources to reach these populations.

Also, despite the recent advances, reimbursement for telemedicine remains a challenge in many countries, with resistance from insurance health providers. In order for there to be further developments in teleophthalmology, there must be financial support for these efforts, otherwise few clinicians will adapt to this new method of providing ophthalmic care.

Last, but not least, there are some legal barriers. As a relatively new practice modality, legal frameworks have struggled to keep up with the demands placed by the pandemic. For example, countries such as Brazil did not even have regulations for telemedicine before the COVID-19 pandemic [46]. Many of the policy changes in the United States to support telemedicine reimbursement are legislated to only be in effect for the duration of the public health emergency, and it is unclear if these changes will be continued after the pandemic is over. As regulations are developed that may require certain levels of confidentiality and documentation for patient protection, they may also place a burden on low-cost, grassroots initiatives like Oncophone. Telemedicine should be held to high standards to ensure high-quality patient care, but regulators should be sure to balance those needs with the flexibility and local adaptability that telemedicine offers.

8 Conclusions

As this chapter goes to press, telemedicine is being deployed by many patients and clinicians who likely never imagined they would be in this position. Other forms of interprofessional education and communication, like meetings, conferences, lectures, and courses have been transitioned to virtual events. Ophthalmology has already been changed by the COVID-19 pandemic to adopt many telemedicine approaches, and as our chapter has reviewed, there is significant evidence to suggest that these practices can lead to high-quality outcomes for patient care and provider development. While there are many barriers to successful adoption of telemedicine for ophthalmology, the perfect should not be the enemy of the good. While our team believes that every patient with an ocular malignancy should be treated by a specialized eye doctor, initiatives such as OncoPhone can be of great value for patients and doctors in underserved areas. As technology develops, attitudes, financing, and regulation will change as well, and there are many promising areas for teleophthalmology to help provide high-quality ophthalmic care for patients worldwide.

References

1. Sood S, Mbarika V, Jugoo S, et al. What is telemedicine? A collection of 104 peer-reviewed perspectives and theoretical underpinnings. Telemed J E Health. 2007;13(5):573–90.
2. World Health Organization. mHealth: new horizons for health through mobile technologies second global survey on eHealth. In: mHealth: New Horizons for Health through Mobile Technologies: Second Global Survey on eHealth (Global Observatory for eHealth). Switzerland: World Health Organization; 2011.
3. Einthoven W. Le télécardiogramme. Arch Int Physiol. 1906;4:132–64.
4. World Health Organization. Telemedicine: opportunities and developments in member states: report on the second global survey on eHealth. Switzerland: World Health organization; 2009.
5. International Telecommunication Union. Measuring digital developments: facts and figures. Switzerland: International Telecommunication Union; 2020.
6. Rathi S, Tsui E, Mehta N, Zahid S, Schuman JS. The current state of Teleophthalmology in the United States. Ophthalmology. 2017;124(12):1729–34.
7. De Lott LB, Newman-Casey PA, Lee PP, Ballouz D, Azzouz L, Cho J, Valicevic AN, Woodward MA. Change in ophthalmic clinicians' attitudes toward telemedicine during the coronavirus 2019 pandemic. Telemed J E Health. 2021;27(2):231–5.
8. Saleem SM, Pasquale LR, Sidoti PA, Tsai JC. Virtual ophthalmology: telemedicine in a COVID-19 era. Am J Ophthalmol. 2020;216:237–42.
9. Skalet AH, Allen RC, Shields CL, Wilson MW, Mruthyunjaya P, Gombos DS. Considerations for the management and triage of ocular oncology cases during the COVID-19 pandemic. Ocul Oncol Pathol. 2020;6(3):1–4.
10. Langer PD, Bernardini FP. Oculofacial plastic surgery and the COVID-19 pandemic: current reactions and implications for the future. Ophthalmology. 2020;127(9):e70–1.

11. Grossman SN, Calix R, Tow S, Odel JG, Sun LD, Balcer LJ, Galetta SL, Rucker JC. Neuro-ophthalmology in the era of COVID-19: future implications of a public health crisis. Ophthalmology. 2020;127(9):e72–4.
12. Manjandavida FP, Honavar SG, Kim U, Singh U, Menon V, Das S, Kaliki S, Palanivelu MS, Khetan V, Shah PK, Rishi P, Mulay K, Gandhi A, Vadhiraja BM, Reddy VA, Bhat S, Rao V. Ocular oncology practice guidelines during COVID-19 pandemic-an expert consensus. Indian J Ophthalmol. 2020;68(7):1281–91.
13. Sommer AC, Blumenthal EZ. Telemedicine in ophthalmology in view of the emerging COVID-19 outbreak. Graefes Arch Clin Exp Ophthalmol. 2020;258(11):2341–52.
14. World Health Organization. Global diffusion of eHealth: making universal health coverage achievable. Switzerland: World Health organization; 2016.
15. Resnikoff S, Felch W, Gauthier TM, Spivey B. The number of ophthalmologists in practice and training worldwide: a growing gap despite more than 200,000 practitioners. Br J Ophthalmol. 2012;96(6):783–7.
16. ConselhoBrasileiro de Oftalmologia. As condições de saúde ocular no Brasil 2019. ConselhoBrasileiro de Oftalmologia: São Paulo; 2019.
17. ConselhoBrasileiro de Oftalmologia. Censo 2014. ConselhoBrasileiro de Oftalmologia: São Paulo; 2014.
18. Bellan L, Buske L, Wang S, Buys YM. The landscape of ophthalmologists in Canada: present and future. Can J Ophthalmol. 2013;48(3):160–6.
19. Ray KN, Chari AV, Engberg J, Bertolet M, Mehrotra A. Disparities in time spent seeking medical care in the United States. JAMA Intern Med. 2015;175(12):1983–6.
20. Parikh D, Armstrong G, Liou V, Husain D. Advances in telemedicine in ophthalmology. Semin Ophthalmol. 2020;35(4):210–5.
21. Lee R, Wong TY, Sabanayagam C. Epidemiology of diabetic retinopathy, diabetic macular edema and related vision loss. Eye Vis (Lond). 2015;2:17.
22. Bastos de Carvalho A, Ware SL, Lei F, Bush HM, Sprang R, Higgins EB. Implementation and sustainment of a statewide telemedicine diabetic retinopathy screening network for federally designated safety-net clinics. PLoS One. 2020;15(11):e0241767.
23. Li HK, Horton M, Bursell SE, Cavallerano J, Zimmer-Galler I, Tennant M, Abramoff M, Chaum E, Debuc DC, Leonard-Martin T, Winchester M, Lawrence MG, Bauman W, Gardner WK, Hildebran L, Federman J, American Telemedicine Association Diabetic Retinopathy Telehealth Practice Recommendations Working Group. Telehealth practice recommendations for diabetic retinopathy, second edition. Telemed J E Health. 2011;17(10):814–37.
24. Gao X, Park CH, Dedrick K, Borkar DS, Obeid A, Reber S, Federman J. Use of telehealth screening to detect diabetic retinopathy and other ocular findings in primary care settings. Telemed J E Health. 2019;25(9):802–7.
25. Owsley C, McGwin G Jr, Lee DJ, Lam BL, Friedman DS, Gower EW, Haller JA, Hark LA, Saaddine J, Innovative Network for Sight (INSIGHT) Research Group. Diabetes eye screening in urban settings serving minority populations: detection of diabetic retinopathy and other ocular findings using telemedicine. JAMA Ophthalmol. 2015;133(2):174–81.
26. Cavallerano AA, Cavallerano JD, Katalinic P, Blake B, Rynne M, Conlin PR, Hock K, Tolson AM, Aiello LP, Aiello LM, Joslin vision network research team. A telemedicine program for diabetic retinopathy in a veterans affairs medical center—the Joslin vision network eye health care model. Am J Ophthalmol. 2005;139(4):597–604.
27. Zimmer-Galler IE, Kimura AE, Gupta S. Diabetic retinopathy screening and the use of telemedicine. Curr Opin Ophthalmol. 2015;26(3):167–72.
28. Kirkizlar E, Serban N, Sisson JA, Swann JL, Barnes CS, Williams MD. Evaluation of telemedicine for screening of diabetic retinopathy in the veterans health administration. Ophthalmology. 2013;120(12):2604–10.
29. Souza GF, Figueira RM, Alkmim MB, Sousa LAP, Bonisson L, Ribeiro ALP, Vasconcelos-Santos DV. Teleophthalmology screening for diabetic retinopathy in Brazil: applicability and economic assessment. Telemed J E Health. 2020;26(3):341–6.
30. Shah PK, Ramya A, Narendran V. Telemedicine for ROP. Asia Pac J Ophthalmol (Phila). 2018;7(1):52–5.
31. Quinn GE, Ells A, Capone A Jr, Hubbard GB, Daniel E, Hildebrand PL, Ying GS, e-ROP (Telemedicine Approaches to Evaluating Acute-Phase Retinopathy of Prematurity) Cooperative Group. Analysis of discrepancy between diagnostic clinical examination findings and corresponding evaluation of digital images in the telemedicine approaches to evaluating acute-phase retinopathy of prematurity study. JAMA Ophthalmol. 2016;134(11):1263–70.
32. Murakami Y, Jain A, Silva RA, Lad EM, Gandhi J, Moshfeghi DM. Stanford University network for diagnosis of retinopathy of prematurity (SUNDROP): 12-month experience with telemedicine screening. Br J Ophthalmol. 2008 Nov;92(11):1456–60.
33. Fijalkowski N, Zheng LL, Henderson MT, Wang SK, Wallenstein MB, Leng T, Moshfeghi DM. Stanford University network for diagnosis of retinopathy of prematurity (SUNDROP): five years of screening with telemedicine. Ophthalmic Surg Lasers Imaging Retina. 2014;45(2):106–13.
34. Hark LA, Adeghate J, Katz LJ, Ulas M, Waisbourd M, Maity A, Zhan T, Hegarty S, Leiby BE, Pasquale LR, Leite S, Saaddine JB, Haller JA, Myers JS. Philadelphia telemedicine glaucoma detection and follow-up study: cataract classifications following eye screening. Telemed J E Health. 2020;26(8):992–1000.
35. Balaskas K, Gray J, Blows P, Rajai A, Flaye D, Peto T, Sagoo MS. Management of choroidal naevomelanocytic lesions: feasibility and safety of a virtual clinic model. Br J Ophthalmol. 2016;100(5):665–70.
36. Lapere S, Weis E. Tele-ophthalmology for the monitoring of choroidal and iris nevi: a pilot study. Can J Ophthalmol. 2018;53(5):471–3.
37. Roelofs K, Weis E. Tele-oncology: a validation study of choroidal and iris nevi. Ocul Oncol Pathol. 2019;5(4):298–302.
38. Yousef YA, Al-Nawaiseh I, Mehyar M, Sultan I, Al-Hussaini M, Jaradat I, Mohammad M, AlJabari R, Abu-Yaghi N, Rodriguez-Galindo C, Qaddoumi I, Wilson M. How telemedicine and centralized care changed the natural history of retinoblastoma in a developing country: analysis of 478 patients. Ophthalmology. 2021;128(1):130–7.
39. Belfort NR. Public health strategy vs. golden standard for ocular cancer care in Brazil. Arq Bras Oftalmol. 2020;83(1):V–VI.
40. Giordano V, Koch H, Godoy-Santos A, Dias Belangero W, Esteves Santos Pires R, Labronici P. WhatsApp messenger as an adjunctive tool for telemedicine: an overview. Interact J Med Res. 2017;6(2):e11.
41. Johnston MJ, King D, Arora S, et al. Smartphones let surgeons know WhatsApp: an analysis of communication in emergency surgical teams. Am J Surg. 2015;209:45–51.
42. Wani SA, Rabah SM, Alfadil S, Dewanjee N, Najmi Y. Efficacy of communication amongst staff members at plastic and reconstructive surgery section using smartphone and mobile WhatsApp. Indian J Plast Surg. 2013;46(3):502–5.
43. Giordano V, Koch HA, Mendes CH, Bergamin A, de Souza FS. Do Amaral NP. WhatsApp messenger is useful and reproducible in the assessment of tibial plateau fractures: inter- and intra-observer agreement study. Int J Med Inform. 2015;84(2):141–8.
44. Holekamp NM, Moving from clinic to home: what the future holds for ophthalmic telemedicine. Am J Ophthalmol. 2018;187:xxviii–xxxv.

45. Kitamura C, Zurawel-Balaura L, Wong RK. How effective is video consultation in clinical oncology? A systematic review. CurrOncol. 2010;17(3):17–27.

46. Brasil, Ministério da Saúde. Portaria n 467, de 20 de março de 2020. Dispõe, emcaráterexcepcional e temporário, sobre as ações de Telemedicina, com o objetivo de regulamentar e operacionalizar as medidas de enfrentamento da emergência de saúdepública de importânciainternacionalprevistas no art. 3° da Lei n° 13.979, de 6 de fevereiro de 2020, decorrente da epidemia de COVID-19. DiárioOficial da União, 23/03/2020. Edição 56-B, seção 1. http://www.in.gov.br/en/web/dou/-/portaria-n-467-de-20-de-marco-de-2020-249312996.

Harnessing the Power of Artificial Intelligence

Zelia M. Correa and T. Y. Alvin Liu

1 Introduction

The recent evolution of computer graphic processing units, advances in mathematical models, and availability of big data have allowed artificial intelligence (AI) using machine learning (ML) and deep learning (DL) techniques to reach unprecedented, robust performance for broad applications and has generated immense interest in the medical field in recent years (Fig. 1). Although these terms are used in an interexchangeable manner, it marks an evolution that started with early computing in the 1950s. Machine learning can be used in many different areas from business and marketing to informatics and technology and medicine. Deep learning (or reinforcement learning) is a subset of machine learning and a technique that autonomously learns features and tasks from a training dataset. "Deep" refers to the multiple layers of algorithms that the presented data pass through during computation, and a network of interconnected algorithms is called a neural network [1]. The performance DL systems can be enhanced using backpropagation algorithms to change reiteratively the internal parameters [2]. DL has been widely adopted in image recognition, speech recognition, and natural language processing, but is only beginning to impact health care. With well-annotated, large datasets, DL can be used to classify medical images accurately, and it has been applied in a wide variety of medical disciplines, including pathology [3], dermatology [4], radiology [5–7], and ophthalmology [8–12]. Often times, the performance of these DL algorithms has been found to be on par with if not superior to that of human clinicians.

A variety of articles concerning AI, ML, and DL automated applications in diagnosing ophthalmic diseases have been published recently [1, 10, 11, 13, 14]. The majority of these studies are related to diabetic retinopathy, macular degeneration, and glaucoma, which are the 3 most prevalent causes of irreversible blindness worldwide. In many recent studies, AI, ML, and DL techniques have been shown to be an effective diagnostic tool for detecting and identifying various eye diseases in ophthalmic health-care services. These applications can make a great contribution to providing support to patients in remote areas where there are no experts, medical devices, and adequate infrastructure. These studies have indicated that AI, ML, and DL applications with high accuracy are capable of detecting and diagnosing multiple retina disorders with promising results in automated image analysis [9, 10].

2 Applications of AI in Ocular Oncology

Basically, DL can be applied in the field of ocular oncology in 3 scenarios—tumor diagnosis, tumor prognosis, and management decisions [15]. There are other instances in which DL can be used such as analysis of big data, disease segmentation and grouping, and learning tasks/skills acquisition (Fig. 2). The latter is exemplified by the use of surgical simulators currently available for cataract surgery and vitrectomy.

The process of automatically detect a disease includes three basic steps [14]. The first step is collecting a large number of images of patients with characteristic lesions, known history, and outcomes that are labeled by experts. This is the essence of machine learning. The second step is creating an algorithm/program through which the computer can extract the features of a disease based on the input of marked images. The third and last step is validation of the algorithm by feeding other images that can be distinguished from other kind of

Z. M. Correa (✉)
Department of Ophthalmology, Retina Service, Ocular Oncology Program, Bascom Palmer Eye Institute, University of Miami, Miami, FL, USA
e-mail: zcorrea@med.miami.edu

T. Y. A. Liu
Department of Ophthalmology, Retina Service, Wilmer Eye Institute, Johns Hopkins Medicine, Baltimore, MD, USA
e-mail: tliu25@jhmi.edu

B. V. Chawla, M. E. Aronow (eds.), *Global Perspectives in Ocular Oncology*, https://doi.org/10.1007/978-3-031-08250-4_25

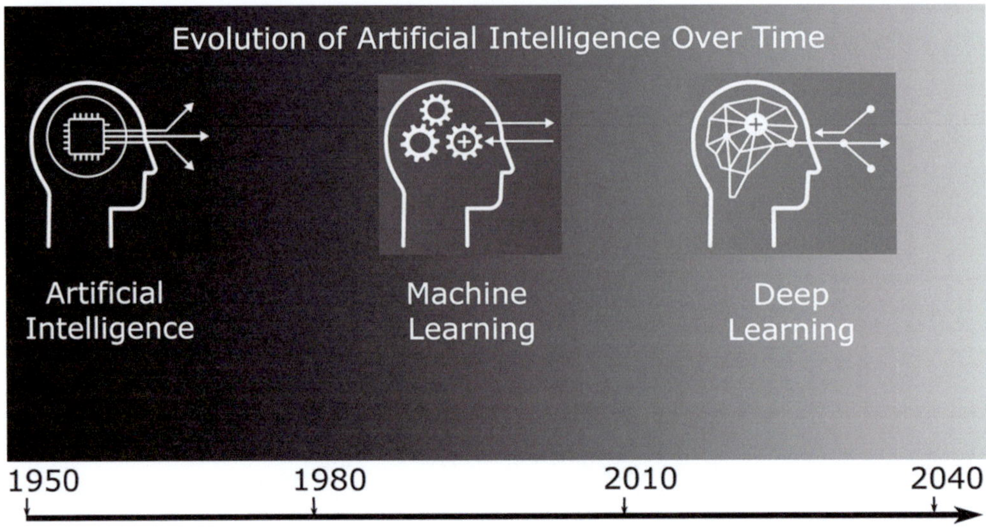

Fig. 1 Evolution of artificial intelligence over time. Artificial intelligence started to be used in the 1950s with early engineering of machines that mimic cognitive functions. Machine learning was an evolution in the 1980s marked by advances in computing ability to perform tasks without explicit instructions by relying on patterns. Deep learning is a more sophisticated mode of machine learning based on neural networks in which the computer uses algorithms to perform tasks surpassing human performance

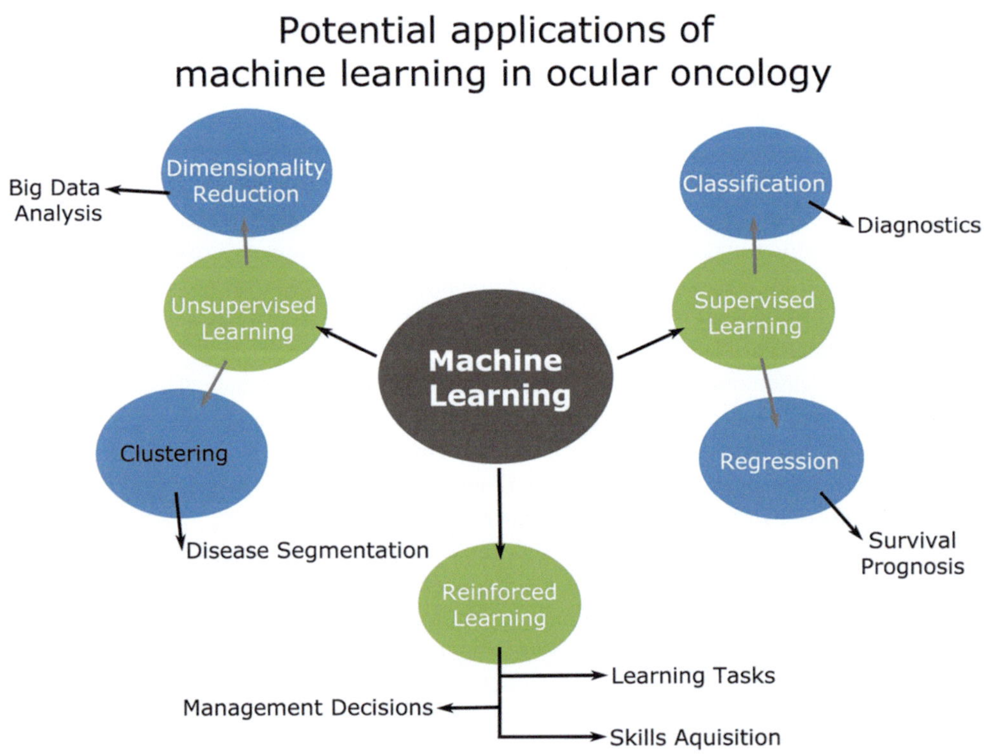

Fig. 2 Simplified chart explaining the different potential applications of machine learning in ocular oncology

disease by the computer. Limiting factors for this technology are incorrect labeling of images, extensive variability of disease presentation, limited number of cases to train the machine, and poor quality of information provided to the computer both during training as well as validation.

2.1 AI-Assisted Diagnosis

AI-assisted diagnosis uses supervised learning to create an algorithm [16]. There are essentially 3 methods of imaging that can be used for diagnosis in ocular oncology: digital slit lamp or external photos [17], digital fundus photography and autofluorescence, grayscale imaging such as optical coherence tomography (OCT) or high-resolution ultrasound, and cytology or histopathology.

The deep learning model has demonstrated a significant improvement in the classification accuracy of conjunctival lesions using synthetic images generated by two generative adversarial networks [17].

Digital fundus photography and autofluorescence are the easiest modalities to assess and currently the most studied in other areas of ophthalmology and likely in oncology. As one would imagine, color photos (slit lamp, external, or fundus) have a potential limitation if different cameras are being used since the output images will display varying magnifications and color tones. Digital fundus auto-fluorescence provides sharper contrast and less variation due to its grayscale images. Similarly, other grayscale photos seem to have an advantage over color photos. OCT has been widely adopted because it produces standardized images that can be easily reproduced. Although high-resolution ultrasound can produce digital images that can be analyzed through the computer, examiner variation and size overlay between tumors may pose an issue in smaller datasets and may be a limiting reason to incorporate this technology in AI studies.

Computational pathology has been shown to add value to clinical practice as well as to medical research. Computational pathology requires standardization and digital slide scanning of good quality and resolution [18]. Whole slide scanners available commercially have been used with remarkable result. For these reasons, the use of AI for pathology diagnosis could potentially fulfill an area of significant unmet need throughout the world. Despite the diagnostic power of histopathology, the field of ocular oncology is moving toward more conservative management for intraocular tumors leading researchers to consider other alternatives such as digital cytology obtained as aspirates [19], exfoliation, and imprint. The use of computational pathology has unraveled information integration and advanced digital communication networks that have the potential to improve clinical workflow efficiency, diagnostic quality, and ultimately create personalized diagnosis and treatment plans for patients [20].

3 Prognosis

AI has the potential to contribute to nearly all aspects of the clinical workflow including in ocular oncology ranging from more accurate diagnosis to prognosis, and personalized treatment [21]. One of the earliest uses of machine learning in ocular oncology was the development of gene expression profile assay to assess prognosis of patients with uveal melanoma [22]. Since then, multiple other attempts at estimating prognosis have been made [23].

Digital image analysis of BAP-1 expression in histopathology slides of enucleated eyes with uveal melanoma has been used to predict prognosis showing that the automated method outperformed the manual method in interobserver concordance and time required for classification [24]. Recently, two separate publications have explored the possibility of estimating survival prognosis of patients with uveal melanoma using DL. One of them looked at enucleated eyes and used BAP1 immunohistochemistry as a poor prognosis indicator [25]. The issue with this model is that ocular oncology is moving away from enucleation making this model difficult to translate in clinical practice. In addition, immunohistochemistry carries many technical variables decreasing the reliability of this model. This is the first study we published showing the algorythm and training set for the machine learning [19]. This model is more translatable since FNAB is part of ocular oncology practice and gene expression profile is the prognostic "ground truth" in uveal melanoma since it is the most robust prognostic test for this disease and it has been prospectively validated. Such algorithm could potentially allow the development of a digital pathology software available globally for prognostication, guidance to appropriate surveillance testing, and possible adjuvant clinical trials for patients with uveal melanoma.

4 Management Decisions

As in other areas of ophthalmology, multiple sources of clinical data can be incorporated into mathematic models to generate diagnostic inferences and predictions, to allow physicians to make the best possible medical decisions [21]. Recent research has shown that DL algorithms in classifying ophthalmic imaging data such as color fundus photography for various eye diseases prove to have an acceptable clinical performance [11]. The influence of AI in OCT analysis is rapidly advancing and it is now being applied to several retinal diseases [1]. However, despite its potential to improve clinical practice and standardize clinical care, DL has not been explored to its full potential in management decisions for ocular tumors using standardized color photos or OCT.

5 Future Perspectives

It is believed that AI is the fourth industrial revolution in mankind's history [12]. Technological innovation in health care is growing at an increasing pace while being integrated into both our lives, such as smart health tracker, and diagnostic algorithm in medical practice. According to experts driving AI into medicine, there are at least 3 potential areas where AI may transform patient care as we know it. The first is in reducing medical errors that lead to misdiagnosis, particularly in reducing false-negative results of tests assuming the technology will reach a point where AI will detect things the human eye cannot. Second, AI will allow globalization of medical knowledge reaching physicians and patients everywhere and permitting broader access to care. New applications are being developed to help patients self-assess their health throughout life thus seeking medical help earlier in the course of their disease. Third, AI holds the promise of "making health care human again" by unburdening the physician and bringing them closer to the patient. AI can potentially lessen or eliminate the chore of data entry that leads to doctor fatigue and steals precious time with the patient.

Surprisingly, there is hope that placing humanity back into the profession will be AI's most important contribution to medicine.

With the rapid development of digital, molecular, and informatics within the field of pathology, computational pathology is increasingly involved in many subspecialties such as pulmonary, renal, gastrointestinal, neurology, gynecology, and ophthalmic pathology [18, 20].

It is believed that the initial phase of AI encompasses specific tasks such as the diagnosis of a particular cancer and classification of tissue types, which require limited and simple criteria. However, the growing medical data, including genomics, proteomics, informatics, and whole-slide images, are expected to integrate together to become a data-rich pathomics and lead to rapid development and prosperity of an AI-assisted computational pathology. Although AI has shown tremendous promise, many challenges remain before we are able to fully integrate this technology into clinical practice. These challenges include clinical validation to translation with increasing technology readiness level, ethical use of DL considering patient variables, confidentiality as well as medical-legal responsibility, and integration of AI solutions in clinical care pathways and health-care systems. It is possible that low-cost, simpler digital solutions, such as smart phone-based systems in resource-limited settings, may facilitate the implementation of AI. Considering the different facets of AI and its potential use in ocular oncology, it doesn't seem far-fetched to see that its translation and implementation will likely revolutionize eye care in the twenty-first century.

References

1. Kapoor R, Whigham BT, Al-Aswad LA. Artificial intelligence and optical coherence tomography imaging. Asia Pac J Ophthalmol (Phila). 2019;8(2):187–94.
2. LeCun Y, Bengio Y, Hinton G. Deep learning. Nature. 2015;521(7553):436–44.
3. Ehteshami Bejnordi B, Veta M, Johannes van Diest P, van Ginneken B, Karssemeijer N, Litjens G, et al. Diagnostic assessment of deep learning algorithms for detection of lymph node metastases in women with breast cancer. JAMA. 2017;318(22):2199–210.
4. Esteva A, Kuprel B, Novoa RA, Ko J, Swetter SM, Blau HM, et al. Dermatologist-level classification of skin cancer with deep neural networks. Nature. 2017;542(7639):115–8.
5. Chung SW, Han SS, Lee JW, Oh KS, Kim NR, Yoon JP, et al. Automated detection and classification of the proximal humerus fracture by using deep learning algorithm. Acta Orthop. 2018;89(4):468–73.
6. Lakhani P, Sundaram B. Deep learning at chest radiography: automated classification of pulmonary tuberculosis by using convolutional neural networks. Radiology. 2017;284(2):574–82.
7. Lakhani P. Deep convolutional neural networks for endotracheal tube position and X-ray image classification: challenges and opportunities. J Digit Imaging. 2017;30(4):460–8.
8. Brown JM, Campbell JP, Beers A, Chang K, Ostmo S, Chan RVP, et al. Automated diagnosis of plus disease in retinopathy of prematurity using deep convolutional neural networks. JAMA Ophthalmol. 2018;136(7):803–10.
9. Burlina P, Pacheco KD, Joshi N, Freund DE, Bressler NM. Comparing humans and deep learning performance for grading AMD: a study in using universal deep features and transfer learning for automated AMD analysis. Comput Biol Med. 2017;82:80–6.
10. Burlina PM, Joshi N, Pekala M, Pacheco KD, Freund DE, Bressler NM. Automated grading of age-related macular degeneration from color fundus images using deep convolutional neural networks. JAMA Ophthalmol. 2017;135(11):1170–6.
11. Gulshan V, Peng L, Coram M, Stumpe MC, Wu D, Narayanaswamy A, et al. Development and validation of a deep learning algorithm for detection of diabetic retinopathy in retinal fundus photographs. JAMA. 2016;316(22):2402–10.
12. Ting DSW, Cheung CY, Lim G, Tan GSW, Quang ND, Gan A, et al. Development and validation of a deep learning system for diabetic retinopathy and related eye diseases using retinal images from multiethnic populations with diabetes. JAMA. 2017;318(22):2211–23.
13. Kapoor R, Walters SP, Al-Aswad LA. The current state of artificial intelligence in ophthalmology. Surv Ophthalmol. 2019;64(2):233–40.
14. Du XL, Li WB, Hu BJ. Application of artificial intelligence in ophthalmology. Int J Ophthalmol. 2018;11(9):1555–61.
15. Chen H, Alvin Liu TY, Correa Z, Unberath M. An interactive approach to region of interest selection in cytologic analysis of uveal melanoma based on unsupervised clustering. In: Fu HGMK, MacGillivray T, Xu Y, Zheng Y, editors. Ophthalmic medical image analysis OMIA 2020 lecture notes in computer science. 12069. Cham: Springer; 2020. p. 114–24.
16. Chen H, Liu TYA, Gomez C, Correa Z, Unberath M An interpretable algorithm for uveal melanoma subtyping from whole slide cytology images. Proceedings of the 38 th International Conference on Machine Learning - PMLR; 2021: 139.
17. Yoo TK, Choi JY, Kim HK. Feasibility study to improve deep learning in OCT diagnosis of rare retinal diseases with few-shot classification. Med Biol Eng Comput. 2021;59(2):401–15.
18. Campanella G, Hanna MG, Geneslaw L, Miraflor A, Werneck Krauss Silva V, Busam KJ, et al. Clinical-grade computational pathology using weakly supervised deep learning on whole slide images. Nat Med. 2019;25(8):1301–9.
19. Liu TYA, Zhu H, Chen H, Arevalo JF, Hui FK, Yi PH, et al. Gene expression profile prediction in uveal melanoma using deep learning: a pilot study for the development of an alternative survival prediction tool. Ophthalmol Retina. 2020;4(12):1213–5.
20. Cui M, Zhang DY. Artificial intelligence and computational pathology. Lab Investig. 2021;101(4):412–22.
21. Ting DSW, Pasquale LR, Peng L, Campbell JP, Lee AY, Raman R, et al. Artificial intelligence and deep learning in ophthalmology. Br J Ophthalmol. 2019;103(2):167–75.
22. Onken MD, Worley LA, Tuscan MD, Harbour JW. An accurate, clinically feasible multi-gene expression assay for predicting metastasis in uveal melanoma. J Mol Diagn. 2010;12(4):461–8.
23. Correa ZM. Assessing prognosis in uveal melanoma. Cancer Control. 2016;23(2):93–8.
24. Stalhammar G, See TRO, Phillips S, Seregard S, Grossniklaus HE. Digital image analysis of BAP-1 accurately predicts uveal melanoma metastasis. Transl Vis Sci Technol. 2019;8(3):11.
25. Zhang H, Kalirai H, Acha-Sagredo A, Yang X, Zheng Y, Coupland SE. Piloting a deep learning model for predicting nuclear BAP1 Immunohistochemical expression of uveal melanoma from hematoxylin-and-eosin sections. Transl Vis Sci Technol. 2020;9(2):50.

Developing Animal Models in Ocular Oncology

Ilyse S. Kornblau, Rachel C. Brennan, and Matthew W. Wilson

1 Introduction

Retinoblastoma (Rb) and uveal melanoma (UM) are the two most common primary intraocular malignancies in children and adults. Both diseases are relatively rare, with Rb occurring in 1 in 15,000–20,000 live births [1] at an estimated rate of 250–300 in the United States of America (USA) [2] and 7000–8000 new cases worldwide per year [3–5]. UM occurs at a rate of 5–6 per one million people in the USA [6–9]. Historically, these low incidence rates have limited the ability to conduct large clinical trials. Additionally, as Rb typically occurs in young children under 5 years of age, conducting clinical trials in this age group has ethical implications. To overcome this barrier, pre-clinical models have been developed to assist with elucidating tumorigenesis characteristics, metastatic progression, and therapeutic evaluation. In this chapter, we will highlight the different models currently published with an emphasis on the specific characteristics of each model and its use in tumor evaluation, focusing on Rb and UM. We will briefly touch on a novel model being used for adenoid cystic carcinoma of the lacrimal gland and preclinical models for evaluating therapeutic methodology in animals with and without induced intraocular tumors.

There are several human cell lines derived directly from patients which have been used in both Rb and UM. These models are useful for testing cellular characteristics but lack the 3-D structure and surrounding extracellular framework seen in human tumors. Furthermore, these models lack the ability to test therapeutics in an immunoprivileged setting mimicking natural formation within the human eye. Additionally, metastatic potential cannot be assessed from cell lines.

Animal models can be divided into three primary types: (1) xenografts, (2) genetically modified models including knock-out (KO) models, and (3) transgenic models. A xenograft uses human tumor cell lines and implants the cells within the animal model, frequently in a subcutaneous location for better monitoring. However, if the tumor is not induced within the eye, then the model is less representative of human tumor growth patterns and metastatic potential. To avoid this issue, orthotopic xenograft models directly implant human Rb and UM tumor cells within the eye (via anterior chamber, intravitreal, subretinal, or suprachoroidal injections) of the species to be used, most commonly mice or rabbits. Orthotopic xenograft models reproduce the tumor microenvironment, specifically the sequestered nature of the eye in Rb and UM. These models frequently require immunosuppression to allow for tumor growth, which limits observations of immune response to tumor presence. Xenograft models are best for evaluating pre-clinical treatments as the tumors grow quickly, allowing for rapid testing of therapeutics in a shorter amount of time.

Genetically modified models including knock-out models are created by selectively breeding animals without certain genomic features to induce tumor development. Transgenic models are created by promoting oncogene expression using viral mediators. Both knock-out and transgenic models are ideal for elucidating which proteins are involved in tumor development, progression, high risk characteristics, and metastasis. Additionally, therapeutic trials utilizing these models can assist with targeted treatment plans based on underlying tumor genomic features. One downside to transgenic models is the artificial induction of tumors via viral mediators, which may not mimic human tumor genetics.

I. S. Kornblau (✉)
Department of Surgical Services, Division of Ophthalmology, Veteran's Health Administration, Memphis, TN, USA
e-mail: Ilyse.kornblau@va.gov

R. C. Brennan
Department of Oncology, St. Jude Children's Research Hospital, Memphis, TN, USA
e-mail: Rachel.brennan@stjude.org

M. W. Wilson
Department of Ophthalmology, Hamilton Eye Institute, University of Tennessee Health Science Center, Memphis, TN, USA
e-mail: Mwilson5@uthsc.edu

B. V. Chawla, M. E. Aronow (eds.), *Global Perspectives in Ocular Oncology*, https://doi.org/10.1007/978-3-031-08250-4_26

Considerations in selecting an animal model include ocular size, immune status, gestation time, lifespan, median time to tumor growth, and cost. Larger animals such as rabbits and primates are closer in size to the human eye, however they are more expensive to develop and maintain. Additionally, these models take many months for tumor development. Smaller animals including zebrafish, frogs, and mice are less expensive and tend to develop tumors within weeks. However, the tumor development and growth patterns do not necessarily reflect the progression in their human counterparts. Therefore, each model should be carefully selected to best answer the research question being addressed.

The goal in utilizing pre-clinical animal models is to better understand tumor growth and development, direct and metastatic spread, test therapeutics targeting these genetic events, and ultimately test therapeutics prior to development of clinical trials. By testing in pre-clinical models, only the most effective treatments will proceed to clinical trial, reducing the time for discovery and potential patient harm.

2 Retinoblastoma

2.1 Transgenic Models

Transgenic models are utilized to both elucidate the pathway of tumor formation and test therapeutics prior to clinical trials. In Rb models, the goal is to create an animal model with tumor formation within the retina with similar histological characteristics, focal or multifocal formation, and a photoreceptor origin. Models which metastasize via local extension to the central nervous system, develop pineal gland tumors, or distant metastasis are useful for understanding the tumor characteristics which led to metastasis and exploring treatment modalities for metastasis.

The original Rb murine model was a transgenic mouse created by Windle [1, 10, 11] in 1990 using the oncogenic T antigen from the simian virus 40 (SV40) inserted at the luteinizing hormone β-subunit (LHβ) promoter. Predominant expression occurred in gonadotroph cells of the anterior pituitary with a single subpopulation of mice developing multifocal bilateral ocular tumors starting at 1–2 months after transfection [10]. The T antigen inhibits both the Rb protein (pRb) and p53, as well as murine Rb proteins p107 and p103. On histology, the tumors displayed neuronal characteristics of human Rb including Homer-Wright and Flexner-Wintersteiner rosettes. However, the tumors appeared to originate from the amacrine and Müller cells, rather than photoreceptors as seen in human Rb. Some tumors showed necrosis and early photoreceptor structural differentiation. The tumors were locally invasive into the choroid, vitreous, and optic nerve. Additionally, 15–27% developed midline intracranial tumors in the midbrain, rather than the pineal gland as in human Rb. Interestingly, this model shows no response to cryotherapy and a lack of focal or clonal tumor formation as is frequently found in human Rb [10].

Subsequently, a series of models using SV40 transfection were created to better localize tumor formation within the retina. A second SV40 mediated model utilizes the inter photoreceptor retinoid binding protein (IRBP Tag) [10]. Unlike LHβ, all mice in this model developed outer retinal tumors around 1 week after transfection and pineal gland tumors. On histology, Homer-Wright rosettes without Flexner-Wintersteiner rosettes were seen. The tumor appeared as a continuous sheet-like structure throughout the retinal layers rather than focal tumors. A third SV40 murine model used the opsin Tag to target developing photoreceptors; opsin being a pigment protein found in photoreceptors. Unfortunately, these models only develop CNS tumors without intraocular tumor formation [10]. This is believed to occur because the well-differentiated retinal cells and photoreceptors present at the time of transfection lack the mitotic potential needed for tumor formation. Interestingly, late expression of the opsin Tag caused photoreceptor cells death, emphasizing the importance of the opsin protein in phototransduction and cell maintenance [10].

A similar model utilizing PAX6-driven T-antigens includes a subpopulation of tumor initiation cells in the form of neurospheres. These spheres can be transplanted to retinal tissue to induce tumor formation and show characteristic histology identical to the parent tumor. This model expresses CD133+, Nestin+, and Sox2+ stem cell markers. Finally, Alpha-crystalline Tag mice develop microphthalmia, cataracts, and lens tumors, but fail to form retinal tumors [10].

Other viral vectors including adenovirus 12 and human papilloma virus (HPV) have also been used to determine additional proteins involved in Rb formation in rodent models. Hamsters transfected with adenovirus 12 develop retinal tumors, believed to occur from the interaction between with adenovirus E1A protein and pRb. However, no hamster Rb transgenic models have been developed for clinical use. Human papilloma virus viral oncogenes E6 and E7 cause malignant transformation of cells [10]. In vitro, E6 causes functional inactivation of p53 and E7 binds pRb. Both inactivation by E6 and E7 are specific without effect on the other protein (pRb and p53 respectively), in contrast to the LHβ Tag model, which affects both p53 and pRb simultaneously. A combination model using E6/E7 inserted at the alpha-crystallin promoter causes the formation of epidermal cancers resembling cervical carcinoma with the additional features of the alpha-crystalline Tag models described above. A single murine line expressing E6 and E7 within the retina developed Rb-like tumors from the bipolar cells. Histologically, these tumors formed Homer-Wright rosettes. This model also developed direct metastasis to the CNS via the optic nerve and distant metastasis to the cervical lymph nodes [1, 10].

To better understand the importance of p53 within Rb formation, models utilizing E7 to selectively inactivate pRb were crossed with p53 −/− mice. Combinations of the above models have had mixed results in Rb formation. The IRBP-E7 model caused photoreceptor death without tumor formation following transfection on day 1 and complete photoreceptor loss by week 4. IRBP-E7 crossed with p53−/− mice led to tumor formation at an early age, confirming that pRb inactivation leads to p53-dependent apoptosis. If p53 is inactivated as well, tumorigenesis occurs. Interestingly, IRBP-E7 xp53−/− retinas still showed apoptosis early on prior to tumor development, with subsequent tumor development occurring within the degenerating retinal tissue. Additional non-neuronal tumors form within the retinal pigment epithelium (RPE), ciliary body, and anterior uveal pigmented epithelium within 2–3 months (compared to 6–12 months in other models). Such tumors are not seen in the p53 −/− murine models and possibly represent reactive hyperplasia rather than tumorigenesis [10]. The inhibitor of DNA binding (Id) proteins consists of 4 subtypes (Id1–4) which are dominant-negative inhibitors of basic helix-loop-helix transcription factors involved in cellular proliferation, differentiation, angiogenesis, and tumorigenesis [12]. Id2 has been previously identified to act as an oncogene, which Rb proteins Rb1, p107, and p130 can bind and inhibit. To elucidate the role of Id2, if any, in the Rb development pathway, Y79, WERI-Rb, and CHLA223 Rb cell lines were measured for Id2 expression by qPCR and western blot [12]. All three cell lines expressed low levels of Id2 mRNA and protein. LHβ-Tag mice were then crossed with Id2 heterozygotes to express the three Id2 genotypes (LHβ-Tag/Id2 +/+, LHβ-Tag/Id2 +/−, and LHβ-Tag/Id2 −/−) and mice were sacrificed at 15 weeks of age. While all three models developed Rb, tumors in the LHβ-Tag/Id2 −/− model tended to be larger, less differentiated, and with greater vascular density. There was no significant difference between the LHβ-Tag/Id2 +/+ and LHβ-Tag/Id2 +/− models. None of the three groups developed metastasis [12]. Id2 may represent a tumor suppressor in Rb, which when lost following Rb inactivation can lead to increased vascularity and growth.

To date, the LHβ-Tag model remains the most utilized transgenic model in current Rb research. The numerous viral oncogene induced models are useful in determining protein involvement in tumorigenesis and have been used to test chemotherapy and brachytherapy response. Limitations of transgenic models include the need for viral oncogene induction, which does not mimic human tumor formation and the potential for viral oncogenes to bind multiple cellular proteins in addition to the intended target protein. Thus, the resultant phenotype may not be due to targeted protein inactivation, but rather a series of protein interactions.

2.2 Genetically Modified and Knockout (KO) Models

Genetically modified models, including knock-out models, are animal models involving selective breeding to remove specific genes. Genes are targeted in embryonic stem cells lines and then incorporated into animal germ cell lines. Based on the 1971 Knudson two-hit hypothesis, loss of heterozygosity at 13q14 should lead to the initiation of tumorigenesis in Rb [13]. Beginning in 1992, a second group of murine models were created to determine the genetic pathway leading to the formation of Rb [13]. Initial models of RB1(+/−) KO mice were found to develop pituitary intermediate lobe adenomas and medullary thyroid carcinomas, but no intraocular tumors. RB1(−/−) KO mutations were lethal between embryonic day 13.5–15.5 [10]. To solve this issue, chimeras of Rb1-deficient and wild-type mice were bred, however these failed to develop intraocular tumors despite high levels of Rb1-deficient retinal cells [10]. Thus, Rb1 deficiency alone was determined to be insufficient to cause Rb formation in mice.

Several years later, Burns [13] and Robanus-Maandag et al. [11] determined that another murine protein, p107, was upregulated in Rb1 (−/−) mice and acts in a protective mechanism when Rb1 is deficient. The murinep107 protein appears to act similarly to pRb1 in humans and is expressed in embryonic stages of development [11, 13]. However, further creation of Rb-/Rb- p107−/p107- models proved to be lethal [11]. The first successful knock-out murine models for Rb were published in 2004, using conditional inactivation of Rb^{Lox} in p107-deficient mice using Nestin-Cre, Pax6-Cre, and Chx10-Cre promoters, all crucial in the formation and development of retinal progenitor cells [11, 13]. Rb-like tumors form in these models (Nestin-Cre and Pax6-Cre) within 3–9 months and originate from retinal progenitor, amacrine, and Müller cells [11]. Nestin-Cre KO models develop tumors with similar histologic characteristics to human Rb including Homer-Wright rosettes, high levels of mitosis, and apoptosis. Tumors arise from the inner nuclear layer and fill the vitreous. Tumors may invade the extraocular muscles through direct extension. Nestin-Cre KO x p107 KO develop tumors which better resemble human Rb, while Chx10-Cre $Rb^{Lox/Lox}$ lack bipolar cells. A similarly created model, alpha-Cre$Rb^{Lox/Lox}$, shows rod, bipolar, and ganglion cell degeneration [11]. Crucially, murine models which only possess a single copy loss of p107 (+/−) can re-enter the cell cycle and frequently develop distant metastasis to the bone marrow. A second protein, p130, also known as Rb-like protein 2 (Rbl2), was subsequently identified in murine models. P130 is expressed in post-natal stages of development and is involved in retinal development, cell cycle regulation, and tumor suppression [11, 13]. Rb/p130 double knock-out (DKO) models form Rb-like tumors from horizontal and amacrine cells with Homer-Wright rosettes. These tumors grow rapidly to fill the vitreous cavity with CNS extension. As such, they can be used to mimic late-stage Rb. Notably an attempt to use IRBP-Cre; $Rb^{Lox/Lox}$; $p107^{-/-}$ mice failed to yield intraocular tumor. This difference in tumor creation versus the other Cre models may be due to the presence of IRBP in cells committed to become photoreceptors rather than expression in precursor retinal cells [13]. The numerous Cre-lox combination models forming Rb allow the study of how individual genetic modifications influence Rb development and progression. Unfortunately, the significant delay to tumor development and low penetrance limits the use of these KO models.

A recent novel model utilizes CRISPR/Cas9 technology on the frog, *Xenopus tropicalis,* to create a rapidly forming Rb model [14]. *X. tropicalis* were injected unilaterally at the 2-cell stage with rb1 coding region 1 gRNA ($rb1^{cr1}$) to create unilateral mosaics with the other side being wild-type for direct comparison. Specimens were followed up for 16 months without development of Rb demonstrating that biallelic Rb1 inactivation is insufficient for Rb formation, unlike their human counterparts. The same experiment was repeated using the rbl1 coding region ($rbl1^{cr1}$). Next, using multiplex genome editing, combination rb1/rbl1 gRNAs were injected unilaterally ($rb1^{cr1}$ with $rbl1^{cr1}$ and $rb1^{cr2}$ with $rbl1^{cr2}$) with recombinant Cas9 protein. The Cr1 locus is a non-specific target causing a small in-frame deletion/insertion which leads to decreased protein function. Cr2 targets a pocket domain on the rbl1 protein responsible for binding E2F transcription factor. The mosaic double knockout (MDKO) tadpoles and frogs developed externally visible Rb tumors. In the $rb1^{cr1}/rbl1^{cr1}$ model, 53% developed unilateral tumors with 11% developing brain metastasis. The $rb1^{cr2}/rbl1^{cr2}$ model yielded 73% with unilateral tumors and 13% with brain metastasis. Tumor formation occurred within 69 days post-injection, with tumors doubling in size every 7 days. Tumor development led to leukocoria, ectopialentis, and neovascularization. On histology, tumors were both endophytic and exophytic arising from the outer retina with potential to seed into the vitreous. There was also local tumor invasion of the optic nerve and direct local spread [14]. This is the first non-mammalian model of Rb formation. Advantages include fast development (69 days post-fertilization vs. 100 +/− 42 days plus 21 days gestation for murine models), large brood, internal control with other side wild-type eye to allow for toxicity comparison during drug testing, and low cost. Furthermore, multiplex genome editing allows for the modification of multiple genes to create high-throughput target testing within a few weeks. Unfortunately, the rapid tumor development and growth does limit longer follow-up.

2.3 Xenograft Models

The third group of models use existing human cell lines transplanted into animal models either in a different location (heterotopic) or similar location to the origin tumor (orthotopic). The animal models used are frequently immunocompromised, which limits the assessment of tumor progression and treatment as well as natural immune cell response. When directly linked to a single patient, these models are known as patient-derived xenografts (PDX) [15].

Y79 is a human Rb cell line originating from a 2.5-year-old female with a strong family history of Rb [16]. WERI-RB-1 is a human Rb cell line originating from a 1-year old female [17]. Both cell lines are routinely used to study in vitro response to therapeutics and form the basis for xenograft models in Rb.

The earliest xenograft models in Rb were performed by McFall [1], who injected Y79 and WERI-RB-1 cells into the anterior chamber of rabbit models. These animals developed tumor growth within 17–22 days. More recently, athymic nude mice were injected with Y79 (RB −/−) cells via intraocular injection into the vitreous cavity [3]. Tumor developed in 67.5% of eyes by 12 weeks with progression from visible tumor to diffuse vitreous seeding and complete ocular invasion in a matter of weeks. These tumors histologically resembled the tumor of origin with rosette-like growth, high mitosis, and necrotic activity. Tumors were transplantable to other murine models. One mouse developed brain metastasis at 35 days via direct scleral extension, however no distant metastasis developed in this group [3].

A similar set of models were created by Chevez-Barrios et al. using intravitreal Y79 cells and WERI-Rb-1 cells injected into the right eye of Rag2 KO immunodeficient mice. The Y79 mice developed vitreous tumors within 2 weeks post-injection, which progressed to focal retinal invasion, with subsequent subretinal, choroidal, and optic nerve invasion within a few weeks. By 5–7 weeks post-injection, tumor filled the eye with scleral involvement. One third of the Y79 mice developed focal brain metastasis via direct invasion by 5 weeks. The WERI-Rb-1 model also developed tumors by 2 weeks, with anterior chamber involvement by 5 weeks. No local or distant metastasis occurred. On histology, there was focal retinal invasion without rosette formation or optic nerve involvement. The anterior chamber, uvea, and lens were frequently involved [18].

Aerts et al. utilized surgically derived patient-derived Rb xenografts implanted subcutaneously in adult nude mice (Swiss nu/nu) to create a Rb panel [2]. These models were then exposed to chemotherapeutic combinations to determine the best individualized response. All tumors responded, but were not intraocular, limiting comparison to human Rb. Utilizing this panel of Rb tumors, Cassoux et al. created orthotopic xenograft murine models through injection into the subretinal space [2]. Mice were imaged weekly and sacrificed at the time of tumor appearance within the vitreous. Tumors developed within 4–6 weeks on average. Using the Rb-200 xenograft model, intravitreal chemotherapeutics were injected weekly over 4 weeks following vitreous involvement to assess tumor response. There was a 33% clearance with Melphalan, 83% with carboplatin, and continued growth with both bevacizumab and saline injections [2].

The type of murine model can affect rates of tumor engraftment. In a highly efficient model, tumors would form with each xenograft injection. Lemaitre et al. examined which murine model of four commonly used mouse lines, both immunodeficient (Swiss nude Rb −/− and severe combined immunodeficient mice or SCID) and immunocompetent (B6 albino mice and C57BL/60 mice), yielded the best Rb model [19]. Rb-200 cell line (Institute Curie) was injected into the subretinal space and the mice were imaged weekly. Rates of engraftment were 28.6% for the Swiss nude mice, 68.8% for the SCID mice, 50.0% for the B6 Albino mice, and no engraftment for the C57BL/60 mice. The Swiss nude model showed retinal thickening and tumor growth by day 20 with progressive growth over time. The SCID model had early pre-retinal seeding by day 13 with progressive growth as a white retinal mass over the next month. One mouse had anterior chamber involvement. The B6 albino model had vitreous seeds and a localized retinal detachment. Retinal detachment was common with this methodology occurring in 33% of Swiss nude mice and 14 and 15% respectively for the SCID and B6 albino models respectively. On histology, central necrosis was present within the tumors without calcification or rosettes [19].

Kang and Grossniklaus [1, 20] developed a rabbit model utilizing WERI-Rb-1 cells injected into the sub-retinal space. The rabbits were immunosuppressed using cyclosporin A (10–15 mg/kg) injected intramuscularly daily for the entire 8 weeks of the experiment. On day 3, 30 μL of cultured WERI-Rb-1 cells (1.5×10^6) were injected into the subretinal space of the right eye [20]. Tumor formation was seen in all animals within 1 week. By week 5, tumors were vascularized and reached maximum growth by 8 weeks. These tumors resembled an exophytic pattern, centering on the posterior pole and extending into the vitreous cavity. No extrascleral extension was seen [20]. Advantages of the rabbit model included larger eyes for easier tumor visualization (fundoscopy and imaging), and better resemblance to the size of a human infant. This model also allows for treatment testing, particularly intraocular therapy for vitreous seeding. Limitations include the use of WERI-Rb-1 cells which come from a non-hereditary tumor sample and are traditionally less aggressive, and tumor location in the subretinal rather than intraretinal space.

A smaller orthotopic model injected RNVOT-RB1 human RB cells into the vitreous cavity of *Danio rerio*, zebrafish, 48 h after fertilization [21]. Zebrafish are a rapidly grown organism frequently used in genetic research with a classic pigment pattern that completes by day 6 post-fertilization. To improve visualization of Rb on confocal microscopy, phenylthiourea was injected on day 1 to prevent pigmentation. At 48 h post-fertilization, 20 or 100 Rb cells tagged with GFP (green florescent protein) were injected. Unsurprisingly, the greater the number of cells injected, the greater the tumor size. GFP intensity was measured and rated. To test tumor response to chemotherapeutics, Zebrafish were cultured in 200 μm of carboplatin or melphalan following the injection of 100 Rb cells. GFP signal expression decreased by 30% with both chemotherapeutics. Additionally, cells were dispersed throughout the vitreous rather than clumped in tumor formation. Given the low cost and rapid development of tumor, the authors propose this model for high throughput testing of new therapeutics [21].

Xenograft models have the advantage of faster growth and human origin of the tumor cells. Limitations include the use of immunocompromised animals which limits observation of immune cell response to tumor presence. Additionally, orthotopic xenografts better mimic tumor location than heterotopic xenografts. The location of cell injection may lead to tumor development which is not representative of human tumor growth patterns and should be carefully considered when creating and developing new model systems.

3 Uveal Melanoma

Like Rb, there are several different pre-clinical animal models currently used in the study of UM. Induced animal models are created by exposing an animal to chemical agents, radiation, virus, cells, or tissues to create the desired disease. In UM, the most common method is direct inoculation of tumor cells to form xenografts [22]. Zebrafish models have been created using both xenograft and transgenic methods. Given their small size, low cost, and rapid growth and development, zebrafish are ideal for high throughput pharmacologic screening. Unfortunately, the zebrafish require a p53 mutation to develop UM [6]. This leads to the formation of additional tumors throughout the organism, making it hard to distinguish between primary and metastatic lesions. Murine models remain the most cost-effective, although their small eye size limits direct tumor visualization and ophthalmic imaging [6]. Rabbit models have larger eyes allowing for easier ophthalmic examination, ophthalmic imaging, and intravitreal injections [6], but are more costly than mice. A few additional rodent and small mammal models which are less frequently used are also discussed below.

3.1 Xenograft Models

3.1.1 Hamsters

The earliest animal models in UM are the Greene melanoma cell line developed in 1949 [22]. Greene used an epidermoid carcinoma of the scrotal skin (Brown-Pearce tumor) in rabbits, and injected cells into the anterior chamber of rabbits, hamsters, and rats as well as the testicle and subcutaneous space of hamsters and rats. Tumors in these early experiments failed to grow or spontaneously regressed. Greene was able to grow a progressive cutaneous melanoma during a second attempt in 1958 using Syrian golden hamsters. After six serial passages, the tumors became amelanotic and this tissue was successfully transplanted to other organs including the eyes of rabbits and guinea pigs. The greater the number of passages, the better the tumor spread. Journee-de-Korver et al. implanted 1 mm^3 Greene melanoma tissue into the abdomen of hamsters and treated with transpupillary thermotherapy (TTT). Tumors showed necrosis within 1-day post-treatment. This early experiment led to the use of TTT in UM. Advantages of the Greene melanoma hamster model include the presence of both a melanocytic and amelanotic variant, intense vascularization of the tumor, response to TTT, immunocompetent animals, and histopathologic appearance similar to human UM [22].

A similar spontaneous cutaneous melanotic hamster melanoma, the Bomirski Melanoma cell line, has been used for allograft transplant using small fragments of tissue into the anterior chamber of hamsters. Unfortunately, this tissue is hard to obtain and must come directly from laboratories in Poland [22].

3.1.2 Rats

Like mice, rats can also be used as xenograft models. Braun et al. used an athymic albino mutant rat strain WAG/RijHs-rnu to develop an UM orthotopic xenograft [22]. Melanotic human OCM1 cell line was subcutaneously implanted into a rat. Tumor tissue was harvested and transplanted into the eye of a second rat via scleral tunnel. Tumor growth occurred at 6–8 weeks within the choroid. No metastasis developed. Braun et al. repeated the experiment, but implanted spheroids rather than smashed tumor into the suprachoroidal space. UM developed in 96% of the rats within 4–41 days after inoculation, without evidence of metastasis. Using the C918 cell line yields similar results [22]. Since athymic rats do not have B or T cells, immunosuppression is unnecessary. This model is inexpensive and provides a primary intraocular tumor model, however immune response to tumor presence cannot be observed.

3.1.3 Rabbits

Rabbits have larger eyes than other rodent models, making direct fundoscopic examination and imaging easier. Three cell line models exist in UM: B16, Greene cell line, and human UM cell lines. Minced tumor fragments from the B16F10 cell line in C57UBU6 or C57BL/6 mice are inoculated trans-sclerally into the subchoroidal space of rabbits. These models do not develop liver metastasis and require cyclosporin A immunosuppression, preventing the study of immunologic response. Additionally, the rabbits only live 12 weeks. The above-mentioned Greene melanoma hamster cell line can be inoculated into rabbits without immunosuppression. These tumors grow quickly, limiting follow-up to 7 days as tumors begin to necrose at day 8–10. Finally, human cell lines can be directly transplanted into cyclosporin A suppressed rabbits, via subchoroidal injection. Liggett et al. used solid tumor fragments, with 67% tumor development. Blanco et al. used MKT-BR cell line in albino rabbits. These rabbits developed lung metastasis. Bonicel et al. used IPC 227 cell lines inoculated into the anterior chamber, with 100% ciliary body tumor development. Finally, Lopez-Velasco et al. studied suprachoroidal implantation of 4 human UM cell lines (MKT-BR, OCM1, 92.1, and SP6.5) and found that 92.1 and SP6.5 were the most aggressive with 100% developing lung metastasis and 18% developing liver micrometastasis [22].

3.1.4 Mice

The first murine UM model was created in 1984 by Niederkorn [6]. UM cells were injected into the anterior chamber and formed iris melanoma. Interestingly, this model did develop metastasis. To better mimic choroidal and ciliary body tumors, a second murine model was formed via suprachoroidal injection into the posterior compartment. These mice developed distant metastasis. Inoculation technique determined extraocular extension, with trans-conjunctival injection causing higher rates of extension than suprachoroidal injection. A third murine model using intravitreal inoculation led to tumor formation invading the uveal tract [6]. This is however inconsistent with human UM formation, which starts in the uveal tract and can proceed to break through Bruch's membrane into the retina.

To create UM metastasis models, cells were injected in other parts of mice to achieve the desired tumor location, specifically the liver and lungs. These models include: (1) direct liver inoculation, (2) splenic inoculation causing liver metastasis, and (3) hematogenous spread via retro-orbital sinus or tail vein injection causing both liver and lung metastasis [6].

Older models of syngeneic cutaneous melanoma use cutaneous melanoma cells transplanted to a second mouse of similar genetic background (for example, C57BL/6 mice with B16L59 cell line). These models allow for the study of local invasion, extravasation, and metastasis in an immunocompetent animal. One syngeneic cutaneous melanoma line, the HCmel12 mouse, reportedly carries a GNA11^{Q209L} variation also seen in human UM tumors. The main disadvantage of these models is that they are of cutaneous melanoma origin, which may not directly mimic the molecular changes seen in UM [6, 22].

There are at least 10 different traditional xenograft models using both primary and metastatic human tumor cells inoculated in murine models via the various above-mentioned injection sites. These models retain the molecular features of the original human tumor, are highly reproducible between mice, and frequently metastasize. Many of the cell lines include known UM genetic markers such as GNAQ^{Q209L}, GNAQ^{Q209P}, GNA11^{Q209L}, EIF1AX^{G6D}, and SF3B1^{R625Q} [6]. Such xenografts are good for studying tumor signaling and treatment response [6].

The most recent models developed are patient-derived xenografts (PDX), as first presented by Didier Decaudin. In these models, freshly harvested primary or metastatic tumor is inoculated into immunocompromised mice (SCID). These models maintain the mutations, chromosomal imbalances, and histopathological features of the original tumor. Decaudin et al. created a panel of 25 PDX mice from 90 available UM tumor samples [22]. They reported a rate of 28% engraftment with interscapular fat pad inoculation of primary UM cells [6, 22]. Interestingly, PDX created from metastatic UM cells had a significantly higher engraftment rate and tended to harbor known genetic mutations (GNAQ^{Q209L}, GNAQ^{Q209P}, GNA11^{Q209L}, EIF1AX^{G6D}, and SF3B1^{R625Q}). Histologically, 11 of the 25 tumors had complete concordance with their parent tumor, with good maintenance of concordance through serial passage over time. Tumors with GNA11 mutations grew better than GNAQ mutations, while BAP1 mutations and monosomy 3 did not affect tumor growth. Genomic analysis of 17 of the tumors created revealed GNAQ mutation in 35%, GNA11 in 65%, BAP1 in 47%, and SF3B1 in 18% mirroring known prevalence of these mutations in human UM. An additional 14 tumors tested with gene expression profiling (GEP) showed 10 GEP class 2 and 4 GEP class 1 tumors, consistent with the skew toward higher risk lesions having a higher rate of engraftment [22]. This is likely due to acquired gain of function mutations in engraftment, angiogenesis, and overall cell survival in high-risk tumors.

The main disadvantage of both traditional xenograft models and PDX are the need for immunocompromised mice which prevents the study of the immune system on tumor development and metastasis. Additionally, many of the tumor models spontaneously regress. When mice with humanized immune systems are used to attempt to study immune response, graft-vs-host-disease (GVHD) frequently develops. Finally, PDX are very costly and at present have a low engraftment rate, requiring many wasted mice to develop enough animals for experimentation [6].

3.2 Transgenic Models and Knock-Out/In Models

Genetically engineered murine models (GEMMs) are mice designed to spontaneously produce a desired tumor. The first transgenic UM model was created in 1991 by Bradl et al. These early UM transgenic mice used pigment cell-specific promotes (Tyrosinase) to drive expression of SV40 large-T antigens or HRAS (Tyr-SV40E, TySV40, Tyr-Tag, Tyr-RAS+Ink4a/Arf−/−) [22]. Unfortunately, most tumors arose from the RPE or a mixed uveal/RPE cell line rather than the uveal tract alone. They did not develop metastasis unless cells were directly transferred to the target organ. The Tg(Grm1) model uses the Dopachrometautomase (Dct) promoter to control expression of the metabotropic glutamate receptor, leading to uveal and cutaneous melanoma development [6]. Eyes in this model show choroidal thickening and ciliary body tumors [6, 22]. A third model, using RET, develops uveal and systemic melanocytic tumors. One common issue with these models is the reliance on molecular drivers which are not found in human tumors [6].

Currently, three models exist using the GNAQ and GNA11 mutations seen in human UM as drivers. The first model uses a Tet-on system to induce GNAQ^{Q209L} expression in p16^{Ink4a} and p19^{Ink4b} deficient mice. While 50% develop cutaneous melanoma within 9 months, UM is not seen. The lox-stop-lox conditional knock-in of GNAQ^{Q209L} at the Rosa26 locus model develop UM within 3 months with 100% penetrance as well as cutaneous melanomas. Oncogene expression is initiated by Mitf-cre. These tumors can enter blood vessels and hematogenously metastasize to the lungs. A third model uses conditional knock-in allele for GNA11^{Q209L} via inducible Tyrosinase-creER^{T2} activation to create UM. Combining this model with a Bap1 deletion yields smaller UM, with greater cutaneous melanomas. While these models utilize known human molecular drivers and develop UM with high penetrance, tumor progression is slower than xenograft models. Additionally, the Mitf-cre model develop microphthalmia, limiting ocular examination. Melanocytic tumor development outside the eye can affect experiments by causing the need for earlier euthanasia prior to UM development and difficulty distinguishing primary melanomas from metastasis [6].

One recent model by Li et al. utilized adenovirus delivery of Cre-recombinase to the uveal tract. Adult mice with conditional null alleles for Hippo kinases Lats1 and Lats2 (YAP/TAX suppressors) that received a suprachoroidal injection of AAV5-CMV-Cre vector produced ocular melanocytic tumor around 6 months post-injection. Tumors from this model stain for Melan-A/Mart1 and HMB45 indicating a uveal melanocytic origin, but are negative for RPE65, implying they are not of retinal origin. This novel system could allow for study of UM in vivo throughout the disease process [6].

While UM GEMMs have been developed using known human UM genetic driver mutations, the lengthy time to tumor development and limited number of GEMM models currently available have limited their use. At present, GEMMs present an area for continued exploration of genetic drivers and new animal model development.

4 Adenoid Cystic Carcinoma

Adenoid cystic carcinoma (ACC) of the lacrimal gland is a malignant tumor accounting for 1.6% of orbital tumors, 4.8% of primary orbital neoplasms, and 25–30% of epithelial neoplasms of the lacrimal gland [23]. Prior xenograft models have utilized salivary gland tumor specimens which have a better prognosis than those of lacrimal gland origin. A novel lacrimal gland tumor cell line from a 35-year-old female patient with solid ACC was created [23]. Tumor sample was cultured with serial subcultures over a 2-year period. ACC clones formed at 69 days after each subsequent subculture. The 84th generation of LACC-1 cell line was injected into the subaxillary space (1×10^6 cells) of 10 nude mice (BALB/c nu/nu). Tumor developed within 7 days of injection in all 10 mice (100% tumor development). Two mice were sacrificed at day 14, 28, 35, 42, and 49 days. Target organs (lung, liver, and alar lymph nodes) were harvested for metastatic surveillance. By day 14, tumors were round or oval with a thin capsule, but were not adherent to the adjacent tissue. At day 49, tumor had intruded into the chest wall and thoracic cavity, indicating local invasion. No metastasis developed. On histology, tumor was pale with a capsule in a solid pattern. Those tumors allowed to progress developed central necrotic tissue. Tissue stained positively for cytoskeletal proteins, including α-SMA, and S100 confirming lacrimal gland origin [23]. This represents the first direct heterotopic xenograft model of ACC from human lacrimal gland tissue. Ideally, a model utilizing injection in the orbital space would better capitulate tumor growth and behavior. Like other xenograft models, this murine model utilizes an immunocompromised line limiting observation of the immune response.

5 Animal Models Exploring Interventional Pathways

Two notable models have explored intra-arterial chemotherapy (IAC), as presently used in Rb treatment, and the effects of both technique and chemotherapeutic agents on animal models with and without induced disease.

Wilson et al. developed a primate model using adult Rhesus macaque monkeys to look at the effects of IAC on retinal vessels and retina histology [24–26]. Six adult Rhesus macaque monkeys were randomized to undergo 3 sessions of supra-selective intra-arterial chemotherapy (SSIAC) with either melphalan 5 mg/30 mL or carboplatin 3 mg/30 mL. Monkeys were euthanized 6 h after the third SSIAC, with subsequent bilateral enucleation and orbital histologic examination [24–26]. Ophthalmic findings included: choroidal blanching (100%), choroidal hypoperfusion on intravenous fluorescein angiography (IVFA) (100%), retinal artery narrowing (100%), retinal edema (100%), retinal artery sheathing (94%), and retinal artery precipitates (56%) [26]. On histology, birefringent foreign bodies were noted in the choroidal and short posterior ciliary arteries. One central retinal artery had a thrombosis with associated ganglion cell layer and retinal thinning consistent with a central retinal artery occlusion. Vessels were noted to be occluded by red blood cell aggregates, macrophages, and membranous debris, with pericyte swelling, and organelle disorganization. Endothelial cells stained positively for human intercellular adhesion molecule 1 protein (ICAM-1) and interleukin-8, both known inflammatory markers. One monkey had persistent right upper eyelid swelling following SSIAC. Histology showed medium sized vessel thrombosis with inflammatory cells in the tarsal conjunctiva. Based on these findings, Wilson et al. concluded that SSIAC is associated with drug-induced retinal endothelial cell inflammatory response with secondary leukocytosis causing vascular occlusion [25].

To assess the comparability of Rhesus macaque monkeys as suitable large animal model for SSIAC, angiographic vessel diameters were measured 2–4 mm from the ophthalmic artery origin in 8 of 12 eyes. These measurements were compared to angiographic measurements on computed tomography (CT) and magnetic resonance imaging (MRI) in 98 children under 6 (186 eyes) without orbital or intraocular tumors. An additional 20 adolescents were measured using the same technique to serve as adult representative measurements. Median ophthalmic artery size in the non-human primate model was 1.06 mm on angiography, 1.09 mm on histology vs. 1.28 mm in children, and 1.45 mm in the adolescents. There was no statistically significant difference in size between the non-human primates and children. The

Rhesus macaque is anatomically and physiologically like a toddler, with similar eye size, and almost identical cephalic arterial system including ophthalmic artery origin [24]. Unfortunately, while chemotherapeutic toxicity can be tested, there are no current Rb models in this animal, limiting direct therapeutic evaluation.

A more recent model was developed by Daniels et al. using New Zealand white rabbits. In a series of successive studies, Daniels created a SSIAC rabbit model and subsequently tested retinal and vitreous penetration of melphalan [5]. Using the model mentioned above by Kang and Grossniklaus to create Rb in rabbits, Daniels then examined the ability of this model to kill Rb cells using SSIAC [5, 20]. Normal rabbits underwent SSIAC via femoral catheterization through the common carotid artery. As rabbits have dual retinal circulation of the ophthalmic artery emanating from the internal and external carotid arteries, fluoroscopic angiography was used to determine the dominant arterial system in each rabbit. The dominant arterial supply was canalized, and 10% fluorescein angiography performed to demonstrate arterial patency. Melphalan 0.4 mg/kg was injected in a pulsatile fashion over 5 min followed by a saline flush. A repeat IVFA was performed to demonstrate continued retinal vascular patency. No occlusion was seen on IVFA pre- or post-SSIAC. Rabbits were euthanized at 30 min, 1, 2, 4, and 6 h post-SSIAC. Peripheral blood serum, vitreous tap samples, and enucleated retina were all snap frozen to assess pharmacodynamics [5].

A subset of 5 rabbits were immunosuppressed with daily subcutaneous cyclosporin A injections. WERI-Rb-1 cells were injected into the subretinal and intravitreal spaces as previously described by Kang et al. to generate Rb [20]. Rabbits were monitored weekly for tumor growth. Two weeks after tumor development, rabbits were randomized to undergo SSIAC with melphalan 3.6 mg or saline. Rabbits were euthanized 2 weeks after SSIAC [5].

All eyes were successfully cannulated (79 eyes in 47 rabbits), with melphalan successfully delivered in all 31 designated eyes. Max concentration in the retina was 4.95 μm with a T_{max} of 0.5 h and a half-life of 1.16 h. Max concentration from a mid-vitreous sample was 2.24 μm, with a T_{max} of 1 h, and half-life of 0.83 h. Peripheral blood max concentration was 1.04 μm with a T_{max} of 0.5 h, and a half-life of 1.08 h. Vitreous melphalan concentration was 100 times higher in the treated vs. the untreated eye. Given the low level of melphalan concentration in peripheral blood, less than 2% of the vitreous and retinal melphalan concentration in treated eyes was attributed to recirculation. Tumor grew as vitreous spheres and intraretinal lesions and showed evidence of apoptosis following melphalan SSAIC as demonstrated by elevated cleaved caspase 3 levels, a marker of apoptosis. From these initial studies, Daniels et al. concluded that the New Zealand white rabbit model could effectively be used to compare Rb response to chemotherapeutic treatment, specifically SSIAC with different agents [5].

Daniels et al. next tested the effect of cannulation technique and chemotherapeutic agent administered utilizing the above rabbit model. Rabbits were administered melphalan 1.2 mg or 2.4 mg using a standard cannulation technique, melphalan 1.2 mg using a continuous flow technique, carboplatin 25 mg or 50 mg using a standard cannulation technique, or a saline control. Rabbits underwent pre-operative testing and testing 5–6 weeks post-IAC including: dark-adapted electroretinography (ERG), fundus photos, optical coherence tomography (OCT), OCT-angiography (OCT-A), IVFA, and a clinical exam. Toxicity was defined as a 25% reduction in ERG amplitude or prolonged average implicit time compared to baseline. The rabbits were euthanized at 5–6 weeks, unless indicated earlier, with subsequent enucleation. Rabbits in the carboplatin group were sacrificed within hours to a few days of intervention due to severe orbital swelling and underwent exenteration including surrounding bone. Systemic toxicity was also measured including baseline and weekly complete blood count (CBC) examining hemoglobin levels, white blood cell count, absolute neutrophil count, and platelet count [27].

Standard cannulation technique involved the occlusion of the ophthalmic artery just prior to medication injection. Rabbits in the saline infusion control group did not demonstrate any retinal toxicity, indicating that the minimal time occluding the ophthalmic artery does not cause retinal damage. Melphalan was dosed at a standard rate of 0.4 mg/kg (1.2 mg) and a higher 0.8 mg/kg (2.4 mg) dose. In the 1.2 mg group, there was no change in OCT, OCT-A, or IVFA. ERG however showed a 30% reduction in the 10,000 mcd a wave scotopic amplitude. The 2.4 mg group had a 49–72% reduction in the scotopic 3000 mcd a wave amplitude, scotopic 10,000 mcd a wave amplitude, scotopic 10,000 mcd b wave amplitude, photopic 3000 mcd b wave amplitude, and 30-Hz flicker b wave amplitude. Retinal arterial damage was seen in 25%. On histology, there was retinal thinning, photoreceptor damage, and ganglion cell degeneration. These two groups show a dose-dependent toxicity related to melphalan injection. When the same dose of melphalan was used (1.2 mg) in either a standard occlusive infusion or with pulse dosing with continuous saline infusion, no difference in toxicity was found. This suggested that toxicity is drug and dose related, rather than related to technique. Carboplatin produced severe periocular swelling within hours of administration at both the 25 mg and 50 mg dose. On histology, swelling was seen in the orbit, extra-ocular muscles, conjunctiva, episclera, and choroid. No long-term systemic toxicity was found on CBC in any rabbit group [27].

Limitations of this rabbit model include the dual ophthalmic artery supply not seen in humans, small vessels in a rabbit which creates a learning curve for initial SSIAC technique, and a merangiotic vascular system above the internal limiting membrane which is not seen in humans [5].

6 Conclusion

Pre-clinical animal models for Rb, UM, and adenoid cystic carcinoma of the lacrimal gland allow for the exploration of genetic driver mutations leading to tumor formation and metastasis, and tumor response to chemotherapeutics and other treatment modalities. Models include xenografts, transgenic models, and genetically modified models (knock-in/out models). Selection of an animal model for experimentation should consider ease of tumor monitoring, characteristics of the tumor formed in relation to its human counterpart including location and genetic driver mutations, cost, and speed of tumor growth. While no ideal pre-clinical animal models exist for any intraocular tumors, selecting the correct model from those currently available can facilitate answering the research question at hand.

References

1. Nair RM, Kaliki S, Vemuganti GK. Animal models in retinoblastoma research. Saudi J Ophthalmol. 2013;27(3):141–6.
2. Cassoux N, Thuleau A, Assayag F, Aerts I, Decaudin D. Establishment of an orthotopic xenograft mice model of retinoblastoma suitable for preclinical testing. Ocul Oncol Pathol. 2015;1(3):200–6.
3. Tschulakow AV, Schraermeyer U, Rodemann HP, Julien-Schraermeyer S. Establishment of a novel retinoblastoma (Rb) nude mouse model by intravitreal injection of human Rb Y79 cells - comparison of in vivo analysis versus histological follow up. Biol Open. 2016;5(11):1625–30.
4. Broaddus E, Topham A, Singh AD. Incidence of retinoblastoma in the USA: 1975-2004. Br J Ophthalmol. 2009;93(1):21–3.
5. Daniels AB, Froehler MT, Pierce JM, Nunnally AH, Calcutt MW, Bridges TM, et al. Pharmacokinetics, tissue localization, toxicity, and treatment efficacy in the first small animal (rabbit) model of intra-arterial chemotherapy for retinoblastoma. Invest Ophthalmol Vis Sci. 2018;59(1):446–54.
6. Richards JR, Yoo JH, Shin D, Odelberg SJ. Mouse models of uveal melanoma: strengths, weaknesses, and future directions. Pigment Cell Melanoma Res. 2020;33(2):264–78.
7. McLaughlin CC, Wu XC, Jemal A, Martin HJ, Roche LM, Chen VW. Incidence of noncutaneous melanomas in the U.S. Cancer. 2005;103(5):1000–7.
8. Damato EM, Damato BE. Detection and time to treatment of uveal melanoma in the United Kingdom: an evaluation of 2,384 patients. Ophthalmology. 2012;119(8):1582–9.
9. Singh AD, Turell ME, Topham AK. Uveal melanoma: trends in incidence, treatment, and survival. Ophthalmology. 2011;118(9):1881–5.
10. Mills MD, Windle JJ, Albert DM. Retinoblastoma in transgenic mice: models of hereditary retinoblastoma. Surv Ophthalmol. 1999;43(6):508–18.
11. Nair RM, Vemuganti GK. Transgenic models in retinoblastoma research. Ocul Oncol Pathol. 2015;1(3):207–13.
12. Landreville S, Ma D, Wu J, Harbour JW. Loss of Id2 potentiates the tumorigenic effect of Rb inactivation in a mouse model of retinoblastoma. Curr Eye Res. 2010;35(5):435–9.
13. MacPherson D, Dyer MA. Retinoblastoma: from the two-hit hypothesis to targeted chemotherapy. Cancer Res. 2007;67(16):7547–50.
14. Naert T, Colpaert R, Van Nieuwenhuysen T, Dimitrakopoulou D, Leoen J, Haustraete J, et al. CRISPR/Cas9 mediated knockout of rb1 and rbl1 leads to rapid and penetrant retinoblastoma development in Xenopus tropicalis. Sci Rep. 2016;6:35264.
15. Carita G, Nemati F, Decaudin D. Uveal melanoma patient-derived xenografts. Ocul Oncol Pathol. 2015;1(3):161–9.
16. Reid TW, Albert DM, Rabson AS, Russell P, Craft J, Chu EW, et al. Characteristics of an established cell line of retinoblastoma. J Natl Cancer Inst. 1974;53(2):347–60.
17. McFall RC, Sery TW, Makadon M. Characterization of a new continuous cell line derived from a human retinoblastoma. Cancer Res. 1977;37(4):1003–10.
18. Chevez-Barrios P, Hurwitz MY, Louie K, Marcus KT, Holcombe VN, Schafer P, et al. Metastatic and nonmetastatic models of retinoblastoma. Am J Pathol. 2000;157(4):1405–12.
19. Lemaitre S, Poyer F, Marco S, Freneaux P, Doz F, Aerts I, et al. Looking for the most suitable orthotopic retinoblastoma mouse model in order to characterize the tumoral development. Invest Ophthalmol Vis Sci. 2017;58(7):3055–64.
20. Kang SJ, Grossniklaus HE. Rabbit model of retinoblastoma. J Biomed Biotechnol. 2011;2011:394730.
21. Jo DH, Son D, Na Y, Jang M, Choi JH, Kim JH, et al. Orthotopic transplantation of retinoblastoma cells into vitreous cavity of zebrafish for screening of anticancer drugs. Mol Cancer. 2013;12:71.
22. Cao J, Jager MJ. Animal eye models for uveal melanoma. Ocul Oncol Pathol. 2015;1(3):141–50.
23. Lin T, Zhu L, Zhou B, Xie L, Lv J, Dong L, et al. Establishment and characterization of a cell line from human adenoid cystic carcinoma of the lacrimal glands and a nude mouse transplantable model. Oncol Rep. 2015;33(6):2797–806.
24. Ditta LC, Choudhri AF, Tse BC, Landers MM, Haik BG, Steinle JJ, et al. Validating a nonhuman primate model of super-selective intraophthalmic artery chemotherapy: comparing ophthalmic artery diameters. Invest Ophthalmol Vis Sci. 2012;53(12):7791–4.
25. Tse BC, Steinle JJ, Johnson D, Haik BG, Wilson MW. Superselective intraophthalmic artery chemotherapy in a nonhuman primate model: histopathologic findings. JAMA Ophthalmol. 2013;131(7):903–11.
26. Wilson MW, Jackson JS, Phillips BX, Buchanan J, Frase S, Wang F, et al. Real-time ophthalmoscopic findings of superselective intraophthalmic artery chemotherapy in a nonhuman primate model. Arch Ophthalmol. 2011;129(11):1458–65.
27. Daniels AB, Froehler MT, Nunnally AH, Pierce JM, Bozic I, Stone CA, et al. Rabbit model of intra-arterial chemotherapy toxicity demonstrates retinopathy and vasculopathy related to drug and dose, not procedure or approach. Invest Ophthalmol Vis Sci. 2019;60(4):954–64.

Part V

Novel Treatment Strategies

Iris Melanoma: Advanced Surgical Techniques

Janani Singaravelu, Alexander Melendez Moreno, Jacquelyn M. Wrenn, and Arun D. Singh

1 Introduction

The surgical management of iris melanoma has evolved over the last century. Traditionally, iris melanoma has been treated by tumor resection or enucleation, with radiation therapy as an alternative [1–3]. More recently, biopsy techniques and minimally invasive tumor resection techniques have been described. We review surgical techniques for management of iris melanoma.

2 Biopsy Techniques

2.1 Fine-Needle Aspiration Biopsy

While this fine-needle aspiration biopsy (FNAB) has been a mainstay in other specialties throughout the modern medical era, FNAB utilization in ophthalmology is relatively recent. The first intraocular biopsy was performed by Hirschberg in 1868; however, it was not until a century later in 1979 that FNAB was used by Jakobiec to diagnose intraocular tumors [4]. This is likely due to the fact that most intraocular tumors can be diagnosed noninvasively with the use of ancillary imaging techniques. It is estimated that only 1–2% of tumors require diagnostic FNAB [5, 6].

2.1.1 Technique

FNAB of iris tumors is generally performed under an operating microscope. A limbal entry with transaqueous approach using a 25- to 30- gauge needle connected to a syringe is typically used (Fig. 1a). The lesion is then approached from a 45- to 90-degree angle. Two methods of sampling have been described: (1) "vacuum cleaner" technique in which gentle aspiration of 0.5 mL aqueous humor, while the needle is swept over the tumor surface [7] and (2) direct insertion of the needle into the tumor [8].

2.1.2 Instrumentation

Twenty-five- to thirty-gauge needles are commonly used for ocular FNAB. Smaller gauge needles are associated with higher chance of obtaining an insufficient sample [5, 9]. Additionally, the beveled end design of all 25–30-gauge needles may lead to partial entry when sampling shallow tumors. Bending the needle tip to 90° has been recommended since it allows for tangential instead of radial entry [10]. Needle design modifications with a shorter bevel and millimeter graduations have also been proposed [11].

2.1.3 Indications

While a consensus on specific indications for intraocular FNAB is absent [12], it is primarily utilized when a definitive diagnosis cannot be made based on clinical examination and ancillary testing alone [5, 13, 14]. FNAB may be particularly useful in atypical cases, situations where patients request histopathological confirmation prior to proceeding with therapy, and where there is concern for uveal metastasis in the setting of unknown primary. With respect to uveal melanoma, FNAB can be used to confirm or rule out melanoma [10, 15].

FNAB can consistently and accurately achieve a diagnosis, even in very unusual cases. When examining 100 cases of iris tumors that underwent FNAB, adequate tumor sample was achieved in 99% [16]. With regard to diagnostic FNAB, numerous studies have demonstrated the >90% accuracy rate (Fig. 1b) [5, 14, 17]. Specifically, FNAB can be used to determine the predominant cell type of a lesion (spindle vs. epithelioid) [18]. Char et al. showed that FNAB is a useful implementation to accurately diagnose all cases of iris ring melanoma in a series of 22 patients [19]. FNAB was also used to diagnose an atypical case of diffuse iris melanoma by Demirci and Finger [20].

J. Singaravelu · A. M. Moreno · J. M. Wrenn · A. D. Singh (✉)
Department of Ophthalmic Oncology, Cole Eye Institute, Cleveland Clinic, Cleveland, OH, USA
e-mail: singha@ccf.org; melenda3@ccf.org; davanzj@ccf.org

B. V. Chawla, M. E. Aronow (eds.), *Global Perspectives in Ocular Oncology*, https://doi.org/10.1007/978-3-031-08250-4_27

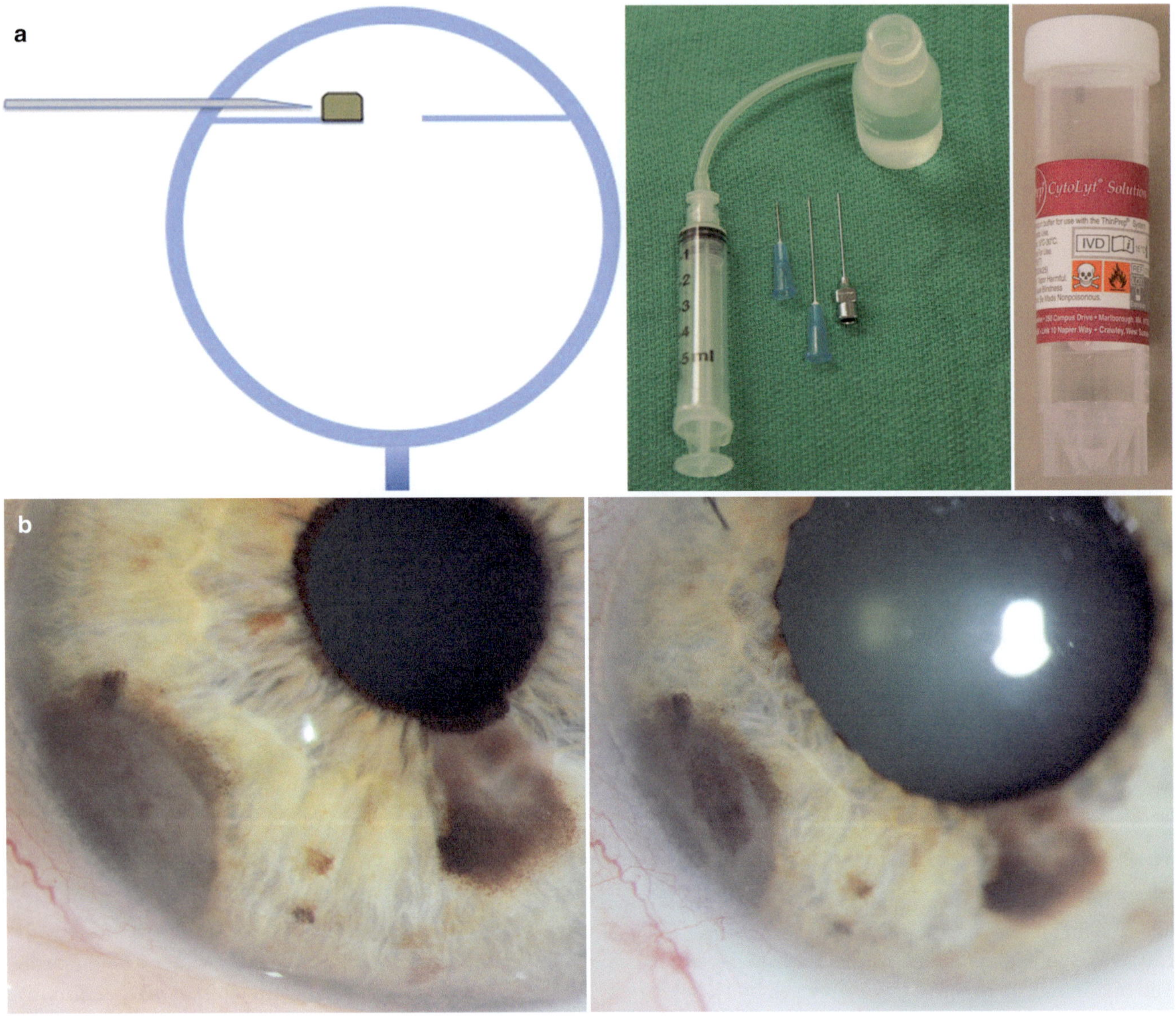

Fig. 1 FNAB technique. Schematic representation of approach for iris tumors. (**a**) The needle bevel is up, parallel to the iris plane, and not going across the pupil [Reprinted from Singh AD, Pelayes DE, Brainard JA, Biscotti CV. History, indications, techniques and limitations. Monographs in clinical cytology 2012;21:1–9. With permission from Karger Publishers. Copyright © 2011, Karger Publishers.] A short 25-gauge needle attached to short tube is used for aspiration. The aspirate sample is placed in a preservative solution, such as CytoLyt® and the needle rinsed to optimize cell yield. A 25-gauge needle with a calibrated tip can also be used. [Reprinted from Singh AD, Pelayes DE, Brainard JA, Biscotti CV. History, indications, techniques and limitations. Monographs in clinical cytology 2012;21:1–9. With permission from Karger Publishers. Copyright © 2011, Karger Publishers.] (**b**) Appearance of the tumor before and after FNAB. Note the crater within the aspirated tumor

FNAB can also be used for prognostic purposes by using various techniques, including cytological indicators of poor prognosis, such as presence of epithelioid cells, mitotic figures, and high number of tumor infiltrating lymphocytes. FNAB can also allow for cytogenetic testing of iris melanoma including the determination of monosomy 3 [21]. Gene expression profiling (GEP) is a recent prognostic test for uveal melanoma which can be performed with FNAB samples. This model stratifies tumors into two major subtypes, class 1 and class 2, corresponding with low and high rate of metastasis respectively [22–24]. Similarly, multiplex ligation-dependent probe amplification (MLPA) testing serves as a prognostication test in uveal melanoma. In this test, chromosome 3 loss (monosomy 3) and chromosome 8q gain portend poor prognosis, whereas chromosome 6p gain is a cytogenetic marker of good prognosis [25, 26].

2.1.4 Limitations

The primary limitation of FNAB is insufficient sampling which may lead to a false-negative interpretation. Diagnostic potential of ocular aspirate samples is diminished by limited cellularity [19].

Adopting the following can reduce the likelihood of a nondiagnostic FNAB:

- Avoid small tumors less than 2.5 mm in height.
- Avoid thinner needles (30 gauge).
- Refrain from plunger retraction following aspiration.
- Avoid dry smears.

Experience is also integral to the successful outcome of FNAB—both with respect to the proceduralist and the cytopathologist [27]. Due to this, cases of negative cytological diagnosis of malignancy should not be used to definitively rule out intraocular malignancy [28].

2.1.5 Complications

With respect to iris biopsy, complications such as persistent hyphema, prolonged hypotony, lens damage, or endophthalmitis are rare (<1%) [8, 16]. Concern for tumor seeding is one of the principal factors which led to the delayed adoption of FNAB for the diagnosis of intraocular tumors, and remains a concern for many clinicians. Indeed, it has been demonstrated that melanoma cells are present in needle tracks of 53% (indirect aspiration) and 67% (direct aspiration) of enucleated eyes that were sampled using FNAB. However, local dissemination and local tumor extension are rare, and it has been established that seeding primarily occurs with the use of large needles [29]. Reviews of approximately 200,000 cases have not shown evidence of local or systemic spread when using 25-gauge or smaller diameter needles to perform transocular FNAB [5, 14, 16, 30–33]. In the setting of transcorneal FNAB for iris tumors, the risk of seeding is extremely low [34].

2.1.6 Conclusions

Diagnostic ocular FNAB is reserved for a minority of iris tumors since most can be diagnosed based on clinical examination and ancillary testing. In cases where ocular FNAB is indicated, there is high diagnostic accuracy. FNAB can be used for both diagnostic and prognostic purposes. The primary limitation of this technique is low cellularity which can be minimized by appropriate case selection and technique. Complications are infrequent.

2.2 Cutter Biopsy

Minimally invasive iridectomy can be performed using a 20- or 25-gauge vitrector to obtain tissue [35]. The use of a 25-gauge aspiration cutter has been described as the Finger iridectomy technique and can be performed through a 1 mm incision. In this series, the diagnostic yield was 90% with minimal need for rehabilitation due to the small incision approach [36]. A series by Milman et al. included 55 eyes of iris and iridociliary tumors who underwent aspiration cutter-assisted biopsy. Nearly all biopsies (55/56) yielded cellular material and 41% yielded diagnostic tissue in cell block preparation. Though the yield of aspiration cutter-assisted biopsy is lower (98%) compared to incisional or excisional biopsy, it remains a useful strategy for anterior segment tumors [37].

2.3 Forceps

Intraocular forceps such as the 23-gauge Essen cavernous sampling forceps have been modified to improve sample yield. This technique was initially developed to sample posterior pole subretinal tumors and was used in conjunction with retinotomy and 23-gauge 3-port vitrectomy [38]. It has since been adapted for use in iris tumors and has subsequently shown to have a low rate of procedure-related complications. In this setting, the Essen forceps are introduced through a clear corneal incision after which the tissue is grasped and pulled out through the incision. A bimanual approach is used as vitrectomy scissors are inserted through a second corneal wound to cut the lesion. Histological and immunohistochemical diagnosis was achieved in 85% of these cases [39].

2.4 Punch Biopsy

Several techniques for incisional biopsy have been described. Pe'er et al. describe the use of a Kelly Descemet membrane punch to isolate tissue sample for histological analysis. The Kelly punch is introduced into the anterior chamber through a clear corneal incision after which the lesion is sampled, yielding a 0.8 × 0.6 mm piece of tissue [40].

2.5 Cannula Aspiration

A transcorneal fine cannula aspiration technique using a 25-gauge Rycroft cannula has been described by Matthews et al. Tumor specimens ranging from 1 to 1.5 mm were obtained and histological diagnosis of all 12 cases included in this series was made [34].

The advantage of these tissue biopsy techniques when compared to FNAB is the ability to perform morphological interpretation and ancillary testing (immunohistochemistry). Furthermore, this method includes sampling of deeper portions of the lesion and not just the surface as commonly seen with FNAB. Equivocal interpretations have been noted in cases where the surface of the lesion alone is sampled.

3 Excisional Techniques

3.1 Standard Iridectomy

3.1.1 Technique

After a conjunctival peritomy is performed, a partial thickness scleral flap (2/3 to 3/4 scleral thickness) is raised. Two

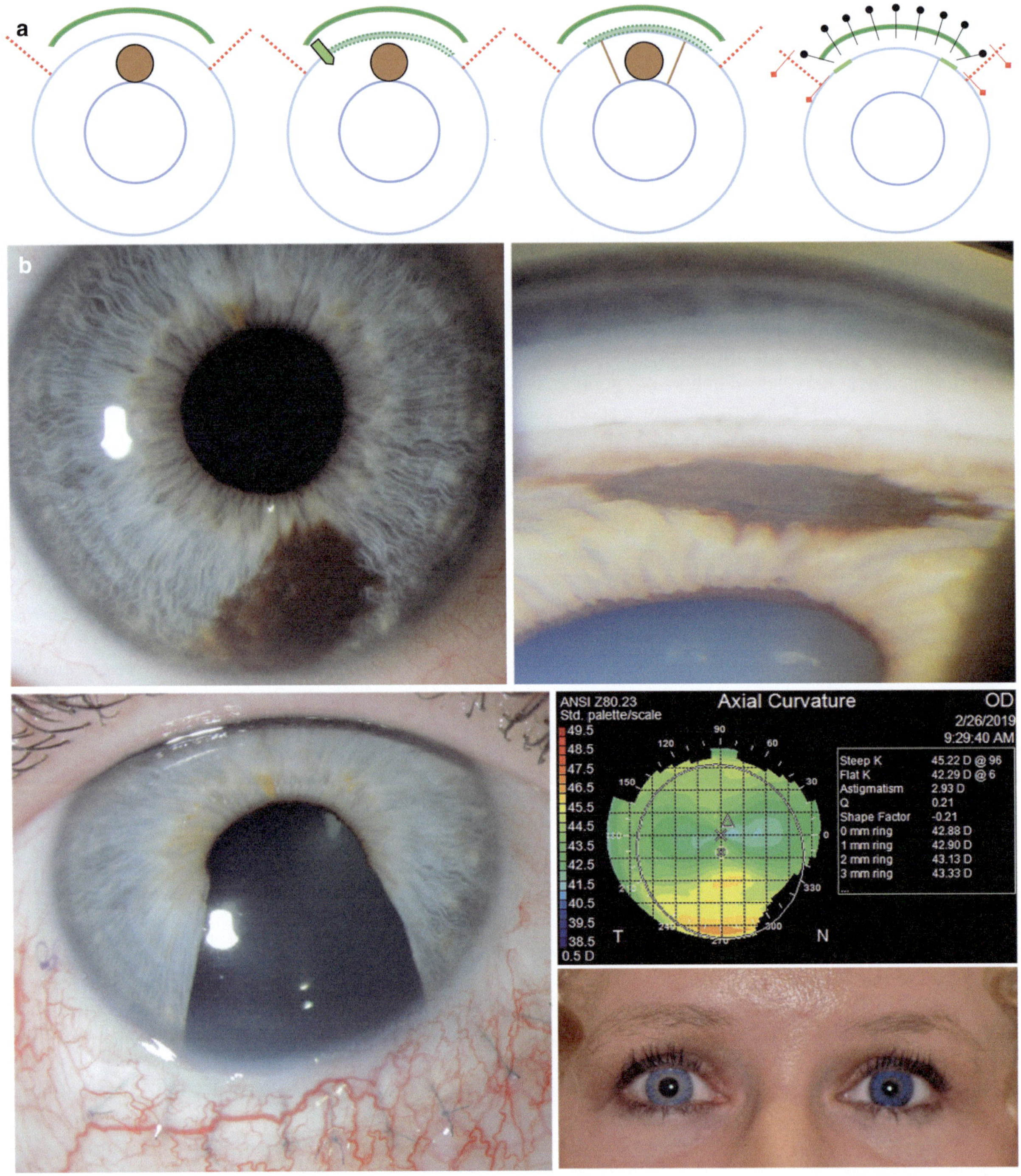

Fig. 2 Standard Iridectomy. Surgical steps. After 120 degrees conjunctival peritomy, the conjunctiva is reflected towards fornix exposing the sclera. (**a**) A partial-thickness scleral flap to thickness of 50% that is 2 mm or beyond tumor margins at limbus) is fashioned. The curvilinear limbus parallel incision is located 2 mm behind the limbus (**a**, solid green). The flap is reflected towards the limbus and extended into the clear cornea. Anterior chamber is entered (blade) and internal corneal incision is extended along the limbus with corneal scissors (**a**, green dots). At this point anterior chamber can be easily accessed by lifting the corneoscleral flap to perform radial (solid brown) and the basal iris incision (dotted brown). Following aspiration of any viscoelastic that may have been used, the anterior chamber is deepened prior to suturing the corneoscleral wound with 10–0 nylon sutures and conjunctiva with 8–0 absorbable sutures. A 41-year-old female who had been for iris nevus was noted to have growth of the nevus. The visual acuity was 20/15 OU and intraocular pressure was 15 mmHg OU. (**b**) Anterior segment examination of the right eye was remarkable for a 3.5 mm × 2.0 mm × flat iris lesion at the 5:30 o'clock position. This lesion was located peripherally and did not involve the pupillary margins or extend to the iris root. Gonioscopy revealed absence angle involvement without evidence of seeding or tumor dispersion. These exam findings in the setting of documented growth were highly suggestive of melanoma rather than iris nevus. Given that the lesion was approaching the iris root, standard iridectomy with scleral incision was performed. It was elected not to perform pupilloplasty because of the large defect of the iris. Pathology confirmed malignant melanoma, arising in spindle cell nevus with surface plaque. Notre persistent inflammation at the wound site even 6 weeks after surgery with 3 Dcyl of astigmatism. Patient managed to overcome photophobia with the use of tinted contact lenses with excellent visual, functional, and cosmetic outcome

parallel incisions are extended 2–3 mm posterior to the limbus and the radial incision is made about 2 mm outside of the tumor border. An incision is made to expose the tumor and the tumor is then resected with 1–2 mm margins. The scleral and corneal wounds are then closed (Fig. 2a) [41].

A variation in sector iridectomy is described by Pe'er and Frankel where extraocular incisions are made through the eye wall to isolate the tumor. Viscoelastic material is then injected through a second incision contralateral to the tumor, thereby prolapsing the lesion through the limbal incision. The tumor is then excised externally and the wounds are closed. The proposed advantage of this technique is that instruments are not introduced into the anterior chamber, thereby minimizing treatment related complications [42].

Early experience with iridectomy was reported by Reese and Cleasby which included 63 cases [1]. Photophobia is an expected sequelae of treatment and can be managed with pupilloplasty or contact lens (Fig. 2b). Complications of iridectomy include cataract as there can be contact between the lens and instrumentation during surgery. Hyphema, wound leak, wound dehiscence, vitreous loss, and episcleral seeding of the tumor have also been reported [43].

3.2 Small Incision Iridectomy

In recent years, minimally invasive surgical techniques for iris tumors resection have been developed. Hood et al. initially described a method in which guarded hydroaspiration was used. In this technique, vitrectomy scissors are introduced through a small clear corneal incision and a sector iridectomy is performed with radial incisions. The lesion is excised with tumor free margins. Sterile tubing or a modified Jones tube primed with a viscoelastic agent is then attached to a syringe. It is inserted into the anterior chamber and the tumor is aspirated into the lumen of the tube using gentle hydroaspiration. The tube is withdrawn from the anterior chamber and the lesion is expressed and unfolded onto filter paper. An additional paracentesis wound can be made to aid with manipulation of the iris. Concurrent pupilloplasty is then performed to minimize postoperative photophobia [44]. The small corneal wound is then closed with interrupted sutures (Fig. 3a).

A series including 22 cases of small, localized iris lesions resected using the aforementioned technique highlights its advantages. When compared to large corneoscleral incisions, this minimally invasive technique has decreased postoperative morbidity and hastens recovery. There were no reported occurrences of hyphema, hypotony, or wound leak. Visual acuity was preserved with low degrees of astigmatism within the immediate postoperative period (Fig. 3b) [45]. Since tumor retrieval is performed in a guarded fashion as it is withdrawn from the anterior chamber, there is also decreased theoretical risk of tumor seeding [44]. Local recurrence and metastasis were not observed [45]. Furthermore, it is important to recognize that the tumor sample is isolated by a "no touch" method. The sample is not manipulated or compressed as it is removed, and it thereby maintains its architecture for accurate histopathological assessment and its margins.

Meyer and Krishnan have used similar technique and have modified it slightly to use an empty intraocular lens cartridge instead of modified Jones tube. This series also reports minimal procedure related complications. They highlight the efficiency of this technique as only a single suture is used to close the wound [46].

3.3 Iridocyclectomy

Iridocyclectomy is indicated when iris melanoma extends into the iris root or ciliary body and includes removal of the tumor with peripheral iridectomy and cyclectomy with a 2 mm margin [47]. It is primarily recommended for well defined, small tumors with less than 3 clock hours of ciliary body involvement (Fig. 4a).

3.3.1 Anteroposterior Approach

The conventional method describes an anteroposterior approach that begins with dissection at the pupil margin known as "irido-cyclectomy" [3]. It may be combined with preoperative pharmacologic mydriasis.

3.3.2 Posteroanterior Approach

A "cyclo-iridectomy" technique has also been described by Damato which involves a posteroanterior or circumferential approach starting with the iris root. The advantage of this technique is preservation of the iris sphincter.

With the posteroanterior approach, a conjunctival peritomy is performed and sclerocorneal flap is created over the tumor. A T-shaped incision centered over the tumor is made and two posterior scleral flaps are created. The anterior chamber is opened and iris incisions outside the borders of the tumor are made. The radial cuts are continued through the chamber angle into the ciliary sulcus. A suture is placed in the corneal flap and the radial cuts are deepened into the floor of the sclera and pars plicata. A similar incision is made posterior to the tumor. The radial portions of the incision are sutured and the tumor is extracted through the slit [41]. The vitreous is examined to ensure that there is no prolapse after which the sclera and conjunctiva are closed.

Complications of iridocyclectomy include hypotony due to ciliary body excision, hyphema, cataract, cyclodialysis, wound dehiscence, and bullous keratopathy [48]. Vail reviewed a series of 244 cases of iridocyclectomy for iris and ciliary body tumors [49]. Photophobia also results from this surgery and symptoms can be mitigated by concurrent pupilloplasty or use of cosmetic contact lenses (Fig. 4b).

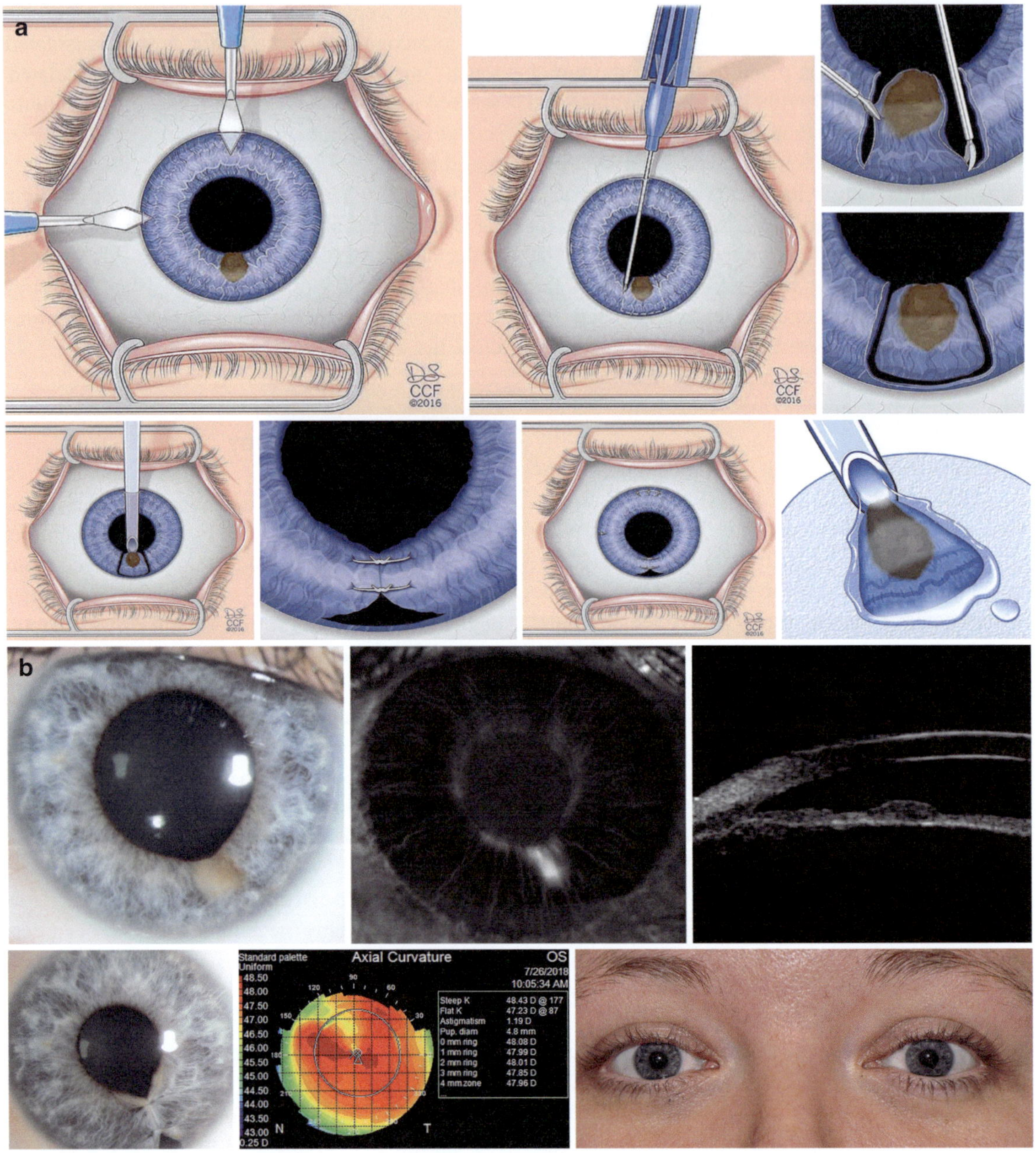

Fig. 3 (**a**) Small incision iridectomy. Surgical steps. Corneal incisions. One primary, small, self-sealing corneal incision was fashioned with keratome in a quadrant opposite to the tumor location. Secondary corneal incisions were also created to facilitate iris incisions. Iris resection. Two linear iris incisions were made by the straight 23-gauge or 25-gauge horizontal vitrectomy scissors about 1.0 mm beyond the tumor margins entering from the pupillary margin. The resected section of the iris was then either grasped by forceps or displaced sideways with use of a viscoelastic agent to facilitate basal iris incision with curved vitrectomy scissors. Guarded hydroaspiration of the excised lesion. A clear plastic tubing (diameter 3.5 mm) with a beveled tip that had been primed with viscoelastic agent was then inserted into the anterior chamber through one of the enlarged corneal incisions (2.75–5.2 mm) and placed next to the free wedge of the iris. By slow retraction of the plunger (3.0 cc or 5.0 cc syringe), the iris wedge was aspirated into the tubing. The tubing was then withdrawn from the anterior chamber with the excised lesion within. Pupilloplasty. Repair of the iris defect, when feasible, was undertaken with 10–0 Prolene suture using a modified Siepser slip-knot technique. Wound closure. The corneal wound was closed with standard interrupted 10–0 nylon sutures. Sample handling. The tumor sample was expressed onto the filter paper for routine histopathological processing. [Illustration by David Schumick, BS, CMI. Reprinted with permission, Cleveland Clinic Center for Medical Art & Photography © 2016–2019. All Rights Reserved]. A 30-year-old woman had been found to have an iris lesion in the left eye at 5:00 which had not been previously observed in her prior visit 1 year ago. The visual acuity was measured at 20/20 in both eyes with normal intraocular pressures OU. (**b**) A nodular translucent partially pigmented iris mass located at 5:30 touching the pupillary margin and measuring 2 mm × 2 mm × 1.6 mm was observed OS . The lesion contained an intrinsic vascularity as well as feeder vessels further characterized by anterior segment fluorescein angiography. The lesion thickness was confirmed by ultrasound biomicroscopy. Because if recent onset, our clinical impression was of iris melanoma. We therefore recommend excisional biopsy. There was minimal postop astigmatism which was corrected with glasses. The small iris defect could be closed with pupilloplasty resulting in equal pupils in ambient light. Pathology confirmed malignant melanoma (spindle cell type)

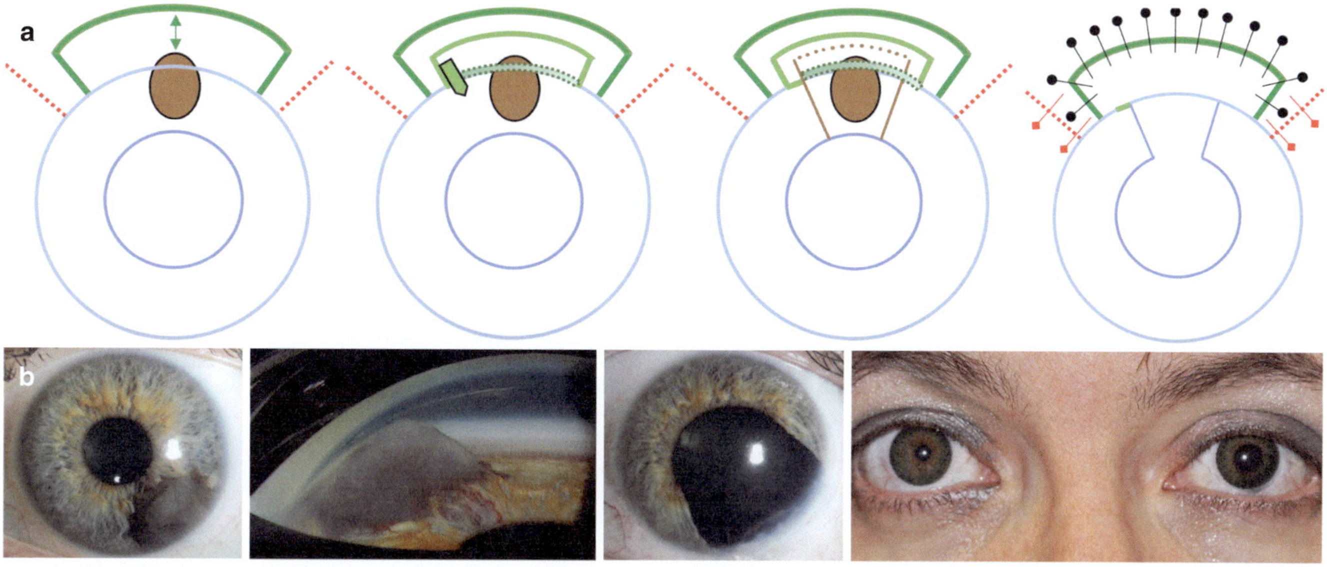

Fig. 4 Iridocyclectomy. Surgical steps. After 120 degrees conjunctival peritomy, the conjunctiva is reflected towards fornix exposing the sclera. A partial-thickness scleral flap to thickness of 50% that is located 2 mm behind the posterior tumor margin is fashioned (**a**, solid green). The flap is reflected towards the limbus and extended into the clear cornea. The inner scleral incision is 1 mm inside the outer incision (**a**, light green). Anterior chamber is entered (blade) and internal corneal incision is extended along the limbus with corneal scissors (**a**, green dots). At this point anterior chamber can be easily accessed by lifting the corneoscleral flap to perform radial iris incision (**a**, solid brown) followed by ciliary body incision after it has been cauterized (**a**, dotted brown). (**a**) Following aspiration of any viscoelastic that may have been used, the anterior chamber is deepened prior to suturing the scleral wound with 10–0 nylon sutures and conjunctiva with 8–0 absorbable sutures. A 40-year-old woman presented with a growing iris nevus. The visual acuity was 20/20 in both eyes and her intraocular pressures were 19 mmHg in both eyes. (**b**) On the left eye examination attention was drawn to the pigmented multinodular iris tumor at present 4o'clock to 5:45 extending from the pupillary margin to the iris root. The tumor was associated with intrinsic vasculature and feeder vessels. Ciliary body extension was excluded by ultrasound biomicroscopy. After a detailed discussion about treatment options that included surgical excision, radiation, and enucleation the patient agreed to proceed with our recommendation of surgical excision of the tumor via iridocyclectomy. Pathology confirmed malignant melanoma of the iris (mixed cell type) involving the trabecular meshwork with negative margins. At 5 years follow up, the patient has not developed local recurrence or systemic metastasis and maintains visual acuity of 20/25 with tinted contact lens

4 Block Resection

A more radical surgical technique known as "block resection" for iridociliary tumors has been described by Naumann and Rummelt. It is been used to treat uveal melanoma with less than 4 clock hours of angle involvement as well as adenomas of the nonpigmented ciliary epithelium [50]. With this method, the entire tumor with adjacent full-thickness cornea and sclera is removed in one block and tectonic corneoscleral grafting is performed. This is in comparison to iridocyclectomy techniques where local en bloc excision is performed and a superficial lamellar scleral flap is preserved. The rationale for this more aggressive approach is that 90% of uveal melanomas invade the sclera histopathologically [51] and 45% reveal invasion of >30% scleral thickness [52]. This suggests that the remaining scleral flap poses a risk for local tumor recurrence. Furthermore, it preserves the globe by avoiding enucleation and allows for satisfactory visual acuity [50]. Given the extensive nature of surgery, it is not surprising that there are significant complications. As reported by Heindl et al., block resection allows for molecular profiling and provides tissue for immune-based vaccination therapy in addition to histopathologic diagnosis [53]. Complications include vitreous hemorrhage, cataract, corneal endothelial decompensation, and retinal detachment [52].

5 Outcomes

Visual acuity is largely preserved after surgical resection. Stability of preoperative and postoperative visual acuity has been demonstrated [42, 54, 55]. In cases of progressive vision loss, the authors identified cataracts as the causative etiology [56].

Overall, recurrence is rare following surgical resection with reported rates of 0–8% [42, 55, 56]. Of the 51 patients in the Conway study, none of them developed metastasis [56]. A recent series reported four cases of subconjunctival recurrence without intraocular component in patients who underwent surgical resection [57]. Rones and Zimmerman reported three cases in a series of 125 iris melanoma cases treated with iridocyclectomy who later developed concurrent intraocular and extraocular relapse [2]. Klauber et al. reviewed 47 cases of iris and iridociliary melanoma who were treated with surgical resection (iridectomy and iridocyclectomy). Within this cohort, one patient had local recurrence and none of the patients had metastatic disease [41]. This suggests that surgical resection as a safe and effective mode of treatment when strict diagnostic and surgical procedures are followed.

Some studies have described late recurrence after surgical resection that occurs 10–30 years after primary treatment [58]. The earliest reports date back to 1964 when local resection alone was recommended for iris melanoma without adjuvant radiotherapy, even in the setting of incomplete resection [59]. We now know that incomplete excision is a risk factor for local recurrence due to the presence of subclinical microscopic disease [60].

6 Conclusions

Significant advancements have been made with regard to surgical management of iris melanoma. As our techniques and instrumentation improve, there is greater emphasis on utilizing a minimally invasive approach. Ultimately, our goal is to successfully diagnose and treat iris melanoma while reducing treatment related morbidity, complications, and local recurrence.

References

1. Reese AB, Cleasby GW. The treatment of iris melanoma. Trans Am Acad Ophthalmol Otolaryngol. 1959;63(3):296–304; discussion –5
2. Rones B, Zimmerman LE. The prognosis of primary tumors of the iris treated by iridectomy. AMA Arch Ophthalmol. 1958;60(2):193–205.
3. Stallard HB. Surgery of malignant melanoma of the iris. Br J Ophthalmol. 1951;35(12):774–83.
4. Jakobiec FA, Coleman DJ, Chattock A, Smith M. Ultrasonically guided needle biopsy and cytologic diagnosis of solid intraocular tumors. Ophthalmology. 1979;86(9):1662–81.
5. Shields JA, Shields CL, Ehya H, et al. Fine-needle aspiration biopsy of suspected intraocular tumors. The 1992 Urwick lecture. Ophthalmology. 1993;100(11):1677–84.
6. Char DH, Miller T. Accuracy of presumed uveal melanoma diagnosis before alternative therapy. Br J Ophthalmol. 1995;79(7):692–6.
7. Grossniklaus HE. Fine-needle aspiration biopsy of the iris. Arch Ophthalmol. 1992;110(7):969–76.
8. Shields JA. Treating some small melanocytic choroidal lesions without waiting for growth. Arch Ophthalmol. 2006;124(9):1344–6.
9. Young TA, Burgess BL, Rao NP, et al. Transscleral fine-needle aspiration biopsy of macular choroidal melanoma. Am J Ophthalmol. 2008;145(2):297–302.
10. Augsburger JJ, Shields JA. Fine needle aspiration biopsy of solid intraocular tumors: indications, instrumentation and techniques. Ophthalmic Surg. 1984;15(1):34–40.
11. Pelayes DE, Zarate JO, Biscotti CV, Singh AD. Calibrated needle for ophthalmic fine needle aspiration biopsy. Br J Ophthalmol. 2012;96(8):1147–8.
12. Seregard S. To biopsy or not to biopsy? Acta Ophthalmol. 2009;87(6):586–7.
13. Eide N, Syrdalen P, Walaas L, Hagmar B. Fine needle aspiration biopsy in selecting treatment for inconclusive intraocular disease. Acta Ophthalmol Scand. 1999;77(4):448–52.
14. Pelayes DE, Zarate JO. Fine needle aspiration biopsy with liquid-based cytology and adjunct immunohistochemistry in intraocular melanocytic tumors. Eur J Ophthalmol. 2010;20(6):1059–65.
15. Gupta M, Puri P, Jacques R, Rennie IG. Fine needle aspiration biopsy: an investigative tool for iris metastasis. Eye (Lond). 2001;15(Pt 4):541–2.
16. Shields CL, Manquez ME, Ehya H, et al. Fine-needle aspiration biopsy of iris tumors in 100 consecutive cases: technique and complications. Ophthalmology. 2006;113(11):2080–6.
17. Eide N, Walaas L. Fine-needle aspiration biopsy and other biopsies in suspected intraocular malignant disease: a review. Acta Ophthalmol. 2009;87(6):588–601.
18. Czerniak B, Woyke S, Domagala W, Krzysztolik Z. Fine needle aspiration cytology of intraocular malignant melanoma. Acta Cytol. 1983;27(2):157–65.
19. Char DH, Kemlitz AE, Miller T, Crawford JB. Iris ring melanoma: fine needle biopsy. Br J Ophthalmol. 2006;90(4):420–2.
20. Demirci H, Finger PT, Cocker R, McCormick SA. Unusual presentation of diffuse melanoma of the iris. Br J Ophthalmol. 2000;84(9):1076–8.
21. Shields CL, Ramasubramanian A, Ganguly A, et al. Cytogenetic testing of iris melanoma using fine needle aspiration biopsy in 17 patients. Retina. 2011;31(3):574–80.
22. Harbour JW. Molecular prognostic testing and individualized patient care in uveal melanoma. Am J Ophthalmol. 2009;148(6):823–9 e1.
23. Onken MD, Worley LA, Ehlers JP, Harbour JW. Gene expression profiling in uveal melanoma reveals two molecular classes and predicts metastatic death. Cancer Res. 2004;64(20):7205–9.
24. Onken MD, Worley LA, Char DH, et al. Collaborative ocular oncology group report number 1: prospective validation of a multi-gene prognostic assay in uveal melanoma. Ophthalmology. 2012;119(8):1596–603.
25. Damato B, Dopierala J, Klaasen A, et al. Multiplex ligation-dependent probe amplification of uveal melanoma: correlation with metastatic death. Invest Ophthalmol Vis Sci. 2009;50(7):3048–55.
26. Damato B, Dopierala JA, Coupland SE. Genotypic profiling of 452 choroidal melanomas with multiplex ligation-dependent probe amplification. Clin Cancer Res. 2010;16(24):6083–92.
27. Singh AD, Biscotti CV. Fine needle aspiration biopsy of ophthalmic tumors. Saudi J Ophthalmol. 2012;26(2):117–23.
28. Char DH, Crawford JB, Kroll S. Iris melanomas. Diagnostic problems. Ophthalmology. 1996;103(2):251–5.
29. Wu M, Burstein DE. Fine needle aspiration. Cancer Investig. 2004;22(4):620–8.
30. Augsburger JJ, Shields JA, Folberg R, et al. Fine needle aspiration biopsy in the diagnosis of intraocular cancer. Cytologic-histologic correlations. Ophthalmology. 1985;92(1):39–49.
31. Char DH, Kemlitz AE, Miller T. Intraocular biopsy. Ophthalmol Clin N Am. 2005;18(1):177–85, x
32. Karcioglu ZA, Gordon RA, Karcioglu GL. Tumor seeding in ocular fine needle aspiration biopsy. Ophthalmology. 1985;92(12):1763–7.
33. Glasgow BJ, Brown HH, Zargoza AM, Foos RY. Quantitation of tumor seeding from fine needle aspiration of ocular melanomas. Am J Ophthalmol. 1988;105(5):538–46.

34. Matthews BJMH, Rennie IG. Trans-corneal fine cannula aspiration: rycroft cannula aspiration technique for sampling iris tumours. Br J Ophthalmol. 2012;96:329–31.
35. Bechrakis NE, Foerster MH, Bornfeld N. Biopsy in indeterminate intraocular tumors. Ophthalmology. 2002;109(2):235–42.
36. Finger PT, Latkany P, Kurli M, Iacob C. The Finger iridectomy technique: small incision biopsy of anterior segment tumours. Br J Ophthalmol. 2005;89(8):946–9.
37. Milman T, Petousis V, McCormick SA, Finger PT. Anterior segment tumor aspiration cutter-assisted biopsy: experience with pathology. Am J Ophthalmol. 2011;152(5):776–83.e1.
38. Akgul H, Otterbach F, Bornfeld N, Jurklies B. Intraocular biopsy using special forceps: a new instrument and refined surgical technique. Br J Ophthalmol. 2011;95(1):79–82.
39. Chronopoulos A, Kilic E, Joussen AM, Lipski A. Small incision iris tumour biopsy using a cavernous sampling forceps. Br J Ophthalmol. 2014;98(11):1539–42.
40. Pe'er J, Blumenthal EZ, Frenkel S. Punch biopsy of iris lesions: a novel technique for obtaining histology samples. Br J Ophthalmol. 2007;91(5):660–2.
41. Klauber S, Jensen PK, Prause JU, Kessing SV. Surgical treatment of iris and ciliary body melanoma: follow-up of a 25-year series of patients. Acta Ophthalmol. 2012;90(2):122–6.
42. Pe'er J, Frenkel S. Sector iridectomy of iris melanoma: a novel technique for excising the melanoma extraocularly. Br J Ophthalmol. 2011;95(10):1474–6.
43. Arentsen JJ, Green WR. Melanoma of the iris: report of 72 cases treated surgically. Ophthalmic Surg. 1975;6(2):23–37.
44. Hood CT, Schoenfield LR, Torres V, Singh AD. Iris melanoma. Ophthalmology. 2011;118(1):221–2.
45. Singh AD. Small incision guarded hydroaspiration of iris lesions. Br J Ophthalmol. 2017;101(11):1570–5.
46. Meyer JJ, Krishnan T, McGhee CN. Minimal iris touch excision: a novel surgical technique for local excision of iris melanoma. Clin Exp Ophthalmol. 2018;46(3):298–9.
47. Schmitzer S, Butea-Simionescu C, Gheorghe A, et al. Iridociliary melanoma - clinical case. J Med Life. 2016;9(1):88–91.
48. Rospond-Kubiak I, Damato B. The surgical approach to the management of anterior uveal melanomas. Eye (Lond). 2014;28(6):741–7.
49. Vail DT. Iridocyclectomy. A review. Gleanings from the literature. Am J Ophthalmol. 1971;71(1 Pt 2):161–8.
50. Cursiefen C, Schlötzer-Schrehardt U, Holbach LM, Naumann GO. Adenoma of the nonpigmented ciliary epithelium mimicking a malignant melanoma of the iris. Arch Ophthalmol. 1999;117(1):113–6.
51. Donders PC. Malignant melanoma of the choroid. Trans Ophthalmol Soc U K. 1973;93:745–51.
52. Naumann GO, Rummelt V. Block excision of tumors of the anterior uvea. Report on 68 consecutive patients. Ophthalmology. 1996;103(12):2017–27. discussion 27-8
53. Heindl LM, Koch KR, Hermann MM, et al. Block excision of Iridociliary tumors enables molecular profiling and immune vaccination. Ophthalmology. 2017;124(2):268–70.
54. Cardine S, Labetoulle M, Kirsch O, et al. Iris melanomas. A retrospective study of 11 patients treated by surgical excision. J Fr Ophtalmol. 2003;26(1):31–7.
55. Romanowska-Dixon B. Surgical management of iris melanoma. Klin Ocz. 2005;107(10–12):622–6.
56. Conway RM, Chua WC, Qureshi C, Billson FA. Primary iris melanoma: diagnostic features and outcome of conservative surgical treatment. Br J Ophthalmol. 2001;85(7):848–54.
57. Fabian ID, Thaung C, AlHarby L, et al. Late solitary extraocular recurrence from previously resected iris melanoma. Am J Ophthalmol. 2017;181:97–105.
58. Bosello F, Al-Jamal RT, Cohen VML. Very late recurrence of iris melanoma: 45 years after treatment. Melanoma Res. 2020;30(3):309–12.
59. Cleasby GW. Recurrent malignant melanoma of the iris. Arch Ophthalmol. 1964;72:332–6.
60. Damato BE, Paul J, Foulds WS. Risk factors for metastatic uveal melanoma after trans-scleral local resection. Br J Ophthalmol. 1996;80(2):109–16.

The MOLES Acronym and Scoring System for Estimating Likelihood of Malignancy in Melanocytic Choroidal Tumors

Bertil E. Damato

1 Introduction

Melanocytic choroidal tumors are found in about 6% of the population [1, 2]. Even though they rarely show malignant growth, they are a problem. Many patients with these lesions experience significant distress, because of concerns that their tumor is malignant or at risk of undergoing malignant transformation. All too often, these fears are amplified by practitioners who lack the confidence or skill to reassure patients about the minimal risk of malignancy and who are unduly worried about the medico-legal consequences of missing a melanoma. As a result, large numbers of patients are referred to specialist clinics, which they may have to attend repeatedly, possibly for a lifetime (Fig. 1). A significant proportion of these patients will be referred for expert care to a supra-regional ocular oncology center, where they may be subjected to long-term monitoring, possibly far from home. They and their families may experience considerable financial hardship even if their medical care is covered by insurance, because of loss of earnings as well as the cost of travel, accommodation, and other expenses, such as childcare. The management of patients with pigmented fundus lesions is also burdensome for healthcare services, taking up precious clinic space, medical staff time, and imaging equipment, possibly lengthening waiting times for clinic appointments. In some healthcare systems, such diversion of limited resources may delay the care of patients needing urgent treatment, such as those with choroidal melanoma. Coronavirus disease 2019 (Covid-19) has exacerbated these difficulties, because of measures to prevent nosocomial coronavirus infection and the healthcare constraints these precautions have caused [3]. Treatment of small melanomas may also be delayed because they are mis-diagnosed as "suspicious nevi" and monitored for growth for months or years, possibly missing any opportunities for preventing metastatic spread (Fig. 2). Although many choroidal melanomas have already developed lethal mutations and metastasized by the time the ocular tumor is detected and treated, there is some tentative evidence that these events can occur late so that they are preventable in some patients [4–6].

To mitigate these problems, the author has devised the MOLES acronym and scoring system for estimating the likelihood of malignancy in melanocytic choroidal tumors. These are described in this chapter together with a discussion on their impact on patient care at Oxford Eye Hospital.

2 Pathophysiology

As melanocytic choroidal tumors grow, they become thicker so that they develop a dome shape. The overlying choriocapillaris is disturbed and retinal pigment epithelium (RPE) becomes multilayered and dysfunctional, so that there is accumulation of subretinal fluid and lipofuscin as well as the formation of drusen and RPE detachments [7, 8]. Intraretinal cystoid edema and outer retinal degeneration can occur. Some tumors develop a choroidal neovascular membrane, which can cause visual loss, treatable with anti-angiogenic agents [9]. In some tumors, the RPE atrophies, usually over the thickest part of the lesion. Bruch's membrane over the tumor becomes deficient, allowing the tumor to bulge into the retina, then forming a knuckle of tumor tissue, and eventually a mushroom shape. This distinctive shape develops when Bruch's membrane obstructs venous drainage to cause interstitial edema and tissue swelling (Fig. 3).

B. E. Damato (✉)
Nuffield Laboratory of Ophthalmology, University of Oxford, Oxford, UK

Ocular Oncology Service, Moorfields Eye Hospital, London, UK

Department of Ocular Oncology, Royal Liverpool University Hospital, Liverpool, UK

University of California, San Francisco, CA, USA
e-mail: Bertil.Damato@NHS.UK

B. V. Chawla, M. E. Aronow (eds.), *Global Perspectives in Ocular Oncology*, https://doi.org/10.1007/978-3-031-08250-4_28

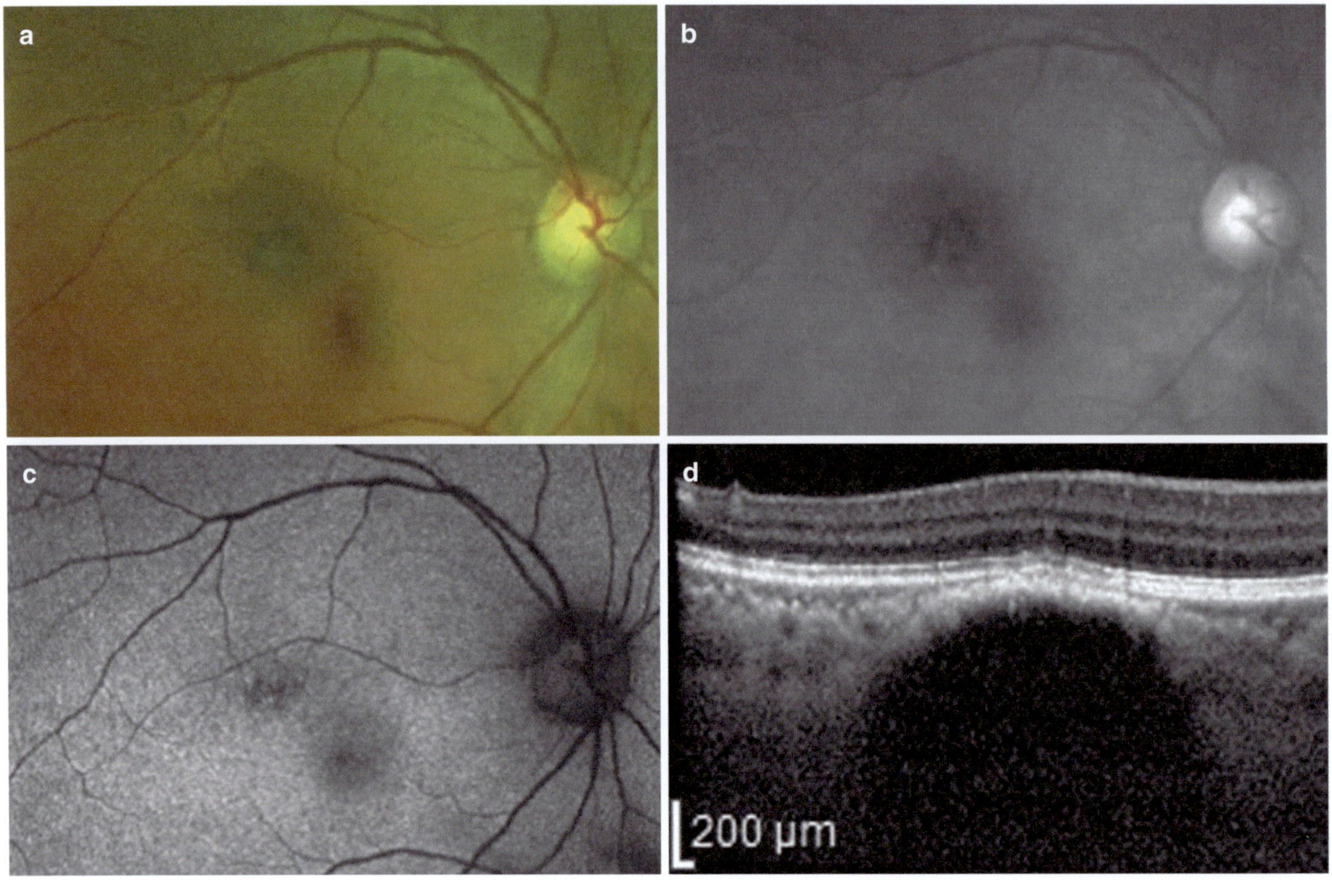

Fig. 1 Common choroidal nevus in the right eye of a 65-year-old woman who underwent 12 assessments at a hospital eye clinic over a 5-year period, with ultrasonography, indocyanine-green angiography and fluorescein angiography. (**a**) color photograph showing a gray lesion supero-temporal to the fovea, with a diameter of 2.3 mm; (**b**) green-free image showing the lateral extent of the lesion; (**c**) fundus autofluorescence image showing no hyper-autofluorescent lipofuscin pigment; and (**d**) optical coherence tomography showing the nevus to have a thickness of 0.5 mm and no sub-retinal fluid (MOLES score = 00000 = 0 = "common nevus")

3 Clinical Signs

3.1 Ophthalmoscopy and Color Photography

On ophthalmoscopy, the RPE multilayering makes the nevi and melanomas appear gray or brown, even if they are amelanotic. The tumor color may vary with the camera that is used to image the lesion. Lipofuscin looks orange over dark lesions, hence the term "orange pigment," but appears brown or black over amelanotic tumors when the RPE is otherwise absent (Fig. 4). The lipofuscin can desquamate off the tumor surface to precipitate within an area of retinal detachment, beyond the tumor margins (Fig. 2) [10]. Some tumors appear to have orange pigment, which on autofluorescence imaging is found not to be present (Fig. 5). Drusen and RPE detachments can develop, especially over thickened lesions and are a sign of chronicity. Subretinal fluid can gravitate inferiorly to cause a pale, vertical band of atrophy of the RPE and outer retina; this feature persisting even after subretinal fluid subsides (Fig. 6). When the tumor expands through the RPE and Bruch's membrane, it can be surrounded by a ring of hemorrhages, possibly as a result of choriocapillaris damage. When outflow of blood in the intraretinal part of the tumor is obstructed, the veins in this part of the tumor become dilated and tortuous, giving rise to the appearance of a "double circulation" (Fig. 3). Although choroidal melanomas tend to be larger than nevi, there is significant overlap [11]. Some nevi are more than 10 mm in diameter (i.e., "giant nevi") [12]. Conversely, melanomas can be detected when they are small and flat, so as to be indistinguishable from common nevi (Fig. 7). The apparent tumor size can vary with eye position, because of distortion of the image [13]. Tumor growth can be detected by comparing sequential photographs and noting extension of its margins closer to adjacent landmarks, such as retinal blood vessels and optic disc (Fig. 8) [14]. Red-light

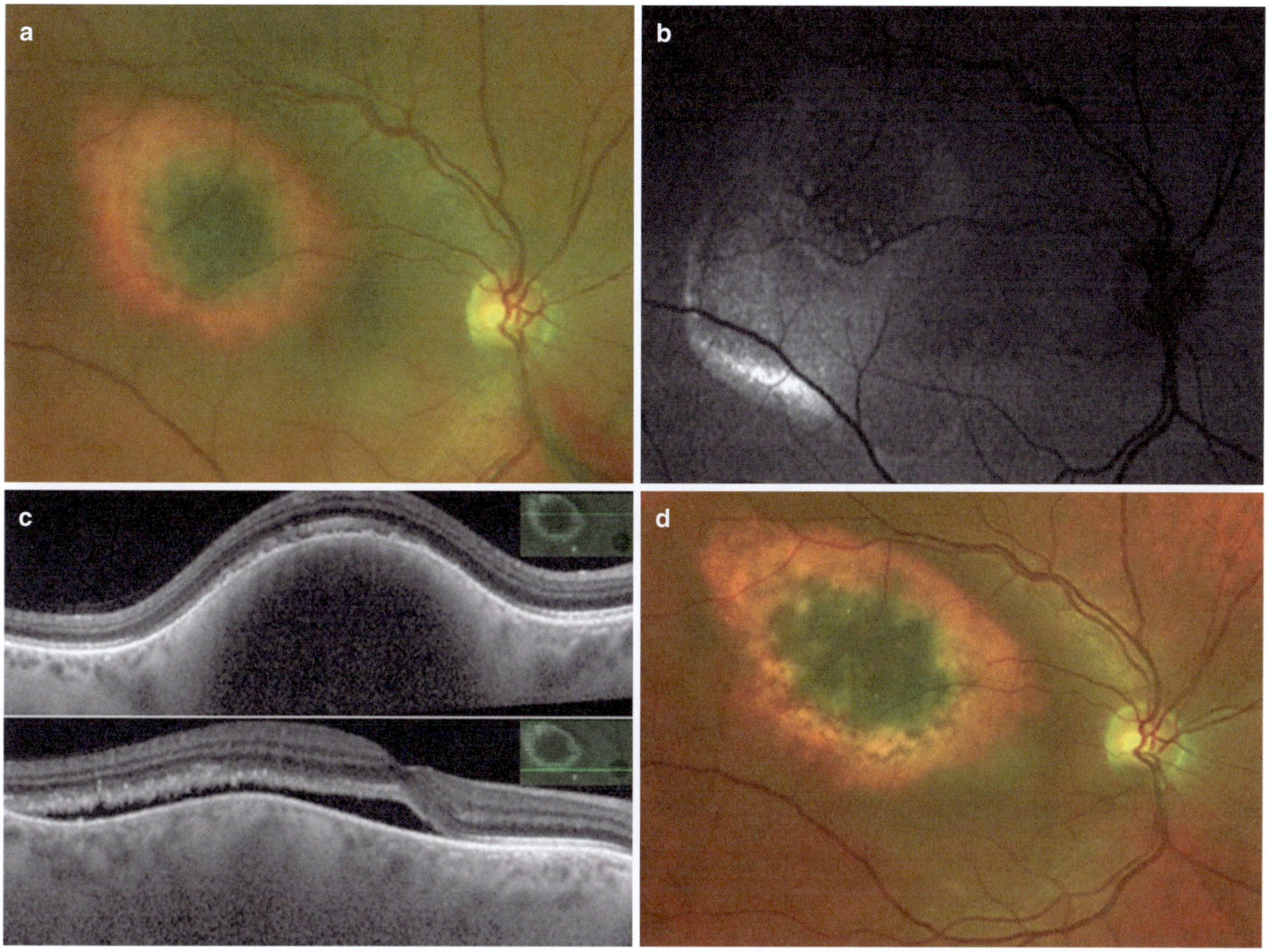

Fig. 2 Right fundus of a 54-year-old man in August 2017, who presented with photopsia and blurred vision. (**a**) Color photograph showing a supero-temporal choroidal tumor, with a central gray area surrounded by a pale halo; (**b**) fundus autofluorescence image showing a few clumps of hyper-autofluorescent lipofuscin on the tumor surface and precipitates of desquamated lipofuscin inferior to the tumor, in an area of detached retina; (**c**) OCT scans showing the tumor with subretinal fluid and lipofuscin clumps on the anterior surface of the retinal pigment epithelium. On ultrasonography, the basal tumor diameter was 5.0 mm and the thickness was 1.6 mm. If given a MOLES score at that time, this would have been 02102 (i.e., 5; "probable melanoma"); however, it was diagnosed (elsewhere) as a "leaky halo naevus" and treated with photodynamic therapy, to improve vision. (**d**) Fundus photograph 34 months later showing tumor growth, increasing the MOLES score to 02222. The patient was treated with ruthenium plaque radiotherapy. (Reprinted with permission from Damato B. Clinical Atlas of Ocular Oncology. New York: Springer; 2022)

photography may define the tumor extent more accurately than color photography [15]. Other signs of tumor progression include greater convexity of its surface on stereoscopic examination, intraretinal tumor growth, and accumulation of lipofuscin and/or subretinal fluid.

3.2 Autofluorescence Imaging

The normal RPE shows moderate autofluorescence, so that areas of RPE atrophy are hypo-autofluorescent (Figs. 3 and 4) [16]. Conversely, lipofuscin deposits are hyper-autofluorescent (Figs. 3 and 4) [17, 18]. Drusen tends to show little or no hyper-autofluorescence. Fundus Autofluorescence (FAF) may underestimate tumor extent if the RPE overlying tapering margins is normal.

3.3 Optical Coherence Tomography (OCT)

RPE thickening or atrophy, choriocapillaris narrowing or occlusion, retinal abnormality, intraretinal edema, outer-retinal degeneration, and subretinal fluid are all demonstrated by OCT [19, 20]. This imaging also helps to distinguish lipo-

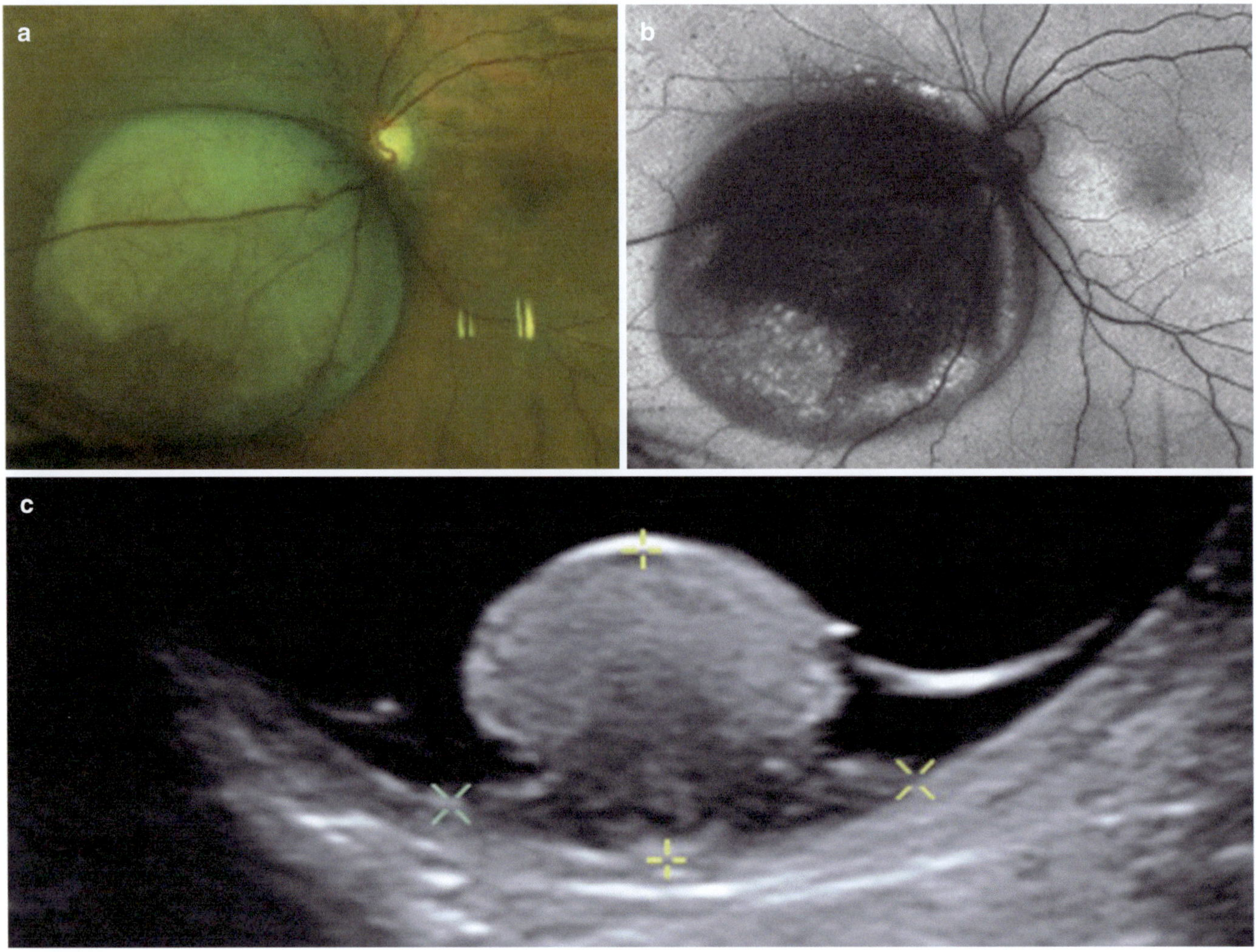

Fig. 3 Mushroom-shaped choroidal melanoma (**a**) Pseudo-color photograph showing the nodular apex, where dilated tumor vessels are visible, except where RPE is still present. Part of the base is visible superiorly. (**b**) Fundus auto-fluorescence image showing (i) hypo-autofluorescence in the apical part of the tumor where RPE is absent, (ii) normal auto-fluorescence where RPE persists, and (iii) hyper-autofluorescent clumps of confluent lipofuscin, within residual RPE overlying the base of the tumor and the intraretinal nodule. (**c**) Ultrasound B-scan showing the mushroom shape, the high acoustic reflectivity in the intraretinal part of the tumor and the low acoustic reflectivity in the tumor base (MOLES score = 22,202 = 8 = "probable melanoma"). (Reprinted with permission from Damato B. Clinical Atlas of Ocular Oncology. New York: Springer; 2022)

fuscin from drusen, the former depositing on the retinal surface of the RPE and the latter developing between RPE and Bruch's membrane. OCT can also show bulging or growth of the tumor through a defect in RPE and Bruch's membrane (Fig. 8). Melanin and hemoglobin cause shadowing. If the tissues are sufficiently transparent, the interface between tumor and sclera is visible so that the tumor thickness can be measured [21]. Some tumors, particularly halo nevi, show posterior "bowing" of the sclera despite having a flat anterior surface (Fig. 9) [22]. On optical coherence tomography angiography (OCTA), melanomas are more likely than nevi to show indistinct margins, avascular areas and abnormalities such as vascular loops [23, 24].

3.4 Ultrasonography (US)

Internal acoustic reflectivity tends to be lower in melanomas than in nevi [25]. This feature is more evident in thicker tumors and when assessed with high-resolution ultrasonography [26]. Acoustic reflectivity is increased by melanin, so that deeply pigmented tumors, such as melanocytomas, are highly reflective, while amelanotic tumors, including some nevi, show low reflectivity. With mushroom-shaped melanomas, the intraretinal part of the tumor shows high reflectivity, probably because of the interstitial edema, whereas the uveal base of the tumor shows low reflectivity, presumably because the tumor cells are packed

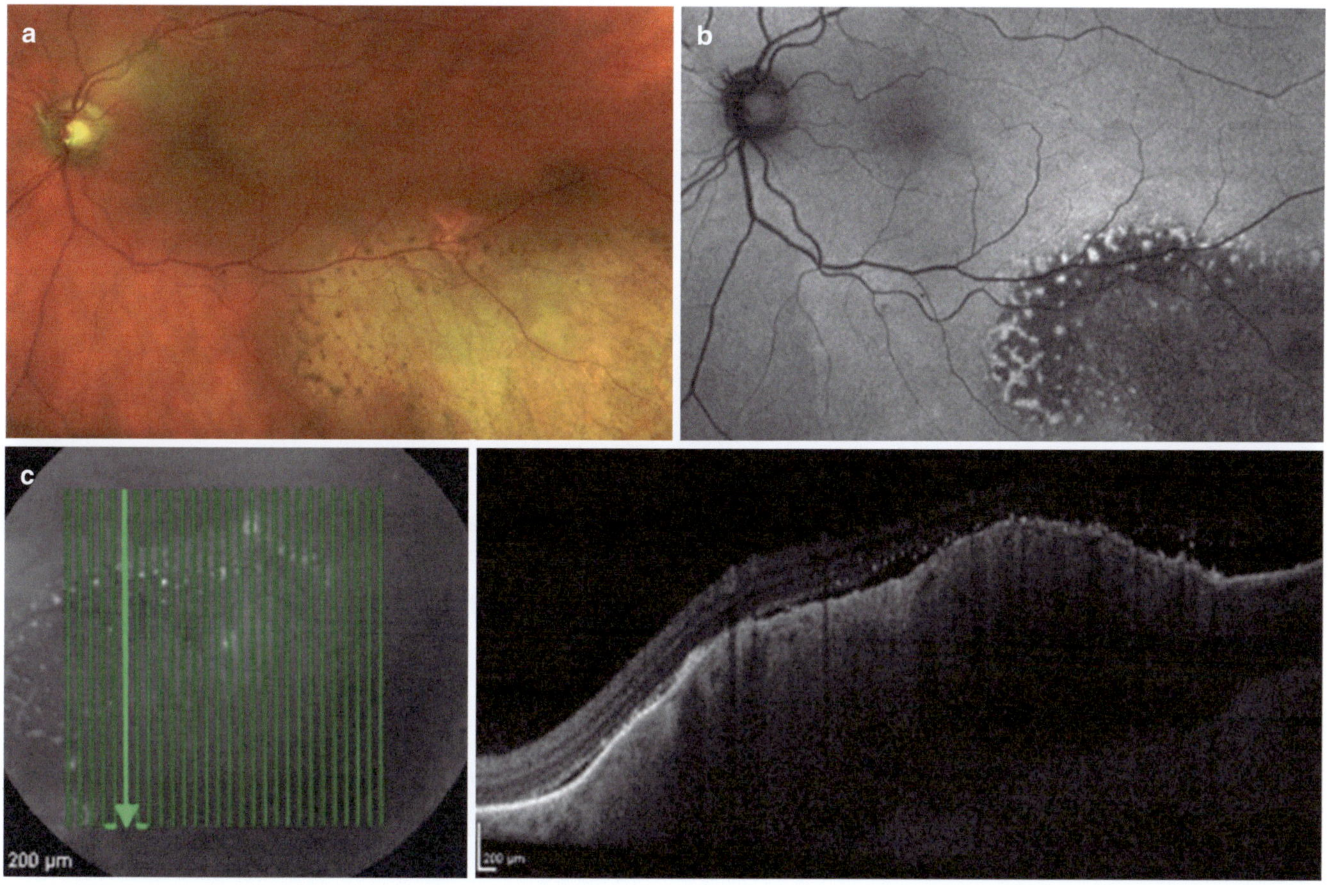

Fig. 4 Choroidal melanoma (biopsy proven) in the left eye of a 65-year-old woman. (**a**) Color photograph showing an amelanotic tumor with black clumps of lipofuscin ("leopard skin appearance") and visible tumor vessels, (**b**) fundus autofluorescence image showing hyper-autofluorescent lipofuscin over a tumor that is hypo-autofluorescent because of the RPE atrophy, and (**c**) OCT showing clumps of lipofuscin on the tumor surface and in the outer surface of the detached neuro-sensory retina. The OCT also shows the tumor to have a lumpy surface where it has eroded through RPE and Bruch's membrane (i.e., "incipient mushroom") (MOLES score = 12,202 = 7 = "probable melanoma"). (Reprinted with permission from Damato B. Clinical Atlas of Ocular Oncology. New York: Springer; 2022)

tightly together (Fig. 3). Ultrasonography is also useful for demonstrating the tumor shape, also identifying extraocular spread, and measuring tumor dimensions. Thickness measurements tend to be slightly greater than those obtained with OCT [27]. Most (but not all) examiners measure tumor thickness from the internal scleral surface, which is best seen when the probe is at right angles to the sclera. Similarly, most exclude retina and subretinal fluid from tumor thickness measurements. Because of measurement variation, differences in tumor thickness in sequential measurements are not considered significant unless they exceed 0.5 mm. Measurement of basal tumor dimensions can be inaccurate if the tumor has tapering margins, which can be difficult to define (Fig. 8). This can result in false impression of tumor growth if basal dimensions are measured inconsistently. Roelofs et al. have found that US is less sensitive at detecting tumor progression than sequential color photography, especially if combined with OCT and FAF imaging [14].

3.5 Fluorescein and Indocyanine-Green Angiography

Melanocytic choroidal tumors tend to be hypo-fluorescent relative to the choroid, especially if pigmented [28]. Any hyperfluorescence caused by these lesions therefore arises overlying RPE abnormalities, such as RPE detachments, drusen, neovascular membranes, subretinal fluid, and cystoid edema. Some authors have reported pinpoint, hyperfluorescent "hot spots" to indicate an increased risk of tumor growth [25]. With ICG angiography, obliteration of choroidal vasculature is more evident.

4 MOLES Acronym

The MOLES acronym refers to Mushroom shape, Orange pigment, Large size, Enlargement, and Subretinal fluid (SRF). These are all well known to be indicators of choroidal melanoma [25, 29, 30].

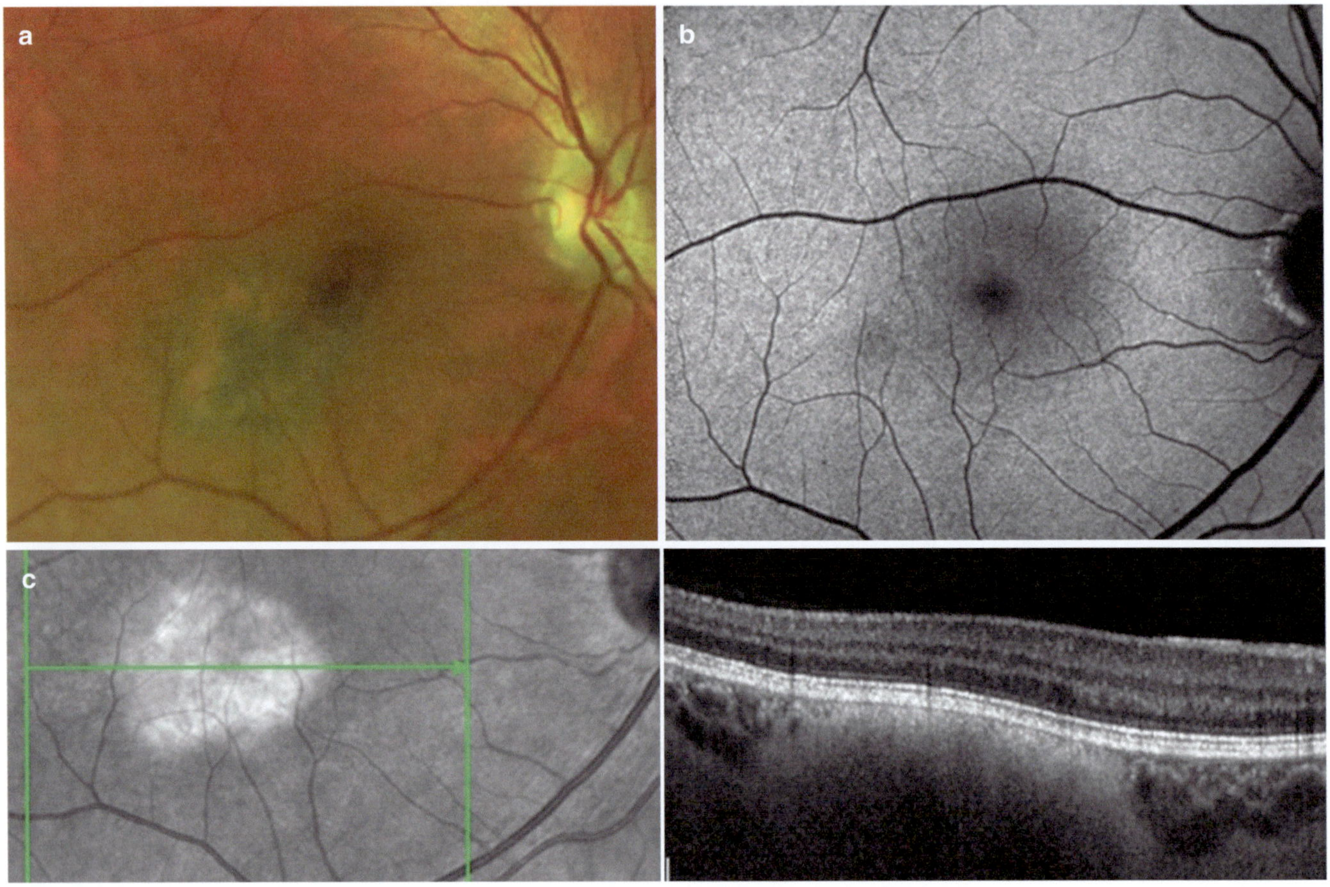

Fig. 5 Pseudo-orange pigment overlying a choroidal nevus. (**a**) Optos photograph showing orange areas suggestive of confluent lipofuscin, (**b**) fundus autofluorescence image showing absence of lipofuscin accumulation, (**c**) OCT showing no lipofuscin deposits on the RPE, which is normal. (MOLES score = 00000 = "common nevus"). (Reprinted with permission from Damato B. Clinical Atlas of Ocular Oncology. New York: Springer; 2022)

4.1 Mushroom Shape

This feature is almost pathognomonic for melanomas, only rarely developing in metastases. Some nevi can show extension through Bruch's membrane and RPE, but this is not extensive enough for a mushroom shape to develop (Fig. 10) [31].

4.2 Orange Pigment

Orange pigment accumulation is more abundant over melanomas than nevi. Clumps of confluent orange pigment can also form over metastases and choroidal hemangiomas; however, MOLES is not designed to differentiate these from melanoma. Lipofuscin can develop over choroidal nevi, but only in trace amounts.

4.3 Large Size

Choroidal melanomas tend to be larger than nevi, although there is significant size overlap between these two conditions. Thickness of small, posterior tumors is best measured with OCT, if the tumor–scleral interface is visible, which is more likely with amelanotic lesions [21]. If the tumor is too thick and/or peripheral for OCT, then US can be useful for measuring thickness. When neither OCT nor US is available, an approximate assessment should suffice as thickness usually increases with basal dimensions. With thin tumors having tapering margins, basal dimensions can be defined in millimeters using calipers provided by the imaging software or by using horizontal disc diameter as a measure (1 DD = 1.5 mm). It must be emphasized that these methods of estimating tumor size are approximate, because of variation in disc diameter and photographic distortion [20].

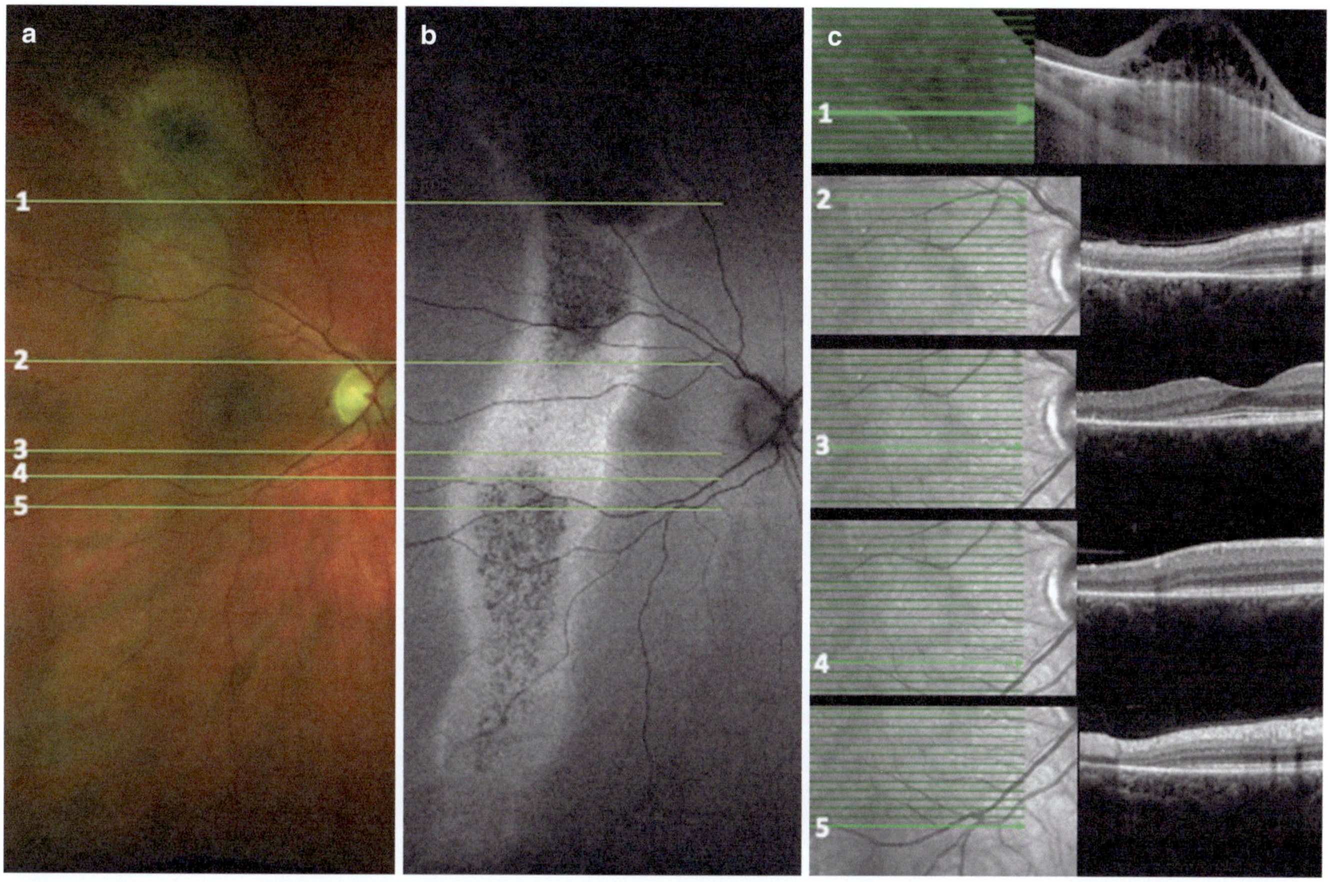

Fig. 6 Choroidal nevus. (**a**) Color photograph showing a pale band, extending inferiorly from the lesion, (**b**) fundus autofluorescence image showing RPE abnormality, with hyper- and hypo-autofluorescent areas, and (**c**) OCT showing cystoid edema on the tumor surface and outer retinal atrophy inferior to the tumor, corresponding to the abnormality caused by previous or intermittent retinal detachment. (MOLES score = 00100 = low-risk nevus). (Reprinted with permission from Damato B. Clinical Atlas of Ocular Oncology. New York: Springer; 2022)

4.4 Enlargement

Enlargement of choroidal naevi is rare after the age of 25 years, and when it occurs, it is minimal and slow. Mashayekhi et al. reported growth in 31% of 278 nevi, with a mean growth rate of growth of 0.06 mm/year. (range, 0.01–0.36) in tumors with a median basal diameter of 5 mm (range, 0.5–14.0) [32]. The author believes that examiners should take account of tumor diameter when assessing lateral extension, by considering such an enlargement in percentage terms instead of millimeters. Intuitively, lateral extension exceeding 5% of the tumor diameter would seem suspicious; however, this needs to be defined by further studies.

4.5 Subretinal Fluid

Retinal detachment tends to be more extensive in melanomas than choroidal nevi, which usually show minimal or no retinal detachment, unless a choroidal neovascular membrane has developed.

4.6 Omitted Features

Several clinical signs have been omitted, because they lack sufficient sensitivity and specificity. Visual symptoms are omitted because many melanomas are asymptomatic and because visual symptoms are often caused by other condi-

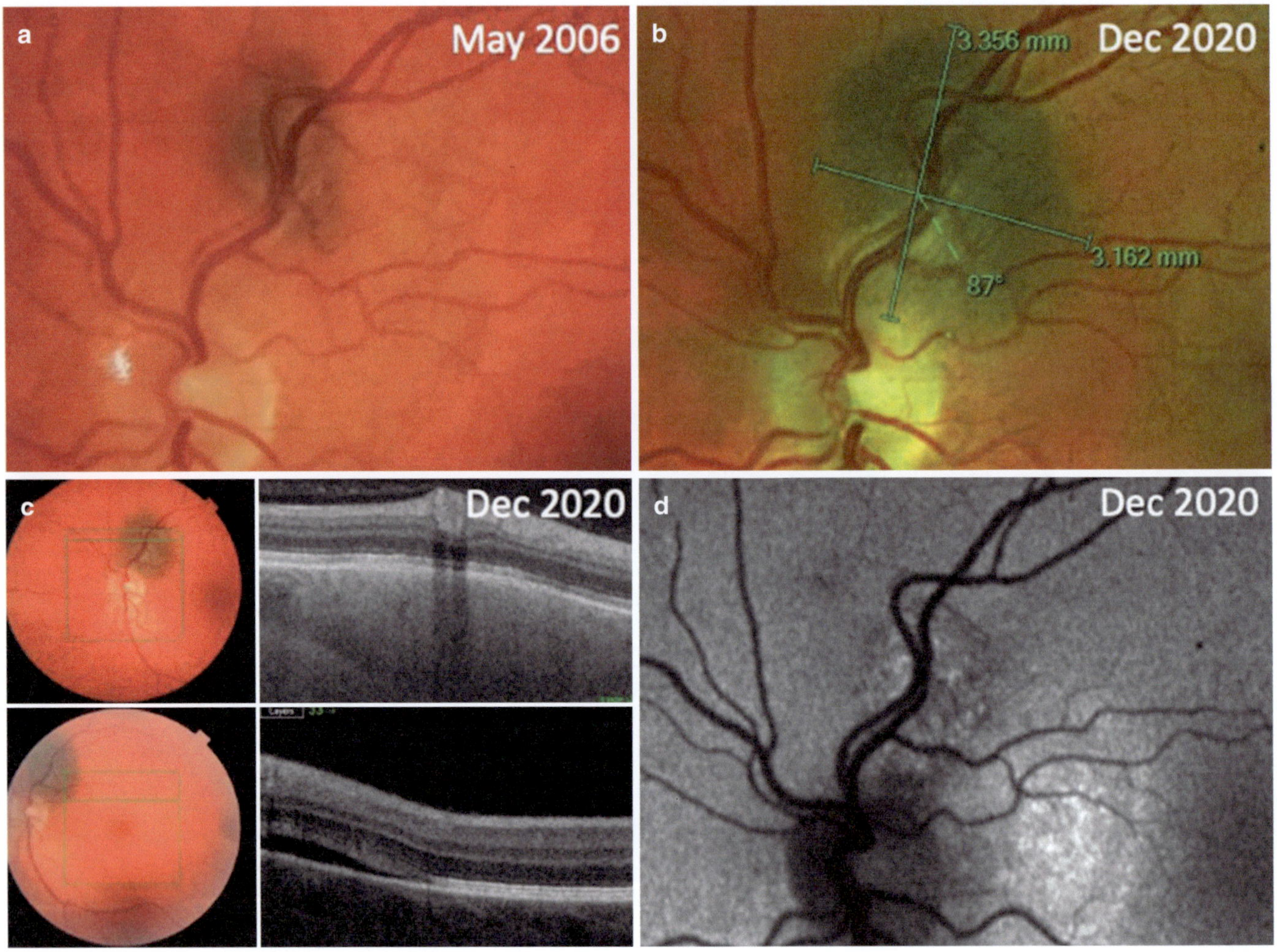

Fig. 7 Melanocytic choroidal tumor in the left eye. (**a**) Color photograph in May 2006, when the patient was 22 years old and when the tumor was flat, with a largest basal diameter of 1.7 mm, no orange pigment, and no subretinal fluid (MOLES = 00000 = 0 = common nevus). (**b**) Color photograph in December 2020 showing that the tumor had a largest basal diameter of 3.4 mm, with (**c**) OCT showing a trace of subretinal fluid, and (**d**) fundus autofluorescence imaging showing faint accumulations of lipofuscin (MOLES = 01021 = 4). If the tumor had not been photographed in 2006, the MOLES score in 2020 would have been 01001 (i.e., 2; high-risk nevus), indicating close monitoring. Whether, in 2006, the tumor was a nevus that later underwent malignant transformation or whether it was already malignant at that time is debatable

tions, such as migraine, vitreoretinal traction, and age-related macular degeneration. Few nevi are surrounded by a de-pigmented halo. Tumor proximity to the optic disc was found to lack statistical significance in predicting malignant growth [33]. Acoustic hollowness is omitted because many clinicians lack the expertise and/or sensitive ultrasonography equipment necessary to assess this feature. Furthermore, it is the author's impression that some deeply pigmented melanomas show high internal reflectivity, whereas some amelanotic nevi show acoustic hollowness.

5 Moles Score

Each of these five MOLES features is scored from 0 to 2 according to whether it is absent, uncertain/borderline, or present (Table 1).

5.1 Mushroom Shape

This feature is given a score of 1 if the tumor is bulging or showing early growth through the RPE and Bruch's mem-

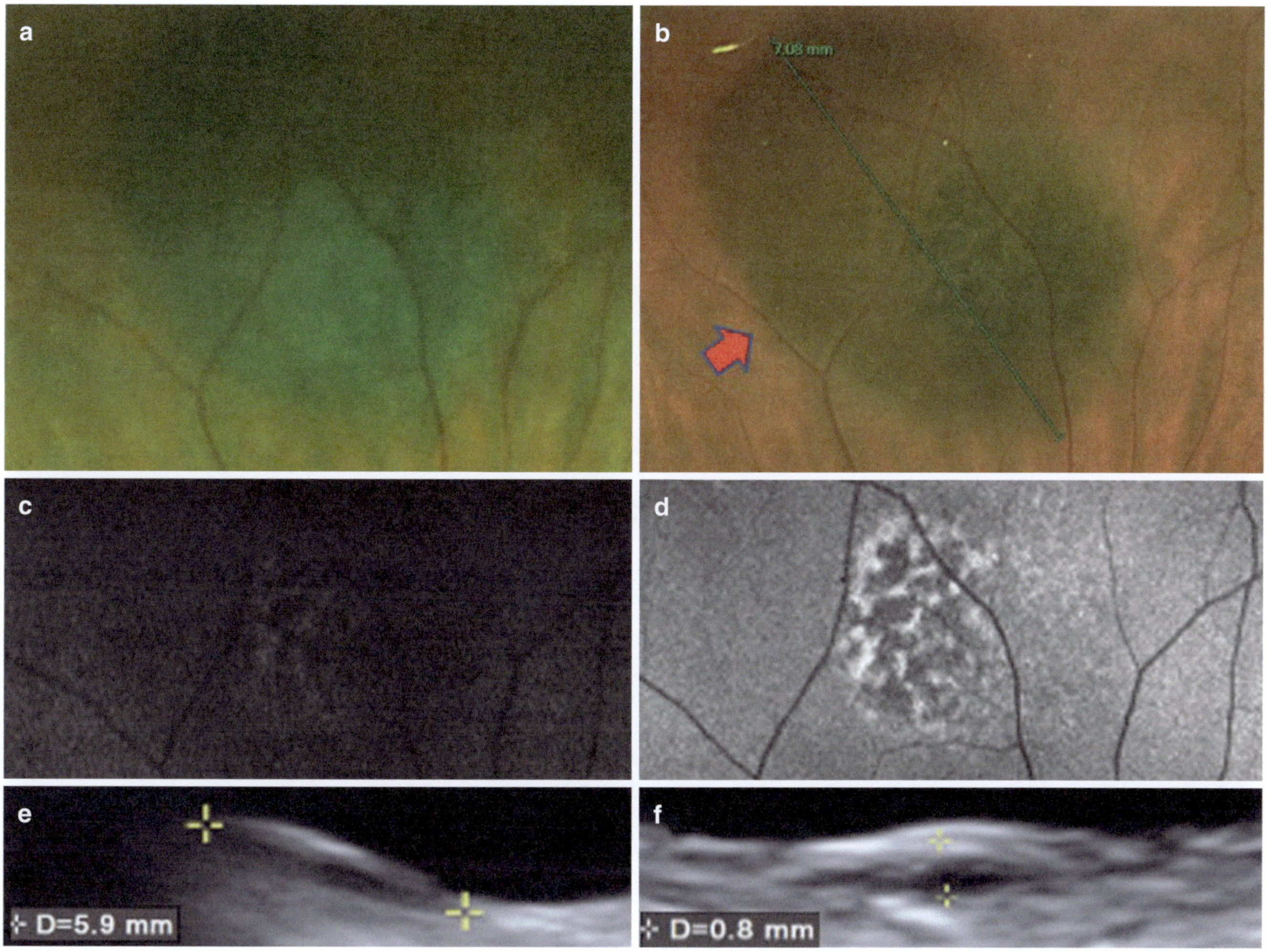

Fig. 8 Choroidal tumor in the left eye of a 60-year-old man. (**a**) Color photograph showing appearance in January 2019. (**b**) Appearance 23 months later, in December 2020, when the tumor had extended closer to an adjacent retinal blood vessel (arrow). The largest basal diameter showed no definite increase during this time. (**c**) Autofluorescence image in 2019 showing clumps of confluent lipofuscin. (**d**) Autofluorescence image in 2020 showing more extensive lipofuscin accumulation. (**e**) B-scan ultrasound in 2020 showing a longitudinal basal diameter of only 5.9 mm as compared to 7.1 mm measured on the color photograph. This discrepancy could have occurred because the tumor had tapering margins or because the longitudinal dimension was less than the largest basal dimension. (**f**) B-scan in December 2020 showing an area of retinal detachment that could not be demonstrated with OCT, because of the peripheral tumor location. The MOLES score increased from 02200 (i.e., 4; probable melanoma) in January 2019 to 02221 (i.e., 7; probable melanoma) in December 2020. This case demonstrates how (a) assessment of distances between tumor margins and adjacent landmarks can be more sensitive than sequential measurement of basal tumor diameter, (b) increasing amounts of lipofuscin can be indicative of tumor progression, and how (c) sequential assessment is more difficult if any of the images are sub-optimal

brane (i.e., "incipient mushroom") and attributed a score of 2 if definite mushroom shape has developed, with an overhang (i.e., "mature mushroom"). Although a mature mushroom shape (i.e., with overhang) strongly suggests melanoma, it is given a score of only 2 in order to simplify the MOLES scoring system. Since such intraretinal growth is likely to increase tumor thickness, the tumor is likely to have a minimum score of 3 in any case.

5.2 Orange Pigment

Accumulation of lipofuscin is given a score of 1 if it consists only of fine dusting and a score of 2 if forming confluent clumps. Further studies are needed to define the minimum number and size of any clumps of lipofuscin that are required for this feature to be given a score of 2. In the meantime, this score would be given if there is even just one clump having a diameter similar to that of a major retinal vein.

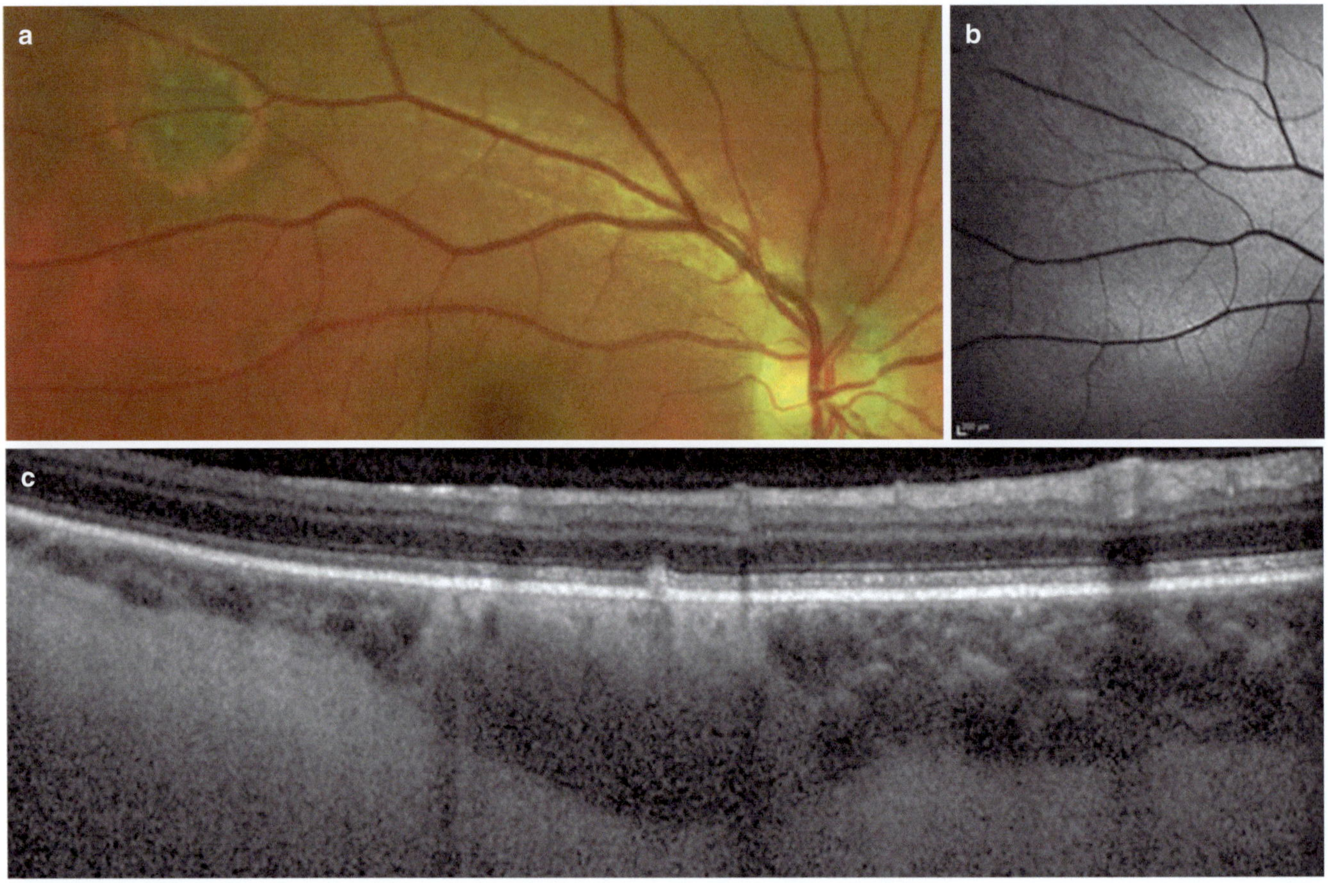

Fig. 9 Halo nevus (**a**) color photograph, and (**b**) Autofluorescence image showing normal RPE; and (**c**) OCT showing posterior "bowing" of the sclera. (MOLES score = 00000 = 0 = common nevus) (Reprinted with permission from Damato B. Clinical Atlas of Ocular Oncology. New York: Springer; 2022)

5.3 Large Size

Tumor size is given a score of 0 if the thickness is less than 1 mm and if the largest basal diameter is less than 3 DD. This feature is given a score of 2 if the thickness exceeds 2 mm or if the largest basal dimension is greater than 4 DD. Intermediate measurements are given a score of 1. These criteria are largely based on a study by Augsburger et al., which found 125 choroidal nevi for every melanoma in the thickness range of 1.5–2 mm, 25 nevi for every melanoma in the thickness range of 2–2.5 mm, and 5 nevi for every melanoma in the thickness range of 2.5–3 mm, approximately [11]. Augsburger et al. also found that there are 70 nevi for every choroidal melanoma in the basal diameter range of 5–6 mm, 10 nevi for every melanoma in the diameter range of 6–7 mm, and 3 nevi for every melanoma in the range 7 to 8 mm, approximately [11].

5.4 Enlargement

Tumor enlargement with basal diameter exceeding approximately 0.1 mm or 5% of basal diameter per year is given a score of 2 if confirmed by sequential imaging. In the absence of such imaging, this feature is scored as 0. Suspected growth is given a score of 1 if uncertain because of poor quality imaging (e.g., variation in light exposure). Even though nevi are known to grow in the first two decades of life, tumor enlargement at this age is given a score of 2 because some melanomas develop before adulthood.

In the absence of any other indicators of malignancy, the discovery of a new pigmented tumor is given a score of 0 the patient has not previously undergone ophthalmoscopy, 1 if the lesion was documented after previous ophthalmoscopy, but without imaging, and 2 if sequential imaging confirms that the lesion was not previously present.

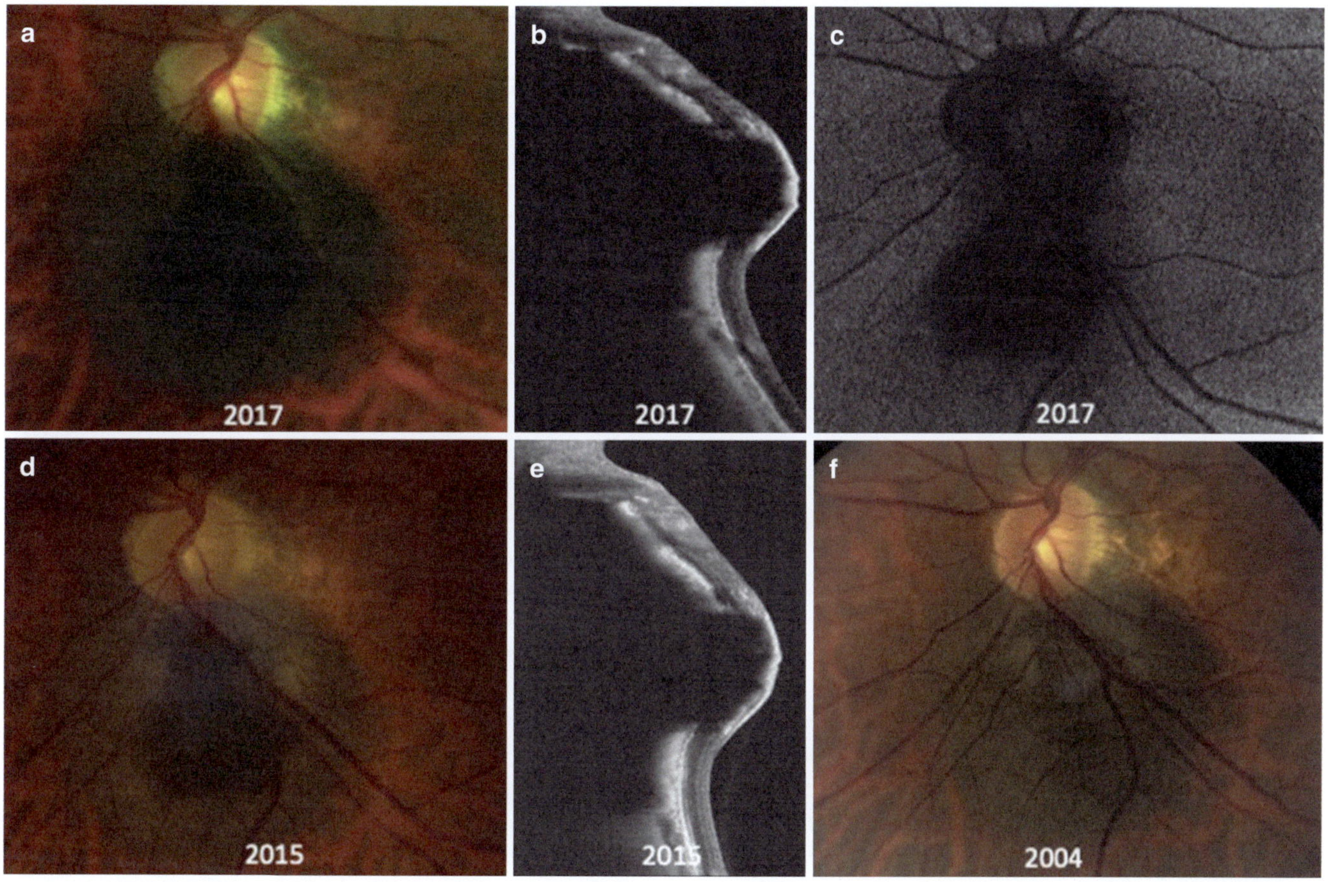

Fig. 10 Juxtapapillary choroidal nevus in the left eye. (**a**) Color photograph in 2017 showing tumor extension through RPE, (**b**) OCT showing extension into retina; (**c**) fundus autofluorescence image showing hypo-autofluorescence where the tumor has perforated RPE, (**d**) color photograph in 2015 showing similar appearance (MOLES score = 10,100 = 2 = high-risk nevus), (**e**) OCT showing similar appearance in 2015, and (**f**) color photograph in 2004 showing less extension through RPE but similar tumor size. (Reprinted with permission from Damato B. Clinical Atlas of Ocular Oncology. New York: Springer; 2022)

Table 1 The MOLES acronym and scoring system for categorizing melanocytic choroidal tumors according to likelihood of malignancy

Risk factor	Severity	Score
Mushroom shape	Absent	0
	Unsure/early growth through RPE	1
	Present	2
Orange pigment	Absent	0
	Unsure/trace (i.e., dusting)	1
	Confluent clumps	2
Large size	**Thickness and diameter**	
	Thickness < 1.0 mm ('flat/minimal thickening') ***and*** diameter < 3 DD	0
	Thickness = 1.0–2.0 mm ('subtle dome shape') and/or diameter = 3–4 DD	1
	Thickness > 2.0 mm ('significant thickening') and/or diameter > 4 DD	2
Enlargement	None (or lesion not documented or mentioned to patient previously)	0
	Unsure (e.g., poor image quality or lesion noted previously but without imaging)	1
	Definite (confirmed with sequential imaging)	2
Subretinal fluid	Absent	0
	Trace (if minimal and detected only with OCT)	1
	Definite (if seen without OCT))	2
	[a]**Total score:**	

DD = disc diameter (=1.5 mm)

[a]Tumors are categorized according to total score as: (0) common nevus; (1) low-risk nevus; (2) high-risk nevus and (>2) probable melanoma

5.5 Subretinal Fluid

Subretinal fluid is given a score of 1 if present in only trace amounts, so that it is detected only with OCT, and a score of 2 if copious enough to be seen ophthalmoscopically or in color photographs. Examiners vary in their ability to detect subretinal fluid without OCT. There is scope for studies aimed at scoring this feature more precisely, possibly according to distance between tumor surface and retina and extent of retinal detachment beyond the tumor margins. Intraretinal cystoid edema is given a score of 0 because it is a sign of chronicity [34]. A band of RPE and retinal atrophy inferior to the tumor is given a score of 2 if the retina is flat, even though this may have been caused by previous gravitation of subretinal fluid from the tumor. Subretinal fluid is scored as 0 if arising from a neovascular membrane, which is generally believed to indicate that the tumor is benign.

5.6 Multivariable Scoring

Several features show significant overlap between nevi and melanomas and, further, some features may be scored or assessed inaccurately by inexpert examiners, especially if such clinicians lack sensitive imaging equipment. The multivariable scoring and the intermediate score of 1 should compensate for these shortcomings.

6 Tumor Categorization

Tumors are categorized as common nevus, low-risk nevus, high-risk nevus and probable melanoma according to whether the sum of these scores is 0, 1, 2, or >2, respectively (Table 1). The reason for categorizing tumors with a score of 3 or more as "probable melanoma" and not simply as "melanoma" is that inexpert examiners may lack the confidence to diagnose this tumor definitively and to distinguish it from other tumors. Further, not all melanomas with a MOLES score >2 grow. In such cases, it can be difficult to decide between monitoring, treatment, and biopsy for tumor analysis by cytology and genetic typing, using methods such as next-generation sequencing [35]. Systemic metastasis without apparent growth of the ocular tumor has been reported [36].

The MOLES system has also made it possible to describe lesions succinctly by means of a 5-digit code. For example, a tumor with a diameter of 3–4 DD and/or a thickness of 1–2 mm, with clumps of confluent orange pigment and traces of subretinal fluid on OCT would be described with the code "02101."

7 Other Diagnosis Aids

7.1 TFSOM-DIM

The mnemonic "To Find Small Ocular Melanoma (TFSOM)" has been devised by Shields to represent Thickness greater than 2 mm, Subretinal Fluid, Symptoms, Orange pigment, and Margin less than 3.1 mm from optic disc [37]. This mnemonic was later expanded to include "Using Helpful Hints Daily (UHHD)" to represent Ultrasound Height, Halo absence and Drusen absence. The TFSOM_UHHD was later revised, with M representing melanoma hollowness on ultrasonography, and UHHD replaced by "Doing Imaging (DIM)"," which represents diameter greater than 5 mm. The likelihood of malignant growth is estimated according to the number of risk factors, the 5-year Kaplan-Meier rate of growth ranging from 1% in the absence of any risk factors to 55% when five predictors are present [30, 38]. The TFSOM-DIM mnemonic is based on extensive statistical studies, with large numbers of patients monitored over many years and has proved extremely useful in guiding the management of patients with melanocytic choroidal tumors.

Unlike TFSOM-DIM, MOLES does not rely on ultrasonography so that it can be used in situations where TFSOM is not applicable. Further, unlike TFSOM, MOLES gives each of the five indicators an intermediate score of 1 for the benefit of practitioners who lack the confidence or expertise to determine whether a risk factor is absent or present and to adjust for inaccuracies in measurements of tumor dimensions. Another difference is that TFSOM predicts growth, whereas MOLES includes this as an indicator of malignancy.

7.2 DOCTOR GASS

Harbour and associates have devised the mnemonic "DOCTOR GASS" to represent Drusen, Overlying retinal degeneration, Chronic RPE changes, Thickness > 2 mm, Orange lipofuscin pigment, Reflectivity (low), Girth (diameter), Angiographic hot spots, Subretinal fluid, and Symptom [39].

8 Validation

MOLES has been validated externally. At the Naevus Clinic of Moorfields Eye Hospital, Al Harby et al. found that MOLES scores indicated melanoma in 100% of 81 patients with this diagnosis and nevus in 95.7% of 141 patients with diagnosis [40]. Of the six tumors with discordant diagnosis, four had basal diameters exceeding 6 mm, all with SRF and/or orange pigment; and two small tumors showed either significant SRF with traces of orange pigment, or vice versa. At the same hospital, Roelofs et al. found that 99.8% of 451 patients treated for choroidal melanoma at Moorfields Eye Hospital (MEH) had MOLES scores of >2 [41].

It must be emphasized that MOLES (and TFSOM-DIM) give only an approximate indication of prognosis. A tumor with no suspicious features may show malignant growth (Fig. 7). Conversely, a tumor with multiple suspicious signs may remain unchanged for several years, perhaps permanently (Fig. 11).

9 Impact on Clinical Practice

At Oxford Eye Hospital, where the author devised MOLES, a clinical audit was performed to assess the management of patients with melanocytic choroidal nevi. The cohort comprised 178 patients referred to the Author between September 2018 and December 2019. Most tumors were categorized retrospectively as common nevus (52.8%) or low-risk nevus (18.0%) with only a minority comprising high-risk nevus (19.1%) or probable melanoma (10.1%). There were 41 patients referred with a common nevus by an ophthalmologist; of these patients, 13 (32%) were referred after one hos-

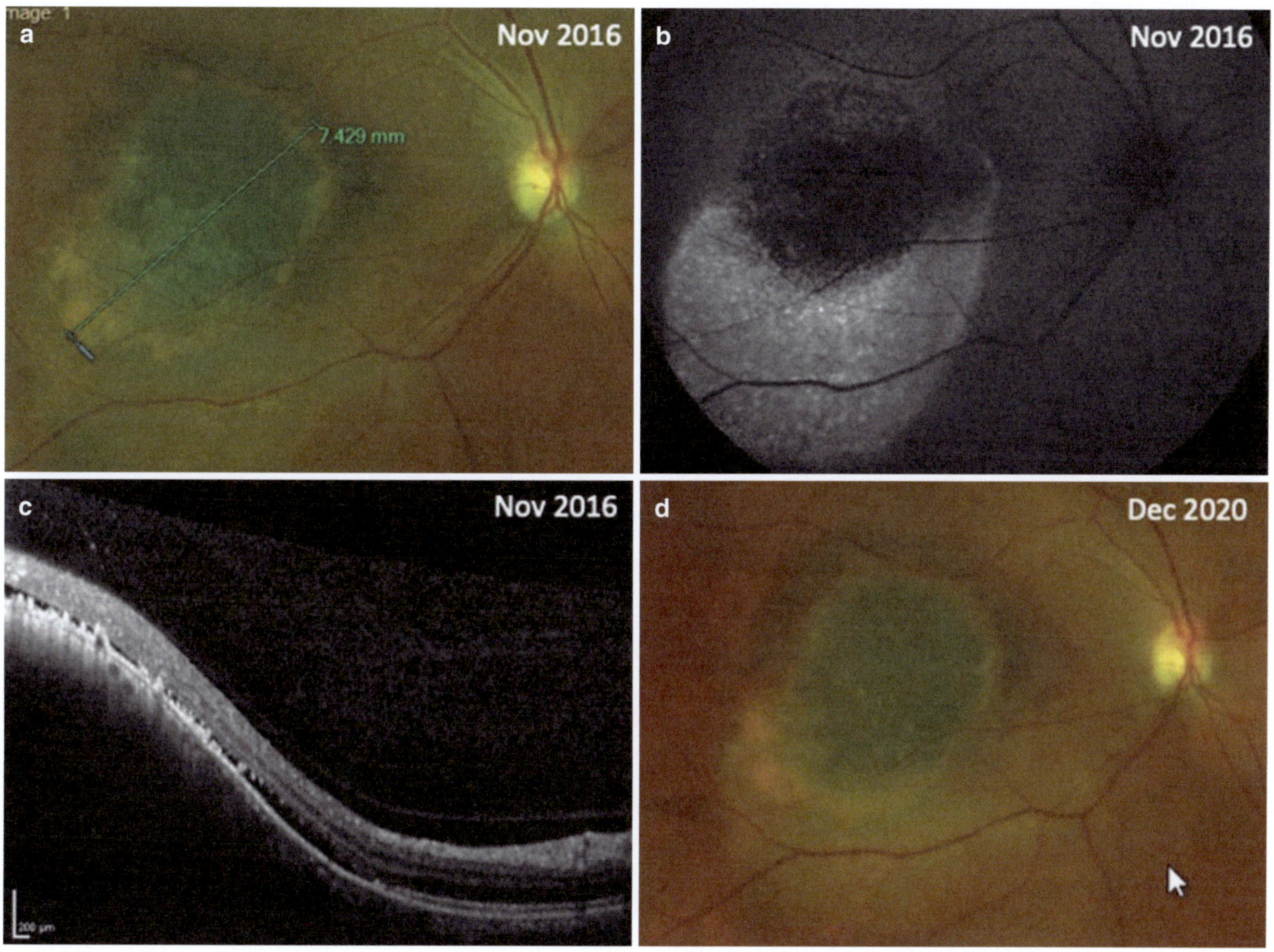

Fig. 11 Melanocytic choroidal tumor in the right of a 49-year-old woman in 2016. (**a**) Color photograph showing the tumor to have a diffuse margin involving fovea; a central gray area, indicating RPE atrophy; and appearances suggestive of inferior retinal detachment, where clumps of orange pigment had precipitated; (**b**) autofluorescence image showing a central hypo-autofluorescent area of RPE atrophy, and inferior hyper-autofluorescence caused by retinal detachment, with intensely hyper-autofluorescent clumps of lipofuscin; (**c**) OCT showing subretinal fluid with clumps of lipofuscin. (**d**) Color photograph 49 months later, with no evidence of progression. The tumor has a thickness of 2.2 mm and a basal diameter of 7.3 mm. The visual acuity is 20/30, with intermittent blurring. The MOLES score of 02202 suggests that the tumor is malignant, despite the lack of growth. The patient is aware of this but prefers not to undergo treatment unless growth is documented, in view of the loss of vision that this would cause. In some centers, trans-retinal biopsy would be performed, using a vitreous cutter, with cytology and genetic analysis using next-generation sequencing [35, 44]

pital visit, 22 (44%) after 2–5 visits and 4 (10%) after 7–12 visits. Several of these patients had undergone repeated ultrasonography, fluorescein angiography and/or indocyanine green angiography. This study revealed the large scale of unnecessary, in-person, hospital clinic assessments for patients with choroidal nevi having minimal risk of malignancy.

To prevent such excessive and wasteful medical care, the author devised a referral form that incorporates the MOLES scoring system, which automatically provides the total score, diagnosis and recommended management, as well as providing instructions and links to useful websites and e-mail addresses [42]. Referring practitioners are instructed to submit images of the lesion so that a diagnosis and advice on management can be provided without the patient having to attend a hospital clinic. When such images are inadequate or unavailable, arrangements are made for the patient to attend the photography unit (i.e., "imaging hub") for wide-field color photography, fundus autofluorescence imaging, and OCT. These images are reviewed remotely by an in-house ocular oncologist in a "virtual clinic"; however, others have shown that nonmedical graders can reliably perform this role [43]. Ultrasonography is performed only if the lesion is too thick or peripheral for OCT and if the MOLES score exceeds 1. Patients with common nevi are given a color photograph of their lesion and referred back to their community optometrist for monitoring. Currently, those with low-risk and high-risk nevi are monitored at the hospital's virtual clinic, with remote reporting by the ocular oncologist. Studies are planned to determine whether patients with low-risk nevi can safely be discharged to their community optometrist. Patients with probable melanoma are urgently referred to one of four supra-regional ocular oncology centers in the UK for treatment. Moorfields Eye Hospital, which is one of these centers, has devised a referral form that is similar to the Oxford form, also triaging patients according to images submitted with this form. After treatment for melanoma at the ocular oncology center, surveillance is subsequently undertaken at Oxford Eye Hospital.

These measures have greatly reduced the number of in-person consultations with ophthalmologists and ocular oncologists, saving time and money both for patients and healthcare services. This has proved especially useful during the Covid-19 pandemic, when patients are reluctant to attend hospital, for fear of catching coronavirus, and because of the way in which this infection has disrupted healthcare, at least in the UK.

10 Conclusions

The management of patients with suspicious choroidal nevi and suspected melanomas requires nuance, which practitioners may not have time for. The TFSOM-DIM mnemonic has been developed to simplify assessing risk of malignant growth but requires measurement of internal acoustic tumor reflectivity. The MOLES acronym, scoring system and protocol remove the need for sensitive ultrasonography and can therefore be used more widely, as well as in tele-ocular oncology. However, the clinician must be able to identify lipofuscin and subretinal fluid. There is scope for further studies to refine MOLES and to evaluate its use in a variety of healthcare systems.

References

1. Sumich P, Mitchell P, Wang JJ. Choroidal nevi in a white population: the Blue Mountains eye study. Arch Ophthalmol. 1998;116(5):645–50.
2. Chien JL, Sioufi K, Surakiatchanukul T, Shields JA, Shields CL. Choroidal nevus: a review of prevalence, features, genetics, risks, and outcomes. Curr Opin Ophthalmol. 2017;28(3):228–37.
3. Damato B. Managing patients with choroidal melanoma in the COVID-19 era: a personal perspective. Br J Ophthalmol. 2020;104(7):885–6.
4. Callejo SA, Dopierala J, Coupland SE, Damato B. Sudden growth of a choroidal melanoma and multiplex ligation-dependent probe amplification findings suggesting late transformation to monosomy 3 type. Arch Ophthalmol. 2011;129(7):958–60.
5. Damato BE, Heimann H, Kalirai H, Coupland SE. Age, survival predictors, and metastatic death in patients with choroidal melanoma: tentative evidence of a therapeutic effect on survival. JAMA Ophthalmol. 2014;132(5):605–13.
6. Damato B. Ocular treatment of choroidal melanoma in relation to the prevention of metastatic death - a personal view. Prog Retin Eye Res. 2018;66:187–99.
7. Smith LT, Irvine AR. Diagnostic significance of orange pigment accumulation over choroidal tumors. Am J Ophthalmol. 1973;76(2):212–6.
8. Shields CL, Furuta M, Mashayekhi A, Berman EL, Zahler JD, Hoberman DM, et al. Clinical spectrum of choroidal nevi based on age at presentation in 3422 consecutive eyes. Ophthalmology. 2008;115(3):546–52 e2.
9. Papastefanou VP, Nogueira V, Hay G, Andrews RM, Harris M, Cohen VM, et al. Choroidal naevi complicated by choroidal neovascular membrane and outer retinal tubulation. Br J Ophthalmol. 2013;97(8):1014–9.
10. Naseripour M, Shields CL, Shields JA, Guyer DR. Pseudohypopyon of orange pigment overlying a stable choroidal nevus. Am J Ophthalmol. 2001;132(3):416–7.
11. Augsburger JJ, Correa ZM, Trichopoulos N, Shaikh A. Size overlap between benign melanocytic choroidal nevi and choroidal malignant melanomas. Invest Ophthalmol Vis Sci. 2008;49(7):2823–8.
12. Li HK, Shields CL, Mashayekhi A, Randolph JD, Bailey T, Burnbaum J, et al. Giant choroidal nevus clinical features and natural course in 322 cases. Ophthalmology. 2010;117(2):324–33.
13. Paul Brett J, Lake A, Downes S. Colour imaging in the monitoring and documentation of choroidal naevi. Are Optomap colour images adequate for this purpose? J Vis Commun Med. 2016;39(1–2):10–7.
14. Roelofs KA, O'Day R, Al Harby L, Hay G, Arora AK, Cohen VML, et al. Detecting progression of melanocytic choroidal tumors by sequential imaging: is ultrasonography necessary? Cancers (Basel). 2020;12(7)
15. Saari JM, Kivelä T, Summanen P, Nummelin K, Saari KM. Digital imaging in differential diagnosis of small choroidal melanoma. Graefes Arch Clin Exp Ophthalmol. 2006;244(12):1581–90.

16. Lavinsky D, Belfort RN, Navajas E, Torres V, Martins MC, Belfort R Jr. Fundus autofluorescence of choroidal nevus and melanoma. Br J Ophthalmol. 2007;91(10):1299–302.
17. Chin K, Finger PT. Autofluorescence characteristics of suspicious choroidal nevi. Optometry. 2009;80(3):126–30.
18. Shields CL, Pirondini C, Bianciotto C, Materin MA, Harmon SA, Shields JA. Autofluorescence of choroidal nevus in 64 cases. Retina. 2008;28(8):1035–43.
19. Shah SU, Kaliki S, Shields CL, Ferenczy SR, Harmon SA, Shields JA. Enhanced depth imaging optical coherence tomography of choroidal nevus in 104 cases. Ophthalmology. 2012;119(5):1066–72.
20. Espinoza G, Rosenblatt B, Harbour JW. Optical coherence tomography in the evaluation of retinal changes associated with suspicious choroidal melanocytic tumors. Am J Ophthalmol. 2004;137(1):90–5.
21. Francis JH, Pang CE, Abramson DH, Milman T, Folberg R, Mrejen S, et al. Swept-source optical coherence tomography features of choroidal nevi. Am J Ophthalmol. 2015;159(1):169–76 e1.
22. Dolz-Marco R, Hasanreisoglu M, Shields JA, Shields CL. Posterior scleral bowing with choroidal nevus on enhanced-depth imaging optical coherence tomography. JAMA Ophthalmol. 2015;133(10):1165–70.
23. Garcia-Arumi Fuste C, Peralta Iturburu F, Garcia-Arumi J. Is optical coherence tomography angiography helpful in the differential diagnosis of choroidal nevus versus melanoma? Eur J Ophthalmol. 2020;30(4):723–9.
24. Mueller AJ, Freeman WR, Schaller UC, Kampik A, Folberg R. Complex microcirculation patterns detected by confocal indocyanine green angiography predict time to growth of small choroidal melanocytic tumors: MuSIC report II. Ophthalmology. 2002;109(12):2207–14.
25. Butler P, Char DH, Zarbin M, Kroll S. Natural history of indeterminate pigmented choroidal tumors. Ophthalmology. 1994;101(4):710–6. discussion 7
26. Pineiro-Ces A, Rodriguez Alvarez MJ, Santiago M, Bande M, Pardo M, Capeans C, et al. Detecting ultrasonographic hollowness in small choroidal melanocytic tumors using 10 MHz and 20 MHz ultrasonography: a comparative study. Graefes Arch Clin Exp Ophthalmol. 2014;252(12):2005–11.
27. Martins MF, Kiefer K, Kanecadan LAA, Garcia PN, Belfort RN, Allemann N. Comparisons of choroidal nevus measurements obtained using 10- and 20-MHz ultrasound and spectral domain optical coherence tomography. Arq Bras Oftalmol. 2017;80(2):78–83.
28. Damato BE. Tumour fluorescence and tumour-associated fluorescence of choroidal melanomas. Eye. 1992;6(Pt 6):587–93.
29. The Collaborative Ocular Melanoma Study Group. Factors predictive of growth and treatment of small choroidal melanoma: COMS Report No. 5. Arch Ophthalmol. 1997;115(12):1537–44.
30. Dalvin LA, Shields CL, Ancona-Lezama DA, Yu MD, Di Nicola M, Williams BK Jr, et al. Combination of multimodal imaging features predictive of choroidal nevus transformation into melanoma. Br J Ophthalmol. 2019;103(10):1441–7.
31. Weiss SJ, Stathopoulos C, Shields CL. Choroidal nevus with retinal invasion in 8 cases. Ocul Oncol Pathol. 2019;5(5):369–78.
32. Mashayekhi A, Siu S, Shields CL, Shields JA. Slow enlargement of choroidal nevi: a long-term follow-up study. Ophthalmology. 2011;118(2):382–8.
33. Shields CL, Dalvin LA, Yu MD, Ancona-Lezama D, Di Nicola M, Williams BK, et al. Choroidal nevus transformation into melanoma per millimeter increment in thickness using multimodal imaging in 2355 CASES: the 2019 Wendell L. Hughes Lecture. Retina. 2019;39(10):1852–60.
34. Gass JD. Problems in the differential diagnosis of choroidal nevi and malignant melanomas. The XXXIII Edward Jackson memorial lecture. Am J Ophthalmol. 1977;83(3):299–323.
35. Afshar AR, Damato BE, Stewart JM, Zablotska LB, Roy R, Olshen AB, et al. Next-generation sequencing of uveal melanoma for detection of genetic alterations predicting metastasis. Transl Vis Sci Technol. 2019;8(2):18.
36. McKnight SJ, Christensen GR. Metastasis of a very small choroidal melanoma without apparent clinical change. Ann Ophthalmol. 1984;16(11):1016–21.
37. Shields CL, Shields JA, Kiratli H, De Potter P, Cater JR. Risk factors for growth and metastasis of small choroidal melanocytic lesions. Ophthalmology. 1995;102(9):1351–61.
38. Shields CL, Furuta M, Berman EL, Zahler JD, Hoberman DM, Dinh DH, et al. Choroidal nevus transformation into melanoma: analysis of 2514 consecutive cases. Arch Ophthalmol. 2009;127(8):981–7.
39. Harbour JW, Paez-Escamilla M, Cai L, Walter SD, Augsburger JJ, Correa ZM. Are risk factors for growth of choroidal nevi associated with malignant transformation? Assessment with a validated genomic biomarker. Am J Ophthalmol. 2019;197:168–79.
40. Al Harby L, Sagoo MS, O'Day R, Hay G, Arora AK, Keane PA, et al. Distinguishing choroidal nevi from melanomas using the MOLES algorithm: evaluation in an ocular nevus clinic. Ocul Oncol Pathol. 2021;7(4):294–302.
41. Roelofs KA, O'Day R, Harby LA, Arora AK, Cohen VML, Sagoo MS, et al. The MOLES system for planning management of melanocytic choroidal tumors: is it safe? Cancers (Basel). 2020;12(5)
42. Oxford Eye Hospital. Ocular MOLES Service - Guidelines. https://www.ouh.nhs.uk/eye-hospital/work/ocular-moles-guidelines.aspx 2020. https://www.ouh.nhs.uk/eye-hospital/work/ocular-moles-guidelines.aspx
43. Balaskas K, Gray J, Blows P, Rajai A, Flaye D, Peto T, et al. Management of choroidal naevomelanocytic lesions: feasibility and safety of a virtual clinic model. Br J Ophthalmol. 2016;100(5):665–70.
44. Sen J, Groenewald C, Hiscott PS, Smith PA, Damato BE. Transretinal choroidal tumor biopsy with a 25-gauge vitrector. Ophthalmology. 2006;113(6):1028–31.

Novel Therapies for Choroidal Melanoma

Hannah J. Yu and Amy C. Schefler

1 Introduction

Uveal melanoma is an intraocular cancer that may affect the choroid, ciliary body, or iris. Although rare, uveal melanoma is the most common intraocular cancer in adults with an approximate annual incidence of 2500 people in North America and 7095 worldwide [1, 2] with 90% of tumors primarily involving the choroid [3]. Overall, uveal melanoma has an estimated 80.9% 5-year survival rate [4].

Choroidal melanoma generally presents as either a dome, mushroom, or diffuse tumor with symptoms including flashes, floaters, or visual acuity loss. Management of primary choroidal melanoma may include radiation therapy or enucleation, depending on the size, location, features, and metastatic status of the tumor. Among patients treated with radiation therapy, side effects to key ocular structures are common and often devastating to visual acuity, resulting in the need for ongoing treatment for years. Thus, there remains a need for a non-surgical treatment method for this population that allows patients to retain good long-term visual acuity while also providing effective local tumor control.

The novel therapeutic, AU-011, is currently under investigation in phase 2 human trials to treat choroidal melanoma with intravitreal or suprachoroidal injections followed by laser photoactivation administered in an office setting. This treatment would target malignant cells with high specificity in addition to initiating immune responses against the tumors. Preclinical studies offered promising results, although the optimal administration route, treatment frequency, and safety outcomes still require ongoing evaluation.

2 Current Treatments for Choroidal Melanoma

Until the late 1980s, the management of choroidal melanoma was controversial among physicians [5]. Before then, the primary method of treatment for ocular melanomas was enucleation, with no prospective literature demonstrating the safety and efficacy of other therapeutic methods such as radiation therapy. However, radiation provided an attractive alternative to enucleation, potentially allowing patients the option to keep their eye and retain some level of visual acuity following treatment. Finally, in the 1990s, the Collaborative Ocular Melanoma Study (COMS) began to provide data from large, prospective randomized trials assessing the efficacy of enucleation versus radiation plaque brachytherapy for choroidal melanoma [6].

2.1 Enucleation Versus Radiation Therapy

Patients treated in the COMS studies had either medium- or large-sized treatment-naïve choroidal melanomas without apparent metastases [7]. Subjects with medium-sized tumors, defined as 2.5–10 mm in apical height and ≤16 mm in largest basal diameter (LBD), were randomized equally to one of two cohorts. The first cohort was enucleated in a single surgical session. The second cohort had a gold, iodine-125 radiation plaque surgically placed on the sclera over the location of the tumor base for 5–7 days; a total 85 Gy of radiation was delivered to the tumor apex over the treatment period. Following the completion of radiation treatment, the plaque was surgically removed. Through 5 years of follow-up, the COMS trial for medium-sized choroidal melanoma demon-

H. J. Yu
Retina Consultants of Texas, Retina Consultants of America, Houston, TX, USA
e-mail: hannah.yu@retinaconsultantstexas.com

A. C. Schefler (✉)
Retina Consultants of Texas, Retina Consultants of America, Houston, TX, USA

Blanton Eye Institute, Houston Methodist Hospital, Houston, TX, USA
e-mail: acsmd@retinaconsultantstexas.com

B. V. Chawla, M. E. Aronow (eds.), *Global Perspectives in Ocular Oncology*, https://doi.org/10.1007/978-3-031-08250-4_29

strated no statistically significant difference in mortality or metastasis rate between subjects treated with enucleation versus radiation plaque therapy, with an estimated 81–82% survival rate [6].

Following these results, the treatment of choroidal melanomas began to shift away from enucleation and towards radiation plaque therapy, although there are still indications and contraindications for each. Tumor characteristics, such as size and location, as well as genetic profiles must be critically evaluated by treating physicians to determine the best management plan for patients.

Today, most ocular oncologists will use plaque therapy as a first-line treatment for patients with medium-sized melanomas as well as small-sized melanomas that are demonstrating recent rapid growth indicative of metastatic potential [5]. Furthermore, at the time of the COMS trials, large-sized tumors, defined as tumors >10 mm in apical height or >16 mm in diameter at the base, could not effectively be treated with radiation plaque therapy due to size constraints of the plaques themselves. Since then, however, newer plaques have been designed and have allowed for the treatment of some larger tumors (Eye Physics Plaques; IsoAid, Port Richley, Florida), although this method of treatment is still controversial among physicians. New notched plaques have also been created to allow for the treatment of tumors close to or touching the optic nerve.

Generally, patients with large-sized tumors that cannot be covered by plaque therapy or proton beam irradiation or those with gross extrascleral extension or optic nerve invasion are treated with enucleation. The COMS trials investigated the treatment of large-sized tumors with enucleation alone versus pre-enucleation external beam radiation. There were no statistically significant nor clinically meaningful differences observed in survival rates or local complication rates between cohorts through 5 and 10 years of follow-up [8], so pre-enucleation radiation is not part of a standard treatment regimen today. Enucleation may also be indicated for patients with ocular pain/neovascular glaucoma, a low probability of visual acuity recovery, and neovascular glaucoma—for this population, radiation therapy simply may not provide enough therapeutic benefit compared to enucleation.

Additionally, some patients may elect to have enucleation over radiation therapy to decrease their own anxiety over concerns of recurrence or the long-term side effects of radiation therapy. In addition to their large, interventional trials, the COMS group also conducted a quality-of-life study following their trials to investigate any significant differences in quality of life between patients treated with enucleation versus radiation therapy [9]. Radiation allows patients to retain some level of visual acuity, which was reflected in better scores on vision-related quality of life measures among subjects treated with plaque therapy. Nevertheless, this group of subjects also had more anxiety about cancer recurrence in the first few years following treatment [10]. Notably, these differences in vision-related quality of life and anxiety decreased in the long term, especially following the publication of the mortality results of the COMS studies. Regardless, these factors are still important for physicians to assess with patients before determining a course of treatment.

2.2 Side Effects of Radiation Therapy

While plaque brachytherapy undoubtedly revolutionized the treatment of choroidal melanoma, it also resulted in its own set of complications for patients (Table 1). Radiation therapy treats malignant tumors directly by damaging the DNA of the rapidly dividing tumor cells and indirectly through the formation of free radicals that damages cell structures. Although this radiation is centered on the cancerous cells in plaque brachytherapy, it can also damage other important ocular structures and tissues in the process, leading to several devastating ocular side effects.

In the COMS study, among eyes treated with I-125 brachytherapy, 10% had a visual acuity of 20/200 or worse before treatment [11]; 3 years after treatment, however, 45% of eyes had a visual acuity of 20/200 or worse. Additionally, 49% of eyes lost 6 lines or more of visual acuity through 3 years of follow-up, with only 4.1% recovering to within 6 lines of pre-treatment acuity. Larger baseline tumors and shorter distance between the tumor and the foveal avascular zone were strongly associated with loss of 6 or more lines of visual acuity, along with patient history of diabetes, presence of tumor-associated retinal detachment, and tumors that were not dome shaped. These risk factors have been confirmed in several studies since the COMS trials, along with additional risk factors of types of radiation, radioactive isotopes, radiation dosimetry, and other patient-level demographics [12–16].

The most common ocular side effect of radiation damage is known as radiation retinopathy, a slowly progressive dis-

Table 1 Potential side effects of radiation therapy for choroidal melanoma

Ocular structure	Side effect	Potential treatment
Retina	Radiation retinopathy	Anti-VEGF
Iris	Atrophy Neovascularization/neovascular glaucoma	Unknown Anti-VEGF
Lens	Cataracts	Cataract surgery
Sclera	Scleral necrosis	Observation or scleral graft
Optic nerve	Radiation optic neuropathy	Steroids or anti-VEGF

VEGF vascular endothelial growth factor

ease that results from loss of retinal vascular endothelial cells and inflammation that may cause irreversible damage to visual function [13, 17–19]. This disease has a delayed onset, typically presenting between 6 months and 3 years following treatment with clinical features of intraretinal hard exudates, cotton wool spots, macular edema, microaneurysms, and retinal ischemia [19]. Atrophy of the retinal pigment epithelial (RPE) cells may also occur. The majority of radiation retinopathy patients present with nonproliferative disease, with a portion of severe cases advancing to proliferative disease, when growth factors are upregulated, resulting in choroidal neovascularization [20, 21].

Currently, there are no U.S. Food and Drug Administration (FDA)-approved therapies for radiation retinopathy, although several retrospective and prospective studies have demonstrated the benefits of intravitreal anti-vascular endothelial growth factor (VEGF) injections in both the anatomic and visual outcomes of the disease [10, 22–25]. Multiple studies have also shown the possible use of prophylactic anti-VEGF for radiation retinopathy [26]. Physician's opinions still differ on the optimal treatment frequency for patients to minimize financial, emotional, and physical burden while maximizing visual and anatomic gains. Further large, multicenter, prospective studies still need to be conducted to confirm and elucidate the best practices for the treatment of radiation retinopathy.

Other important ocular structures may also be damaged during plaque brachytherapy. Tumors closer to the anterior portion of the eye may result in damage to the iris, including thinning and atrophy of the structure [27, 28]. Damage to the posterior portion of the eye may also indirectly damage the iris through the upregulation of VEGF molecules in the vitreous, resulting in neovascularization of the iris [17, 29–31]. Similarly to radiation retinopathy, neovascularization of the iris may be treated with anti-VEGF agents, although few prospective trials have studied the safety and efficacy of this treatment [32–34].

Radiation-induced cataracts are another common side effect of plaque brachytherapy and other radiation treatment. In the COMS studies, 83% of study eyes reported some level of cataract formation through 5 years of follow-up, with 12% undergoing cataract surgery [35]. Cataract surgery did appear to improve the visual acuity of these patients, when visual acuity loss was primarily caused by the cataract formation and not other side effects.

Radiation optic neuropathy is also seen in patients treated with ocular radiation, and is characterized by sudden, painless vision loss within months or years of radiation therapy [14, 36, 37]. Optic neuropathy may present with atrophy and optic nerve edema, although it may be difficult to visualize on a fundus examination if the majority of the damage to the optic nerve is posterior to the globe. Treatment for radiation optic neuropathy is controversial, with some studies using intravitreal steroids or anti-VEGF agents [38–41]. Large, multicenter prospective trials are needed to clarify the best treatment approach for radiation retinopathy and optic neuropathy. Such trials are currently being planned through the Diabetic Retinopathy Clinical Research Network (DRCR).

Side effects to the sclera may also be observed, although the sclera is surprisingly resistant to radiation damage [28, 42–45]. Scleral necrosis is most often seen among eyes with large, anterior tumors that are treated with high doses of radiation. Nevertheless, many cases of scleral necrosis can simply be observed, with severe cases generally treated with scleral grafts.

2.3 Future of Treatment for Choroidal Melanoma

While both enucleation and radiation therapy have been successful treatment options that have increased the survival rate of patients with choroidal melanoma, neither option is perfect. As described, both management options have benefits and risks, with visual acuity loss occurring with either treatment. Therefore, there is a need in the field for a better therapeutic option that is as effective at achieving local control for patients while also protecting the critical ocular anatomic structures and preserving vision in the long term.

3 AU-011 Technology and Preclinical Trials

In recent years, researchers have become very interested in the use of human papillomavirus (HPV) virus-like particles (VLPs) in targeting and treating a variety of cancer cell types. HPV VLPs are 55 nm capsids formed by the major HPV capsid proteins, L1 and L2 [46]. These have been used as gene delivery vectors in the vaginal mucosa, respiratory tract, muscle, and skin, but are nonreplicative as they are recombinantly derived and do not contain viral DNA. HPV VLPs bind with high specificity to basement membrane modified heparan sulfate proteoglycans (HSPGs) commonly found on many solid tumor cancer cells, including melanoma cells, both in vivo and in vitro, resulting in epithelial cell binding and permeation of the cell membrane [46].

In 2018, a study was published introducing the specific use of HPV VLPs for ocular melanomas [47]. AU-011 (Aura Biosciences, Cambridge, Massachusetts, USA) is a novel, recombinant virus-like particle bioconjugate (VPB), that is currently being investigated as a first-in-class therapy for primary uveal melanoma. AU-011 is a VLP conjugated with approximately 200 phthalocyanine photosensitizer (IRDye®700DX) molecules and is activated by near infrared (IR) laser excitation at 689 nm, causing cytotoxic effects on

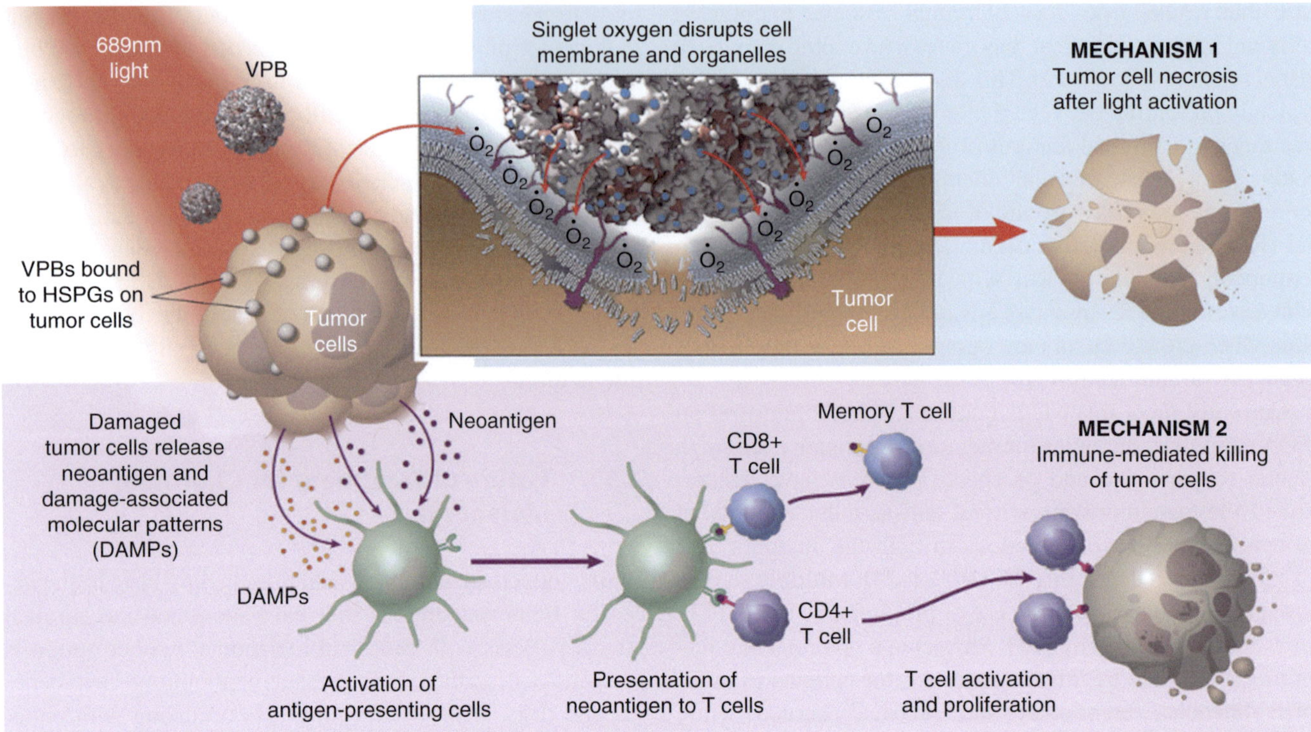

Fig. 1 Mechanisms of action of AU-011, the virus-like particle bioconjugate (VPB). Figure courtesy of Aura Biosciences (Cambridge, Massachusetts, USA)

the tumor (Fig. 1). These cytotoxic effects are thought to be due to the release of reactive oxygen species on the cell membrane and organelles, triggering cell membrane disruption and acute tumor cell necrosis. In contrast to traditional bivalency of antibody cancer treatments, the binding of AU-011 to tumor cells is multivalent due to the large and three-dimensional shape of the VLP, which increases the affinity to the target tumor cells considerably. While antibody-drug conjugate technology typically delivers 3–8 dye molecules, each VLP delivers approximately 200 molecules of IRDye®700DX enabling high amounts of the light sensitizer to the tumor. Additionally, a dual mechanism of action is thought to occur when acutely damaged tumor cells release neoantigens and damage-associated molecular patterns (DAMPs). These neoantigens are then presented by antigen-presenting cells to T cells, triggering the formation of memory T-cells and T-cell activation and proliferation, resulting in immune-mediated tumor cell killing [48].

The clinical use of AU-011 is attractive for its specificity to tumor cells, its ease of use, and its favorable, low-burden outcomes for patients, including improved long-term visual acuity with little collateral damage to surrounding structures. In theory, injection of AU-011 in eyes with choroidal melanoma using an appropriate route of administration should allow for its distribution to the tumor and targeted binding to modified HSPGs on malignant tumor cells and subsequent activation through laser stimulation, allowing for specific treatment of the tumor without damage to other ocular structures. AU-011 could also allow patients to be treated in an outpatient setting without need for surgical intervention or other health care professionals such as radiation oncologists without the burden of the visual side effects seen with radiation therapy.

In preclinical studies, the specificity of AU-011 binding was studied in vitro and in vivo through the use of a panel of human cancer cell lines, HSPG-deficient cells, and the inclusion of soluble heparin in the in vitro studies [47]. In the in vitro studies, human cancer cells were incubated with AU-011 or free IR700 dye and exposed to 690 nm light. Only the cells that had AU-011 bound to their cell membrane and were exposed to light were affected and began to round and detach. The inclusion of heparin in these experiments blocked the effect of AU-011, confirming that the HSPG dependence for binding of the VLP was not affected by the dye conjugation. Additionally, cells only exposed to an equivalent amount of free IR700 dye with or without laser did not show any demonstrable killing highlighting the importance of AU-011 binding for cytotoxic activity of AU-011. AU-011-mediated cell binding and killing were consistent across a panel of human tumor cell lines (ovarian, lung, breast, cervical, cutaneous melanoma, head and neck, bladder, oropharyngeal, renal, bladder urothelium, prostate and uveal melanoma), but were not seen in the presence of heparin or in HSPG-deficient cells, further reinforcing the specificity of AU-011 and the role of HSPG in targeted binding of tumor cells.

For in vivo studies, researchers used murine subcutaneous and rabbit orthotopic xenograft models of uveal melanoma [47]. Murine models supported subcutaneous AU-011 activity against the uveal melanoma line in vivo, and the rabbit orthotopic xenograft model was then used to determine tumor uptake and the pharmacokinetics of AU-011 through intravitreal injection. In rabbit orthotopic xenograft model, 92.1MEL human tumor cells are implanted in the choroid, and treatment is administered after tumor growth. Tumor response is evaluated using clinical exams and histopathology. Results indicated localization of AU-011 in the tumor tissue with a potent dose-dependent necrotic effect in the tumors following photoactivation. Notably, none of the murine or rabbit models demonstrated any evidence of retinal damage after AU-011 treatment.

4 Clinical Trials

The promising in vivo and in vitro preclinical results for AU-011 have led to the currently ongoing human clinical trials investigating the safety and efficacy of AU-011 in patients diagnosed with primary indeterminate lesions and small choroidal melanomas. Two methods of administration are being assessed in these trials: intravitreal injection and suprachoroidal injection. Intravitreal injection is a well-understood method of drug delivery to the eye, in which pharmacotherapies are injected directly into the vitreous, and is used in the treatment of multiple retinal exudative diseases.

Suprachoroidal injection is a novel method of drug delivery that targets the choroid with high bioavailability to the posterior portion of the eye [49, 50], while maintaining low levels of the drug in the vitreous and the anterior portion of the eye. Preclinical studies with AU-011 have confirmed the safety, efficacy, and biodistribution of the pharmaceutical [51]; suprachoroidal drug delivery is also being studied as a method of delivery for triamcinolone acetonide for uveitis with recent positive results [52].

4.1 Intravitreal Treatment

In 2017, a non-randomized, open label phase 1b/2 trial was initiated to investigate the safety, immunogenicity, and efficacy of AU-011 in patients with choroidal melanoma [53]. A total 57 subjects were enrolled in the study and sorted into one of several cohorts, listed in Table 2. Laser applications occurred 6–8 h after injection; in cohorts that had more than one laser treatment, the second laser was applied approximately 30 min following the first. Preliminary data for the study was recently presented at the 2020 American Academy of Ophthalmology Annual Meeting (Virtual; [54]). Through the data cutoff date of July 22, 2020, 56 subjects had been treated. The safety profile of AU-011 was reported with treatment-related adverse events (AEs) that occurred in ≥15% of subjects. AEs included anterior chamber inflammation (69.6% of subjects, 1.8% considered severe), vitreous inflammation (85.7% of subjects, 7.1% considered severe), increase in intraocular pressure (41.1% of subjects, 0% considered severe), and floaters/vitreous opacities (16.1% of subjects, 1.8% considered severe). These events were manageable with steroid treatment and ocular anti-hypertensives and were transient in the vast majority of subjects; one subject with severe vitreous opacities was treated with vitrectomy. Intraocular inflammation was expected based on the secondary mechanism of action of AU-011 and steroid treat-

Table 2 Cohorts enrolled in the phase 1b/2 intravitreal AU-011 clinical trial

Phase	Cohort	N	Dose (μg)	Number of treatments[a]	Laser applications per treatment	Cycles[b]
Single dose	Cohort 1	3	20	1	1	–
	Cohort 2	3	40	1	1	–
	Cohort 3	3	80	1	1	–
	Cohort 6	3	80	1	2	–
Multiple dose	Cohort 4	3	40	2	1	–
	Cohort 5	3	40	3	1	–
	Cohort 7	3	80	3	1	–
	Cohort 8	3	80	3	2	1
First expansion	Cohort 9	12	80	3	2	1[c]
Second expansion	Cohort 10[d]	3	80	3	2	2
	Cohort 11	5	80	3	2	2
	Cohort 12[e]	13	80	3	2	2

[a] Treatments administered by intravitreal injections followed by laser applications; multiple treatments were administered weekly
[b] One cycle comprised of 3 weekly treatments of highest administered dose (80 μg × 2 laser applications)
[c] Potential for 2 treatment cycles
[d] Observation until documented growth of tumor
[e] Required evidence of growth prior to entry

Table 3 Cohorts enrolled in the phase 2 suprachoroidal AU-011 clinical trial

Phase	Cohort	N[a]	Dose (μg)	Number of treatments[b]	Laser applications per treatment	Cycles[c]
Dose escalation	Cohort 1	1–5	20	1	1	–
	Cohort 2	2–5	40	1	2	–
	Cohort 3	2–5	40	1	2	–
	Cohort 4	3–6	MTD (1–3)	2	MTD (1–3)	–
	Cohort 5	3–6	MTD (1–3)	3	MTD (1–3)	1–2
Dose expansion	Cohort 6	10	MTD (1–5)	MTD (1–5)	MTD (1–5)	MTD (1–5)
		10	Sham	Sham	Sham	Sham

MTD (1-#)—Maximum tolerated dose (from Cohort 1 to Cohort #)
[a] Number of subjects are approximate and dependent on results of dose escalation study
[b] Treatments administered by suprachoroidal injections followed by laser applications; multiple treatments were administered weekly
[c] One cycle will be comprised of up to 3 weekly treatments of highest administered dose

ment was not started with initial treatment until the inflammation was observed to increase the chance that a secondary immune response would occur. Two subjects with juxtafoveal tumors also experienced treatment-related serious adverse events (SAEs) of vision loss.

Through 6 months of follow-up, 73% of treated subjects experienced tumor control, defined as any subject that did not meet the definition of tumor progression (growth in tumor height >0.5 mm; LBD >1 mm due to definitive tumor growth) and not treated with standard care. Through a median 12 months of follow-up, 55% of subjects experienced tumor control. Among subjects with any level of documented growth in tumor thickness prior to treatment (n = 32), a growth rate reduction of −0.532 mm/year was observed from a historical growth rate of 0.718 mm/year to an on-study growth rate of 0.185 mm/year (p = 0.0316). Among subjects eligible for a phase 3 trial (n = 22)—defined as any subject with a document growth of ≥0.3 mm within 2 years, tumor thickness 0.5–3.0 mm, LBD ≤13.0 mm, and tumor volume ≤50 mm^3—a tumor growth rate of 0.77 mm/year was projected based on mean documented growth rate before treatment; following treatment, the mean tumor growth rate was significantly decreased to −0.065 mm/year (p = 0.007).

As for visual acuity, among all subjects treated with AU-011, a vision preservation rate of 91% was observed at 6 months and with 12 months median of follow-up. Among subjects eligible for a phase 3 trial and at high-risk for vision loss (n = 19)—defined as subjects with tumors ≤3.0 mm from the fovea and/or optic nerve—89% experienced vision preservation at 6 months and with 9 months median follow-up.

A potential phase 3 randomized trial is also being designed for intravitreal injection of AU-011 with over 90% power with an estimated 67 subjects. Inclusion criteria will be listed as described above, and subjects will be randomized 2:1:2 to a therapeutic high-dose regimen, a low-dose regimen, and a sham group for two treatment cycles. The primary efficacy endpoint will occur at 12 months evaluating disease progression and/or visual acuity failure. Safety and durability will be evaluated through 24 months.

4.2 Suprachoroidal Treatment

A randomized phase 2 trial is also currently recruiting to evaluate the safety and efficacy of AU-011 via suprachoroidal administration in subjects with treatment-naïve, non-metastatic primary indeterminate lesions and small choroidal melanomas [55]. The study is planned to occur in two parts; the first part is an open-label dose escalation phase, and the second is a subject, assessor and sponsor masked randomized dose expansion phase. The dose escalation phase will consist of five cohorts receiving varied doses, number of doses, number of laser applications, and treatment cycles; the randomized dose expansion phase will consist of subjects randomized 1:1 to either the maximum tolerated dose regimen from the dose escalation cohorts or to sham treatment (sham injection and sham laser). These cohorts are described in detail in Table 3. The primary outcome will be tumor thickness growth rate over 52 weeks with additional safety and efficacy endpoints through 104 weeks. This study has an estimated primary completion in September 2023. The safety profile in subjects enrolled in the single dose cohorts is favorable with no SAEs reported to date [56, 57].

5 Conclusions

While the treatment of choroidal melanoma was transformed by the results of the COMS trials, there still remains devastating side effects among patients treated with enucleation and radiation therapy. However, recent developments in the use of VLPs hold great promise for the treatment of multiple types of cancer. Specifically, the development of AU-011 for choroidal melanoma has provided the opportunity for patients to be treated with non-surgical intervention with higher probability of retaining their eye and long-term visual acuity post-therapy. Additionally, AU-011 has the potential to be the first targeted therapy for the treatment of primary indeterminate lesions and small choroidal melanoma. Although this treatment still requires safety and efficacy validation in larger, confirmatory clinical trials, initial results are encouraging and promising for the future of choroidal melanoma treatment.

References

1. Kivelä T. The epidemiological challenge of the most frequent eye cancer: retinoblastoma, an issue of birth and death. Br J Ophthalmol. 2009;93(9):1129–31.
2. Singh AD, Topham A. Incidence of uveal melanoma in the United States: 1973-1997. Ophthalmology. 2003;110(5):956–61.
3. Shields CL, Kaliki S, Furuta M, Mashayekhi A, Shields JA. Clinical spectrum and prognosis of uveal melanoma based on age at presentation in 8,033 cases. Retina. 2012;32(7):1363–72.
4. Aronow ME, Topham AK, Singh AD. Uveal melanoma: 5-year update on incidence, treatment, and survival (SEER 1973-2013). Ocul Oncol Pathol. 2018;4(3):145–51.
5. Yang J, Manson DK, Marr BP, Carvajal RD. Treatment of uveal melanoma: where are we now? Ther Adv Med Oncol. 2018;10:1758834018757175.
6. Diener-West M, Earle JD, Fine SL, Hawkins BS, Moy CS, Reynolds SM, et al. The COMS randomized trial of iodine 125 brachytherapy for choroidal melanoma, III: initial mortality findings. COMS Report No. 18. Arch Ophthalmol. 2001;119(7):969–82.
7. Collaborative Ocular Melanoma Study Group. Design and methods of a clinical trial for a rare condition: the Collaborative Ocular Melanoma Study. COMS Report No. 3. Control Clin Trials. 1993;14(5):362–91.
8. Collaborative Ocular Melanoma Study Group. The Collaborative Ocular Melanoma Study (COMS) randomized trial of pre-enucleation radiation of large choroidal melanoma II: initial mortality findings COMS Report No. 10. Am J Ophthalmol. 1998;125(6):779–96.
9. COMS Quality of Life Study Group. Quality of life assessment in the collaborative ocular melanoma study: design and methods. COMS-QOLS Report No. 1. COMS Quality of Life Study Group. Ophthalmic Epidemiol. 1999;6(1):5–17.
10. Melia M, Moy CS, Reynolds SM, Hayman JA, Murray TG, Hovland KR, et al. Quality of life after iodine 125 brachytherapy vs enucleation for choroidal melanoma: 5-year results from the Collaborative Ocular Melanoma Study: COMS QOLS Report No. 3. Arch Ophthalmol. 2006;124(2):226–38.
11. Melia BM, Abramson DH, Albert DM, Boldt HC, Earle JD, Hanson WF, et al. Collaborative ocular melanoma study (COMS) randomized trial of I-125 brachytherapy for medium choroidal melanoma. I. Visual acuity after 3 years COMS Report No. 16. Ophthalmology. 2001;108(2):348–66.
12. Bernicker EH, Schefler AC. Uveal melanoma: biology and management; 2021. https://doi.org/10.1007/978-3-030-78117-0.
13. Haas A, Pinter O, Papaefthymiou G, Weger M, Berghold A, Schröttner O, et al. Incidence of radiation retinopathy after high-dosage single-fraction gamma knife radiosurgery for choroidal melanoma. Ophthalmology. 2002;109(5):909–13.
14. Kim IK, Lane AM, Egan KM, Munzenrider J, Gragoudas ES. Natural history of radiation papillopathy after proton beam irradiation of parapapillary melanoma. Ophthalmology. 2010;117(8):1617–22.
15. Monroe AT, Bhandare N, Morris CG, Mendenhall WM. Preventing radiation retinopathy with hyperfractionation. Int J Radiat Oncol Biol Phys. 2005;61(3):856–64.
16. Parsons JT, Bova FJ, Fitzgerald CR, Mendenhall WM, Million RR. Radiation retinopathy after external-beam irradiation: analysis of time-dose factors. Int J Radiat Oncol Biol Phys. 1994;30(4):765–73.
17. Finger PT, Chin KJ, Duvall G, Palladium-103 for Choroidal Melanoma Study Group. Palladium-103 ophthalmic plaque radiation therapy for choroidal melanoma: 400 treated patients. Ophthalmology 2009;116(4):790–6, 796.e1.
18. Krema H, Somani S, Sahgal A, Xu W, Heydarian M, Payne D, et al. Stereotactic radiotherapy for treatment of juxtapapillary choroidal melanoma: 3-year follow-up. Br J Ophthalmol. 2009;93(9):1172–6.
19. Schachat AP, editor. Ryan's retina. 6th ed. Edinburgh; New York: Elsevier; 2018.
20. Bianciotto C, Shields CL, Pirondini C, Mashayekhi A, Furuta M, Shields JA. Proliferative radiation retinopathy after plaque radiotherapy for uveal melanoma. Ophthalmology. 2010;117(5):1005–12.
21. Kinyoun JL, Lawrence BS, Barlow WE. Proliferative radiation retinopathy. Arch Ophthalmol. 1996;114(9):1097–100.
22. Fallico M, Reibaldi M, Avitabile T, Longo A, Bonfiglio V, Chronopoulos A, et al. Intravitreal aflibercept for the treatment of radiation-induced macular edema after ruthenium 106 plaque radiotherapy for choroidal melanoma. Graefes Arch Clin Exp Ophthalmol. 2019;257(7):1547–54.
23. Finger PT, Chin KJ. High-dose (2.0 mg) intravitreal ranibizumab for recalcitrant radiation retinopathy. Eur J Ophthalmol. 2013;23(6):850–6.
24. Murray TG, Latiff A, Villegas VM, Gold AS. Aflibercept for radiation maculopathy study: a prospective, randomized clinical study. Ophthalmol Retina. 2019;3(7):561–6.
25. Schefler AC, Fuller D, Anand R, Fuller T, Moore C, Munoz J, et al. Randomized trial of monthly versus as-needed intravitreal ranibizumab for radiation retinopathy-related macular edema: 1 year outcomes. Am J Ophthalmol. 2020;216:165–73.
26. Kim IK, Lane AM, Jain P, Awh C, Gragoudas ES. Ranibizumab for the prevention of radiation complications in patients treated with proton beam irradiation for choroidal melanoma. Trans Am Ophthalmol Soc. 2016;114:T2.
27. Finger PT. Plaque radiation therapy for malignant melanoma of the iris and ciliary body. Am J Ophthalmol. 2001;132(3):328–35.
28. Groenewald C, Konstantinidis L, Damato B. Effects of radiotherapy on uveal melanomas and adjacent tissues. Eye (Lond). 2013;27(2):163–71.
29. Cappin JM. Malignant melanoma and rubeosis iridis. Histopathological and statistical study. Br J Ophthalmol. 1973;57(11):815–24.
30. Foss AJ, Whelehan I, Hungerford JL, Anderson DF, Errington RD, Kacperek A, et al. Predictive factors for the development of rubeosis following proton beam radiotherapy for uveal melanoma. Br J Ophthalmol. 1997;81(9):748–54.
31. Tarr KH, Constable IJ. Late complications of pterygium treatment. Br J Ophthalmol. 1980;64(7):496–505.
32. Liu L, Xu Y, Huang Z, Wang X. Intravitreal ranibizumab injection combined trabeculectomy versus Ahmed valve surgery in the treatment of neovascular glaucoma: assessment of efficacy and complications. BMC Ophthalmol. 2016;16:65.
33. Wittström E, Holmberg H, Hvarfner C, Andréasson S. Clinical and electrophysiologic outcome in patients with neovascular glaucoma treated with and without bevacizumab. Eur J Ophthalmol. 2012;22(4):563–74.
34. Yazdani S, Hendi K, Pakravan M, Mahdavi M, Yaseri M. Intravitreal bevacizumab for neovascular glaucoma: a randomized controlled trial. J Glaucoma. 2009;18(8):632–7.
35. Collaborative Ocular Melanoma Study Group. Incidence of cataract and outcomes after cataract surgery in the first 5 years after iodine 125 brachytherapy in the Collaborative Ocular Melanoma Study: COMS Report No. 27. Ophthalmology. 2007;114(7):1363–71.
36. Danesh-Meyer HV. Radiation-induced optic neuropathy. J Clin Neurosci. 2008;15(2):95–100.
37. Levin LA, Gragoudas ES, Lessell S. Endothelial cell loss in irradiated optic nerves. Ophthalmology. 2000;107(2):370–4.

38. Eckstein D, Riechardt AI, Heufelder J, Zeitz O, Böker A, Brockmann C, et al. Radiation-induced optic neuropathy: observation versus intravitreal treatment: can visual acuity be maintained by intravitreal treatment? Am J Ophthalmol. 2019;208:289–94.
39. Finger PT, Chin KJ. Antivascular endothelial growth factor bevacizumab for radiation optic neuropathy: secondary to plaque radiotherapy. Int J Radiat Oncol Biol Phys. 2012;82(2):789–98.
40. Roelofs K, Larocque MP, Murtha A, Weis E. The use of intravitreal anti-VEGF and triamcinolone in the treatment of radiation papillopathy. Ocul Oncol Pathol. 2018;4(6):395–400.
41. Shields CL, Demirci H, Marr BP, Mashayekhi A, Dai VV, Materin MA, et al. Intravitreal triamcinolone acetonide for acute radiation papillopathy. Retina (Philadelphia, Pa.). 2006;26(5):537–44.
42. Chaudhry IA, Liu M, Shamsi FA, Arat YO, Shetlar DJ, Boniuk M. Corneoscleral necrosis after episcleral Au-198 brachytherapy of uveal melanoma. Retina (Philadelphia, Pa). 2009;29(1):73–9.
43. Corrêa ZM, Augsburger JJ, Freire J, Eagle RC. Early-onset scleral necrosis after iodine I 125 plaque radiotherapy for ciliochoroidal melanoma. Arch Ophthalmol. 1999;117(2):259–61.
44. Gündüz K, Shields CL, Shields JA, Cater J, Freire JE, Brady LW. Radiation retinopathy following plaque radiotherapy for posterior uveal melanoma. Arch Ophthalmol. 1999;117(5):609–14.
45. Radin PP, Lumbroso-Le Rouic L, Levy-Gabriel C, Dendale R, Sastre X, Desjardins L. Scleral necrosis after radiation therapy for uveal melanomas: report of 23 cases. Graefes Arch Clin Exp Ophthalmol. 2008;246(12):1731–6.
46. Kines RC, Cerio RJ, Roberts JN, Thompson CD, de Los Pinos E, Lowy DR, et al. Human papillomavirus capsids preferentially bind and infect tumor cells. Int J Cancer. 2016;138(4):901–11.
47. Kines RC, Varsavsky I, Choudhary S, Bhattacharya D, Spring S, McLaughlin R, et al. An infrared dye-conjugated virus-like particle for the treatment of primary uveal melanoma. Mol Cancer Ther. 2018;17(2):565–74.
48. Ogawa M, Tomita Y, Nakamura Y, Lee M-J, Lee S, Tomita S, et al. Immunogenic cancer cell death selectively induced by near infrared photoimmunotherapy initiates host tumor immunity. Oncotarget. 2017;8(6):10425–36.
49. Chiang B, Jung JH, Prausnitz MR. The suprachoroidal space as a route of administration to the posterior segment of the eye. Adv Drug Deliv Rev. 2018;126:58–66.
50. Habot-Wilner Z, Noronha G, Wykoff CC. Suprachoroidally injected pharmacological agents for the treatment of chorio-retinal diseases: a targeted approach. Acta Ophthalmol. 2019;97(5):460–72.
51. Savinainen A. Ocular distribution and efficacy after suprachoroidal injection of AU-011 for treatment of ocular melanoma. Virtual; 2020.
52. Yeh S, Khurana RN, Shah M, Henry CR, Wang RC, Kissner JM, et al. Efficacy and safety of suprachoroidal CLS-TA for macular edema secondary to noninfectious uveitis. Ophthalmology. 2020;127(7):948–55.
53. Study in subjects with small primary choroidal melanoma. ClinicalTrials.gov. 2020. https://clinicaltrials.gov/ct2/show/NCT03052127.
54. Kim I. Update from an ongoing phase 1B/2 open-label trial with intravitreal AU-011 for choroidal melanoma and further development plan. Virtual; 2020.
55. Phase 2 trial to evaluate safety and efficacy of AU-011 via suprachoroidal administration in subjects with primary indeterminate lesions and small choroidal melanoma. ClinicalTrials.gov. 2021. https://clinicaltrials.gov/ct2/show/NCT04417530.
56. Mruthyunjaya P. An ongoing phase 1B/2 open-label clinical trial to evaluate the safety and efficacy of AU-011 for the treatment of choroidal melanoma—study update. Virtual; 2020.
57. Shields CL, Lim L-AS, Dalvin LA, Shields JA. Small choroidal melanoma: detection with multimodal imaging and management with plaque radiotherapy or AU-011 nanoparticle therapy. Curr Opin Ophthalmol. 2019;30(3):206–14.

Novel Treatment Strategies for Malignant Anterior Segment Tumors

Jane S. Kim, Emily Chang, and Hakan Demirci

1 Introduction

Malignant anterior segment tumors are relatively uncommon tumors of the ocular surface and iris. Classically, complete surgical resection using a no-touch technique is recommended and is often followed by topical therapy for ocular surface tumors. Depending on the extent of local and systemic involvement, other treatment modalities, such as radiation and chemotherapy, may be recommended. In certain cases, exenteration may be the only hope for locoregional control and disease-specific survival, but can be disfiguring and undesirable. With the recent arrival of targeted molecular therapies (e.g., BRAF/MEK inhibitors) and immunotherapies (e.g., immune checkpoint inhibitors [ICIs]), however, globe-sparing treatment has become a viable option for patients with advanced disease. Intralesional injections of rituximab have also been reported with good response in patients with low-grade conjunctival and iris lymphomas, but also in those with relapsed or refractory disease. Here, we review novel treatment strategies for malignant anterior segment tumors, with an emphasis on targeted molecular therapy for advanced conjunctival melanoma, immunotherapy for advanced conjunctival melanoma and squamous cell carcinoma (SCC), intralesional rituximab injections for conjunctival and iris lymphoma, and small-incision guarded hydroaspiration for small iris melanoma.

J. S. Kim
Eye Plastic, Orbital and Facial Cosmetic Surgery, Kellogg Eye Center, University of Michigan, Ann Arbor, MI, USA

E. Chang · H. Demirci (✉)
Eye Plastic, Orbital and Facial Cosmetic Surgery, Kellogg Eye Center, University of Michigan, Ann Arbor, MI, USA

Ocular Oncology, Kellogg Eye Center, University of Michigan, Ann Arbor, MI, USA
e-mail: emicha@med.umich.edu; hdemirci@med.umich.edu

2 Conjunctival Melanoma

Conjunctival melanomas are rare primary ocular surface tumors that account for 2% of all ocular malignancies [1]. They typically originate from primary acquired melanosis (PAM) with atypia, but can arise from benign conjunctival nevi or de novo [2]. Five- and 10-year overall survival rates for conjunctival melanoma were reported to be 74% and 41%, respectively [3]. Tumor recurrence has been estimated to occur in approximately 26% and 51% of cases at 5 and 10 years after treatment, respectively [2]. Regional lymph node metastasis and distant metastasis can be seen in approximately 41% and 26% of cases, respectively [2, 3]. Current treatment guidelines recommend wide local excision with double freeze-thaw cryotherapy to the margins for resectable tumors and exenteration for locally advanced disease [4]. Adjuvant therapies with topical mitomycin-C and interferon-α2b are also options. More recently, systemic molecular therapies targeting BRAF and MEK, kinases in the mitogen-activated protein kinase (MAPK) pathway, as well as systemic ICIs against programmed cell death protein 1 (PD-1) and cytotoxic T-lymphocyte-associated antigen 4 (CTLA-4), negative regulators of T-cell immune function, have been utilized off-label to treat advanced conjunctival melanomas.

2.1 Targeted Molecular Therapy with Selective BRAF/MEK Inhibitors

Unlike uveal melanomas, which are associated with *GNAQ* and *GNA11* mutations, up to half of conjunctival melanomas have been found to harbor activating *BRAF V600E* or *V600F* mutations, which are also commonly found in cutaneous melanomas [4]. Selective BRAF inhibitors (e.g., dabrafenib, vemurafenib) as well as MEK inhibitors (e.g., trametinib, cobimetinib) have been approved by the U.S. Food and Drug Administration (FDA) for the treatment of unresectable, metastatic cutaneous melanomas. However, given the rarity

B. V. Chawla, M. E. Aronow (eds.), *Global Perspectives in Ocular Oncology*, https://doi.org/10.1007/978-3-031-08250-4_30

of conjunctival melanomas, there are no clinical trials to date investigating the use of these targeted molecular inhibitors in advanced, unresectable conjunctival disease. Table 1 summarizes the clinical characteristics and outcomes of case reports or small case series with advanced conjunctival melanoma treated with selective BRAF/MEK inhibitors as single-agent or dual therapy [5–15].

Weber et al. first described the off-label, single-agent use of vemurafenib, a *BRAF* inhibitor, for the treatment of *BRAF V600E*-positive conjunctival melanoma in a 45-year-old man with nodal, subcutaneous, pulmonary, and osseous metastases [5]. Despite subjective improvement in pain, there was predominantly progressive disease, and vemurafenib was discontinued at 2 months. Maleka et al. also described a case of a 53-year-old woman with metastatic *BRAF V600E*-positive conjunctival melanoma treated with vemurafenib as single agent [6]. Despite enucleation, she developed orbital recurrence and metastatic disease in the parotid gland, lung, and brain. Within 4 weeks of treatment with vemurafenib, there was no clinically apparent disease within the orbit or parotid gland, but, at 4 months, there was orbital recurrence, with a greater number of intracranial lesions. Vemurafenib was discontinued, and the patient died approximately 1 month later.

Multiple case reports of patients with advanced, recurrent conjunctival melanomas were reported to benefit from tumor regression and improved survival with single-agent MAPK inhibition following other treatments. Because resistance typically develops within 6–8 months of treatment initiation, long-term efficacy of single-agent MAPK inhibition can be limited [4]. Pahlitzsch et al. described a case of an 80-year-old woman who had multiple recurrences of conjunctival melanoma previously excised with negative margins and treated with adjuvant plaque brachytherapy [7]. Instead of exenteration, the patient was treated with vemurafenib for 16 months, which allowed for complete globe-sparing surgical resection. Vemurafenib was discontinued due to significant side effects approximately 1 month after complete local excision. The patient has remained in clinical remission for over 3 years. Pinto Torres et al. also reported on a 56-year-old woman with unresectable, metastatic conjunctival melanoma, who was treated with vemurafenib after palliative radiation [8]. After 34 months of treatment, complete remission was noted, and the dose was halved due to drug intolerance. She remained in complete remission 40 months following initiation of vemurafenib.

Compared to monotherapy, combined BRAF/MEK inhibition has been shown to be more effective in reducing tumor burden and prolonging survival in patients with unresectable, metastatic cutaneous melanomas harboring *BRAF V600* mutations, with response rates of 64–68% (compared to 45–51%) and median progression-free survival of 9.9–11.4 months (compared to 6.2–7.3 months) [9, 10]. In clinical trials for advanced cutaneous melanomas, adverse effects were more frequently observed with combined BRAF/MEK inhibition than with single-agent BRAF inhibition; yet, the rate of grade III or IV events was still considered to be low overall for both single-agent and combination therapy [4]. Interestingly, the rate of development of keratoacanthoma or squamous cell carcinoma (SCC) of the skin, an adverse effect of BRAF inhibitors, was significantly lower in patients who received combined BRAF/MEK inhibition than with single-agent BRAF inhibition [4]. Thus, combination therapy, if tolerated, can be more effective and beneficial than monotherapy alone for cutaneous melanomas with *BRAF*-activating mutations.

Combined BRAF/MEK therapy has also been effectively utilized off-label to treat advanced *BRAF V600*-positive, recurrent, metastatic conjunctival melanomas. Kim et al. described a case of a 52-year-old man with multifocal recurrence of *BRAF V600*-positive conjunctival melanoma, without nodal or systemic metastasis, treated with combined dabrafenib/trametinib therapy [11]. Complete resolution was noted within 10 months. There was no evidence of disease (NED) at 15 months. Rossi et al. reported on a 70-year-old male with recurrent, metastatic *BRAF V600E*-positive conjunctival melanoma treated with combined dabrafenib/trametinib therapy [12]. After 8 months, there was reduced metabolic activity of cervical nodal metastases, but the mesenteric nodule remained the same size. There was no evidence of tumor progression or ocular recurrence at 11 months.

Demirci et al. reported the first case of a 72-year-old woman with extensive, multifocal *BRAF V600E*-positive conjunctival melanoma treated with combined dabrafenib/trametinib therapy as a neoadjuvant therapy [13]. This case was therapy-naïve and had no metastasis at presentation. After 3 months, there was sufficient tumor response to allow for globe-sparing surgical resection with sentinel lymph node biopsy. Although she did not have local recurrence, she developed pulmonary and intracranial metastases after 13 months.

Detecting the presence of certain genetic mutations in primary conjunctival melanomas, such as *BRAF V600* mutations, may allow for targeted molecular therapy in advanced and unresectable diseases. Although not FDA-approved for conjunctival disease, single-agent or combined BRAF/MEK inhibition can reduce tumor burden and promote survival in patients with locally advanced conjunctival melanomas harboring *BRAF V600* mutations. BRAF/MEK inhibition may also permit globe-sparing resection for patients whose tumors were previously unresectable or would otherwise require exenteration for locoregional control, but close surveillance is required, as disease recurrence and distant metastasis can still occur.

Table 1 Clinical characteristics and outcomes of patients with advanced conjunctival melanoma treated with selective BRAF/MEK inhibitors

Study	Age (y)	Gender	Orbital involvement	AJCC stage	Prior resection	Prior topical therapy	Prior radiation	Prior systemic therapy	BRAF/MEK inhibitor (treatment duration)	Tumor response	Adverse events	Status after cessation of targeted molecular therapy (follow-up since treatment initiation)	Comments
Weber et al. [5]	45	M	No	TXN1M1[a]	Yes	No	No	No	Vemurafenib (2 mo)	Mixed, but predominantly PD	None	AWD (2 mo)	Subjective improvement in pain at 1 mo, progression of axillary and peripancreatic LAD and significant growth of a paraspinal mass, despite modest regression of a mesenteric mass at 2 mo
Maleka et al. [6]	53	F	Yes	TXNXM1[a]	Yes, with cryotherapy, then enucleation	Yes—MMC	Whole-brain radiation	Temozolomide, investigational AdCD40L gene therapy, and low-dose cyclophosphamide	Vemurafenib (4 mo)	Partial, then PD	Grade II maculopapular rash requiring temporary cessation and dose reduction	Died, 1 mo (5 mo)	Orbital recurrence with new metastases at 4 mo, treatment discontinued due to PD and worsened general condition
Pahlitzsch et al. [7]	80	F	No	T3bN0M0[a]	Yes	No	Plaque brachytherapy (ruthenium)	No	Vemurafenib (16 mo)	Partial, allowing for complete surgical resection	Weight loss, nausea/vomiting, headaches requiring treatment cessation	NED, >3 y??	
Pinto Torres et al. [8]	56	F	No	T1N1M0[a]	Yes	No	Regional at site of nodal metastasis	No	Vemurafenib (34 mo)	Complete	Grade II arthralgia, grade II diarrhea, grade I rash requiring dose reduction	NED (~40 mo)	Diagnosed with early-stage, grade-2, invasive ductal carcinoma of left breast and was treated with mastectomy, SLNB, and tamoxifen at 34 mo
Kim et al. [11]	52	M	No	T2N0M0[a]	Yes, with EtOH and cryotherapy	No	No	No	Dabrafenib and trametinib (15 mo)	Complete	Self-limited fevers initially, transaminitis with normalization after 2-week dose reduction	NED (15 mo)	Complete resolution within 10 mo
Rossi et al. [12]	70	M	No	T1N1M1[a]	Yes, with parotidectomy and neck dissection	No	No	No	Dabrafenib and trametinib (~11 mo)	Stable	Self-limited low-grade fever, grade I transaminitis without subsequent dose reduction	AWD (~11 mo)	
Demirci et al. [13]	70s	F	No	T3cN0M0	No	No	No	No	Dabrafenib and trametinib (13 mo)	Partial, allowing for globe-sparing surgical resection with SLNB, then PD with distant metastases	None	AWD (~13 mo)	Globe-sparing surgical resection with SLNB after 3 mo of BRAF/MEK inhibition, distant metastasis to lung and brain at 13 mo

(continued)

Table 1 (continued)

Study	Age (y)	Gender	Orbital involvement	AJCC stage	Prior resection	Prior topical therapy	Prior radiation	Prior systemic therapy	BRAF/MEK inhibitor (treatment duration)	Tumor response	Adverse events	Status after cessation of targeted molecular therapy (follow-up since treatment initiation)	Comments
Kiyohara et al. [14]	72	M	No	T1N1M0	Yes, with cryotherapy, partial parotidectomy, and neck dissection	Yes—MMC	No	No	Dabrafenib and trametinib (6 mo)	No recurrence	None	NED (6 mo)	
	71	M	No	T1NXM1	Yes, with cryotherapy, then enucleation	No	No	No	Vemurafenib (6 mo), then nivolumab (unknown duration), then dabrafenib and trametinib along with radiation (24 mo)	Stable, then distant metastases at 6 mo of single-agent BRAF inhibition	Erythema multiforme-like eruption requiring dose reduction, two keratinous tumors removed by simple excision	Died (>30 mo)	Developed a keratoacanthoma-like tumor on right side of chest and a seborrheic keratosis-like acanthotic tumor on parietal scalp approximately 2 and 3 months of vemurafenib, but neither tumor showed cellular atypia; at 6 months of vemurafenib, there were multiple vertebral and hepatic metastases on restaging scans
Dagi Glass et al. [15]	61	F	No	T3bN1M0[a]	Yes, with cryotherapy, then parotidectomy and neck dissection	No	No	No	Dabrafenib and trametinib (1.5 mo), then vemurafenib (3.5 mo), then pembrolizumab (2 mo), then vemurafenib (4 mo), then vemurafenib and cobimetinib (10 mo)	Stable/stable but still histopathologic evidence of microinvasive melanoma/progression/stable but still histopathologic evidence of microinvasive melanoma/nearly complete clinical response	Nausea and vomiting requiring cessation of dabrafenib/trametinib and change to single-agent BRAF inhibition	AWD (~21 mo)	Multifocal microinvasive melanoma, e/o microinvasive melanoma at 3 and 4 mo of single-agent anti-BRAF therapy, nearly complete clinical response after 1 mo of vemurafenib/cobimetinib

Abbreviations: *AJCC* American Joint Committee on Cancer; *AWD* alive with disease; *F* female; *LAD* lymphadenopathy; *M* male; *mo* month(s); *NED* no evidence of disease; *PD* progressive disease; *SLNB* sentinel lymph node biopsy; *y* years

[a]AJCC classification determined by clinical information provided in published study

2.2 Immunotherapy with Checkpoint Inhibitors

ICIs are a relatively new class of drugs that block cell-surface receptors on activated T-lymphocytes, such as CTLA-4 and PD-1, to facilitate the immune-mediated recognition of cancer cells and have been shown in clinical trials to significantly increase overall and progression-free survival in unresectable and metastatic cutaneous melanomas [16–18]. Consequently, CTLA-4 (e.g., ipilimumab) and PD-1 inhibitors (e.g., nivolumab, pembrolizumab) have been approved by the FDA for the treatment of advanced cutaneous melanomas. Due to the rarity of conjunctival melanomas, however, there are no clinical trials investigating the efficacy of ICIs for the treatment of advanced disease. Given the promising results in cutaneous melanomas and the expression of PD-1 in tumor-infiltrating lymphocytes in conjunctival melanomas [19], immunotherapy has also been used off-label to treat advanced conjunctival melanomas with or without activating *BRAF* mutations. Table 2 summarizes the clinical characteristics and outcomes of patients with advanced conjunctival melanoma treated with ICIs [20–26].

ICIs were used as neoadjuvant or adjuvant therapy for conjunctival melanomas. Kini et al. first described a case of a man in his 60s who presented with recurrent conjunctival melanoma involving the inferior fornix and anterior orbit, despite prior complete resection and cryotherapy [20]. The patient was treated with pembrolizumab for 6 months, without adverse effects. There was sufficient regression to allow for complete surgical resection with negative margins and cryotherapy. The patient tolerated systemic therapy for 1 year, without recurrence. Chaves et al. reported on a 72-year-old man with diffuse multifocal conjunctival melanoma, which was treated with surgical debulking, unshielded brachytherapy, neck dissection, and ultimately ipilimumab as an adjuvant theapy [21]. After 16 months, there was no evidence of locoregional recurrence or distant metastasis. Hong et al. also reported on a 53-year-old woman with diffuse multifocal conjunctival melanoma treated with neoadjuvant pembrolizumab [22]. There was modest pigment reduction by the end of the fourth cycle, after which topical mitomycin-C drops were added in 2-week cycles for a total of four cycles. Pembrolizumab was discontinued after 12 months, with residual faint conjunctival pigmentation remaining, but there was complete histologic response. After 12 months off pembrolizumab, the patient remains NED.

ICIs have also been used for metastatic conjunctival melanoma cases. Chang et al. reported on a 60-year-old woman who presented with locally invasive amelanotic tarsal conjunctival melanoma [23]. Despite complete surgical resection, the patient developed orbital recurrence, with hepatic metastasis. The patient was treated with ipilimumab/nivolumab therapy for two cycles but developed grade II/III hepatitis; she was switched to single-agent nivolumab. However, she developed an infusion reaction with nivolumab and was therefore switched to pembrolizumab. After a total of 14 cycles, the recurrent orbital tumor resolved; her hepatic lesion also regressed and remained stable at 2 years. Hong et al. reported on a 66-year-old man with a large superior forniceal conjunctival melanoma, with pulmonary and hepatic metastases, treated with combined ipilimumab/nivolumab therapy [22]. After 5 months, there was significant reduction in primary tumor size, with only a trace amount of tarsal pigment. The metastatic lesions also responded to immunotherapy, but the patient developed pituitary failure, requiring supplementation with hydrocortisone and levothyroxine. Nine months after presentation, there was stable disease, without progression or recurrence.

Besides case reports, recently small case series have evaluated the effectiveness of ICIs for conjunctival melanoma. Finger and Pavlick reported on three patients with locally advanced conjunctival melanoma and two patients with metastatic conjunctival melanoma treated with PD-1 inhibitors [24]. In this series, a single-agent ICI therapy was started for 3 months, and if there was no clinical response after at least 3 months, another ICI agent or topical interferon was added in an attempt to augment the effect of PD-1 inhibition by increasing tumoral PD-L1 expression or inducing a local inflammatory reaction, respectively. Of five cases, three were treated for residual tumor after multiple local therapies and two for metastatic conjunctival melanoma. All five cases showed response. One patient with systemic metastatic disease and one patient with local disease showed complete response. One patient with systemic metastatic disease was under remission, one patient with local disease was still under treatment due to recurrence, and one patient with local disease passed away due to heart failure. Systemic side effects of adrenal insufficiency, grade-III colitis, grade-II dermatitis, grade-II hepatotoxicity, and grade-II pneumonitis were observed. They concluded that advanced conjunctival melanoma with local or systemic metastatic disease responded to systemic immunotherapy. PD-1 inhibitors in conjunction with other biologic therapies (ipilimumab, topical interferon eye drops, and radiation therapy) achieved durable responses to treatment for locally advanced and metastatic diseases. Sagiv et al. also described five patients with recurrent, metastatic conjunctival melanoma treated with systemic PD-1 inhibitors [25, 26]. Four were treated with nivolumab and had complete response with NED at 1, 7, 9, and 36 months following treatment completion. One patient was treated with pembrolizumab and had stable metastases in the first 6 months of treatment, but, after 11 months, there was evidence of disease progression. The patient was switched to ipilimumab, with partial response after two cycles. Autoimmune colitis and hepatotoxicity were each observed in two patients. In this case series, treatment

Table 2 Clinical characteristics and outcomes of patients with advanced conjunctival melanoma treated with immune checkpoint inhibitor

Study	Age (y)	Gender	Orbital involvement	AJCC stage	Prior resection	Prior topical therapy	Prior radiation	Previous systemic therapy	Checkpoint inhibitor (treatment duration)	Tumor response	Adverse events	Status at completion of immunotherapy (follow-up since initiation of immunotherapy)	Comments
Kini et al. [20]	60s	M	Yes	T3cNXM0[a]	Yes, with cryotherapy	No	No	No	Pembrolizumab (12 mo)	Complete	None	NED(12 mo)	No residual tumor at 6 mo of immunotherapy (complete histologic response)
Pinto Torres et al. [8]	51	M	No	TXN1M1[a]	Yes	No	No	No	Pembrolizumab (~9 mo)	Complete	–	NED (~9 mo)	Remote history of HIV and HCV treated with ART; normal CD4 count and undetectable VL; near complete resolution of SQ lesions after third cycle
Chaves et al. [21]	72	M	No	T3bN1M0	Yes	No	Brachytherapy with custom unshielded I^{125} device	No	Ipilimumab (3 mo)	Complete	Mild fatigue	NED (~16 mo)	Multifocal
Hong et al. [22]	53	F	No	T3bN0M0	No, incisional biopsies only	No	No	No	Pembrolizumab with/without topical MMC (12 mo)	Complete	Mild generalized cutaneous pruritus	NED (~24 mo)	No improvement with concurrent topical MMC, complete histologic response at 12 mo
	66	M	Yes	T3aN0M1	No, incisional biopsies only	No	No	No	Ipilimumab in combination with nivolumab (5 mo)	Partial	Pituitary failure requiring hydrocortisone and thyroxine replacement	AWD (9 mo)	Observation recommended for very small amount of residual pigmentation on tarsal plate

Chang et al. [23]	60	F	Yes	T3cN0M1[a]	Yes, with cryotherapy	No	No	No	Ipilimumab in combination with nivolumab (~2 mo), then nivolumab (2 mo), then pembrolizumab (~10.5 mo)	Partial	Hepatitis on dual therapy requiring change in therapy; infusion reaction to nivolumab requiring change in therapy	AWD (~24 mo)	
Finger and Pavlick [24]	76	M	No	T3bN0M0	Yes	Yes	No	No	Ipilimumab (~2 mo), then pembrolizumab with topical IFN (~18 mo)	No response/ near complete clinical response	Drug-induced adrenal insufficiency on ipilimumab requiring cessation of immunotherapy/ grade II dermatitis on pembrolizumab and topical IFN	NED (36 mo)	Minimal response on pembrolizumab until topical IFN started; continued same dose of topical IFN gtts to eyelid after cessation of pembrolizumab
	94	F	No	cT3bN0M0, pT4b	No	No	No	No	Pembrolizumab (4 mo), then combination with low-dose ipilimumab (~3 mo)	Progression/ partial clinical response	None	Died from CHF at 5 mo after cessation of immunotherapy (~12 mo)	Immunotherapy discontinued for worsening CHF unrelated to immunotherapy
	84	F	No	T3bN0M0	Yes, with cryotherapy	Yes—MMC	Plaque brachytherapy	No	Pembrolizumab (~3 mo), then combination with low-dose ipilimumab (~15 mo, IFN later added)	Minimal/ partial (50%)	None	AWD (~18 mo)	Intralesional IFN was added when new pigmented nodules developed on eyelids while on hiatus from immunotherapy for cataract surgery

(continued)

Study	Age (y)	Gender	Orbital involvement	AJCC stage	Prior resection	Prior topical therapy	Prior radiation	Previous systemic therapy	Checkpoint inhibitor (treatment duration)	Tumor response	Adverse events	Status at completion of immunotherapy (follow-up since initiation of immunotherapy)	Comments
	76	F	No	TXN1M1[a]	Yes, with cryotherapy, then parotidectomy and neck dissection	Yes—MMC	Regional at site of metastases	No	Ipilimumab (~3 mo), then ipilimumab with concurrent radiation (~3 mo), then pembrolizumab with concurrent radiation (concurrent for 6 weeks, single agent for ~10.5 mo)	Complete; later with distant metastases	None	NED (~65 mo)	Developed new subcarinal metastasis after first round of ipilimumab (treated with surgical resection, adjuvant radiation, and concurrent ipilimumab); developed SQ nodule (treated with surgical resection, adjuvant radiation, and concurrent pembrolizumab followed by single-agent pembrolizumab)
	72	F	No	TXNXM1[a]	Yes	Yes	No	No	Ipilimumab in combination with nivolumab (~2 mo)	Partial (75%)	Grade II hepatotoxicity after 2 cycles requiring treatment delay; grade III colitis after third cycle requiring cessation of immunotherapy; grade II delayed-onset pneumonitis	NED (~32 mo)	Resolution of all palpable SQ nodules after 2 cycles (~1.5 mo)

Sagiv et al. [25]	50s	F	Yes	T3cNXM1[a]	Orbital exenteration, and parotidectomy	No	No	No	Nivolumab (3 mo)	Complete	Transaminitis requiring cessation of immunotherapy	NED (12 mo)	Immunotherapy stopped at 3 mo d/t adverse effects; complete resolution of orbital and metastatic lesions 9 mo after cessation of immunotherapy
	28	F	No	T2NXM1[a]	Yes, with cryotherapy	Yes—MMC	No	No	Nivolumab (3.5 mo)	Complete	–	NED (~39.5 mo)	Significant response after first cycle; complete response after 3.5 mo of immunotherapy
	40s	F	No	TXN1M1[a]	Yes, with cryotherapy and parotidectomy	Yes—IFN and MMC	No	No	Nivolumab (5 mo)	Complete	Autoimmune colitis after 10 cycles (5 mo) requiring cessation of immunotherapy	NED (12 mo)	Resolution of lung metastasis after 4 cycles (2 mo)
	60s	F	No	T2N0M1[a]	Yes, with cryotherapy, then orbital exenteration and parotidectomy	Yes—MMC	Yes	No	Pembrolizumab (11 mo), then ipilimumab + dacarbazine (1.5 mo)	Stable at 6 mo, then progression at 11 mo/ partial at 1.5 mo	Grade IV hepatotoxicity on ipilimumab requiring treatment cessation	AWD (~13.5 mo)	Minor progression of pulmonary metastases and development of minor tracheoesophageal and periesophageal LAD after 13 cycles (11 mo) of pembrolizumab
	70s	M	No	T3bNXM1[a]	Yes	Yes—IFN	No	No	Nivolumab (11 mo)	Complete	Immune-related colitis requiring cessation of immunotherapy	NED (12 mo)	Partial response after 6 cycles (3 mo)

Abbreviations: *AJCC* American Joint Committee on Cancer; *ART* antiretroviral therapy; *AWD* alive with disease; *CHF* congestive heart failure; *F* female; *HCV* hepatitis C virus; *HIV* human immunodeficiency virus; *IFN* interferon; *LAD* lymphadenopathy; *M* male; *MMC* mitomycin C; *mo* month(s); *NED* no evidence of disease; *SQ* subcutaneous; *VL* viral load; *y* years

[a]AJCC classification determined by clinical information provided in published study

duration ranged from 3 to 11 months; immunotherapy was most often discontinued for treatment toxicity.

ICIs were used for patients who could not tolerate combined BRAF/MEK inhibitor therapy or who developed recurrence while on the therapy. Kiyohara et al. described another case of a 71-year-old man with *BRAF V600E*-positive conjunctival melanoma, complicated by multiple local recurrences and distant metastatic disease [14]. He underwent enucleation and was started on vemurafenib. At 6 months, multiple vertebral and hepatic metastases were found; trametinib and nivolumab were started in conjunction with dabrafenib and radiation therapy. The patient died 24 months after starting combination therapy. Dagi Glass et al. reported a case of a 61-year-old woman with *BRAF V600E*-positive multifocal conjunctival melanoma with cervical and parotid nodal metastases, who was treated with wide local excision, cryotherapy, parotidectomy, and modified radical neck dissection [15]. Despite negative margins, the patient developed new conjunctival lesions and was started on combination dabrafenib/trametinib therapy. Due to intolerable nausea and vomiting, combination therapy was discontinued at 1.5 months, and vemurafenib was started. After 3.5 months, vemurafenib was discontinued, and pembrolizumab was started because of histopathologic evidence of microinvasive melanoma and known risk of resistance on single-agent BRAF inhibition. However, there was progression at 2 months, so pembrolizumab was discontinued. Vemurafenib was restarted, which appeared to stabilize conjunctival involvement, but repeat biopsy again demonstrated microinvasive melanoma. The patient was restarted on combined BRAF/MEK inhibition by adding cobimetinib. By 1 month, there was nearly complete resolution of conjunctival disease, and the patient continued to demonstrate stable disease, without metastasis at 23 months from presentation.

Immunotherapy with ICIs may be tolerated in patients with concomitant human immunodeficiency virus (HIV) and hepatitis C virus (HCV) infections. Pinto Torres et al. reported on a 51-year-old man with remote history of HIV and HCV infections, both well controlled on antiretroviral therapy, whose previously excised compound melanocytic nevus transformed to malignant conjunctival melanoma [8]. Due to locoregional recurrence with rapid progression, pembrolizumab was started. After the third cycle, there was near complete resolution. Approximately 9 months after initiating immunotherapy, there was NED.

ICIs can extend survival in patients with advanced conjunctival melanomas whose tumors are not amenable to local surgical excision and/or require exenteration. Immunotherapy may also be safe in elderly individuals and in those with well-controlled, chronic viral infections. However, treatment with ICIs may be limited by immune-related adverse effects, such as dermatitis, transaminitis, colitis, and pneumonitis. Of note, ophthalmic complications, mainly dry eye disease, have been reported in early clinical trials for advanced solid tumors [27], but, since their FDA approval, cases of intraocular and orbital inflammation have been reported with ICIs, albeit rare [28, 29]. Although initial reports show significant promise for patients with advanced conjunctival melanomas, these studies are limited by a small number of cases with variable treatment regimens and short follow-up times. All patients with conjunctival melanomas require close surveillance.

3 Conjunctival Squamous Cell Carcinoma

Conjunctival squamous cell carcinoma (cSCC) is part of a spectrum of malignant diseases termed ocular surface squamous neoplasia (OSSN) [30]. Predisposing factors include chronic ultraviolet radiation, tobacco smoking, immunosuppression (e.g., history of HIV infection, status post organ transplantation), and certain genetic conditions (e.g., xeroderma pigmentosum) [31]. There is overall good prognosis, with rare incidence of invasive disease and low risk of distant metastasis [31], but local recurrence is not infrequent, with approximately 10% at 1 year and 17–21% at 5 years despite complete excision and adjuvant therapy [32, 33]. OSSN is typically managed surgically, often with topical (e.g., interferon alpha-2b, 5-fluorouracil, mitomycin-C) or intralesional therapy (e.g., interferon alpha-2b) [30, 31]. When there is evidence of intraocular or intraorbital extension, however, enucleation or exenteration is recommended, respectively. In recent years), ICIs have been used off-label to treat advanced cSCC with orbital extension [34]. Table 3 summarizes the clinical characteristics and outcomes of patients with advanced cSCC treated with immune checkpoint inhibitors [34].

3.1 Immunotherapy with Immune Checkpoint Inhibitors

In cSCC, PD-L1 tumor expression has been shown to correlate with the presence of $CD8^+$ T-lymphocytes within the tumor and surrounding stroma but not with human papilloma virus (HPV) status [35, 36]. Despite its potential application in the management of advanced cSCC, to date, there is only one published case series of five patients with cSCC with orbital extension treated with PD-1 inhibitors (Table 3) [34]. Of these five patients, one patient was immunosuppressed due to chronic inflammatory demyelinating polyneuropathy. Two patients received pembrolizumab, and three had cemiplimab, with treatment duration ranging from 3 to 10 months. Over a mean follow-up duration of 15 months (range, 9–26 months), 4 patients with high tumor mutation

Table 3 Clinical characteristics and outcomes of patients with advanced conjunctival squamous cell carcinoma treated with immune checkpoint inhibitor

Study	Age (y)	Gender	Orbital involvement	AJCC stage	Prior resection	Prior topical therapy	Prior radiation	Previous systemic therapy	Checkpoint inhibitor (treatment duration)	Tumor response	Adverse events	Status at completion of immunotherapy (follow-up since initiation of immunotherapy)	Comments
Demirci et al. [34]	82	M	Yes	T4N0M0	Yes	No	Yes—plaque brachytherapy	No	Pembrolizumab (5.5 mo)	Complete	Colitis requiring temporary cessation and systemic corticosteroids	NED (26 mo)	TMB: 87.5 Mut/Mb
	59	M	Yes	T4N0M0	Yes	No	No	No	Cemiplimab (7 mo)	Complete	None	NED (13 mo)	TMB: 61.5 Mut/Mb
	86	F	Yes	T4N0M0	Yes	No	No	No	Cemiplimab (7.5 mo)	Complete	Mild dermatitis, furuncle, pain	NED (11.5 mo)	TMB: 109.6 Mut/Mb
	71	M	Yes	T4N0M0	Yes	No	Yes	No	Cemiplimab (7.5 mo)	Complete	None	NED (9.5 mo)	TMB: 95.2 Mut/Mb
	61	M	Yes	T4N0M0	Yes	No	No	No	Pembrolizumab, 5-FU, and carboplatin (2 mo); then carboplatin and docetaxel only (2 mo)	PD/PD	None	AWD (13 mo)	History of CIDP treated with chronic immunosuppression; TMB: 8.1 Mut/Mb

Abbreviations: *5-FU* 5-fluorouracil; *AJCC* American Joint Committee on Cancer; *AWD* alive with disease; *CIDP* chronic inflammatory demyelinating polyneuropathy; *mo* month(s); *NED* no evidence of disease; *PD* progressive disease; *y* years

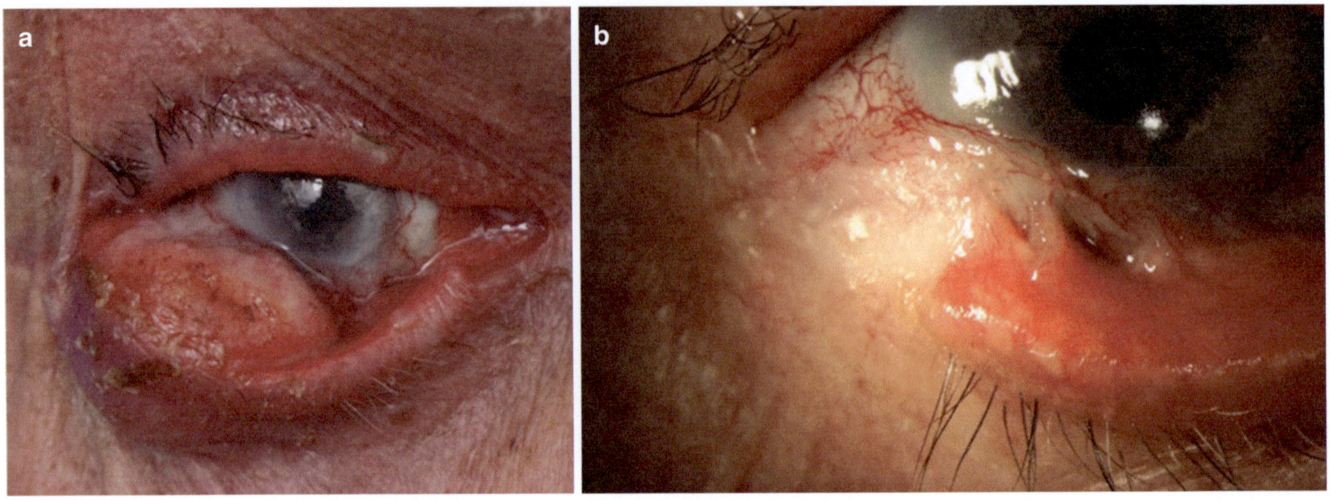

Fig. 1 (**a**) An 86-year-old man who presented with recurrent conjunctival squamous cell carcinoma of the right lateral bulbar conjunctiva. (**b**) After seven cycles of systemic pembrolizumab therapy, his conjunctival tumor responded significantly, and no recurrence observed after 3 years of follow-up

burden (TMB) showed complete response to immune checkpoint inhibitors, without recurrence (Fig. 1). One patient, who had low TMB and therefore supplemented ICI with carboplatin and topical 5-fluorouracil, had progressive disease despite three cycles of combination therapy. There was continued progression even after switching to carboplatin and docetaxel, requiring surgical resection followed by external beam radiotherapy. Of note, one patient developed autoimmune colitis after the first cycle of pembrolizumab, but completed seven cycles without further complications after temporary treatment cessation and systemic corticosteroids. Another patient developed a furuncle and mild dermatitis, but was treated with topical medications and did not require treatment cessation.

ICIs may be considered for first-line therapy in patients with advanced cSCC with orbital extension, but clinical experience with immunotherapy for cSCC is currently quite limited, as durability of treatment response is still unclear. Immunotherapy may be limited by the occurrence of immune-related adverse events, but can be continued in select patients with appropriate treatment and close monitoring. TMB may best predict treatment response to immune checkpoint blockade in cSCC. All patients require long-term surveillance for recurrence.

4 Conjunctival Lymphoma

Conjunctival lymphomas are usually CD20-expressing B-cell non-Hodgkin lymphomas [37]. The most common subtype is mucosa-associated lymphoid tissue (MALT) or extranodal marginal zone lymphoma (EMZL), followed by follicular lymphoma (FL), mantle cell lymphoma (MCL), and diffuse large B-cell lymphoma (DLBCL) [37]. Most patients with conjunctival lymphomas present with unilateral disease without evidence of prior or systemic dissemination and are typically treated with external beam radiation therapy (EBRT) with or without chemotherapy, with overall good success [37, 38]. EBRT is considered to be the gold standard for low-grade, isolated ocular adnexal lymphomas, including conjunctival lymphomas, with 5-year local control rates ranging from 89 to 100% [39]. However, up to 50% of patients who receive EBRT can develop both short- and long-term complications, including conjunctivitis, dry eye syndrome, corneal ulceration, cataract formation, radiation retinopathy, and even orbital fat atrophy [39]. Since its approval in 1997, systemic immunotherapy with rituximab, a chimeric monoclonal antibody directed against cell-surface antigen CD20, has been used as first-line monotherapy for low-grade conjunctival lymphomas as an intralesional injection or systemic therapy or in combination with chemotherapy for high-grade conjunctival lymphomas [38, 40].

4.1 Intralesional Rituximab Injections

CD20 is essential in generating a T-lymphocyte independent antibody response. Rituximab thus depletes both normal and malignant B-cells and has been used systemically to treat a variety of autoimmune diseases and cancers. Because of their indolence and generally good response with cutaneous MALT lymphomas, local therapy with intralesional injections of rituximab has also been used to treat low-grade conjunctival lymphomas [41–44]. Table 4 summarizes the clinical characteristics and outcomes of patients with conjunctival lymphomas treated with intralesional rituximab injections [41–44].

Table 4 Clinical characteristics and outcomes of patients with conjunctival lymphoma treated with intralesional rituximab injections

Study	Age (y)	Gender	Laterality	Tumor type AJCC stage	Prior resection	Prior topical therapy	Prior radiation	Previous systemic therapy	Intralesional rituximab injection (duration)	Tumor response	Adverse events	Status at completion of immunotherapy (follow-up since initiation of immunotherapy)	Comments
Demirci et al. [43]	69	F	OD	MALT T1bN0M0[a]	No	No	No	No	50 mg/5 mL × 3 mo, then EBRT	Partial/?	Fever; chills; fatigue after first injection	NED (68 mo)	
	67	M	OS	MALT T1aN0M0[a]	No	No	No	No	50 mg/5 mL × 2 mo	Complete	None	NED (39 mo)	
	62	F	OD	MALT T1aN0M0[a]	No	No	No	No	50 mg/5 mL × 2 mo	Complete	None	NED (78 mo)	
	86	M	OS	MALT T1aN0M0[a]	Unk	Unk	Unk	Unk	50 mg/5 mL × 2 mo	Complete	None	NED (45 mo)	History of low-grade lymphoma
	78	F	OD	MALT T1aN0M0[a]	Unk	Unk	Unk	Unk	50 mg/5 mL × 2 mo, then EBRT	Partial/?	None	AWD (21 mo)	History of DLBCL
	75	M	OU	MALT T1cN0M0[a]	No	No	No	No	50 mg/5 mL × 2 mo	Complete	None	NED (22 mo)	
	41	F	OD	MALT T1aN0M0[a]	No	No	No	No	50 mg/5 mL × 2 mo	Complete	None	NED (8 mo)	
	96	M	OD	MALT T1aN0M0[a]	No	No	No	No	50 mg/5 mL × 2 mo	Complete	None	NED (23 mo)	
	62	F	OD	MALT T1aN0M0[a]	No	No	No	No	50 mg/5 mL × 1 mo	Partial	Joint pain; tachycardia	AWD (8 mo)	
	23	M	OS	MALT T1cN0M0[a]	No	No	No	No	50 mg/5 mL × 2 mo	Partial	None	AWD (6 mo)	
	39	F	OD	MALT T1cN0M0[a]	No	No	No	No	50 mg/5 mL × 1 mo	Complete	None	NED (60 mo)	
	69	M	OD	Follicular T1aN0M0[a]	No	No	No	No	50 mg/5 mL × 2 mo	Complete	None	NED (21 mo)	
	71	M	OU	Mantle cell T1bN0M0[a]	Unk	Unk	Unk	Unk	50 mg/5 mL × 2 mo	Complete, then recurrence	Periocular swelling and erythema OU	NED, then treated for recurrence (84 mo)	History of MCL; developed orbital and systemic recurrence OD approximately 4 years later; treated with systemic rituximab/ bendamustine

Table 4 (continued)

Study	Age (y)	Gender	Laterality	Tumor type AJCC stage	Prior resection	Prior topical therapy	Prior radiation	Previous systemic therapy	Intralesional rituximab injection (duration)	Tumor response	Adverse events	Status at completion of immunotherapy (follow-up since initiation of immunotherapy)	Comments
Ferreri et al. [44]	48	F	OS	MALT T1aN0M0[a]	No	No	No	Rituximab; chlorambucil; doxycycline	15 mg/2.5 mL × 4 wk, then 6 mo	Complete	Mild pain during injections and local inflammation lasting <24 h after treatment	NED (13 mo)	History of liver transplantation for HBV-related cirrhosis; with chronic immunosuppression; complicated by HCV
	42	M	OU	MALT T1aN0M0[a]	No	Yes—IFN	Yes	Cyclophosphamide, doxorubicin, vincristine, and prednisone for first recurrence, then rituximab for second recurrence	15 mg/2.5 mL × 4 wk, then 6 mo for third recurrence	Complete	Local inflammation lasting <24 h after treatment	NED (10 mo)	First recurrence—OU, second recurrence—OU, third recurrence—OD
	76	F	OD	Follicular T2dN0M0	No	No	No	Doxycycline	6 mg/mL × 4 wk, then 9 mo, with last 6 monthly doses supplemented with AS	Complete	None	NED (11 mo)	History of invasive ductal carcinoma of left breast s/p lumpectomy and adjuvant hormonal therapy; complete response after 3 doses supplemented with AS
Rodríguez Villa et al. [42]	49	F	OD	Follicular T1bN0M0[a]	Yes	No	No	No	8.4 mg/1.4 mL × 4 wk, then 6 mo	Complete	None	NED (10 mo)	

Note: This table does not include details from the phase 2 clinical trial (NCT01514344) as reported by Ferreri et al., 2020[44]

Abbreviations: *AJCC* American Joint Committee on Cancer; *AS* autologous serum; *AWD* alive with disease; *DLBCL* diffuse large B-cell lymphoma; *EBRT* external beam radiation therapy; *F* female; *HBV* hepatitis B virus; *HCV* hepatitis C virus; *IFN* interferon; *M* male; *MALT* mucosa-associated lymphoid tissue lymphoma; *MCL* mantle cell lymphoma; *mo* month(s); *NED* no evidence of disease; *OD* right eye; *OS* left eye; *OU* both eyes; *Unk* unknown; *wk* weeks; *y* years

[a]AJCC classification determined by clinical information provided in published study

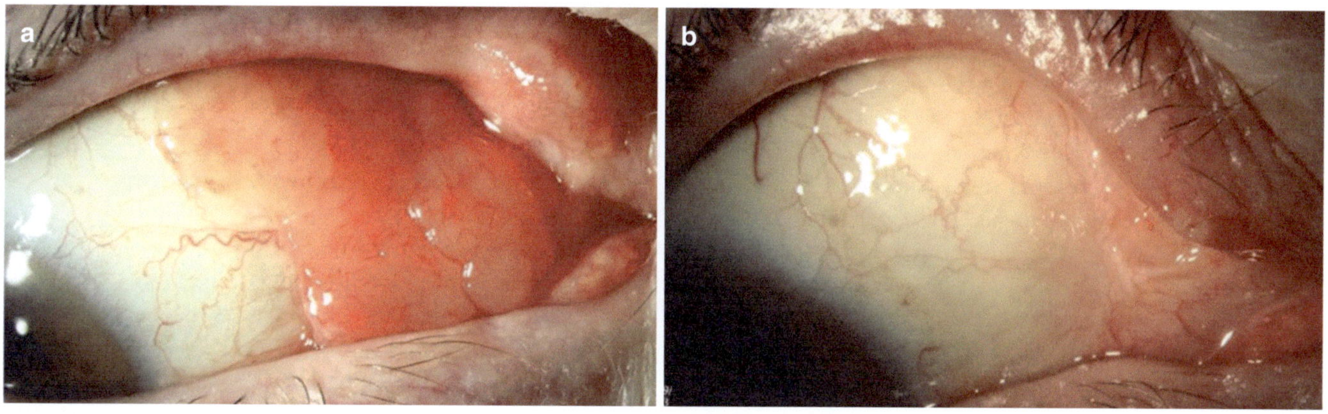

Fig. 2 (**a**) A 69-year-old woman who presented with conjunctival MALT lymphoma in the forniceal conjunctiva of the right eye. (**b**) After two intralesional injection of rituximab (50 mg in 5 cc), complete response was observed and there was no recurrence after 2 years of follow-up

Demirci et al. recently reported on their experience with intralesional rituximab for 15 eyes in 13 patients with conjunctival lymphoma [43]. All except two patients had MALT lymphoma; one had FL, and the other had MCL. Of two patients with conjunctival MALT lymphoma, one had prior history of a low-grade lymphoma, and another had history of DLBCL. For all patients, rituximab (50 mg/5 mL) was injected subconjunctivally adjacent to the tumor, with most receiving 2 monthly injections. Eleven eyes (73%) exhibited complete response, whereas 4 (27%) had partial response, with notable decrease in tumor size (Fig. 2). Two eyes with partial response also underwent adjuvant EBRT. One patient experienced periocular swelling and edema postprocedurally; two others developed systemic symptoms (e.g., fevers, chills, fatigue, joint pain). Over a mean follow-up of 37 months (range, 6–84 months), no patients with low-grade tumors had local recurrence or progression to systemic lymphoma; however, one patient with mantle cell lymphoma had orbital recurrence and systemic dissemination approximately 4 years later, which were treated with intravenous rituximab and bendamustine.

Ferreri et al. and Rodríguez Villa et al. also described the use of intralesional rituximab injections to treat relapsed or refractory low-grade conjunctival lymphomas [41, 42, 44]. In a patient with local relapse of conjunctival FL, Rodríguez Villa et al. reported complete clinical response after treatment with 4 weekly intralesional injections of rituximab (6 mg/mL), followed by 6 monthly injections [42]. The patient remained progression-free after 10 months of follow-up, and no adverse events were observed. Ferreri et al. also described a pilot study of three patients with relapsed or refractory low-grade lymphomas (i.e., two MALT lymphoma, one FL) treated with 4 weekly intralesional injections of rituximab (6 mg/mL), followed by 6 monthly injections [41]. Despite being previously treated with intravenous rituximab, 2 patients with conjunctival MALT lymphoma demonstrated complete response after intralesional rituximab injections, without recurrence at 10 and 13 months of follow-up, respectively. Of note, one of these patients also had concomitant hepatitis B and C viral infections and underwent intralesional rituximab injections without complications. One patient with FL received intralesional rituximab injections for local progression after a period of disease stabilization. After 4 weekly and 3 monthly injections, there were no significant changes in tumor size. This patient then received an additional 6 monthly intralesional rituximab injections that were supplemented with autologous serum to increase local bioavailability of immunologic effectors (e.g., C3 and C4) and thereby improve rituximab's complement-dependent cytotoxic activity within the tumor [45]. After 3 months of these serum-fortified intralesional injections, complete remission was noted. At 11 months of follow-up, there was no evidence of disease recurrence or progression.

Ferreri et al. showed similar results in a phase 2 clinical trial (NCT01514344), in which patients with relapsed or refractory conjunctival MALT lymphomas were treated with 4 weekly intralesional rituximab injections, followed by 6 monthly injections [44]. If a patient did not demonstrate a clinical response after 4 weekly injections, each subsequent monthly rituximab injection was supplemented with autologous serum. Twenty patients enrolled in the study, with a total of 27 eyes. After 4 weekly doses, 11 patients (55%) achieved tumor regression, 8 (40%) demonstrated stable disease, and 1 (5%) had disease progression. Subsequent intralesional injections were supplemented with autologous serum in seven of eight patients with stable disease and in two patients who showed partial clinical response to weekly rituximab injections. At median follow-up of 42 months (range, 10–78 months), 12 (60%) had a complete response without remission, although 2 of these patients underwent palliative radiation of the treated eye for local symptoms after 4 and 22 months, respectively. Two patients with initial partial response who underwent monthly rituximab injections supplemented with autologous serum had complete remission of disease. Of the seven patients with stable disease who received serum-supplemented rituximab injections, only one achieved complete remission; another showed a partial response. The remaining five did not benefit from autologous serum supplementation. Overall, eight patients (40%) experienced progressive disease, although two of three patients who showed local relapse after rituximab-only injections achieved a complete and durable response after having subsequent intralesional injections supplemented with autologous serum. Five-year progression-free survival and time-to-next-treatment rates were 59 ± 11% and 69 ± 11%, respectively. Overall, intralesional rituximab injections were well tolerated, with or without autologous serum supplementation. Grade I edema, grade I hyperemia, and grade II bleeding were the only reported adverse events; the first two were attributed to antitumor activity, and the latter was considered to be self-limited. There were no severe adverse events or deaths reported throughout the follow-up period.

Although the literature is limited by small case series with different treatment protocols, intralesional rituximab injections can be appropriate therapy for patients with both treatment-naïve and relapsed or treatment-refractory indolent conjunctival lymphomas. Intralesional rituximab is also well tolerated in elderly individuals and in those with well-controlled, chronic viral infections. In a proportion of patients, the addition of autologous serum may improve the clinical response to intralesional rituximab injections and can result in complete remission without recurrence or progression of disease over at least 3 years. Favorable responses have also been observed in patients who previously demonstrated progressive disease on intravenous rituximab. Intralesional rituximab injections may be better tolerated than other local therapeutic agents, including topical mitomycin-C drops and intralesional interferon injections, which have been associated with greater incidence and severity of local complications [44, 46, 47].

5 Iris Lymphoma

Iris lymphomas are very rare, with approximately 50 cases described in the literature over the last 40 years [48]. Most cases are secondary manifestations of systemic B-cell non-Hodgkin lymphoma, followed by T-cell lymphoma and multiple myeloma [48]. Unlike its choroidal counterpart, iris lymphomas tend to be high-grade, aggressive tumors (e.g., DLBCL) with systemic involvement [48, 49]. This may be partly due to the delay in diagnosis, as iris lymphomas are often initially misdiagnosed as anterior uveitis and frequently treated with topical corticosteroids prior to diagnosis [49]. Definitive diagnosis requires tissue or aqueous sampling. Depending on the extent and subtype of disease, treatment may include local rituximab injections, complete surgical resection, enucleation, radiation therapy, and/or systemic chemotherapy.

5.1 Intralesional Rituximab Injections

Due to good treatment responses observed in cases of primary ocular adnexal and vitreoretinal lymphomas [50, 51], Demirci et al. reported the novel use of intralesional rituximab for the treatment of primary MALT lymphoma of the iris [52]. In this technique, an anterior chamber tap was first performed to reduce intraocular volume and thus intraocular pressure. Then, 0.1 mL of rituximab (1 mg/0.1 mL) was injected directly into the tumor under slit lamp visualization. A total of 3 monthly injections were performed, with a clinical response noted after the first injection. By 5 months, there was complete resolution on slit lamp examination, gonioscopy, and ultrasound biomicroscopy. At 11 months, there is no evidence of local toxicity, local recurrence, or systemic dissemination. The authors note that there may be limited treatment response in high-grade lymphomas and in tumors with ciliary body and/or choroidal involvement. Furthermore, injection of rituximab into the aqueous or vitreous may simplify and be as effective as direct intralesional injections, which may result in unwanted hyphema, focal cataract, and inadvertent dispersion of tumor cells. Pharmacokinetic studies in rabbits have shown that the half-life of rituximab is 5.3 and 4.7 days in the aqueous and vitreous, respectively: A direct 1 mg intravitreal rituximab injection may deliver vitreous drug levels that would remain above 10 ng/mL for 72 days [53].

6 Iris Melanoma

Of uveal melanomas, iris melanomas are the least common type, constituting only 2–3% of cases [54–56]. Because of their greater visibility, iris melanomas are often diagnosed at earlier stages than ciliary body or choroidal melanomas [55]. As such, 5-, 10-, and 20-year metastasis rates can be as low as 1–3%, 5–6%, and 10%, respectively, for biopsy-proven cases [54, 57]; however, a multicenter international study found that the risk for metastasis may be as high as even 10% at 5 years for biopsy-proven iris melanomas [58].

Depending on tumor size, location, seeding, and other factors, such as secondary glaucoma and cataract formation, observation, fine-needle aspiration biopsy (FNAB), incisional biopsy, excision of the tumor, plaque radiotherapy, or enucleation may be recommended [54, 59]. For the nodular iris melanoma, typically, sector iridectomy via a large corneoscleral or scleral flap incision is performed. Hood et al. described a minimally invasive technique for the complete resection of small, circumscribed melanocytic tumors (≤5.0 mm in size, ≤2.5 mm in thickness) via small corneal incisions and guarded hydroaspiration [60]. If there is evidence of iris root or angle involvement, however, partial iridocyclectomy or iridogoniocyclectomy is recommended, respectively [54]. If there is diffuse seeding or involvement of iris, FNAB of the primary lesion can be first performed to exclude other etiologies (e.g., iris melanocytoma, juvenile xanthogranuloma), but once the diagnosis of iris melanoma is confirmed histologically, plaque brachytherapy, proton beam radiotherapy, or enucleation may be advised [54, 59].

6.1 Small-Incision Guarded Hydroaspiration of Small Iris Melanomas

To reduce the risk of hyphema, hypotony, wound leak, astigmatism, and delayed visual recovery associated with traditional sector iridectomy while avoiding unwanted tumor dissemination, Singh and colleagues developed a minimally invasive surgical technique for the en bloc resection of small, circumscribed melanocytic tumors (≤5.0 mm in size, ≤2.5 mm in thickness) with at least 2.0 mm of uninvolved peripheral iris [60]. In this technique, a single 2–3 mm, beveled, clear corneal incision is created in the quadrant opposite the tumor, and one to three secondary corneal incisions are made using a paracentesis blade [59]. Then, radial iris incisions approximately 1.0 mm beyond the tumor margins and a curvilinear basal iris incision are created using straight and curved vitrectomy scissors, respectively, with viscoelastic stabilizing the anterior chamber. Once the tumor is resected en bloc, the primary corneal incision is enlarged, and clear plastic tubing of 3.5 mm diameter with a beveled tip (previously primed with viscoelastic and attached to a 3.0 mL syringe) is inserted into the anterior chamber to slowly aspirate the excised iris wedge. The tubing, containing the excised lesion, is then carefully withdrawn from the anterior chamber, avoiding unwanted seeding of the wound bed. When feasible, pupilloplasty is then performed with 10-0 prolene suture using a modified Siepser slip-knot technique. Buried interrupted 10-0 nylon sutures are then used to close the primary and secondary corneal incisions, as needed, for watertight closure.

In a review of 22 patients with small, localized iris lesions resected by this technique, Singh reported complete resection with clear surgical margins in all neoplastic cases, 2 of which were benign, 1 borderline, and 16 malignant [59]. Of malignant cases, no local recurrence or metastasis was observed over a mean follow-up period of 33 months (range, 1–90 months), suggesting that the use of guarded aspiration may effectively avoid wound bed contamination at the time of tumor retrieval, although there is still a theoretical risk. Furthermore, the use of multiple small corneal incisions allows for significantly less postoperative morbidity (i.e., hyphema, hypotony, wound leak, corneal astigmatism, >2-line change in best-corrected visual acuity) compared to traditional sector iridectomy. However, traditional excisional approaches may be more suitable for tumors that are large, demonstrate diffuse configuration, extend to the iris root, or involve the ciliary body, but internal radial incisions can still be utilized in these cases to facilitate en bloc tumor removal.

7 Conclusion

Novel treatment strategies have significantly altered which treatment options can be considered first-line in patients with malignant ocular surface and iris tumors. With the advent of BRAF/MEK inhibitors and ICIs in oncotherapeutics, globe-sparing treatment is possible, with overall good response, but can be limited by the development of off-target effects, such as secondary cutaneous malignancies as well as immune-related adverse events (e.g., dermatitis, transaminitis, colitis, and pneumonitis), respectively. Furthermore, these novel systemic therapies may be well tolerated in elderly individuals as well as those with well-controlled, chronic viral infections. Monthly intralesional injections of rituximab have also been reported with durable clinical response in patients with low-grade conjunctival and iris lymphomas. Outcomes are also favorable in those with relapsed or refractory disease, even among patients who previously did not respond to systemic rituximab infusions. Supplementation with autologous serum has also been shown to improve clinical response in select patients. In patients with small iris melanomas, small-incision guarded hydroaspiration can reduce visual morbidity associated with traditional methods of tumor resection, with good outcomes. Given the rarity of these tumors, there are no randomized controlled clinical trials investigating the safety, efficacy, and long-term outcomes of these novel treatment strategies, but targeted molecular therapy for advanced conjunctival melanoma, immunotherapy for advanced conjunctival melanoma and squamous cell carcinoma, intralesional rituximab injections for conjunctival and iris lymphoma, and small-incision guarded hydroaspiration for small iris melanoma should be considered in the appropriate patients.

Acknowledgement It is partially supported by Richard N and Marilyn K Witham Professorship.

Conflicts of Interest HD is in advisory board for Castle Biosiences and investigator for Immunocore.

References

1. Vora GK, Demirci H, Marr B, Mruthyunjaya P. Advances in the management of conjunctival melanoma. Surv Ophthalmol. 2017;62(1):26–42.
2. Shields CL, Shields JA, Gunduz K, et al. Conjunctival melanoma: risk factors for recurrence, exenteration, metastasis, and death in 150 consecutive patients. Arch Ophthalmol. 2000;118(11):1497–507.
3. Esmaeli B, Wang X, Youssef A, Gershenwald JE. Patterns of regional and distant metastasis in patients with conjunctival melanoma: experience at a cancer center over four decades. Ophthalmology. 2001;108(11):2101–5.
4. Mor JM, Heindl LM. Systemic BRAF/MEK inhibitors as a potential treatment option in metastatic conjunctival melanoma. Ocul Oncol Pathol. 2017;3(2):133–41.
5. Weber JL, Smalley KS, Sondak VK, Gibney GT. Conjunctival melanomas harbor BRAF and NRAS mutations—letter. Clin Cancer Res. 2013;19(22):6329–30.
6. Maleka A, Astrom G, Bystrom P, Ullenhag GJ. A case report of a patient with metastatic ocular melanoma who experienced a response to treatment with the BRAF inhibitor vemurafenib. BMC Cancer. 2016;16:634.
7. Pahlitzsch M, Bertelmann E, Mai C. Conjunctival melanoma and BRAF inhibitor therapy. J Clin Exp Ophthalmol. 2014;5(1):322.
8. Pinto Torres S, Andre T, Gouveia E, et al. Systemic treatment of metastatic conjunctival melanoma. Case Rep Oncol Med. 2017;2017:4623964.
9. Larkin J, Ascierto PA, Dreno B, et al. Combined vemurafenib and cobimetinib in BRAF-mutated melanoma. N Engl J Med. 2014;371(20):1867–76.
10. Robert C, Karaszewska B, Schachter J, et al. Improved overall survival in melanoma with combined dabrafenib and trametinib. N Engl J Med. 2015;372(1):30–9.
11. Kim JM, Weiss S, Sinard JH, Pointdujour-Lim R. Dabrafenib and trametinib for BRAF-mutated conjunctival melanoma. Ocul Oncol Pathol. 2020;6(1):35–8.
12. Rossi E, Maiorano BA, Pagliara MM, et al. Dabrafenib and trametinib in BRAF mutant metastatic conjunctival melanoma. Front Oncol. 2019;9:232.
13. Demirci H, Demirci FY, Ciftci S, et al. Integrative exome and transcriptome analysis of conjunctival melanoma and its potential application for personalized therapy. JAMA Ophthalmol. 2019;137(12):1444–8.
14. Kiyohara T, Tanimura H, Miyamoto M, et al. Two cases of BRAF-mutated, bulbar conjunctival melanoma, and review of the published literature. Clin Exp Dermatol. 2020;45(2):207–11.
15. Dagi Glass LR, Lawrence DP, Jakobiec FA, Freitag SK. Conjunctival melanoma responsive to combined systemic BRAF/MEK inhibitors. Ophthalmic Plast Reconstr Surg. 2017;33(5):e114–e6.
16. Schadendorf D, Hodi FS, Robert C, et al. Pooled analysis of long-term survival data from phase II and phase III trials of ipilimumab in unresectable or metastatic melanoma. J Clin Oncol. 2015;33(17):1889–94.
17. Ascierto PA, Long GV, Robert C, et al. Survival outcomes in patients with previously untreated BRAF wild-type advanced melanoma treated with nivolumab therapy: three-year follow-up of a randomized phase 3 trial. JAMA Oncol. 2019;5(2):187–94.
18. Hamid O, Robert C, Daud A, et al. Five-year survival outcomes for patients with advanced melanoma treated with pembrolizumab in KEYNOTE-001. Ann Oncol. 2019;30(4):582–8.
19. Cao J, Brouwer NJ, Richards KE, et al. PD-L1/PD-1 expression and tumor-infiltrating lymphocytes in conjunctival melanoma. Oncotarget. 2017;8(33):54722–34.
20. Kini A, Fu R, Compton C, et al. Pembrolizumab for recurrent conjunctival melanoma. JAMA Ophthalmol. 2017;135(8):891–2.
21. Chaves LJ, Huth B, Augsburger JJ, Correa ZM. Eye-sparing treatment for diffuse invasive conjunctival melanoma. Ocul Oncol Pathol. 2018;4(4):261–6.
22. Hong BY, Ford JR, Glitza IC, et al. Immune checkpoint inhibitor therapy as an eye-preserving treatment for locally advanced conjunctival melanoma. Ophthalmic Plast Reconstr Surg. 2021;37(1):e9–e13.
23. Chang M, Lally SE, Dalvin LA, et al. Conjunctival melanoma with orbital invasion and liver metastasis managed with systemic immune checkpoint inhibitor therapy. Indian J Ophthalmol. 2019;67(12):2071–3.
24. Finger PT, Pavlick AC. Checkpoint inhibition immunotherapy for advanced local and systemic conjunctival melanoma: a clinical case series. J Immunother Cancer. 2019;7(1):83.
25. Sagiv O, Thakar SD, Kandl TJ, et al. Immunotherapy with programmed cell death 1 inhibitors for 5 patients with conjunctival melanoma. JAMA Ophthalmol. 2018;136(11):1236–41.
26. Ford J, Thuro BA, Thakar S, et al. Immune checkpoint inhibitors for treatment of metastatic melanoma of the orbit and ocular adnexa. Ophthalmic Plast Reconstr Surg. 2017;33(4):e82–e5.
27. Brahmer JR, Tykodi SS, Chow LQ, et al. Safety and activity of anti-PD-L1 antibody in patients with advanced cancer. N Engl J Med. 2012;366(26):2455–65.
28. Antoun J, Titah C, Cochereau I. Ocular and orbital side-effects of checkpoint inhibitors: a review article. Curr Opin Oncol. 2016;28(4):288–94.
29. Bitton K, Michot JM, Barreau E, et al. Prevalence and clinical patterns of ocular complications associated with anti-PD-1/PD-L1 anticancer immunotherapy. Am J Ophthalmol. 2019;202:109–17.
30. Shields CL, Chien JL, Surakiatchanukul T, et al. Conjunctival tumors: review of clinical features, risks, biomarkers, and outcomes—the 2017 J. Donald M. Gass Lecture. Asia Pac J Ophthalmol (Phila). 2017;6(2):109–20.
31. Sayed-Ahmed IO, Palioura S, Galor A, Karp CL. Diagnosis and medical management of ocular surface squamous neoplasia. Expert Rev Ophthalmol. 2017;12(1):11–9.
32. Ramberg I, Heegaard S, Prause JU, et al. Squamous cell dysplasia and carcinoma of the conjunctiva. A nationwide, retrospective, epidemiological study of Danish patients. Acta Ophthalmol. 2015;93(7):663–6.
33. Galor A, Karp CL, Oellers P, et al. Predictors of ocular surface squamous neoplasia recurrence after excisional surgery. Ophthalmology. 2012;119(10):1974–81.
34. Demirci H, Elner VM, Demirci FY, et al. Immunotherapy for conjunctival squamous cell carcinoma with orbital extension. Ophthalmology. 2021;128(5):801–4.
35. Nagarajan P, El-Hadad C, Gruschkus SK, et al. PD-L1/PD1 expression, composition of tumor-associated immune infiltrate, and HPV status in conjunctival squamous cell carcinoma. Invest Ophthalmol Vis Sci. 2019;60(6):2388–98.
36. Wolkow N, Jakobiec FA, Afrogheh AH, et al. PD-L1 and PD-L2 expression levels are low in primary and secondary adenoid cystic carcinomas of the orbit: therapeutic implications. Ophthalmic Plast Reconstr Surg. 2020;36(5):444–50.
37. Kirkegaard MM, Rasmussen PK, Coupland SE, et al. Conjunctival lymphoma—an international multicenter retrospective study. JAMA Ophthalmol. 2016;134(4):406–14.
38. Shome D, Esmaeli B. Targeted monoclonal antibody therapy and radioimmunotherapy for lymphoproliferative disorders of the ocular adnexa. Curr Opin Ophthalmol. 2008;19(5):414–21.
39. Tanenbaum RE, Galor A, Dubovy SR, Karp CL. Classification, diagnosis, and management of conjunctival lymphoma. Eye Vis (Lond). 2019;6:22.
40. Tuncer S, Tanyildiz B, Basaran M, et al. Systemic rituximab immunotherapy in the management of primary ocular adnexal lymphoma: single institution experience. Curr Eye Res. 2015;40(8):780–5.

41. Ferreri AJ, Govi S, Colucci A, et al. Intralesional rituximab: a new therapeutic approach for patients with conjunctival lymphomas. Ophthalmology. 2011;118(1):24–8.
42. Rodriguez Villa S, Ruiz Rodriguez MJ, Vargas PM. Intralesional rituximab in primary conjunctival follicular lymphoma relapsed. Arch Soc Esp Oftalmol. 2017;92(7):326–9.
43. Demirci H, Ozgonul C, Diniz Grisolia AB, Elner VM. Intralesional rituximab injection for low-grade conjunctival lymphoma management. Ophthalmology. 2020;127(9):1270–3.
44. Ferreri AJM, Sassone M, Miserocchi E, et al. Treatment of MALT lymphoma of the conjunctiva with intralesional rituximab supplemented with autologous serum. Blood Adv. 2020;4(6):1013–9.
45. Takami A, Hayashi T, Kita D, et al. Treatment of primary central nervous system lymphoma with induction of complement-dependent cytotoxicity by intraventricular administration of autologous-serum-supplemented rituximab. Cancer Sci. 2006;97(1):80–3.
46. Blasi MA, Tiberti AC, Valente P, et al. Intralesional interferon-alpha for conjunctival mucosa-associated lymphoid tissue lymphoma: long-term results. Ophthalmology. 2012;119(3):494–500.
47. Bahrami B, Greenwell T, Muecke JS. Long-term outcomes after adjunctive topical 5-flurouracil or mitomycin C for the treatment of surgically excised, localized ocular surface squamous neoplasia. Clin Exp Ophthalmol. 2014;42(4):317–22.
48. Kakkassery V, Md P, Coupland Se MP, Heindl Lm Md PM. Iris lymphoma-a systematic guide for diagnosis and treatment. Surv Ophthalmol. 2021;66(1):41–53.
49. Mashayekhi A, Shields CL, Shields JA. Iris involvement by lymphoma: a review of 13 cases. Clin Exp Ophthalmol. 2013;41(1):19–26.
50. Savino G, Battendieri R, Gari M, et al. Long-term outcomes of primary ocular adnexal lymphoma treatment with intraorbital rituximab injections. J Cancer Res Clin Oncol. 2013;139(7):1251–5.
51. Larkin KL, Saboo US, Comer GM, et al. Use of intravitreal rituximab for treatment of vitreoretinal lymphoma. Br J Ophthalmol. 2014;98(1):99–103.
52. Demirci H, Grant JS, Elner VM. Intralesional rituximab for primary iris lymphoma. JAMA Ophthalmol. 2015;133(1):104–5.
53. Kim H, Csaky KG, Chan CC, et al. The pharmacokinetics of rituximab following an intravitreal injection. Exp Eye Res. 2006;82(5):760–6.
54. Shields CL, Shields JA, Materin M, et al. Iris melanoma: risk factors for metastasis in 169 consecutive patients. Ophthalmology. 2001;108(1):172–8.
55. Jager MJ, Shields CL, Cebulla CM, et al. Uveal melanoma. Nat Rev Dis Primers. 2020;6(1):24.
56. Jensen OA. Malignant melanomas of the human uvea. Recent follow-up of cases in Denmark, 1943-1952. Acta Ophthalmol. 1970;48(6):1113–28.
57. Rones B, Zimmerman LE. The prognosis of primary tumors of the iris treated by iridectomy. AMA Arch Ophthalmol. 1958;60(2):193–205.
58. Khan S, Finger PT, Yu GP, et al. Clinical and pathologic characteristics of biopsy-proven iris melanoma: a multicenter international study. Arch Ophthalmol. 2012;130(1):57–64.
59. Singh AD. Small incision guarded hydroaspiration of iris lesions. Br J Ophthalmol. 2017;101(11):1570–5.
60. Hood CT, Schoenfield LR, Torres V, Singh AD. Iris melanoma. Ophthalmology. 2011;118(1):221–2.

Recent Developments in the Management of Orbital and Periocular Neoplasms

Jeremy A. Goldfarb and Bita Esmaeli

1 Eyelid and Periocular Melanoma

Melanoma of the periocular region is rare, comprising less than 2% of all eyelid lesions [1, 2]. It may arise on eyelid skin, conjunctiva, or both. Eyelid skin melanoma behaves similarly to cutaneous melanoma in other anatomic sites and thus histologic features such as tumor thickness (Breslow thickness), presence of ulceration (microscopic, histologic ulceration), and mitotic figures are correlated with the risk of nodal and distant metastases and disease-free survival [3, 4]. The status of sentinel lymph node (SLN) is viewed as the single most important prognostic factor for patients with early-stage cutaneous melanoma [5].

The majority of patients with newly diagnosed eyelid melanoma have early-stage disease. In such patients, surgery is the treatment of choice and is curative in most cases [6]. Two significant recent advances that will be highlighted in this section in relation to management of periocular melanomas are sentinel lymph node (SLN) biopsy for identifying microscopic nodal metastasis and availability of targeted therapy and immune checkpoint inhibitors for patients with metastatic or locally advanced melanoma.

1.1 Sentinel Node Biopsy for Conjunctival and Periocular Melanomas

Status of local lymph nodes is a major prognostic factor and is highly correlated with survival in patients with cutaneous and conjunctival melanoma [7–9]. Sentinel lymph node biopsy is a method of biopsying one or two lymph nodes that drain the lymphatics from a given anatomic region. The sentinel lymph node(s) that are biopsied are then carefully evaluated through breadloafing and careful pathologic evaluation, to find microscopic metastasis. The technique used at our center entails the injection of 0.3–0.4 mci of technetium in 0.2 cc volume around the site of the primary lesion by the ophthalmic plastic surgeon 24 h prior to surgery [8]. For conjunctival lesions, the injection is subconjunctival and for periocular skin melanoma, the injection is intradermal. Preoperative lymphoscintigraphy and more recently single-photon emission computerized tomography/computed tomography (SPECT/CT) scans (Fig. 1) are obtained prior to surgery to help with localization of the sentinel lymph node. Intraoperatively, a handheld gamma probe is used transcutaneously to confirm increased radioactivity overlying a lymph node basin. The sentinel lymph nodes are then dissected out and sent for histopathologic evaluation.

In a recent American Academy of Ophthalmology Technology Transfer review article, the authors reported that there have been 127 reported cases of sentinel lymph node biopsy for periocular melanoma; 85 of these are conjunctival and 42 are eyelid cutaneous melanoma [10]. Of these patients, 19 (15%) were found to have tumor-positive sentinel node biopsy result. Included in this group, is the largest single cohort of 51 patients from our institution that had a similar positivity rate of 20%, or 10 patients [8]. The median number of SLN sampled was 2 and the most common lymph node basins sampled were the intraparotid and level 2. This publication also demonstrated that certain key histological features correlate with risk of positive SLN biopsy; tumor thickness, greater number of mitotic figures, and presence of histologic ulceration. Importantly, this study and others, examining SLN biopsy for different periocular cancers, have shown excellent safety profile with adverse events reported in 17 of 197 patients [10]. These included seven cases of transient conjunctival staining with blue dye, seven patients with transient facial nerve weakness, one case of neck hematoma, and one case of suture abscess [10].

The role of positive sentinel node biopsy in further management decisions is evolving, especially in the context of

J. A. Goldfarb · B. Esmaeli (✉)
Orbital Oncology & Ophthalmic Plastic Surgery, Department of Plastic Surgery, The University of Texas MD Anderson Cancer Center, Houston, TX, USA
e-mail: JGoldfarb@mdanderson.org; besmaeli@mdanderson.org

B. V. Chawla, M. E. Aronow (eds.), *Global Perspectives in Ocular Oncology*, https://doi.org/10.1007/978-3-031-08250-4_31

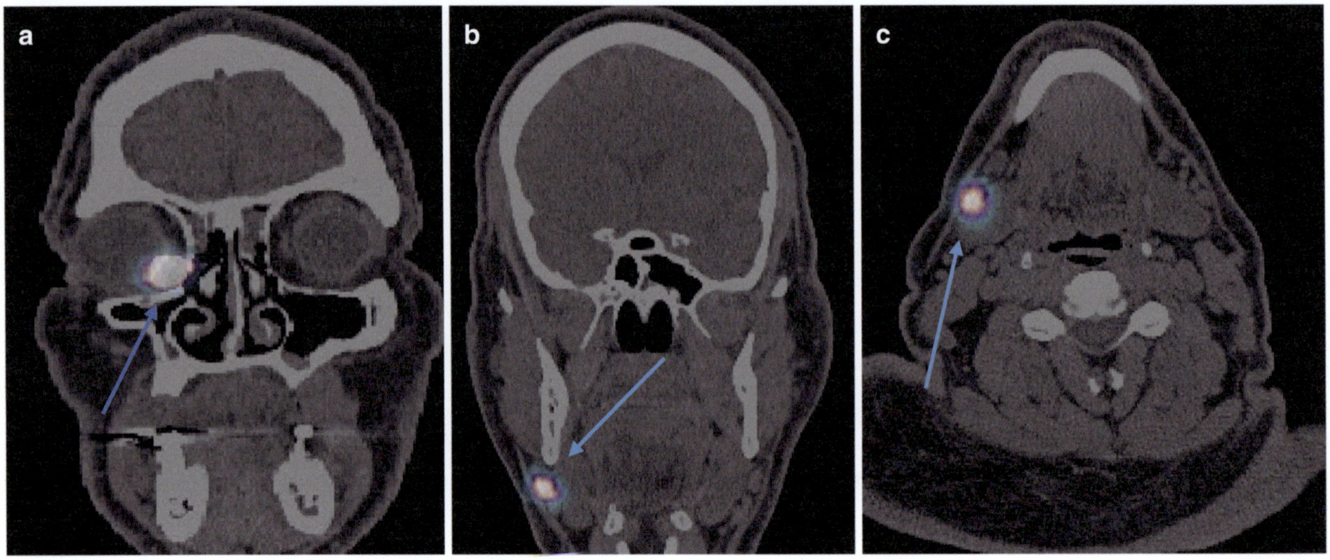

Fig. 1 (**a**) SPECT/CT scan in a patient with caruncular conjunctival melanoma demonstrating the area of injection of technetium in the subconjunctival space in the right caruncular area (arrow). (**b**) A coronal image showing the draining sentinel lymph node in the submandibular basin (arrow). (**c**) An axial image showing the same draining sentinel lymph node (arrow)

emerging therapies. Historically, of the 127 reports of SLN biopsy for periocular melanoma, treatment is reported in 7 cases and includes completion of neck dissection, parotidectomy, radiation therapy, immunotherapy, and experimental melanoma vaccine therapy [10]. Treatments are tailored to the individual patient. The recent availability of effective immune checkpoint inhibitor therapy is rapidly changing the management of patients with positive SLN biopsy results in favor of immune checkpoint inhibitor therapy rather than parotidectomy, neck dissection, or adjuvant radiation therapy [11].

1.2 Targeted and Immunotherapy for Periocular Melanomas

1.2.1 Targeted Therapies

BRAF kinase plays a key role in cell growth and proliferation and is encoded by the BRAF gene. The BRAF mutation is found in 66% of cutaneous melanomas, 90% of which is the specific V600E mutation [12, 13]. This mutated protein results in abnormal activation of the MAPK signaling cascade and results in increased survival and proliferation of affected cells. Currently, there are three U.S. Food and Drug Administration (FDA)-approved BRAF inhibitors. Vemurafenib (Zelboraf®, Genentech) was FDA-approved in 2011 for the treatment of unresectable or metastatic melanoma, in patients with confirmed V600E mutation [14]. Dabrafenib (Tafinlar®, Novartis) was FDA-approved in 2013 for the treatment of V600E-positive, unresectable or metastatic melanoma. It is also approved in combination with trametinib (Mekinist, Novartis), an MEK inhibitor, as adjuvant therapy in patients with positive lymph nodes following complete melanoma resection or as first-line therapy for V600E- or V600K-positive unresectable or metastatic melanoma [15]. The most recently approved BRAF inhibitor is encorafenib (Braftovi®, Array BioPharma Inc), which is approved in combination with binimetinib (Mektovi®, Array BioPharma), an MEK inhibitor, for the treatment of unresectable or metastatic melanoma with V600E or V600K mutation. The addition of MEK inhibitors to BRAF inhibitors improves disease-free survival in patients with metastatic melanoma compared with BRAF inhibitor therapy alone [16].

Clinical trials using BRAF inhibitors alone have shown overall response rate of 40–54%, progression-free survival of 6–9 months, and overall survival of 17–19 months [16]. Patients treated with BRAF inhibitors in combination with an MEK inhibitor show improved outcomes, with a response rate of 63–76%, progression-free survival of 9–15 months, and an overall survival of 22–34 months [16]. Due to the synergistic efficacy of BRAF and MEK inhibitors, combination therapy has largely replaced BRAF inhibitor monotherapy. There are few published case reports investigating BRAF inhibitor therapy for eyelid or conjunctival melanoma [17–20]. All reported cases demonstrated clinical response, with progression-free survival ranging from 4 to 23 months. Yet, despite these encouraging results, resistance to treatment develops in many cases with re-growth of previously responsive metastasis [21].

The most common side effects of BRAF inhibitors include arthralgia, alopecia, nausea, pruritus, photosensitivity, fatigue, and skin rash [22]. The combination of BRAF inhibitors and MEK inhibitors has been found to significantly increase certain adverse events including pyrexia, chills, hypertension, vomiting, liver toxicity, and ocular side effects such as central serous chorioretinopathy and retinal detachment [23]. BRAF inhibitor monotherapy has also been associated with an increased rate of squamous cell carcinoma (SCC) in up to 12.5% of patients versus 3% in patients treated with BRAF and MEK inhibitor combination therapy [24, 25].

1.2.2 Immune Checkpoint Inhibitors

Improved understanding of the pathophysiology of melanoma, coupled with discoveries related to the role of the immune system in tumor control, has yielded a new class of systemic medication for locally advanced and/or metastatic melanoma and for many other cancer types called immune checkpoint inhibitors. Programmed cell death protein 1 (PD-1) and cytotoxic T-lymphocyte antigen 4 (CTLA-4) are proteins found on the surface of activated T-lymphocytes. When these surface proteins are activated, they halt the proliferation of cancer fighting T-cells. It is thought that abnormal activation of these immune checkpoints (PD-1 and CTLA-4) prevents the activation of T-lymphocytes and allows evasion by host immune response and proliferation of cancer cells. Development and now commercial availability of monoclonal antibodies directed against PD-1 and CTLA-4 have revolutionized the management of patients with metastatic melanoma by improving disease-free and overall survivals in such patients. Several immune checkpoint inhibitors have been approved by the U.S. Food and Drug Administration (FDA) over the last 10 years, with expanding indications. Ipilimumab (Yervoy®, Bristol-Myers Squibb) is a CTLA-4 inhibitor approved by the FDA in 2011 [26]. It is indicated for the treatment of adult and pediatric patients with metastatic or unresectable melanoma, as well as an adjuvant therapy for patients with cutaneous melanoma and pathologically confirmed lymph node involvement of more than 1 mm who have undergone complete resection, including lymphadenectomy. Nivolumab (Opdivo®, Bristol-Myers Squibb) and pembrolizumab (Keytruda®, Merck) are two FDA-approved anti-PD-1 agents approved in 2014 and are indicated in the treatment of metastatic or unresectable melanoma, and as adjuvant therapy in patients with metastatic or lymph node involvement after complete resection [27, 28]. Pivotal multicenter, prospective, randomized trials have shown improved survival in patients with unresectable or metastatic melanoma treated with ipilimumab [29, 30], pembrolizumab [31], and nivolumab [32]. Studies show that the combination of ipilimumab with nivolumab or pembrolizumab increases efficacy but is also associated with increased toxicity [33].

There are emerging, promising results in case reports and series that support the use of immune checkpoint inhibitors in the periocular region. Sagiv et al. [34] reported on 5 cases of metastatic conjunctival melanoma treated with nivolumab or pembrolizumab, 4 of which had complete response with no evidence of disease at 1–36 months after treatment completion. Other case reports and series have demonstrated similar partial or complete response with this class of medication [35–38].

It should be noted that immune checkpoint inhibitors are associated with significant immune-related adverse events. Different from traditional chemotherapy reaction, immunotherapy side effects result from over-activation of the immune system. Common adverse events including enterocolitis, dermatitis, hepatitis, thyroiditis, arthritis, and myositis have all been reported but can be mitigated with medical treatment with steroids or similar anti-inflammatory strategies. The incidence of fatal events is between 0.3 and 1.3%, and most fatal events are due to colitis, pneumonitis, or hepatitis. Ten percent of patients will have a grade 3 or worse reaction, and the common side effects include fatigue and rash, diarrhea, and endocrinopathies [40]. Treatment of these side effects is systemic immunosuppression, most commonly steroids, in a targeted fashion, and most resolve without lasting complications [41]. Immunotherapy is also costly. Therefore, the use of immune checkpoint therapy in the periocular region should be reserved for locally advanced, surgically unresectable, and/or metastatic disease (Fig. 2).

2 Eyelid and Periocular Squamous Cell Carcinoma

Cutaneous squamous cell carcinoma (SCC) is the second most common eyelid malignancy accounting for 5–10% of all eyelid cancers [42–44]. SCC has a reported rate of local recurrence that ranges from 6.8 to 36.9% [45–48] and a propensity for perineural invasion (PNI) along cranial nerves in up to 25% of patients [45, 46]. Distant metastasis is rare (0.8–6.2%) [48–51] and regional nodal metastasis ranges from 1.3 to 24% [45, 46, 49, 52].

Surgical excision with histologic confirmation of tumor-free margins on frozen section is the standard treatment for most patients with eyelid and periorbital SCC [52–54]. In locally advanced cases or in the presence of PNI, postoperative adjuvant radiation therapy, concurrent chemo-radiation therapy, or immunotherapy may be considered to improve local control or to treat metastatic disease. In a recent series of 109 patients with eyelid and periorbital SCC from our center, 59 patients (54%) had eye-sparing surgery with frozen section control of margins, and 34 patients (31%) had eye-sparing surgery with frozen section control of margins followed by adjuvant radiotherapy or concurrent chemoradiation. Thirteen additional patients (12%) had orbital exenteration followed by adjuvant radiotherapy or chemoradiation. Thirty-six of the 40 patients with PNI (90%) received adju-

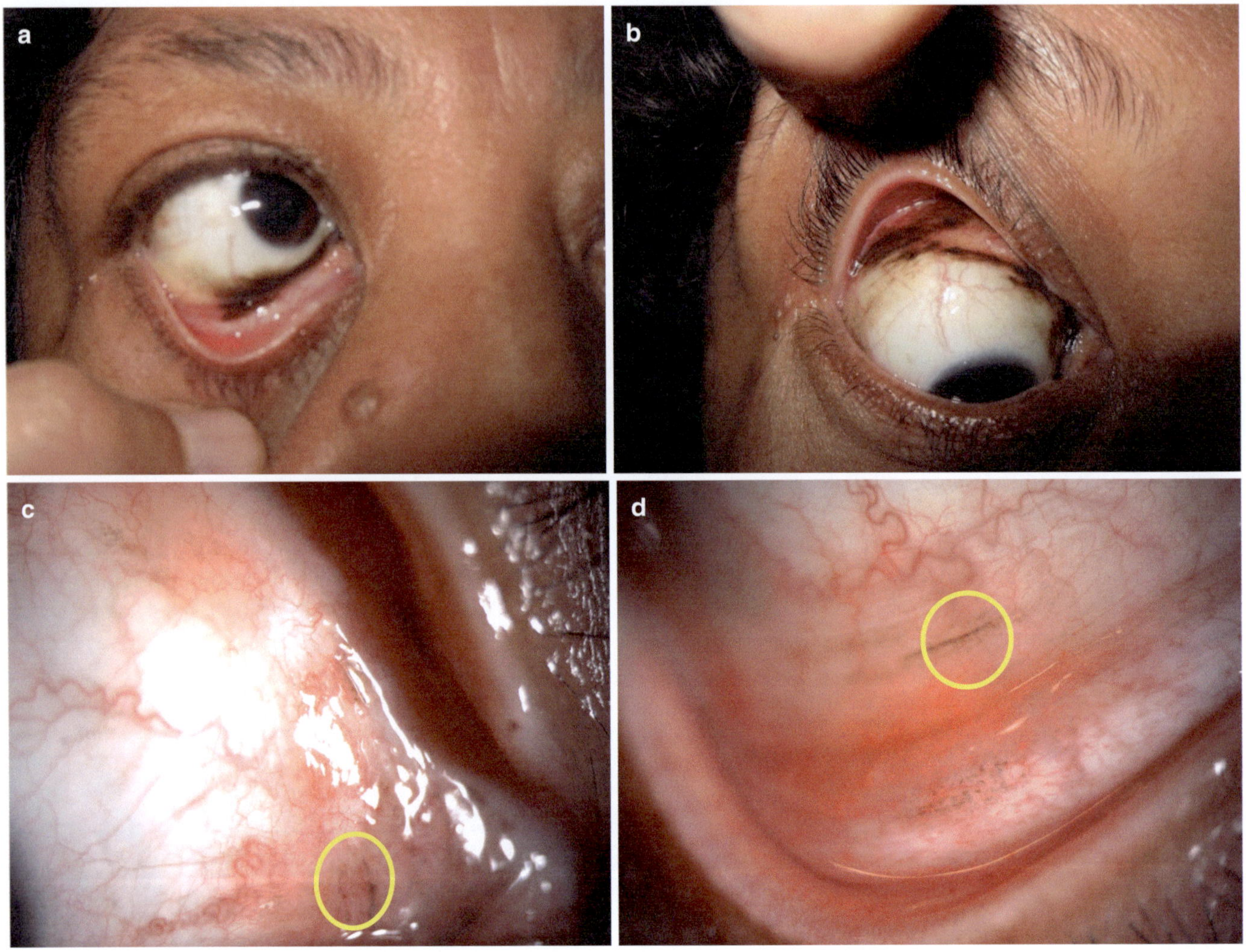

Fig. 2 (**a**, **b**) External photographs of a 58-year-old woman with a biopsy-proven conjunctival melanoma that involved all four quadrants and also both the upper and lower eyelid tarsal and palpebral conjunctiva and caruncle. (**c**, **d**) Slit lamp photographs of the only remaining areas of faint pigmentation (yellow circles) remaining after 12 months of treatment with nivolumab. These areas were biopsied and found to contain macrophages with pigment, and no residual melanoma. Patient has remained without evidence of disease for 2 years after end of treatment with nivolumab

vant radiotherapy [45]. Overall, slightly over 40% of patients had adjuvant radiation or concurrent chemo-radiation therapy.

Historically, cytotoxic chemotherapy (e.g., cisplatin, doxorubicin, bleomycin, peplomycin, methotrexate, 5-fluorouracil) was used for patients with locally advanced or metastatic squamous carcinoma. However, these older drugs have fallen to second- and third-line options in favor of the more recently available targeted therapies such as epidermal growth factor receptor (EGFR) inhibitors and immunotherapy. In this section, we will focus on advances made in the treatment of locally advanced and/or metastatic periocular SCC using EGFR-based targeted therapy and immune checkpoint inhibitor therapy as recent advances in the management of periocular cutaneous SCC.

2.1 Epidermal Growth Factor Receptor (EGFR) Inhibitors for Locally Advanced Periocular SCC

EGFR is a transmembrane receptor protein that is involved in proliferation of keratinocytes, cellular migration, and increased survival and resistance to apoptosis [55, 56]. Overexpression of EGFR has been found in cutaneous SCC [57].

Several EGFR inhibitors (cetuximab, panitumumab, gefitinib, lapatinib, erlotinib) are approved by the U.S. FDA, and are typically used either as single agent or in combination with other chemotherapy for treatment of patients with metastatic or locally advanced head and neck squamous cell carcinoma (HNSCC) [58]. Cetuximab (Erbitux, Lilly) is a monoclonal antibody EGFR inhibitor that is FDA-approved to treat locally or regionally advanced head and neck SCC (HNSCC) in combination with radiation therapy or recurrent or metastatic HNSCC progressing after treatment with platinum-based therapy. Erlotinib (Tarceva, Genentech) is an oral drug, a small-molecule tyrosine kinase EGFR inhibitor, that has been studied as an off-label potential treatment for locally advanced HNSCC [59]. Addition of EGFR inhibitors to radiation therapy as adjuvant therapy has improved locoregional control in patients with locally advanced HNSCC in several large-scale multi-institution phase III trials [59, 60].

EGFR is overexpressed in cutaneous SCC as well as in conjunctival SCC [61]. For patients with recurrent periocular SCC with orbital invasion and/or with regional metastasis secondary to periocular cutaneous SCC, both cetuximab and erlotinib have been used successfully with good responses in a few cases published by our group [62]. Cetuximab in combination with platinum-based chemotherapy can also be used in the neoadjuvant setting to chemo-reduce large periorbital SCC, such as primary lacrimal sac/duct carcinomas, to decrease surgical morbidity (Fig. 3).

The side effects of EGFR inhibitors are relatively minor and include an acneiform rash, pruritus, nail changes, diarrhea, and secondary infections. More specifically, the following ocular side effects have also been reported: mild superficial keratopathy, and notably trichomegaly, and rarely uveitis [63, 64].

2.2 Immune Checkpoint Inhibitors for Locally Advanced or Metastatic Periocular SCC

The discovery of immune checkpoints, specifically programmed cell death protein 1 (PD-1), has revolutionized the management of patients with locally advanced or metastatic squamous carcinoma. This class of drugs was first approved for use in melanoma (please see detailed discussion above in the section on periocular melanoma) but are now also approved for use in patients with locally advanced cutaneous SCC. Cemiplimab (Libtayo, Regeneron Pharmaceuticals, Tarrytown, NY, USA) and Pembrolizumab (Keytruda, Merck, Kenilworth, NJ, USA) are human monoclonal antibodies directed against programmed death 1 (PD-1) receptor, that are specifically FDA-approved in the USA for locally advanced or metastatic cutaneous SCC [65, 66]. Currently, immunotherapy is being employed as first-line treatment for cutaneous SCC that is metastatic, or locally advanced and not amenable to surgery and radiation [67]. For locally advanced cutaneous SCC, cemiplimab treatment has demonstrated a response rate of 12%, 36%, 31%, and 13% for progression, stable disease, partial response, and complete response, respectively [68]. Its role in these and other settings is the subject of 14 current prospective clinical trials at the time of the writing of this chapter [69]. Of these, two are neoadjuvant, seven are primary treatment, two are adjuvant, two are adjuvant and neoadjuvant, and one is for intralesional injection of cemiplimab. While new research supports the cost effectiveness of cemiplimab for advanced SCC when compared to traditional second-line chemotherapy [70], the cost and potential side effects of immunotherapy in the neoadjuvant setting have to be considered carefully in the treatment decisions and patient selection.

Currently, there are only case reports of the off-label use of pembrolizumab for locally advanced periocular SCC and the results have been promising [71]. At the time of this chapter's writing, our group has submitted a cohort of seven patients treated with cemiplimab (in six patients) and pembrolizumab (in one patient) for locally advanced periorbital SCC. Our findings in this cohort suggest that anti-PD-1 immunotherapy can be highly effective at reducing the size of locally advanced periorbital cutaneous SCC (Fig. 4). In all seven patients, measurable clinical and/or radiologic response was observed. In five patients, administration of immunotherapy was followed by surgery with or without postoperative radiation therapy. In two patients with multiple recurrent periorbital SCC heavily pretreated with surgery and radiation and with massive perineural invasion involving the skull base, surgery was not done after immunotherapy as it was felt that the recurrent lesions were not surgically resectable. Both of these patients remained without evidence of disease at last follow-up, 17 months and 14 months, respectively, after completion of immunotherapy. The off-label use of immune checkpoint inhibitors in the neoadjuvant setting is an area of active study [39, 40].

Immune checkpoint inhibitors are generally safe, but serious immune-related adverse events are common and may require prompt management. Please see the section above under immunotherapy for periocular melanoma for a more detailed discussion of expected side effects with immunotherapy.

3 Eyelid and Periocular Basal Cell Carcinoma

Basal cell carcinoma (BCC) is the most common human cancer and comprises 90% of eyelid tumors [72]. Mortality rates from BCCs are rare and metastases rarely occur at a rate of 0.0028–0.5% [73, 74]. Typically, periocular BCC is amenable to surgical excision, with a 5-year recurrence rate of 1–5.3% [75]. Excision with intraoperative frozen sections and Mohs micrographic surgery (MMS) are the most commonly employed techniques for ensuring complete patho-

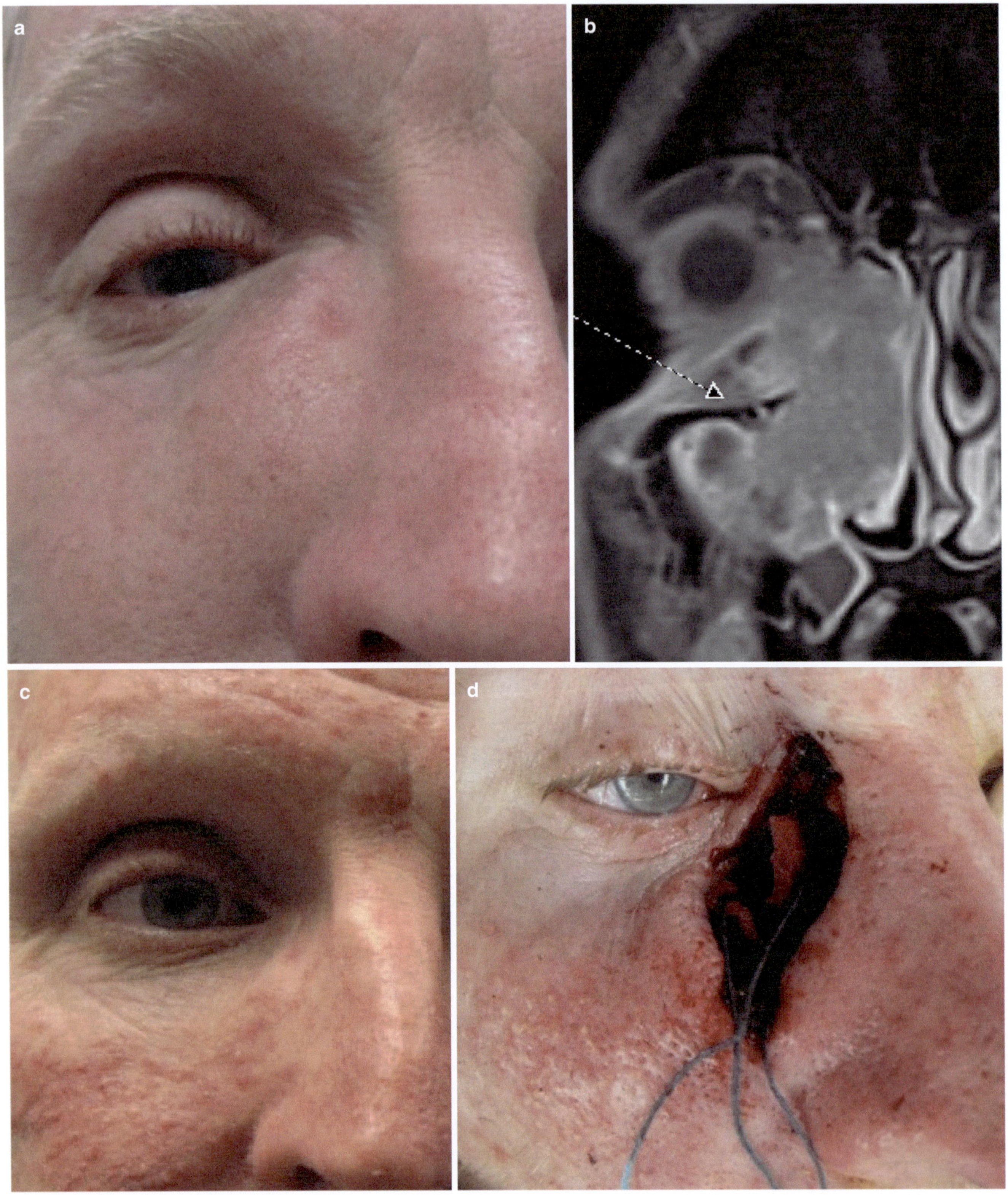

Fig. 3 (**a**) A 53-year-old man presented with a large squamous carcinoma of the right lacrimal sac/duct area. (**b**) Magnetic resonance imaging (MRI) in the same patient shows an infiltrative mass involving the lacrimal sac, nasolacrimal duct, and medial maxilla. (**c**) After three cycles of cetuximab plus carboplatin and paclitaxel, the mass in the medial canthal area is completely resolved; note the maculopapular rash on the face secondary to cetuximab. (**d**) After three cycles of neoadjuvant chemotherapy plus cetuximab, the patient had surgery; the surgical specimen showed a complete pathologic response with no tumor present

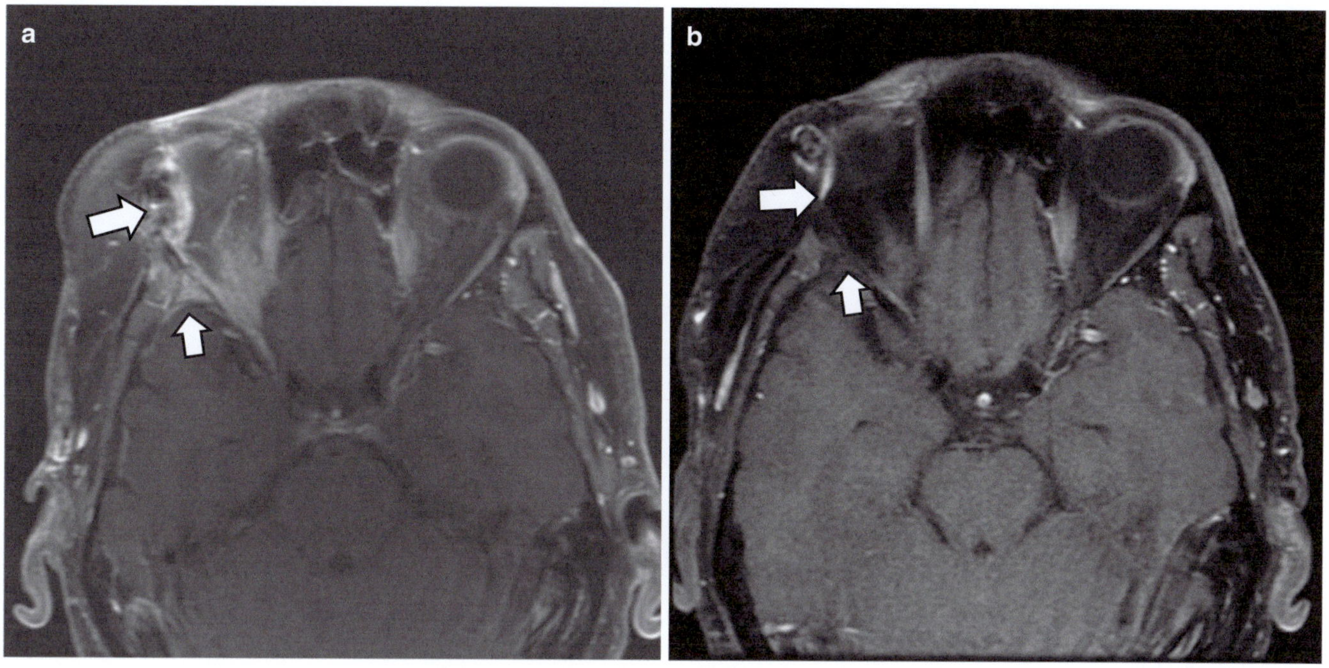

Fig. 4 (**a**) Axial-T1 post-contrast magnetic resonance (MR) image with fat-saturation shows abnormal enhancement at the right orbital apex and superotemporal right orbit (large arrows) as well as involving the right sphenoid bone (small arrow). (**b**) Axial-T1 post-contrast MR with fat-saturation demonstrates near complete resolution of the enhancement

logical excision and are associated with low local recurrence rates of 2.0% and 2.1%, respectively [76, 77]. For locally advanced periocular BCC, characterized by large tumor size or recurrent disease with extension into the orbit or paranasal sinuses, definitive surgical treatment may be impossible without significant ocular morbidity or removal of the eye and orbital contents. While surgery remains the preferred treatment modality, recent advances in the medical management of advanced periocular BCC will be the focus of the following segment.

3.1 Sonic Hedgehog Inhibitors

The discovery of mutations in the hedgehog pathway has enabled the emergence of targeted medical therapy for BCC [78]. The hedgehog pathway includes the Patched-1 transmembrane receptor (Ptch-1), which is a tumor suppressor. Ptch-1 normally inhibits the downstream receptor Smoothened (Smo) [79, 80]. A mutation in the hedgehog pathway leads to hedgehog protein binding to Ptch-1. This leads to a reversal of the normal inhibition of Smo, as well as expression of the downstream product GLI-1, which is thought to lead to the formation of BCC [80]. Medications that target this pathway can cause regression of BCC tumors.

Vismodegib (Erivedge®; Genentech) was the first sonic hedgehog inhibitor to be approved by the U.S. Food and Drug Administration (FDA) in 2012. Vismodegib is a selective hedgehog pathway inhibitor that blocks hedgehog signaling by binding to Smo, inhibiting downstream activation of hedgehog target genes [81]. Its approval was based on results from the ERIVANCE trial, which showed 43% and 30% response in patients with locally advanced BCC and metastatic BCC, respectively [82]. Adverse events were reported in 20% of patients and included muscle spasms, alopecia, dysgeusia, weight loss, fatigue, nausea, decrease in appetite, and diarrhea [82].

Since the ERIVANCE trial was published, the role for vismodegib in the periocular setting has been examined and refined. For periocular BCC treated with vismodegib, most patients show partial response, some have complete response, and a small subset will have stable disease [83]. The neoadjuvant use of vismodegib for locally advanced periocular BCC has been reported by our group at MD Anderson as an effective strategy in patients who would otherwise need an orbital exenteration or major disfiguring surgery (Fig. 5) [84]. In this cohort, patients were treated for a median of 14 months (4–36), underlining the need for long-term treatment to observe response. Also in this group, we observed that over half of patients achieved a complete response with no residual microscopic disease found at the time of surgery. Careful follow-up is needed to confirm long-term disease control.

Sonidegib (ODOMZO®, Novartis) is the second sonic hedgehog inhibitor approved by FDA in 2015 based on results from the phase 2 BOLT trial [85]. Similar to vismo-

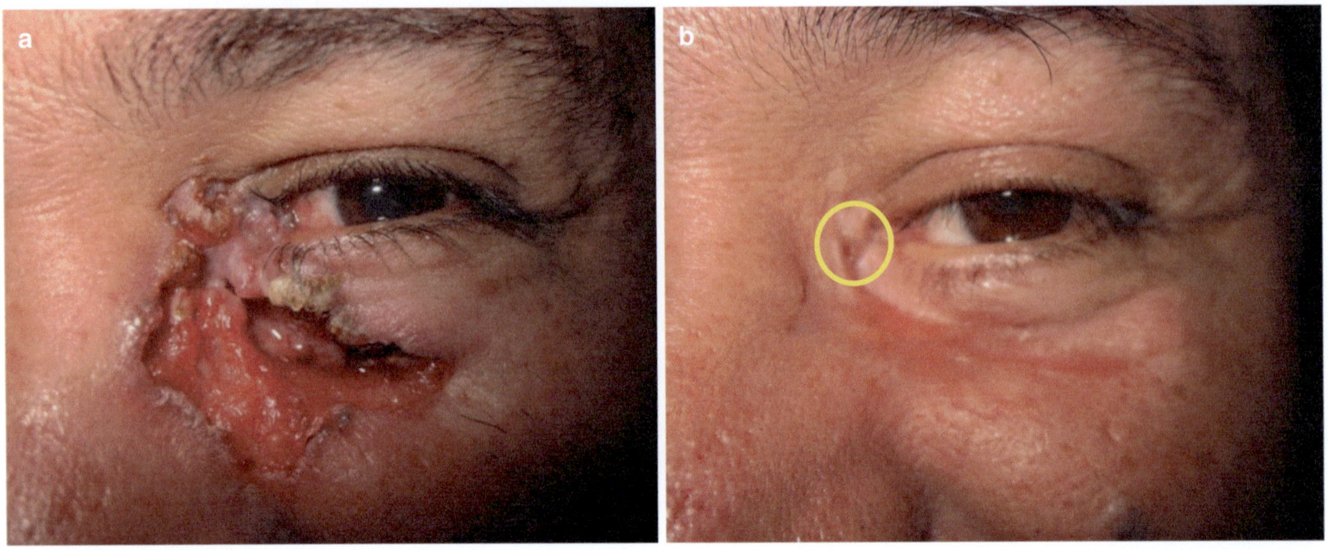

Fig. 5 (**a**) A 45-year-old man with a locally advanced recurrent basal cell carcinoma of the left medial canthus with anterior orbital soft tissue involvement and some bony erosion. (**b**) After 9 months of treatment with daily vismodegib, the lesion has nearly totally resolved based on clinical examination with the exception of a small residual area of ulceration noted (yellow circle). This area was excised surgically with negative margins and the scarred area in the left lower eyelid biopsied in multiple areas and found to have no tumor present

degib, sonidegib also binds Smo, inhibiting downstream activation of hedgehog target genes. Its efficacy in the BOLT trial was 34–36% response rate and it had a similar adverse event profile to vismodegib, including muscle spasms, dysgeusia, alopecia, nausea, elevated serum creatine kinase levels, weight loss, and fatigue [85].

Published reports on the specific use of sonidegib in the periocular region are limited to one published case showing complete response to treatment [86]. However, this is very likely due to the fact that sonidegib became available several years after vismodegib. Both drugs are very similar in their mechanism of action, expected efficacy in treatment of BCC, and their side effect profile.

3.2 Immune Checkpoint Inhibitors for Locally Advanced BCC

Pembrolizumab (Keytruda®, Merck) is a programmed cell death protein-1 (PD-1) inhibitor that has demonstrated efficacy in multiple cancer types, including squamous cell carcinoma and melanoma as mentioned earlier in this chapter. A nonrandomized, open-label study of patients with locally advanced BCC showed a response rate of 38% (6 of 16 patients) with pembrolizumab given with or without vismodegib [87]. Efficacy has also been shown in case reports of pembrolizumab for metastatic BCC that has failed hedgehog pathway inhibitors [88]. Overall, the off-label use of pembrolizumab in patients with locally advanced BCC is reserved for surgically unresectable or metastatic disease that is not responsive to vismodegib or sonidegib.

Cemiplimab (Libtayo®, Regeneron Pharmaceuticals) is a PD-1 inhibitor originally FDA-approved for patients with metastatic or locally advanced squamous cell carcinoma who are not candidates for curative surgery or radiotherapy [89]. Recently, cemiplimab received accelerated approval to expand its indication to include surgically unresectable or metastatic BCC that has failed treatment with a hedgehog inhibitor [89]. This approval was based on interim results of a phase 2 clinical trial for advanced or metastatic BCC that has failed or is intolerant to hedgehog inhibitors. Of 84 patients enrolled in the locally advanced arm of the study, 26 showed an objective response with 5 patients showing a complete response. Of the remaining patients, 41 had stable disease and only 9 had progression at a median follow-up of 15 months [90]. In the metastatic group, of 28 patients treated, 6 patients had partial response and 13 patients had stable disease [91].

4 Ocular Adnexal Lymphoma

The term ocular adnexal lymphoma (OAL) has been used to refer to lymphomas of the conjunctiva, orbit, and eyelid [92]. The vast majority of OAL is non-Hodgkin lymphoma (NHL). NHL is further classified based on its presumed cell of origin as defined by the World Health Organization (WHO) Classification of Tumors of Hematopoietic and Lymphoid Tissue [93]. Greater than 98% of ocular adnexal lymphomas are of B-cell NHL variety [92, 94]. OAL can develop primarily in the ocular adnexal area as the first and only site of manifestation of lymphoma or the ocular adnexal lymphoma may represent relapsed lymphoma with systemic involvement in other extraocular sites in the past [94]. While OAL accounts for only about 2% of all lymphomas, it is the most common primary orbital malignant neoplasm in adults [95]. Of note, OAL is usually low grade with marginal zone lymphoma accounting for 60–70% of cases followed by low-grade follicular lymphoma (FL) and diffuse large B-cell lymphoma (DLBCL) as the next most frequent histologic varieties [96]. OAL must be distinguished from intraocular lymphoma, which are typically a high-grade diffuse large B-cell lymphoma with a distinct therapeutic strategy [96].

Treatment of OAL depends on the histologic variety and stage of OAL at the time of diagnosis. The Ann Arbor Staging and, more recently, the american joint committee on cancer (AJCC) Cancer Staging Manual are the most common methods for staging of ocular adnexal lymphoma [97]. Initial steps in management of OAL entail a fresh tissue biopsy for lymphoma studies to establish the exact histologic subtype followed by staging work-up that usually includes a total body positron emission tomography (PET)/CT scan, a bone marrow biopsy, and an MRI of orbit if the lesion is suspected to have an orbital component on clinical grounds [98, 99].

We herein will highlight two recent advances in the management of OAL that are noteworthy: the "ultra-low-dose" radiation, the so-called "boom-boom" for low-grade OAL; and the use of rituximab in combination with other chemotherapy for management of diffuse large B-cell lymphoma and for low-grade OAL that involves extraocular sites.

4.1 Ultra-Low-Dose External Beam Radiation Therapy

External beam radiation therapy (EBRT) is the most commonly used treatment modality for OAL, particularly low-grade lymphomas such as extranodal marginal zone lymphoma (EMZL), follicular lymphoma (FL), and small lymphocytic lymphoma (SLL) without systemic involvement (i.e., stage IE by Ann Arbor staging criteria) [100, 101]. Historically, OAL was treated with moderate to high radiation doses, from 25 to 54 Gy [102–104]. These dosages yield excellent local control from 90 to 100%; however, there is some risk of ocular toxicity [105]. Late toxic side effects, including keratitis, severe dry eye syndrome, glaucoma, retinopathy, and cataracts, have been reported in up to 47% of patients treated with the higher-dose range of EBRT for OAL [104]. More recently, in a report by Pinnix et al. from our institution, we reported complete response or significant partial response in 100% of 22 patients with low-grade OAL who were treated with only 4 Gy of radiation, and only two sessions of radiotherapy—the so-called "boom-boom" regimen. This is a significantly lower radiation dose compared with "historical standard dose," is delivered over only 2 days (instead of 2–3 weeks), and is associated with negligible radiation-related ocular toxicity to date [106]. Complete response as defined by RECIST criteria [107] was observed in 86% of patients (Fig. 6), while 14% of patients experienced partial response. Only one of the 22 patients had very mild dry eye symptoms; no other ocular toxicity was seen in this report. We have completed a prospective trial of the same regimen of 4 Gy of radiation in 40 patients with low-grade OAL treated to date confirming essentially the same findings as was reported in our retrospective study. A report summarizing the findings in our prospective trial and long-term data on patients treated off-protocol for a total of approximately 70 patients with OAL treated with ultra-low-dose radiotherapy is currently under preparation.

4.2 Rituximab-Based Chemotherapy Regimens (R-CHOP, Rituximab, cyclophosphamide, vincristine sulfate, and prednisone (R-CVP), R-Bendamustine) for High-Grade OAL or Low-Grade OAL with Extraocular Sites of Involvement

Newer chemotherapy regimens add rituximab to well-established combination protocols such as CHOP—cyclophosphamide, hydroxydaunorubicin, oncovin, and prednisone—for diffuse large B-cell lymphoma (DLBCL). Prior to the addition of rituximab, the 3-year complete response rate and overall survival of patients with diffuse large B-cell lymphoma treated with CHOP was 40–50% and 35–40%, respectively [108]. The addition of rituximab increased the rate of complete response and overall survival to 60% and 76%, respectively, at 3 years and has become standard of care for DLBCL [108]. For patients with low-grade lymphomas, rituximab as single-agent monotherapy is associated with about 50% relapse rate [109]. The addition of bendamustine to rituximab as first-line therapy has yielded an overall survival of 96% at 4 years in patients with mucosal associated lymphoid tissue (MALT) lymphoma, which was significantly higher than rituximab alone or rituximab CHOP regimens [110].

5 Lacrimal Gland Carcinoma

Malignant epithelial tumors of the lacrimal gland include adenoid cystic carcinoma (ACC), carcinoma ex pleomorphic adenoma, adenocarcinoma, mucoepidermoid carcinoma, and a number of other rare variants. These cancers are quite rare with an overall incidence estimated at one per one million per year [111], ACC, which accounts for about 60% of cases of lacrimal gland carcinoma, is associated with a high

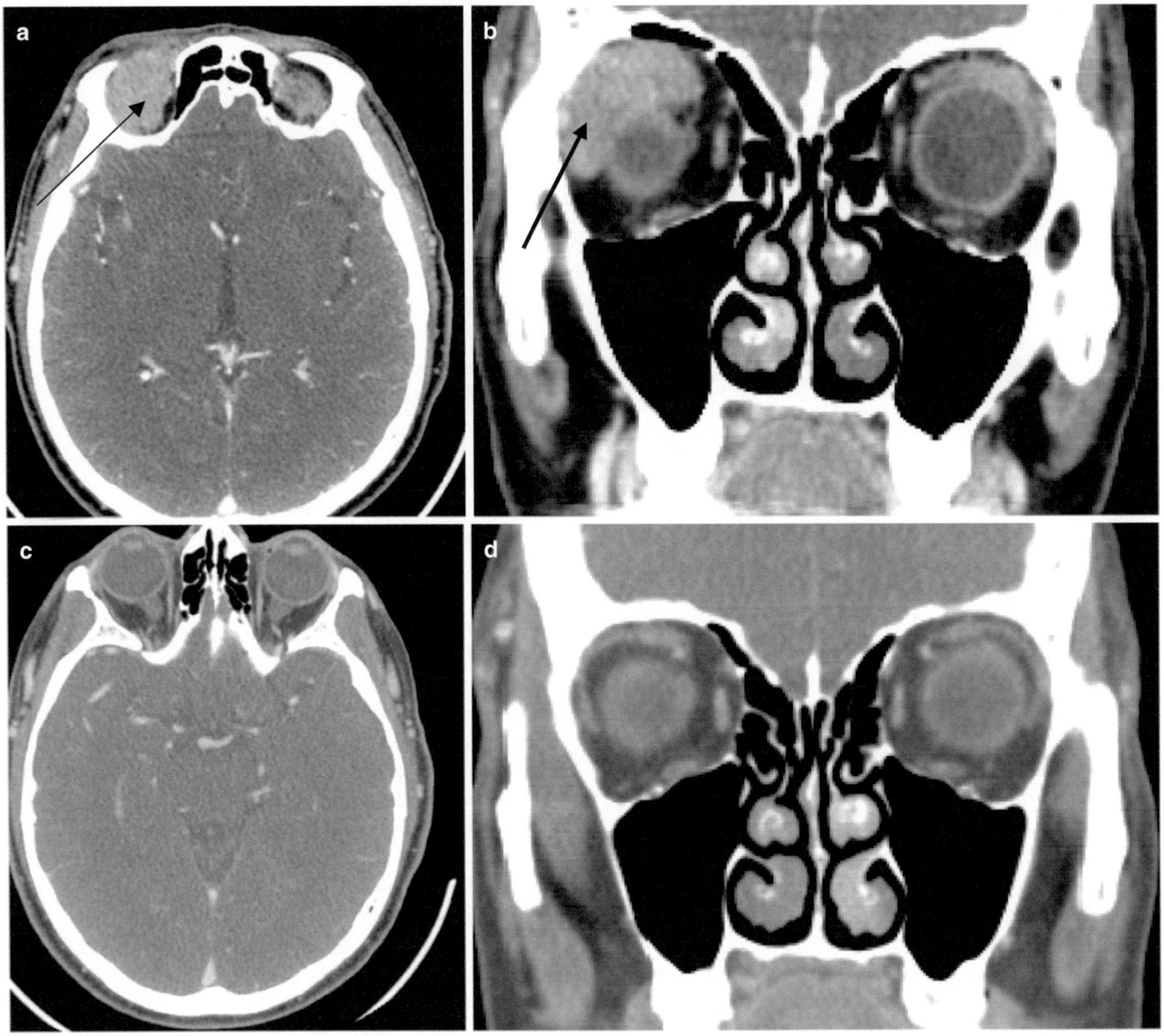

Fig. 6 (**a**) Computed tomography, axial image, in a patient with marginal zone lymphoma of the superolateral orbit (arrow). (**b**) Coronal image in the same patient further delineates the mass (arrow). (**c**) Axial image in the same patient 3 months after delivery of 4 Gy of radiation to the right orbit shows total resolution of the mass. (**d**) Coronal image again confirming complete resolution of the mass

rate of local recurrence and distant metastasis and is associated with death in about half of patients [112]. Carcinoma ex pleomorphic adenoma, which accounts for about 20% of lacrimal gland carcinomas, can occur either de novo or after incomplete excision of a pleomorphic adenoma [113]. Another 10% of cases of lacrimal gland carcinoma are adenocarcinoma and these can be high- or low-grade.

The treatments for lacrimal gland carcinoma have evolved considerably in the last decade or so and there is a shift away from orbital exenteration and toward eye-sparing multidisciplinary strategies [114–120]. Advances in the area of eye-sparing multimodality management of lacrimal gland carcinoma and the use of neoadjuvant intra-arterial chemotherapy specifically in patients with adenoid cystic carcinoma of lacrimal gland will be highlighted in the following section.

5.1 Eye-Sparing Surgery and Adjuvant Radiotherapy

Eye-sparing surgery, followed by adjuvant radiotherapy, is an approach that has gained in popularity in recent years [114–120]. Lacrimal gland carcinomas that are anatomically amenable to gross total resection are candidates for eye-sparing surgery. Outcomes of eye-preserving surgery with or without adjuvant therapy have shown favorable results in several published series [114–120]. One large series of 37 patients by Woo et al., combining patients from two centers including ours, concluded that multimodality eye-sparing treatments are associated with locoregional control rates similar to that of orbital exenteration with a very reasonable ocular toxicity profile and good visual and ocular function for patients who have eye-sparing surgery followed by eye-sparing adjuvant radiation therapy [115]. A visual acuity of 20/40 or better was found in 68% of patients with vision-limiting ocular toxicity most commonly occurring from dry eye and radiation retinopathy. A more recent updated series from MD Anderson reported on 55 patients with lacrimal gland carcinoma that were treated over a recent 20-year period [121]. In this series, orbital exenteration with adjuvant therapy and eye-sparing surgery with adjuvant therapy produced similar recurrence outcomes, although eye-sparing surgery was associated with better disease-specific survival. The reported rates of local recurrence, distant metastasis, and death from disease were 22%, 29%, and 20%, respectively. The reported 5-year local-recurrence-free survival rate was 0.77 (95% confidence interval [CI]: 0.59–1), and the 5- and 10-year distant-metastasis-free survival rates were 0.67 (95% CI: 0.53–0.85) and 0.49 (95% CI: 0.30–0.81), respectively. Five- and 10-year disease-specific survival rates were 0.81 (95% CI: 0.69–0.95) and 0.75 (95% CI: 0.60–0.94), respectively. Other investigators have shown similar local control and survival rates with eye-sparing surgery and adjuvant radiation therapy. For example, Wolkow et al. reported that 4 out of 18 (22%) patients with ACC of the lacrimal gland treated with eye-sparing surgery followed by adjuvant proton radiation therapy experienced local recurrence and 3 (17%) died of metastatic disease [116].

5.2 Neoadjuvant Intra-Arterial Chemotherapy for Adenoid Cystic Carcinoma

In an attempt to improve the outcomes in patients with lacrimal gland ACC, Tse et al. used intra-arterial cytoreductive chemotherapy (IACC) using cisplatin and doxorubicin as a neoadjuvant treatment followed by orbital exenteration followed by radiation therapy and additional adjuvant chemotherapy [122]. Tse et al., in a long-term study using this regimen in 19 patients with lacrimal gland ACC, divided the patients into two groups (patients with the "lacrimal artery intact" and patients with the "lacrimal artery not intact") and concluded that all patients with an intact artery (8/8 patients), and 72% (8/11 patients) of those with the artery not intact, were alive more than 10 years after treatment. The authors did not specifically report the overall 5- and 10-year disease-specific survival for their cohort of 19 patients, but overall close to 80% of patients were still living at 10 years, some with active disease [122].

Subsequent studies from other institutions report cases of late relapse with distant metastasis and disease-specific death after IACC, and also significant morbidity and side effects associated with IACC in patients with lacrimal gland adenoid cystic carcinoma [123, 124].

As a future direction, it may be interesting to study the role of intravenous or intra-arterial chemotherapy in the neoadjuvant setting in patients with large lacrimal gland ACC in an attempt to reduce the size of tumor and make it more surgically resectable and potentially allow for a lesion that would otherwise require an orbital exenteration to be treated with eye-sparing surgery instead.

References

1. Esmaeli B, Wang B, Deavers M, Gillenwater A, Goepfert H, Diaz E, Eicher S. Prognostic factors for survival in malignant melanoma of the eyelid skin. Ophthalmic Plast Reconstr Surg. 2000;16(4):250–7.
2. Wong JR, Nanji AA, Galor A, Karp CL. Management of conjunctival malignant melanoma: a review and update. Expert Rev Ophthalmol. 2014;9(3):185–204.
3. Mancera N, Smalley KS, Margo CE. Melanoma of the eyelid and periocular skin: histopathologic classification and molecular pathology. Surv Ophthalmol. 2019;64(3):272–88.
4. Yin VT, Warneke CL, Merritt HA, Esmaeli B. Number of excisions required to obtain clear surgical margins and prognostic value of AJCC T category for patients with eyelid melanoma. Br J Ophthalmol. 2014;98(12):1681–5.
5. Morton DL, Wanek L, Nizze JA, Elashoff RM, Wong JH. Improved long-term survival after lymphadenectomy of melanoma metastatic to regional nodes. Analysis of prognostic factors in 1134 patients from the John Wayne Cancer Clinic. Ann Surg. 1991;214(4):491.
6. Ross MI, Gershenwald JE. Evidence-based treatment of early-stage melanoma. J Surg Oncol. 2011;104(4):341–53.
7. Esmaeli B, Eicher S, Popp J, Delpassand E, Prieto VG, Gershenwald JE. Sentinel lymph node biopsy for conjunctival melanoma. Ophthalmic Plast Reconstr Surg. 2001;17(6):436–42.
8. Pfeiffer ML, Ozgur OK, Myers JN, Peng A, Ning J, Zafereo ME, Thakar S, Thuro B, Prieto VG, Ross MI, Esmaeli B. Sentinel lymph node biopsy for ocular adnexal melanoma. Acta Ophthalmol. 2017;95(4):e323–8.
9. Cohen VM, Tsimpida M, Hungerford JL, Jan H, Cerio R, Moir G. Prospective study of sentinel lymph node biopsy for conjunctival melanoma. Br J Ophthalmol. 2013;97(12):1525–9.
10. Freitag SK, Aakalu VK, Tao JP, Wladis EJ, Foster JA, Sobel RK, Yen MT. Sentinel lymph node biopsy for eyelid and conjunctival malignancy: a report by the American Academy of Ophthalmology. Ophthalmology. 2020;127(12):1757–65.
11. Herrscher H, Robert C. Immune checkpoint inhibitors in melanoma in the metastatic, neoadjuvant, and adjuvant setting. Curr Opin Oncol. 2020;32(2):106–13.
12. Davies H, Bignell GR, Cox C, Stephens P, Edkins S, Clegg S, Teague J, Woffendin H, Garnett MJ, Bottomley W, Davis N. Mutations of the BRAF gene in human cancer. Nature. 2002;417(6892):949–54.

13. Chapman PB, Hauschild A, Robert C, Haanen JB, Ascierto P, Larkin J, Dummer R, Garbe C, Testori A, Maio M, Hogg D. Improved survival with vemurafenib in melanoma with BRAF V600E mutation. N Engl J Med. 2011;364(26):2507–16.
14. US-FDAFDA labeling information—ZELBORAF.2020FDA. https://www.accessdata.fda.gov/drugsatfda_docs/label/2020/202429s019lbl.pdf. Accessed 14 May 2021.
15. US-FDAFDA labeling information—TAFINLAR.2020FDA. https://www.accessdata.fda.gov/drugsatfda_docs/label/2020/202806s015lbl.pdf. Accessed 14 May 2021.
16. Greco A, Safi D, Swami U, Ginader T, Milhem M, Zakharia Y. Efficacy and adverse events in metastatic melanoma patients treated with combination BRAF plus MEK inhibitors versus BRAF inhibitors: a systematic review. Cancers. 2019;11(12):1950.
17. Pahlitzsch M, Bertelmann E, Mai C. Conjunctival melanoma and BRAF inhibitor therapy. J Clin Exp Ophthalmol. 2014;5(1):322.
18. Maleka A, Åström G, Byström P, Ullenhag GJ. A case report of a patient with metastatic ocular melanoma who experienced a response to treatment with the BRAF inhibitor vemurafenib. BMC Cancer. 2016;16(1):1–5.
19. Glass LR, Lawrence DP, Jakobiec FA, Freitag SK. Conjunctival melanoma responsive to combined systemic BRAF/MEK inhibitors. Ophthalmic Plast Reconstr Surg. 2017;33(5):e114–6.
20. Rossi E, Maiorano BA, Pagliara MM, Sammarco MG, Dosa T, Martini M, Rindi G, Bria E, Blasi MA, Tortora G, Schinzari G. Dabrafenib and trametinib in BRAF mutant metastatic conjunctival melanoma. Front Oncol. 2019;9:232.
21. Ascierto PA, McArthur GA, Dréno B, Atkinson V, Liszkay G, Di Giacomo AM, Mandalà M, Demidov L, Stroyakovskiy D, Thomas L, de la Cruz-Merino L. Cobimetinib combined with vemurafenib in advanced BRAFV600-mutant melanoma (coBRIM): updated efficacy results from a randomised, double-blind, phase 3 trial. Lancet Oncol. 2016;17(9):1248–60.
22. Mackin AG, Pecen PE, Dinsmore AL, Patnaik JL, Gonzalez R, Robinson WA, Palestine AG. Inflammatory side effects of BRAF and MEK inhibitors. Melanoma Res. 2019;29(5):522–6.
23. Liu M, Yang X, Liu J, Zhao B, Cai W, Li Y, Hu D. Efficacy and safety of BRAF inhibition alone versus combined BRAF and MEK inhibition in melanoma: a meta-analysis of randomized controlled trials. Oncotarget. 2017;8(19):32258.
24. Peng L, Wang Y, Hong Y, Ye X, Shi P, Zhang J, Zhao Q. Incidence and relative risk of cutaneous squamous cell carcinoma with single-agent BRAF inhibitor and dual BRAF/MEK inhibitors in cancer patients: a meta-analysis. Oncotarget. 2017;8(47):83280.
25. Yin VT, Wiraszka TA, Tetzlaff M, Curry JL, Esmaeli B. Cutaneous eyelid neoplasms as a toxicity of vemurafenib therapy. Ophthalmic Plast Reconstr Surg. 2015;31(4):e112–5.
26. US-FDAFDA labeling information—YERVOY.2020FDA. https://www.accessdata.fda.gov/drugsatfda_docs/label/2020/125377s074lbl.pdf. Accessed 10 March 2021.
27. US-FDAFDA labeling information—OPDIVO.2019FDA. https://www.accessdata.fda.gov/drugsatfda_docs/label/2019/125554s024lbl.pdf. Accessed 10 March 2021.
28. US-FDAFDA labeling information—KEYTRUDA.2021FDA. https://www.accessdata.fda.gov/drugsatfda_docs/label/2021/125514s015lbl.pdf. Accessed 10 March 2021.
29. Schadendorf D, Hodi FS, Robert C, Weber JS, Margolin K, Hamid O, Patt D, Chen TT, Berman DM, Wolchok JD. Pooled analysis of long-term survival data from phase II and phase III trials of ipilimumab in unresectable or metastatic melanoma. J Clin Oncol. 2015;33(17):1889.
30. Hodi FS, O'Day SJ, McDermott DF, Weber RW, Sosman JA, Haanen JB, Gonzalez R, Robert C, Schadendorf D, Hassel JC, Akerley W. Improved survival with ipilimumab in patients with metastatic melanoma. N Engl J Med. 2010;363(8):711–23.
31. Barone A, Hazarika M, Theoret MR, Mishra-Kalyani P, Chen H, He K, Sridhara R, Subramaniam S, Pfuma E, Wang Y, Li H. FDA approval summary: pembrolizumab for the treatment of patients with unresectable or metastatic melanoma. Clin Cancer Res. 2017;23(19):5661–5.
32. Beaver JA, Theoret MR, Mushti S, He K, Libeg M, Goldberg K, Sridhara R, McKee AE, Keegan P, Pazdur R. FDA approval of nivolumab for the first-line treatment of patients with BRAFV600 wild-type unresectable or metastatic melanoma. Clin Cancer Res. 2017;23(14):3479–83.
33. Larkin J, Chiarion-Sileni V, Gonzalez R, Grob JJ, Cowey CL, Lao CD, Schadendorf D, Dummer R, Smylie M, Rutkowski P, Ferrucci PF. Combined nivolumab and ipilimumab or monotherapy in untreated melanoma. N Engl J Med. 2015;373(1):23–34.
34. Sagiv O, Thakar SD, Kandl TJ, Ford J, Sniegowski MC, Hwu WJ, Esmaeli B. Immunotherapy with programmed cell death 1 inhibitors for 5 patients with conjunctival melanoma. JAMA Ophthalmol. 2018;136(11):1236–41.
35. Finger PT, Pavlick AC. Checkpoint inhibition immunotherapy for advanced local and systemic conjunctival melanoma: a clinical case series. J Immunother Cancer. 2019;7(1):1–7.
36. Kini A, Fu R, Compton C, Miller DM, Ramasubramanian A. Pembrolizumab for recurrent conjunctival melanoma. JAMA Ophthalmol. 2017;135(8):891–2.
37. Chaves LJ, Huth B, Augsburger JJ, Correa ZM. Eye-sparing treatment for diffuse invasive conjunctival melanoma. Ocular Oncol Pathol. 2018;4(4):261–6.
38. Pinto Torres S, André T, Gouveia E, Costa L, Passos MJ. Systemic treatment of metastatic conjunctival melanoma. Case Rep Oncol Med. 2017;2017:4623964.
39. Wang DY, Salem JE, Cohen JV, Chandra S, Menzer C, Ye F, Zhao S, Das S, Beckermann KE, Ha L, Rathmell WK. Fatal toxic effects associated with immune checkpoint inhibitors: a systematic review and meta-analysis. JAMA Oncol. 2018;4(12):1721–8.
40. Martins F, Sofiya L, Sykiotis GP, Lamine F, Maillard M, Fraga M, Shabafrouz K, Ribi C, Cairoli A, Guex-Crosier Y, Kuntzer T. Adverse effects of immune-checkpoint inhibitors: epidemiology, management and surveillance. Nat Rev Clin Oncol. 2019;16(9):563–80.
41. Martins F, Sykiotis GP, Maillard M, Fraga M, Ribi C, Kuntzer T, Michielin O, Peters S, Coukos G, Spertini F, Thompson JA. New therapeutic perspectives to manage refractory immune checkpoint-related toxicities. Lancet Oncol. 2019;20(1):e54–64.
42. Reifler DM, Hornblass A. Squamous cell carcinoma of the eyelid. Surv Ophthalmol. 1986;30(6):349–65.
43. Tanenbaum M, Grove AS Jr, McCord CD Jr. Eyelid tumors: diagnosis and management. Oculoplastic Surgery. 3rd ed. New York: Raven Press Ltd.; 1995. p. 145–74.
44. Wawrzynski J, Tudge I, Fitzgerald E, Collin R, Desai P, Emeriewen K, Saleh GM. Report on the incidence of squamous cell carcinomas affecting the eyelids in England over a 15-year period (2000–2014). Br J Ophthalmol. 2018;102(10):1358–61.
45. Nasser QJ, Roth KG, Warneke CL, Yin VT, El Sawy T, Esmaeli B. Impact of AJCC 'T'designation on risk of regional lymph node metastasis in patients with squamous carcinoma of the eyelid. Br J Ophthalmol. 2014;98(4):498–501.
46. Sun MT, Andrew NH, O'Donnell B, McNab A, Huilgol SC, Selva D. Periocular squamous cell carcinoma: TNM staging and recurrence. Ophthalmology. 2015;122(7):1512–6.
47. Ford J, Thakar S, Thuro B, Esmaeli B. Prognostic value of the staging system for eyelid tumors in the 7th edition of the American Joint Committee on Cancer Staging Manual. Ophthal Plast Reconstr Surg. 2017;33(5):317–24.
48. Faustina M, Diba R, Ahmadi MA, Gutstein BF, Esmaeli B. Patterns of regional and distant metastasis in patients with

eyelid and periocular squamous cell carcinoma. Ophthalmology. 2004;111(10):1930–2.
49. Sullivan TJ. Squamous cell carcinoma of eyelid, periocular, and periorbital skin. Int Ophthalmol Clin. 2009;49(4):17–24.
50. McCord CD Jr, Cavanagh HD. Microscopic features and biologic behavior of eyelid tumors. Ophthalmic Surg. 1980;11(10):671–81.
51. Rowe DE, Carroll RJ, Day CL Jr. Prognostic factors for local recurrence, metastasis, and survival rates in squamous cell carcinoma of the skin, ear, and lip: implications for treatment modality selection. J Am Acad Dermatol. 1992;26(6):976–90.
52. Xu S, Sagiv O, Rubin ML, Sa HS, Tetzlaff MT, Nagarajan P, Ning J, Esmaeli B. Validation study of the AJCC cancer staging manual, staging system for eyelid and periocular squamous cell carcinoma. JAMA Ophthalmol. 2019;137(5):537–42.
53. Cook BE Jr, Bartley GB. Treatment options and future prospects for the management of eyelid malignancies: an evidence-based update. Ophthalmology. 2001;108(11):2088–98.
54. Yin VT, Merritt HA, Sniegowski M, Esmaeli B. Eyelid and ocular surface carcinoma: diagnosis and management. Clin Dermatol. 2015;33(2):159–69.
55. Herbst RS. Review of epidermal growth factor receptor biology. Int J Radiat Oncol Biol Phys. 2004;59(2):S21–6.
56. Yin VT, Pfeiffer ML, Esmaeli B. Targeted therapy for orbital and periocular basal cell carcinoma and squamous cell carcinoma. Ophthal Plast Reconstr Surg. 2013;29(2):87–92.
57. Uribe P, Gonzalez S. Epidermal growth factor receptor (EGFR) and squamous cell carcinoma of the skin: molecular bases for EGFR-targeted therapy. Pathol Res Pract. 2011;207(6):337–42.
58. Moreira J, Tobias A, O'Brien MP, Agulnik M. Targeted therapy in head and neck cancer: an update on current clinical developments in epidermal growth factor receptor-targeted therapy and immunotherapies. Drugs. 2017;77(8):843–57.
59. Bonner JA, Harari PM, Giralt J, Cohen RB, Jones CU, Sur RK, Raben D, Baselga J, Spencer SA, Zhu J, Youssoufian H. Radiotherapy plus cetuximab for locoregionally advanced head and neck cancer: 5-year survival data from a phase 3 randomised trial, and relation between cetuximab-induced rash and survival. Lancet Oncol. 2010;11(1):21–8.
60. Acevedo-Henao CM, Valette G, Miglierini P, Lefur E, Pradier O. Radiotherapy combined with cetuximab for locally advanced head and neck cancer: results and toxicity. Cancer/Radiothérapie. 2012;16(7):601–3.
61. Shepler TR, Prieto VG, Diba R, Neuhaus RW, Shore JW, Esmaeli B. Expression of the epidermal growth factor receptor in conjunctival squamous cell carcinoma. Ophthalmic Plast Reconstr Surg. 2006;22(2):113–5.
62. El-Sawy T, Sabichi AL, Myers JN, Kies MS, William WN, Glisson BS, Lippman S, Esmaeli B. Epidermal growth factor receptor inhibitors for treatment of orbital squamous cell carcinoma. Arch Ophthalmol. 2012;130(12):1608–11.
63. Gellrich FF, Hüning S, Beissert S, Eigentler T, Stockfleth E, Gutzmer R, Meier F. Medical treatment of advanced cutaneous squamous-cell carcinoma. J Eur Acad Dermatol Venereol. 2019;33:38–43.
64. Bindiganavile SH, Bhat N, Lee AG, Gombos DS, Al-Zubidi N. Targeted cancer therapy and its ophthalmic side effects: a review. J Immunother Prec Oncol. 2021;4(1):6–15.
65. Markham A, Duggan S. Cemiplimab: first global approval. Drugs. 2018;78(17):1841–6.
66. Stevenson ML, Wang CQ, Abikhair M, Roudiani N, Felsen D, Krueger JG, Pavlick AC, Carucci JA. Expression of programmed cell death ligand in cutaneous squamous cell carcinoma and treatment of locally advanced disease with pembrolizumab. JAMA Dermatol. 2017;153(4):299–303.
67. Migden MR, Rischin D, Schmults CD, Guminski A, Hauschild A, Lewis KD, Chung CH, Hernandez-Aya L, Lim AM, Chang AL, Rabinowits G. PD-1 blockade with cemiplimab in advanced cutaneous squamous-cell carcinoma. N Engl J Med. 2018;379(4):341–51.
68. Migden MR, Khushalani NI, Chang AL, Lewis KD, Schmults CD, Hernandez-Aya L, Meier F, Schadendorf D, Guminski A, Hauschild A, Wong DJ. Cemiplimab in locally advanced cutaneous squamous cell carcinoma: results from an open-label, phase 2, single-arm trial. Lancet Oncol. 2020;21(2):294–305.
69. ClinicalTrials.gov [Internet]. Bethesda (MD): National Library of Medicine (US).
70. Konidaris G, Paul E, Kuznik A, Keeping S, Chen CI, Sasane M, Xu Y, Atsou K, Ayers D, Ruiz ES, Khushalani NI. Assessing the value of cemiplimab for adults with advanced cutaneous squamous cell carcinoma: a cost-effectiveness analysis. Value Health. 2021;24(3):377–87.
71. Conger JR, Grob SR, Tao J. Massive periocular squamous cell carcinoma with response to pembrolizumab (Keytruda). Ophthalmic Plast Reconstr Surg. 2019;35(5):e127.
72. Cook BE Jr, Bartley GB. Epidemiologic characteristics and clinical course of patients with malignant eyelid tumors in an incidence cohort in Olmsted County, Minnesota. Ophthalmology. 1999;106(4):746–50.
73. Margo CE, Waltz K. Basal cell carcinoma of the eyelid and periocular skin. Surv Ophthalmol. 1993;38(2):169–92.
74. Branson SV, McClintic E, Ozgur O, Esmaeli B, Yeatts RP. Orbitofacial metastatic basal cell carcinoma: report of 10 cases. Ophthal Plast Reconstr Surg. 2017;33(3):213–7.
75. Savar A, Esmaeli B. Management of primary eyelid cancers. Ophthalmic oncology. Boston, MA: Springer; 2010. p. 113–25.
76. Wong VA, Marshall JA, Whitehead KJ, Williamson RM, Sullivan TJ. Management of periocular basal cell carcinoma with modified en face frozen section controlled excision. Ophthalmic Plast Reconstr Surg. 2002;18(6):430–5.
77. Malhotra R, Huilgol SC, Huynh NT, Selva D. The Australian Mohs database, part II: periocular basal cell carcinoma outcome at 5-year follow-up. Ophthalmology. 2004;111(4):631–6.
78. Tang JY, Mackay-Wiggan JM, Aszterbaum M, Yauch RL, Lindgren J, Chang K, Coppola C, Chanana AM, Marji J, Bickers DR, Epstein EH Jr. Inhibiting the hedgehog pathway in patients with the basal-cell nevus syndrome. N Engl J Med. 2012;366(23):2180–8.
79. Marigo V, Davey RA, Zuo Y, Cunningham JM, Tabin CJ. Biochemical evidence that patched is the Hedgehog receptor. Nature. 1996;384(6605):176–9.
80. Von Hoff DD, LoRusso PM, Rudin CM, Reddy JC, Yauch RL, Tibes R, Weiss GJ, Borad MJ, Hann CL, Brahmer JR, Mackey HM. Inhibition of the hedgehog pathway in advanced basal-cell carcinoma. N Engl J Med. 2009;361(12):1164–72.
81. LoRusso PM, Rudin CM, Reddy JC, Tibes R, Weiss GJ, Borad MJ, Hann CL, Brahmer JR, Chang I, Darbonne WC, Graham RA. Phase I trial of hedgehog pathway inhibitor vismodegib (GDC-0449) in patients with refractory, locally advanced or metastatic solid tumors. Clin Cancer Res. 2011;17(8):2502–11.
82. Sekulic A, Migden MR, Oro AE, Dirix L, Lewis KD, Hainsworth JD, Solomon JA, Yoo S, Arron ST, Friedlander PA, Marmur E. Efficacy and safety of vismodegib in advanced basal-cell carcinoma. N Engl J Med. 2012;366(23):2171–9.
83. Ozgur OK, Yin V, Chou E, Ball S, Kies M, William WN, Migden M, Thuro BA, Esmaeli B. Hedgehog pathway inhibition for locally advanced periocular basal cell carcinoma and basal cell nevus syndrome. Am J Ophthalmol. 2015;160(2):220–7.
84. Sagiv O, Nagarajan P, Ferrarotto R, Kandl TJ, Thakar SD, Glisson BS, Altan M, Esmaeli B. Ocular preservation with neoadjuvant vismodegib in patients with locally advanced periocular basal cell carcinoma. Br J Ophthalmol. 2019;103(6):775–80.

85. Migden MR, Guminski A, Gutzmer R, Dirix L, Lewis KD, Combemale P, Herd RM, Kudchadkar R, Trefzer U, Gogov S, Pallaud C. Treatment with two different doses of sonidegib in patients with locally advanced or metastatic basal cell carcinoma (BOLT): a multicentre, randomised, double-blind phase 2 trial. Lancet Oncol. 2015;16(6):716–28.
86. Hou X, Rokohl AC, Ortmann M, Heindl LM. Effective treatment of locally advanced periocular basal cell carcinoma with oral hedgehog pathway inhibitor? Graefes Arch Clin Exp Ophthalmol. 2020;258:2335–7.
87. Chang AL, Tran DC, Cannon JG, Li S, Jeng M, Patel R, Van der Bokke L, Pague A, Brotherton R, Rieger KE, Satpathy AT. Pembrolizumab for advanced basal cell carcinoma: an investigator-initiated, proof-of-concept study. J Am Acad Dermatol. 2019;80(2):564–6.
88. Fischer S, Ali OH, Jochum W, Kluckert T, Flatz L, Siano M. Anti-PD-1 therapy leads to near-complete remission in a patient with metastatic basal cell carcinoma. Oncol Res Treat. 2018;41(6):391–4.
89. US-FDA. FDA labeling information—LIBTAYO. FDA. https://www.accessdata.fda.gov/drugsatfda_docs/label/2021/761097s007lbl.pdf. Accessed 10 May 2021.
90. Stratigos AJ, Sekulic A, Peris K, Bechter O, Kaatz M, Lewis KD, Basset-Seguin N, Chang AL, Dalle S, Orland AF, Licitra L. Primary analysis of phase 2 results for cemiplimab in patients (pts) with locally advanced basal cell carcinoma (laBCC) who progress on or are intolerant to hedgehog inhibitors (HHIs). Head Neck. 2021;89:75.
91. Lewis K, Peris K, Sekulic A, Stratigos A, Dunn L, Eroglu Z, Chang AL, Migden M, Li S, Mohan K, Coates E. 428 Interim analysis of Phase 2 results for cemiplimab in patients with metastatic basal cell carcinoma (mBCC) who progressed on or are intolerant to hedgehog inhibitors (HHIs). J Immunother Cancer. 2021;(5)1.
92. Olsen TG, Holm F, Mikkelsen LH, Rasmussen PK, Coupland SE, Esmaeli B, Finger PT, Graue GF, Grossniklaus HE, Honavar SG, Khong JJ. Orbital lymphoma—an international multicenter retrospective study. Am J Ophthalmol. 2019;199:44–57.
93. Swerdlow SH, Campo E, Pileri SA, Harris NL, Stein H, Siebert R, Advani R, Ghielmini M, Salles GA, Zelenetz AD, Jaffe ES. The 2016 revision of the World Health Organization classification of lymphoid neoplasms. Blood. 2016;127(20):2375–90.
94. Hindsø TG, Esmaeli B, Holm F, Mikkelsen LH, Rasmussen PK, Coupland SE, Finger PT, Graue GF, Grossniklaus HE, Honavar SG, Khong JJ. International multicentre retrospective cohort study of ocular adnexal marginal zone B-cell lymphoma. Br J Ophthalmol. 2020;104(3):357–62.
95. Margo CE, Mulla ZD. Malignant tumors of the orbit: analysis of the Florida Cancer Registry. Ophthalmology. 1998;105(1):185–90.
96. Rubenstein J, Ferreri AJ, Pittaluga S. Primary lymphoma of the central nervous system: epidemiology, pathology and current approaches to diagnosis, prognosis and treatment. Leuk Lymphoma. 2008;49(sup1):43–51.
97. Sniegowski MC, Roberts D, Bakhoum M, Mc Laughlin P, Yin VT, Turturro F, Esmaeli B. Ocular adnexal lymphoma: validation of American Joint Committee on Cancer seventh edition staging guidelines. Br J Ophthalmol. 2014;98(9):1255–60.
98. Thuro BA, Ning J, Peng SA, Pace ST, Dudeja G, Ozgur O, Turturro F, Samaniego F, Hagemeister FB, Fayad LE, Fowler NH. Rates of positive findings on positron emission tomography and bone marrow biopsy in patients with ocular adnexal lymphoma. Ophthal Plast Reconstr Surg. 2017;33(5):355–60.
99. Nasser QJ, Pfeiffer ML, Romaguera J, Fowler N, Debnam JM, Samaniego F, El-Sawy T, McLaughlin P, Bakhoum MF, Esmaeli B. Clinical value of magnetic resonance imaging and other baseline testing for conjunctival mucosa-associated lymphoid tissue lymphoma. Leuk Lymphoma. 2014;55(5):1013–7.
100. Kirkegaard MM, Rasmussen PK, Coupland SE, Esmaeli B, Finger PT, Graue GF, Grossniklaus HE, Honavar SG, Khong JJ, McKelvie PA, Mulay K. Conjunctival lymphoma—an international multicenter retrospective study. JAMA Ophthalmol. 2016;134(4):406–14.
101. Svendsen FH, Rasmussen PK, Coupland SE, Esmaeli B, Finger PT, Graue GF, Grossniklaus HE, Honavar SG, Khong JJ, McKelvie PA, Mulay K. Lymphoma of the eyelid–an international multicenter retrospective study. Am J Ophthalmol. 2017;177:58–68.
102. Bolek TW, Moyses HM, Marcus RB Jr, Gorden L III, Maiese RL, Almasri NM, Mendenhall NP. Radiotherapy in the management of orbital lymphoma. Int J Radiat Oncol Biol Phys. 1999;44(1):31–6.
103. Pelloski CE, Wilder RB, Ha CS, Hess MA, Cabanillas FF, Cox JD. Clinical stage IEA–IIEA orbital lymphomas: outcomes in the era of modern staging and treatment. Radiother Oncol. 2001;59(2):145–51.
104. Stafford SL, Kozelsky TF, Garrity JA, Kurtin PJ, Leavitt JA, Martenson JA, Habermann TM. Orbital lymphoma: radiotherapy outcome and complications. Radiother Oncol. 2001;59(2):139–44.
105. Decaudin D, de Cremoux P, Vincent-Salomon A, Dendale R, Rouic LL. Ocular adnexal lymphoma: a review of clinicopathologic features and treatment options. Blood. 2006;108(5):1451–60.
106. Pinnix CC, Dabaja BS, Milgrom SA, et al. Ultra-low-dose radiotherapy for definitive management of ocular adnexal B-cell lymphoma. Head Neck. 2017;39(6):1095–100.
107. Eisenhauer EA, Therasse P, Bogaerts J, Schwartz LH, Sargent D, Ford R, Dancey J, Arbuck S, Gwyther S, Mooney M, Rubinstein L. New response evaluation criteria in solid tumours: revised RECIST guideline (version 1.1). Eur J Cancer. 2009;45(2):228–47.
108. Coiffier B, Lepage E, Brière J, Herbrecht R, Tilly H, Bouabdallah R, Morel P, Van Den Neste E, Salles G, Gaulard P, Reyes F. CHOP chemotherapy plus rituximab compared with CHOP alone in elderly patients with diffuse large-B-cell lymphoma. N Engl J Med. 2002;346(4):235–42.
109. Keating GM. Spotlight on rituximab in chronic lymphocytic leukemia, low-grade or follicular lymphoma, and diffuse large B-cell lymphoma. BioDrugs. 2011;25(1):55–61.
110. Salar A, Domingo-Domenech E, Panizo C, Nicolás C, Bargay J, Muntañola A, Canales M, Bello JL, Sancho JM, Tomás JF, Rodríguez MJ. First-line response-adapted treatment with the combination of bendamustine and rituximab in patients with mucosa-associated lymphoid tissue lymphoma (MALT2008-01): a multicentre, single-arm, phase 2 trial. Lancet Haematol. 2014;1(3):e104–11.
111. von Holstein SL. Tumours of the lacrimal gland. Epidemiological, clinical and genetic characteristics. Doctoral dissertation. 2013.
112. Shields J, Shields C. Lacrimal gland primary epithelial tumors. In: Shields J, Shields C, editors. Eyelid, conjunctival, and orbital tumors: an atlas and text. Philadelphia: Lippincott Williams and Wilkins; 2011. p. 700–25.
113. Tom A, Bell D, Ford JR, Debnam JM, Guo Y, Frank SJ, Esmaeli B. Malignant mixed tumor (carcinoma ex pleomorphic adenoma) of the lacrimal gland. Ophthal Plast Reconstr Surg. 2020;36(5):497–502.
114. Esmaeli B, Yin VT, Hanna EY, Kies MS, William WN Jr, Bell D, Frank SJ. Eye-sparing multidisciplinary approach for the management of lacrimal gland carcinoma. Head Neck. 2016;38(8):1258–62.
115. Woo KI, Sagiv O, Han J, Frank SJ, Kim YD, Esmaeli B. Eye-preserving surgery followed by adjuvant radiotherapy for lacrimal gland carcinoma: outcomes in 37 patients. Ophthalmic Plast Reconstr Surg. 2018;34(6):570–4.
116. Wolkow N, Jakobiec FA, Lee H. Long-term outcomes of globe-preserving surgery with proton beam radiation for adenoid cystic carcinoma of lacrimal gland. Am J Ophthalmol. 2019;201:84–5.

117. Rose GE, Gore SK, Plowman NP. Cranio-orbital resection does not appear to improve survival of patients with lacrimal gland carcinoma. Ophthalmic Plast Reconstr Surg. 2019;35(1):77–84.
118. Hung JY, Wei YH, Huang CH, Chen LW, Fuh CS, Liao SL. Survival outcomes of eye-sparing surgery for adenoid cystic carcinoma of lacrimal gland. Jpn J Ophthalmol. 2019;63(4):344–51.
119. Han J, Kim YD, Woo KI, Sobti D. Long-term outcomes of eye-sparing surgery for adenoid cystic carcinoma of lacrimal gland. Ophthal Plast Reconstr Surg. 2018;34(1):74–8.
120. Bonavolontà P, Esmaeli B, Donna P, Tranfa F, Iuliano A, Abbate V, Fossataro F, Attanasi F, Bonavolontà G. Outcomes after eye-sparing surgery vs orbital exenteration in patients with lacrimal gland carcinoma. Head Neck. 2020;42(5):988–93.
121. Ford JR, Rubin ML, Frank SJ, Ning J, Debnam JM, Bell D, El-Naggar A, Ferrarotto R, Esmaeli B. Prognostic factors for local recurrence and survival and impact of local treatments on survival in lacrimal gland carcinoma. Br J Ophthalmol. 2021;105(6):768–74.
122. Tse DT, Kossler AL, Feuer WJ, Benedetto PW. Long-term outcomes of neoadjuvant intra-arterial cytoreductive chemotherapy for lacrimal gland adenoid cystic carcinoma. Ophthalmology. 2013;120(7):1313–23.
123. Fellman M, Carter K, Call CB, Esmaeli B. Disease recurrence after intraarterial chemotherapy in 2 patients with adenoid cystic carcinoma of lacrimal gland. Can J Ophthalmol. 2013;48(2):e17–8.
124. Jang SY, Kim DJ, Kim CY, Wu CZ, Yoon JS, Lee SY. Neoadjuvant intra-arterial chemotherapy in patients with primary lacrimal adenoid cystic carcinoma. Cancer Imaging. 2014;14(1):1–8.

Proton Beam Irradiation: Expanding Indications

Mary E. Aronow, Alexei V. Trofimov, Anne Marie Lane, Yen-Lin E. Chen, Florence K. Keane, Shannon M. MacDonald, Helen A. Shih, Evangelos S. Gragoudas, and Ivana K. Kim

1 Introduction

Proton beam irradiation (PBI) has multiple attributes that make it ideally suited for treating ocular tumors. High-energy protons are precisely delivered with minimal scatter; there is tissue sparing at the entry site, maximal ionization density covering the tumor (Bragg peak), and a sharp dose fall-off at the end of the beam. This allows for highly conformal delivery of radiation to the tumor, with the ability in many cases to spare critical ocular structures such as the macula and optic nerve. The result is excellent local tumor control, with minimization of damage to surrounding normal tissue, and retention of vision in many cases. The first patient with uveal melanoma to be treated with PBI was at the Harvard Cyclotron in 1975 [1]. Since that time, PBI protocols for uveal melanoma have become well established and proton centers have been built worldwide. Patients undergoing PBI for uveal melanoma generally require surgical placement of fiducial markers (e.g., tantalum rings) to localize tumor margins and facilitate radiographical setup prior to treatment [2]. A light field setup is an alternative for anterior uveal melanoma (iris and/or ciliary body tumors), and other types of tumors requiring overall lower radiation doses. This chapter describes how PBI using a light field setup can be applied to a spectrum of ocular tumors including: conjunctival melanoma, choroidal hemangioma, retinal hemangioblastoma, and choroidal metastases.

2 Light Field Technique

The light field setup is a technique for delivering PBI without the need for surgical placement of fiducial markers. For anteriorly located intraocular tumors, or those involving the ocular surface, localization is accomplished by utilizing the visible light field on the surface of the eye. The light field is coincident with the proton irradiation field and is used to position the beam over the desired treatment area (Fig. 1).

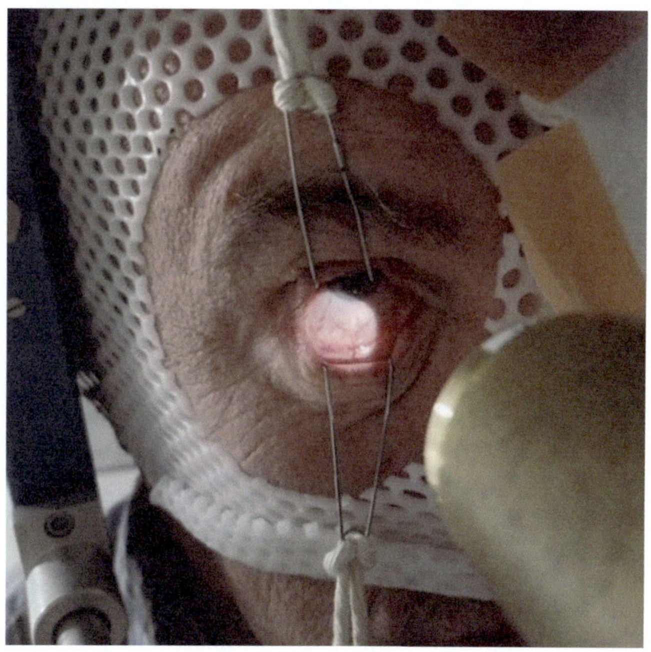

Fig. 1 Light field setup demonstrating head immobilization with the aid of a face mask. The eye is in fixed upward gaze. The incident light field is positioned to coincide with the PBI irradiation field to cover an anteriorly located tumor

M. E. Aronow (✉) · A. M. Lane · E. S. Gragoudas · I. K. Kim
Retina Service, Massachusetts Eye and Ear, Harvard Medical School, Boston, MA, USA
e-mail: mary_aronow@meei.harvard.edu; Anne_Lane2@meei.harvard.edu; Evangelos_Gragoudas@meei.harvard.edu; Ivana_Kim@meei.harvard.edu

A. V. Trofimov · Y.-L. E. Chen · F. K. Keane · S. M. MacDonald · H. A. Shih
Department of Radiation Oncology, Massachusetts General Hospital, Harvard Medical School, Boston, MA, USA
e-mail: atrofimov@mgh.harvard.edu; YCHEN9@mgh.harvard.edu; Florence.Keane@mgh.harvard.edu; SMACDONALD@mgh.harvard.edu; HSHIH@mgh.harvard.edu

B. V. Chawla, M. E. Aronow (eds.), *Global Perspectives in Ocular Oncology*, https://doi.org/10.1007/978-3-031-08250-4_32

At Massachusetts Eye and Ear, this technique has proven to be highly effective. In a recent review of 125 patients with anterior uveal melanoma treated by PBI at the Harvard Cyclotron Laboratory, and more recently at the Massachusetts General Hospital Burr Proton Therapy Center using a light field setup, with the prescription dose of 70 Gy relative biological effectiveness (RBE), the local tumor control rate was 90% at a median follow-up of 4 years [3]. For posteriorly located non-melanoma intraocular tumors that can be treated using a lower dose of radiation (15–35 Gy [RBE]), light field preparation utilizes information from examination, supportive imaging (color fundus photography and ultrasonography), and tumor drawings combined with specialized software for creating radiation plans. At our center, PBI treatment plans are reviewed on a weekly basis in a multidisciplinary radiation treatment planning meeting. In this way, ocular oncologists, medical physicists, and radiation oncologists collaborate to produce individualized treatment plans for optimal patient outcomes.

3 Conjunctival Melanoma

Conjunctival melanoma is rare and comprises <1% of all forms of melanoma [4]. Despite multiple available therapies, local relapse has been reported to exceed 50% [5, 6]. Primary surgical excision with wide margins remains the most common first-line approach [7]. Tumor excision can be combined with adjuvant therapies such as cryotherapy, topical chemotherapy (mitomycin-C), and various forms of radiation (brachytherapy, external beam radiotherapy [EBRT], PBI).

While not a common first-line therapy, PBI has been used to treat conjunctival melanoma in some settings, particularly for advanced cases. It can be used either as primary therapy for unresectable disease or in the adjuvant setting. Wuestemeyer and colleagues used PBI in a series of 20 patients with advanced disease as an alternative to exenteration. These were predominantly American Joint Committee on Cancer (AJCC) stage T3 tumors, 16 (80%) of which were recurrences following primary excision or other therapy. Areas of conjunctiva with suspected microscopic disease received 31 Gy (RBE) delivered in 6 fractions. The clinically observable tumor (primary target volume) received an additional boost given in 2 fractions, bringing the total dose to 45 Gy (RBE). At a median follow-up of 34 months, recurrence developed in 6 individuals (30%), only 1 of which occurred within the primary target volume. Two patients (10%) ultimately underwent exenteration. Six patients (30%) developed metastatic disease [8]. Similarly, Scholz and colleagues treated a series of 89 patients with advanced conjunctival melanoma (AJCC stage ≥T2) or tumors with multifocal bulbar involvement (AJCC stage T1c/d), with PBI using a dose of 45 Gy (RBE) given in 8 fractions. Treatment was delivered using a main field that included regions of suspicious microscopic disease (such as primary acquired melanosis) and a boost field for high-risk areas with clinically and pathologically confirmed tumor. The main field was treated with 31 Gy (RBE) in 6 fractions and the boost field received 14 Gy (RBE) in 2 fractions. At a median follow-up of 4.2 years, local recurrence was observed in 33% and metastatic disease developed in 16% of patients. The main side effects following PBI were dry eye (30%), secondary glaucoma (11%), and limbal stem cell deficiency (8%) [9].

PBI has also been used as an adjuvant therapy in the treatment of earlier stage, localized conjunctival melanoma. In a series of 92 patients (AJCC stage T1 in 71.6% of cases), primary tumor excision was followed by PBI. A total dose of 45 Gy (RBE) was delivered in 8 fractions. After a mean follow-up of 4.7 years, local recurrence was observed in 25 cases (33%). Of these, only 4 recurrences (16%) were within the field of radiation [10]. In another series of 39 patients with localized conjunctival melanoma (AJCC stage T1 in 82% of cases), tumor excision with cryotherapy was performed followed by PBI 2 weeks later. Areas of suspected microscopic disease received 36 Gy (RBE) in 6 fractions and a boost of an additional 16 Gy (RBE) given in 2 fractions (total dose 52 Gy [RBE]) was delivered to higher-risk areas. After a follow-up of 5 years, 69% of patients remained local recurrence-free and 91% were metastasis-free [11].

Local recurrence in the range of 30% was similar to conjunctival melanoma treated with conventional primary excision followed by adjuvant therapies such as cryotherapy or topical chemotherapy [12]. The optimal indications, dose, and timing of PBI are not well established for conjunctival melanoma due to the rarity of this disease and complexity of cases. PBI could have a potential role in primary treatment, for example in patients who are medically unable to undergo surgery, or in unique clinical scenarios, as illustrated in the following case.

3.1 Case

A 28-year-old male was referred for management of conjunctival melanoma of the left eye. He had a remote history of laser-assisted in situ keratomileusis (LASIK) in both eyes. Two years prior to evaluation, the patient noticed a fleshy lesion overlying his left cornea, which gradually increased in size. He was evaluated at an outside institution where incisional biopsy was performed. His pathology was reviewed at Massachusetts Eye and Ear and confirmed invasive conjunctival melanoma. On examination, the uncorrected vision in the affected left eye was 20/25. A pinkish, highly vascularized mass was present overlying the inferotemporal corneal

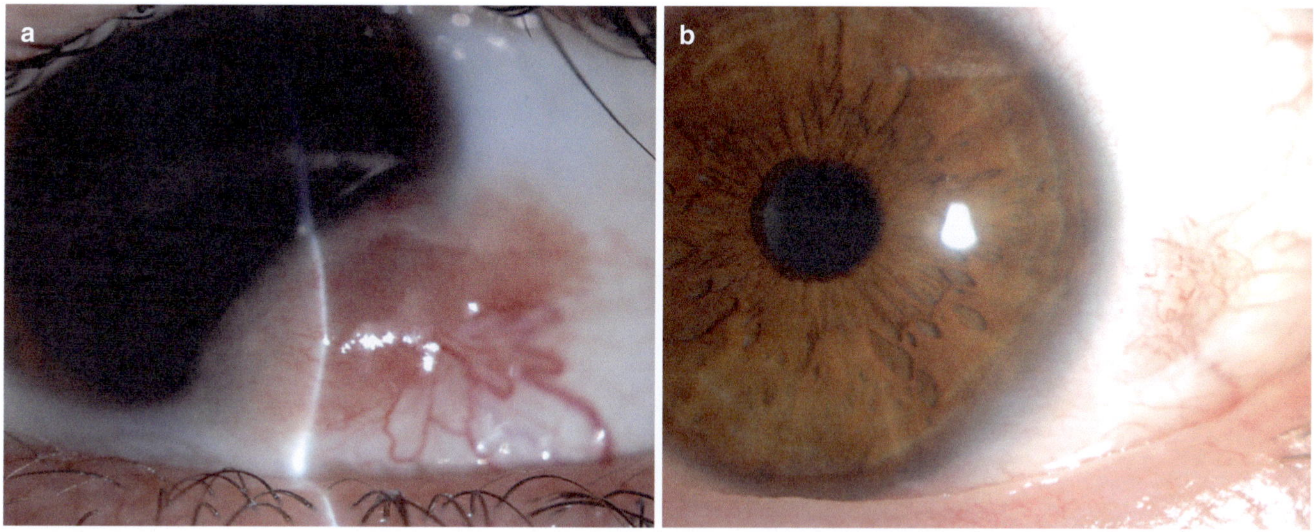

Fig. 2 (**a**) Conjunctival melanoma presenting as a highly vascularized tumor overlying the corneal limbus with LASIK flap invasion. The patient was treated with PBI (70 Gy [RBE] given in 5 fractions). (**b**) He had complete tumor regression and no recurrence at last follow-up 17 months later

limbus (Fig. 2a). Invasion overlying and beneath the LASIK flap was clinically apparent. Traditional excisional biopsy with wide margins was considered. Given the high risk for further tumor dissemination and morbidity following his prior LASIK procedure, a non-invasive approach was chosen. He was treated with PBI using a light field technique with a total dose of 70 Gy (RBE) delivered in 5 fractions (14 Gy [RBE] per fraction). At his last visit, 17 months following PBI, the lesion demonstrated complete regression (Fig. 2b). His vision in the left eye remained 20/25 uncorrected. The LASIK flap was intact without evidence of tumor involvement. He had mild dry eye symptoms that were manageable and responsive to topical artificial tear lubricants.

4 Choroidal Hemangioma

Circumscribed choroidal hemangiomas are sporadic, while diffuse choroidal hemangioma occurs in association with Sturge-Weber or Klippel-Trenaunay-Weber syndrome. Circumscribed choroidal hemangiomas are often asymptomatic. Larger tumors, especially those with macular involvement or with active subretinal or intraretinal fluid, can result in significant vision loss. Diffuse choroidal hemangioma can also be asymptomatic, but these tumors have a propensity for developing extensive, and in some cases, total retinal detachment resulting in severe vision loss. Treatment is aimed at tumor ablation through a variety of techniques, with the goal of resolution of fluid, and ultimately improvement in visual acuity. Several treatment modalities can be used, including photocoagulation, transpupillary thermotherapy (TTT), and photodynamic therapy (PDT). In recent years, PDT has become a common first-line therapy, particularly for circumscribed choroidal hemangioma. Multiple series have demonstrated that PDT is effective in resolving subretinal and intraretinal fluid, and in improving visual acuity [13–16]. A limitation of PDT is the relatively frequent need for multiple treatment sessions and the propensity for recurrence, particularly when tumors have thickness exceeding 3 mm. Multiple PDT sessions can also result in chorioretinal atrophy among other complications [17–19].

PBI is ideal for treating both circumscribed and diffuse choroidal hemangiomas. For young patients, due to high conformality and lack of scatter dose, there is little to no dose to sensitive growth plates of the developing orbit and skull and therefore a decreased risk for secondary malignancies. PBI can therefore be safely delivered in a small number of fractions, reducing the number of treatment sessions. This is particularly advantageous for young children as radiation sessions often require sedation with general anesthesia. PBI can significantly reduce this exposure as it can be administered with fewer fractions (generally 4–10), compared to standard photon-based external beam radiotherapy (EBRT), which generally requires ten or more treatment sessions. PBI has a high success rate, with tumor regression and resolution of subretinal fluid reported in 67–100% of cases [20–22].

At Massachusetts Eye and Ear, protocols for the treatment of choroidal hemangioma have used a light field technique [23]. This setup is currently used for circumscribed choroidal hemangioma and was used in the past for diffuse choroidal hemangioma. More recently, we have treated diffuse choroidal hemangioma using a computed tomography (CT)-based planning setup (Fig. 3) on the gantry to deliver 20 Gy (RBE) in 10 fractions (2 Gy [RBE] per fraction) [24].

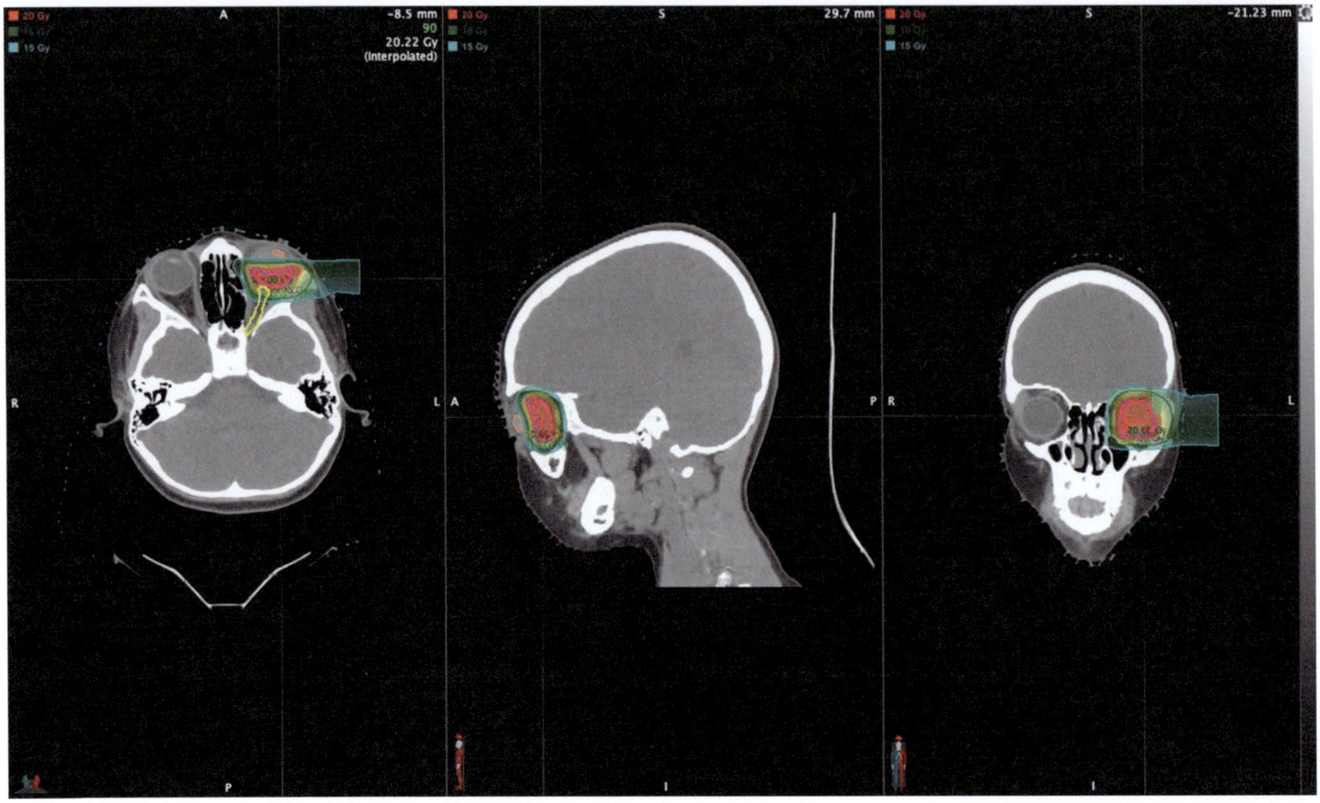

Fig. 3 CT-based PBI scanning plan for a 5-year-old girl with diffuse choroidal hemangioma. The gross tumor volume (GTV) is the choroidal hemangioma as defined by CT. The prescription dose of 20 Gy (RBE) is shown in red and was delivered in 10 fractions

PBI treatment planning begins with color fundus photography and drawings to precisely target the tumor location and ultrasonography to determine tumor diameter and thickness. The optimal dose for choroidal hemangioma has not been well established, but historically doses have ranged from 15 to 30 Gy (RBE). In a recent series of 19 circumscribed choroidal hemangiomas, treated with low doses in the range of 15–30 Gy (RBE), resolution of subretinal fluid was observed in 100% of treated patients and tumor regression occurred in 18 out of 19 eyes (95%) [23]. Our center has observed that doses as low as 15 Gy (RBE) delivered in 4 fractions (3.75 Gy [RBE] per fraction) have successfully maintained visual acuity and induced tumor regression [23]. Additionally, rapid resolution of subretinal fluid reduces the risk of developing chronic, vision-threatening retinal changes such as fibrosis.

4.1 Case

A 54-year-old male was referred for treatment of circumscribed choroidal hemangioma in the right eye. At baseline, his vision measured 20/100 in both eyes due to an inherited macular dystrophy. In the months preceding evaluation, he noted a decrease in vision and metamorphopsia in his right eye. On examination, the vision in the right eye measured 20/150 and an orange-colored circumscribed choroidal hemangioma was present temporal to the macula (Fig. 4a) with subretinal fluid extending into the fovea (Fig. 4b). The tumor measured 2.7 mm in thickness by ultrasonography (Fig. 4c). He was initially treated with PDT using a full dose of verteporfin (6 mg/m^2), standard fluence (50 J/cm^2), and standard treatment time (83 s). The tumor demonstrated a good response with complete resolution of subfoveal fluid (Fig. 4d). Six months later, he developed recurrent subretinal fluid (Fig. 4e) and was treated with a second session of full fluence PDT. The tumor regressed to 2.2 mm in thickness and the subretinal fluid again resolved, but 9 months later, there was recurrence of subretinal fluid. Given his history of multiple recurrences with PDT, he was subsequently treated with PBI using a light field technique with a total dose of 15 Gy (RBE) given in 4 fractions (3.75 Gy [RBE] per fraction). At 15 months of follow-up, the tumor had regressed to 1.4 mm in thickness (Fig. 4f), there was interval resolution of subretinal fluid (Fig. 4g), he had no metamorphopsia, and his vision returned to 20/100 baseline.

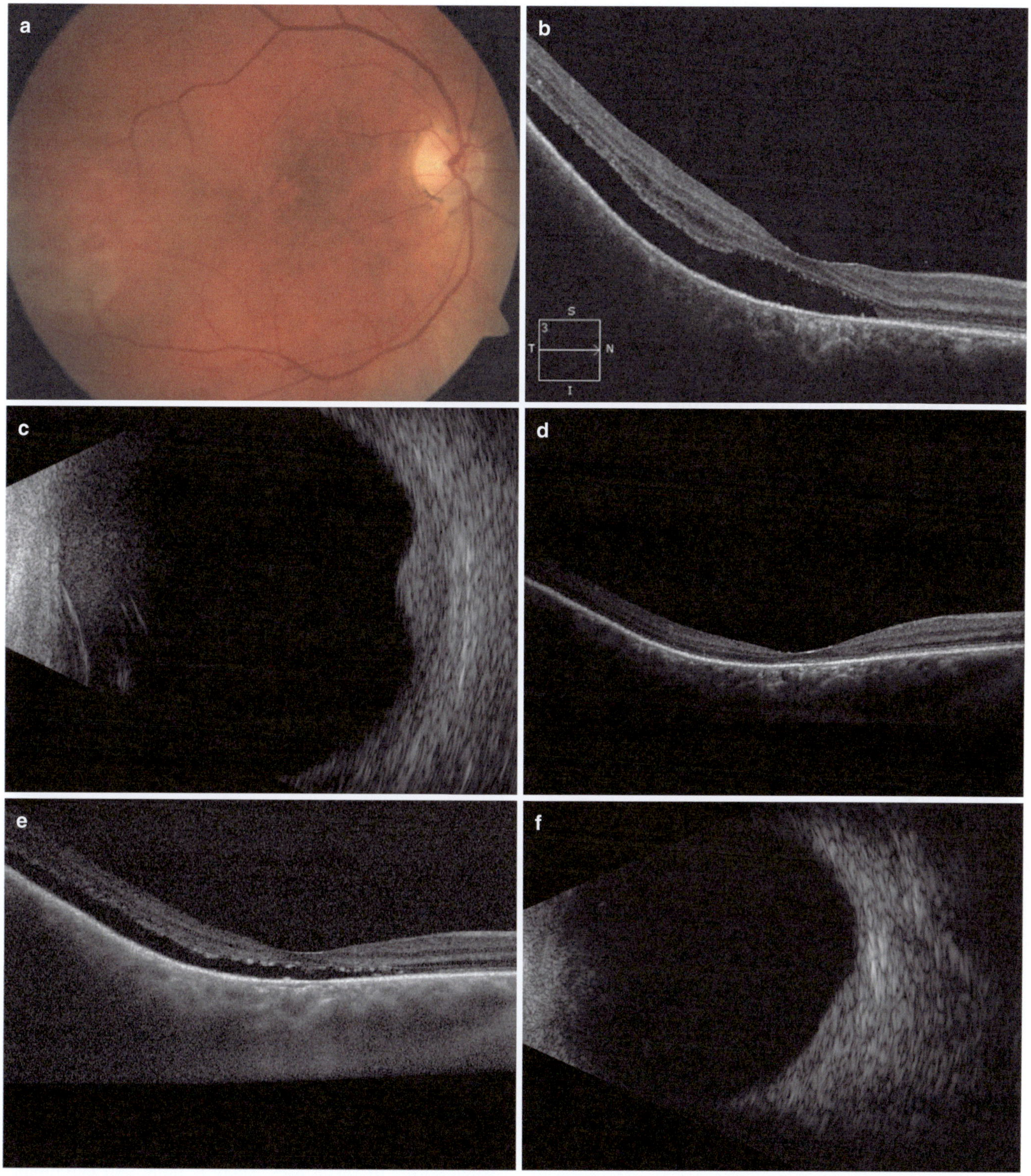

Fig. 4 (**a**) Circumscribed choroidal hemangioma in the right fundus (**b**) with significant overlying subretinal fluid affecting the fovea. (**c**) The tumor measured 2.7 mm in thickness by ultrasonography. (**d**) Full fluence PDT initially resulted in complete resolution of subretinal fluid. (**e**) Unfortunately, the subretinal fluid returned despite a second treatment with full fluence PDT. (**f**) He was subsequently treated with PBI (15 Gy [RBE] given in 4 fractions) and the tumor regressed to 1.4 mm thickness, (**g**) subretinal fluid resolved, and there was no recurrence at last follow-up 15 months later

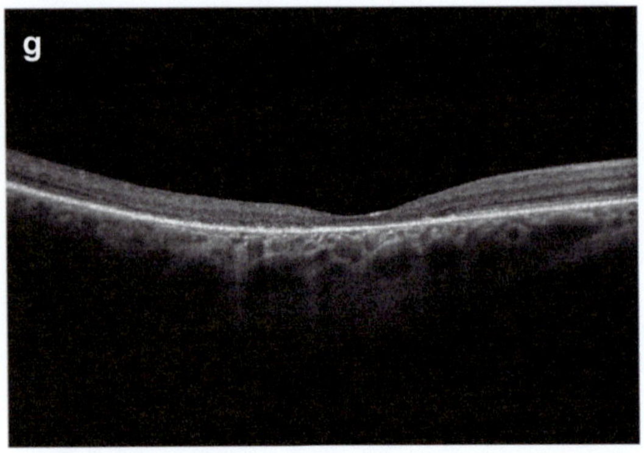

Fig. 4 (continued)

5 Retinal Hemangioblastoma

Retinal hemangioblastoma, whether sporadic or occurring in the setting of von Hippel-Lindau disease, can be managed using a variety of modalities. Thermal laser photocoagulation, cryotherapy, PDT, TTT, and radiotherapy (brachytherapy, EBRT, PBI) have all been employed to treat retinal hemangioblastoma. In general, the goal is to treat tumors while they are small and amenable to thermal laser photocoagulation.

Radiotherapy has a minor role in the treatment of these tumors. PBI may be efficacious for larger retinal hemangioblastomas (>3 mm) not amenable to other forms of treatment, for tumors with extensive subretinal fluid, or for tumors involving the optic nerve [25]. Only a few reports describe the use of PBI to treat retinal hemangioblastoma. While anatomic outcomes have been favorable, corresponding gains in visual acuity have not been observed [26]. In one series of 8 patients with juxtapapillary retinal hemangioblastoma, tumors were treated with PBI using a total dose of 18 Gy (RBE) delivered in 4 fractions. Three years following treatment, all tumors demonstrated regression (mean thickness 1.2 mm compared to 2.4 mm pretreatment). Resolution of subretinal fluid was observed in all cases within 3–6 months following treatment. While vision stabilized, the majority had poor vision at baseline with no further improvement following PBI [27]. While not a common first-line treatment, there are unique circumstances where PBI can be useful such as the case illustrated below of a sizeable exudative retinal hemangioblastoma, not amenable to other standard treatments.

5.1 Case

A 54-year-old male was referred for evaluation of an isolated, exudative retinal hemangioblastoma in the right eye. The vison was 20/60 at baseline. A solitary, highly vascular retinal tumor with associated lipid exudation and subretinal fluid was observed in the temporal mid-periphery (Fig. 5a). Additionally, there was breakthrough vitreous hemorrhage and macular edema. The tumor measured 2.8 mm in thickness by ultrasonography. Given the large size, the decision was made to treat with PBI using a light field technique and a dose of 35 Gy (RBE) in 5 fractions (7 Gy [RBE] per fraction). With the eye positioned in a vertical gaze (Fig. 5b), the isodose curves demonstrate highly conformal tumor coverage while avoiding the fovea and the optic nerve (Fig. 5c). At his last follow-up 6 years later, the tumor remained regressed, with overall thickness measuring 1.4 mm on ultrasonography (Fig. 5d). His vision remained stable at 20/60.

6 Choroidal Metastasis

Multiple options exist for managing choroidal metastases, including close observation while receiving systemic therapy, PDT, and radiation (EBRT, plaque brachytherapy, PBI). Radiation therapy has a prominent role in the management of these tumors, particularly those that are unresponsive to systemic therapy, or for tumors causing significant morbidity due to their location or degree of fluid exudation. PBI is advantageous for the treatment of choroidal metastases as it can simultaneously treat multifocal lesions using a light field technique, thereby avoiding the need for surgical placement of fiducial markers [28]. Due to the high conformality of PBI and lower doses needed for response (most metastases are more radiosensitive than uveal melanoma), PBI generally requires a small number of treatment fractions (two at our institution). In comparison, standard EBRT is administered in daily fractions over 2–3 weeks, a major quality-of-life consideration for individuals with advanced stages of cancer. In a large series of 76 eyes with choroidal metastases treated by PBI, tumor regression was observed in 84% of eyes at 5 months of follow-up. Subretinal fluid resolved in 82% of patients and no tumor recurrence was observed at a mean follow-up of 10 months [29].

At Massachusetts Eye and Ear, patients with choroidal metastases who are treated with PBI receive a total dose of 20 Gy (RBE) delivered in 2 fractions (10 Gy [RBE] per fraction) using the light field setup technique. For more radioresistant forms of metastases, such as renal cell carcinoma, 24 Gy (RBE) is used. In a recent series, results from 77 patients (99 affected eyes) using this approach were analyzed. Local control was achieved in 94% of cases after a median follow-up of 7.7 months. Radiation vasculopathy was noted in 7% of cases and visual acuity decreased compared to pretreatment in 44% [30].

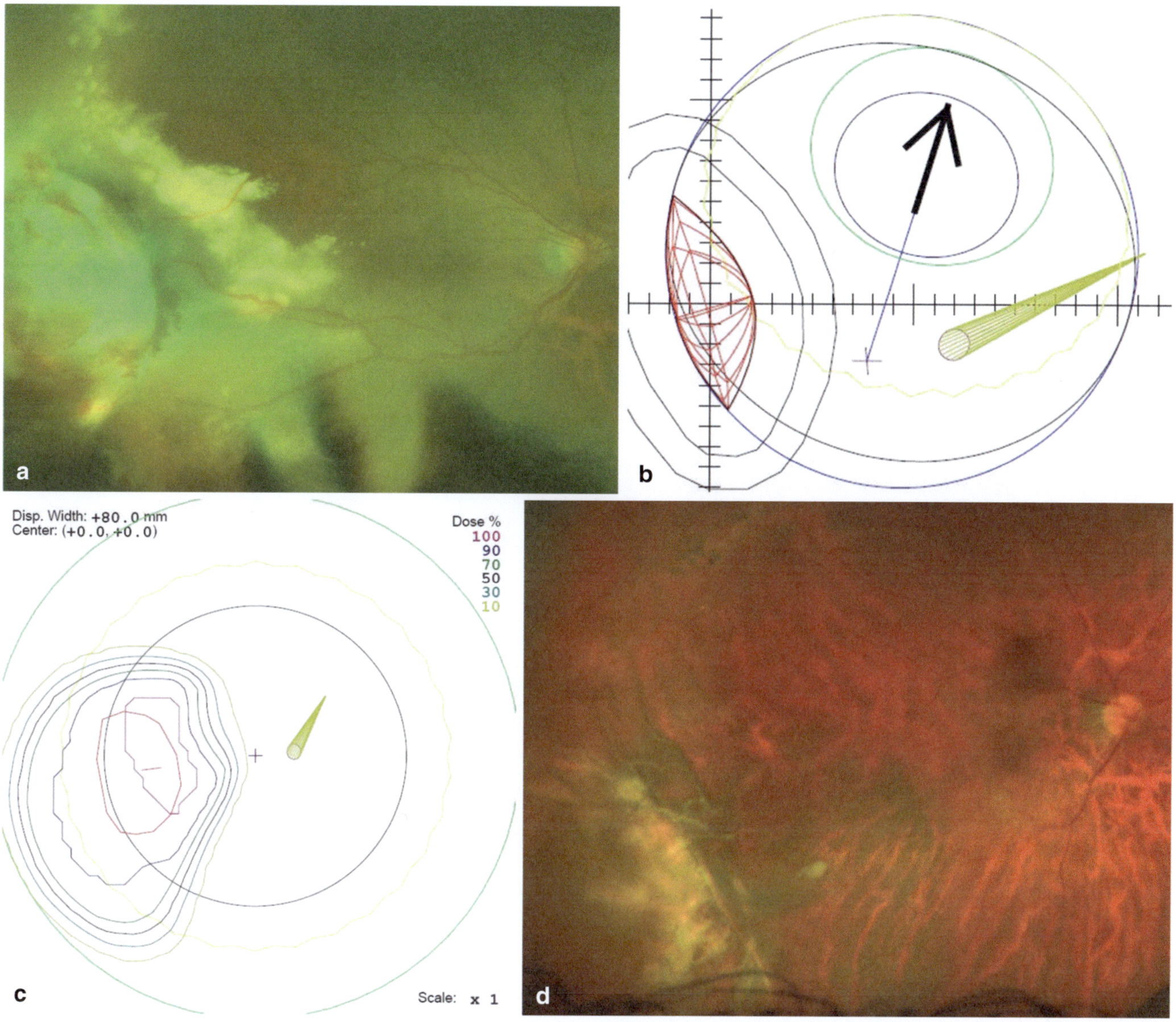

Fig. 5 (**a**) Large, exudative retinal hemangioblastoma in the right fundus. (**b**) The treatment plan shows the eye positioned in an upward gaze (**c**) resulting in highly conformal coverage of the tumor (**c**) and sparing of the fovea (plus sign) and optic nerve (yellow circle). (**d**) He was treated with PBI (35 Gy [RBE] given in 5 fractions) with excellent tumor regression and stable visual acuity at 6 years of follow-up

6.1 Case

A 32-year-old female with metastatic breast carcinoma to the right choroid was referred for management. On examination, her vision was 20/50 in the right eye and 20/20 in the left eye. Dilated fundus examination revealed a solitary choroidal metastasis in the right macula involving the fovea (Fig. 6a) with overlying subfoveal fluid (Fig. 6b). The tumor measured 1.5 mm in thickness by ultrasonography. No metastases were present in the left fundus. Given the macular location of the tumor, presence of subfoveal fluid, and history of worsening symptoms while receiving systemic chemotherapy, the decision was made to proceed with PBI. She received a total of 20 Gy (RBE) delivered in 2 fractions (10 Gy [RBE] per fraction) using the light field technique. At 1-year follow-up, there was complete tumor regression (Fig. 6c), no recurrence of subretinal fluid (Fig. 6d), and her vision in the right eye improved to 20/25.

7 Conclusion

PBI has an established history of providing a high rate of local tumor control for uveal melanoma. While practice patterns are well established for treating uveal melanoma [31], more recent protocols using the light field setup, and CT-guided planning in some cases, have been used to treat a variety of ocular tumors, both benign and malignant. This

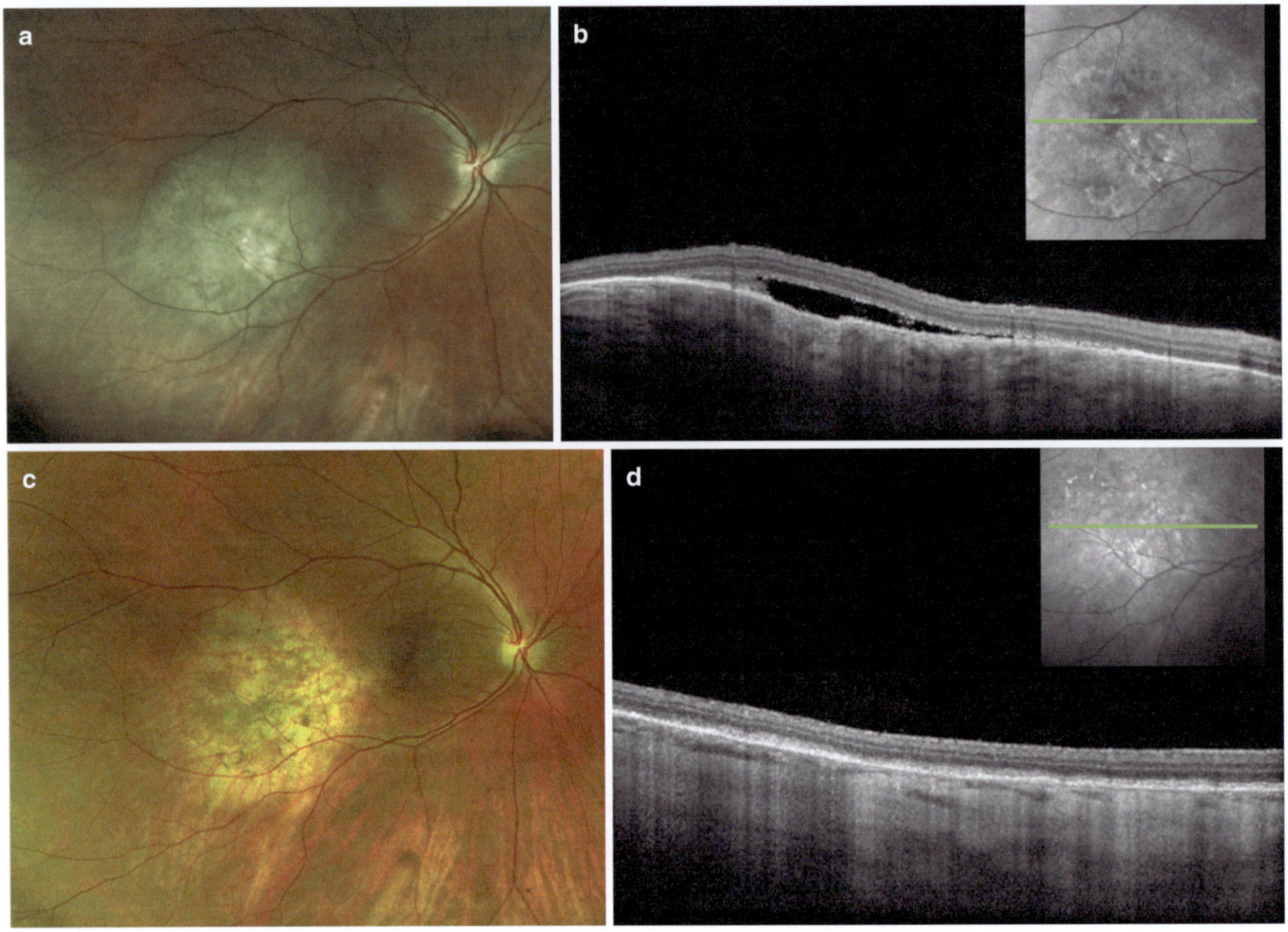

Fig. 6 (**a**) Choroidal metastasis in a patient with metastatic breast carcinoma. (**b**) Visual acuity was declining (20/50) despite systemic therapy due to tumor location involving the fovea and presence of subretinal fluid. She was treated with PBI (20 Gy [RBE] given in 2 fractions). (**c**) At 1-year follow-up, there was complete tumor regression, (**d**) resolution of subretinal fluid, and improvement in vision to 20/25

has expanded the potential indications for PBI and has provided several advantages to patients, including avoiding the need for surgical fiducial marker placement and shorter treatment times (and number of radiation sessions), compared to other conventional forms of radiation (EBRT, plaque brachytherapy). PBI using the light field technique maintains high rates of tumor control and improvement or preservation of vision in many cases.

References

1. Gragoudas ES, Goitein M, Koehler AM, et al. Proton irradiation of small choroidal malignant melanomas. Am J Ophthalmol. 1977;83(5):665–73.
2. Gragoudas ES. Proton beam irradiation of uveal melanomas: the first 30 years. The Weisenfeld Lecture. Invest Ophthalmol Vis Sci. 2006;47(11):4666–73.
3. Oxenreiter MM, Lane AM, Aronow MB, et al. Proton beam irradiation of uveal melanoma involving the iris, ciliary body and anterior choroid without surgical localisation (light field). Br J Ophthalmol. 2022;106(4):518–21.
4. Yu G-P, Hu D-N, McCormick S, et al. Conjunctival melanoma: is it increasing in the United States? Am J Ophthalmol. 2003;135:800–6.
5. Jain P, Finger PT, Fili M, et al. Conjunctival melanoma treatment outcomes in 288 patients: a multicentre international data-sharing study. Br J Ophthalmol. 2021;105(10):1358–64.
6. Ditta LC, Shildkrot Y, Wilson MW. Outcomes in 15 patients with conjunctival melanoma treated with adjuvant topical mitomycin C: complications and recurrences. Ophthalmology. 2011;118:1754–9.
7. Vora GK, Demirci H, Marr B, et al. Advances in the management of conjunctival melanoma. Surv Ophthalmol. 2017;62:26–42.
8. Wuestemeyer H, Sauerwein W, Meller D, et al. Proton radiotherapy as an alternative to exenteration in the management of extended conjunctival melanoma. Graefes Arch Clin Exp Ophthalmol. 2006;244(4):438–46.
9. Scholz SL, Hérault J, Stang A, et al. Proton radiotherapy in advanced malignant melanoma of the conjunctiva. Graefes Arch Clin Exp Ophthalmol. 2019;257(6):1309–18.
10. Thariat J, Salleron J, Maschi C, et al. Oncologic and visual outcomes after postoperative proton therapy of localized conjunctival melanomas. Radiat Oncol. 2019;14(1):239.

11. Maschi-Cayla C, Doyen J, Gastaud P, Caujolle JP. Conjunctival melanomas and proton beam therapy. Acta Ophthalmol. 2013;91(8):e647.
12. Nahon-Estève S, Bertolotto C, Picard-Gauci A, et al. Small but challenging conjunctival melanoma: new insights, paradigms and future perspectives. Cancers (Basel). 2021;13(22):5691.
13. Porrini G, Giovannini A, Amato G, et al. Photodynamic therapy of circumscribed choroidal hemangioma. Ophthalmology. 2003;110(4):674–80.
14. Shields JA. Photodynamic therapy for choroidal hemangioma. Graefes Arch Clin Exp Ophthalmol. 2006;244(9):1071–2.
15. Singh AD, Kaiser PK, Sears JE, et al. Photodynamic therapy of circumscribed choroidal haemangioma. Br J Ophthalmol. 2004;88(11):1414–8.
16. Gupta M, Singh AD, Rundle PA, Rennie IG. Efficacy of photodynamic therapy in circumscribed choroidal 1345 haemangioma. Eye. 2004;18(2):139–42.
17. Verbraak FD, Schlingemann RO, Keunen JE, de Smet MD. Longstanding symptomatic choroidal hemangioma managed with limited PDT as initial or salvage therapy. Graefes Arch Clin Exp Ophthalmol. 2003;241:891–8.
18. Shields CL, Materin MA, Marr BP, et al. Resolution of advanced cystoid macular edema following photodynamic therapy for choroidal hemangioma. Ophthalmic Surg Lasers Imaging. 2005;36:237–9.
19. Tuncer S, Demirci H, Shields CL, Shields JA. Polypoidal choroidal vasculopathy following photodynamic therapy for choroidal hemangioma. Eur J Ophthalmol. 2009;19:159–62.
20. Lee V, Hungerford JL. Proton beam therapy for posterior pole circumscribed choroidal haemangioma. Eye. 1998;12:925–8.
21. Hannouche D, Frau E, Desjardins L, Cassoux N, et al. Efficacy of proton therapy in circumscribed choroidal hemangiomas associated with serious retinal detachment. Ophthalmology. 1997;104(11):1780–4.
22. Zografos L, Egger E, Bercher L, Chamot L, Munkel G. Proton beam irradiation of choroidal hemangiomas. Am J Ophthalmol. 1998;126(2):261–8.
23. Chan RV, Yonekawa Y, Lane AM, et al. Proton beam irradiation using a light-field technique for the treatment of choroidal hemangiomas. Ophthalmologica. 2010;224(4):209–16.
24. Yonekawa Y, MacDonald SM, Shildkrot Y, Mukai S. Standard fractionation low-dose proton radiotherapy for diffuse choroidal hemangiomas in pediatric Sturge-Weber syndrome. J AAPOS. 2013;17(3):318–22.
25. Palmer JD, Gragoudas ES. Advances in treatment of retinal angiomas. Review Int Ophthalmol Clin. 1997;37(4):159–70.
26. Seibel I, Cordini D, Hager A, et al. Long-term results after proton beam therapy for retinal papillary capillary hemangioma. Am J Ophthalmol. 2014 Aug;158(2):381–6.
27. Hussain RN, Hassan S, Ho V, et al. Proton beam radiotherapy (PBR) for the treatment of retinal capillary haemangioblastoma stabilises tumour progression but with poor visual outcomes. Eye (Lond). 2019;33(7):1188–90.
28. Gragoudas ES, Carroll JM. Multiple choroidal metastasis from bronchial carcinoid treated with photocoagulation and proton beam irradiation. Am J Ophthalmol. 1979;87(3):299–304.
29. Tsina EK, Lane AM, Zacks DN, et al. Treatment of metastatic tumors of the choroid with proton beam irradiation. Ophthalmology. 2005;112(2):337–43.
30. Kamran SC, Collier JM, Lane AM, et al. Outcomes of proton therapy for the treatment of uveal metastases. Int J Radiat Oncol Biol Phys. 2014;90(5):1044–50.
31. Hrbacek J, Mishra KK, Kacperek A, et al. Practice patterns analysis of ocular proton therapy centers: the international OPTIC survey. Int J Radiat Oncol Biol Phys. 2016;95(1):336–43.

The Rise in Immunotherapy and Associated Ocular Toxicities

Anam Mazharuddin, Dan S. Gombos, and Nagham Al-Zubidi

1 Introduction

The advent of immune checkpoint inhibitors (ICI) has revolutionized the field of oncology. Immunotherapy harnesses the patient's own immune system to overcome cancer [1]. Many malignancies have had minimal response to traditional therapies such as radiation and chemotherapy [2]. However, these tumors have shown remarkable response to ICI, leading to improved prognosis in advanced or metastatic cancers [2].

The origins of modern immunotherapy date back to the efforts of William Coley in the nineteenth century [3]. Known as the father of immunotherapy, Coley described several cases where cancer patients went into spontaneous remission after developing acute bacterial infections. Summoning the immune system appeared to halt cancer growth and progression. He went on to inoculate his cancer patients with strains of *Streptococcus* and *Serratia* and successfully achieved remission in several malignancies including sarcoma [3]. Years of subsequent research have increased our understanding of the immune system and its relationship to tumor growth. Tumor cells activate immune checkpoint pathways that inhibit the immune system [4]. In 2018, James Allison and Tasuku Honjo were awarded the Nobel Prize in Physiology or Medicine for their discovery of specific proteins involved in suppressing immune checkpoint regulation [5]. The primary targets of checkpoint inhibition are cytotoxic T lymphocyte-associated antigen 4 (CTLA-4), program cell death receptor 1 (PD-1), and programmed cell death ligand 1 (PD-L1) [6]. These ICI interrupt the activation of checkpoint pathways and promote immune-mediated elimination of tumor cells [4]. Thus, ICI enhances the immune system and has significantly improved the prognosis for patients with advanced malignancies [7].

T cell activation requires at least two signals [8]. The first signal comes from an antigen-presenting cell (APC) and occurs when its major histocompatibility complex II (MHC II) interacts with a T cell receptor (TCR) on the surface of a T cell [8]. To complete activation, CD28 on a T cell then binds to a B7 complex on an APC. However, initiation of the first signal also upregulates CTLA-4 [8]. This protein then competes with the stimulatory CD28 binding to the B7 complex and provides a signal to inhibit the T cell's activation. Ipilimumab, a CTLA-4 antibody, was the first ICI approved by the Food and Drug Administration (FDA) in 2010 [9]. Blockade of CTLA-4 results in enhanced T cell response.

PD-1 is commonly found on T cells and normally prevents T cells from attacking other cells in the body when bound to PD-L1 [6]. Tumor cells can evade an immune attack by secreting large amounts of PD-L1 [6]. Monoclonal antibodies that target PD-1 or PD-L1 can block this binding and increase the T cell response [6]. Interestingly, PD-1 and PD-L1 play a role in ocular immune privilege. PD-1 is constitutively expressed in the eye by retinal pigment epithelial cells [4, 5]. When blocked this can trigger an immune response against intraocular tissues [5]. In a mouse model that underwent corneal transplantation, the transplants developed rejection when PD-1 or PD-L1 was blocked [5]. While CTLA-4 inhibition occurs at the time of T cell initiation, PD-1 inhibition occurs downstream to promote T cell function. PD-1 inhibitors include nivolumab, pembrolizumab, and cemiplimab. FDA-approved drugs that target PD-L1 include atezolizumab, avelumab, and durvalumab.

Ipilimumab was approved by the FDA for the management of metastatic melanoma [10]. Nivolumab and pembrolizumab were approved for advanced melanoma and pretreated non-small cell lung cancer (NSCLC) [10]. Atezolizumab may be used for pretreated NSCLC and

A. Mazharuddin
Department of Ophthalmology, University of Texas Medical Branch, Galveston, TX, USA
e-mail: NSAI@mdanderson.org

D. S. Gombos (✉) · N. Al-Zubidi
Department of Head and Neck Surgery, MD Anderson Cancer, Houston, TX, USA
e-mail: dgombos@mdanderson.org; aamazhar@utmb.edu

B. V. Chawla, M. E. Aronow (eds.), *Global Perspectives in Ocular Oncology*, https://doi.org/10.1007/978-3-031-08250-4_33

advanced urothelial carcinoma [10]. Cemiplimab was authorized by the FDA to treat metastatic or unresectable squamous cell cancer [2]. Other indications for ICI are renal cell carcinoma, head and neck squamous cell carcinoma, Hodgkin lymphoma, and Merkel cell carcinoma [7].

2 General Principles

Despite their success, ICI have been associated with a broad spectrum of side effects. These have been coined immune-related adverse events (irAEs) [7]. IrAEs are thought to arise from the enhancement of the immune system [7]. ICI not only allows the T cells to attack tumor cells but also allows them to respond against normal healthy tissue [5]. Common adverse events include rash, diarrhea, and fatigue. Ocular irAEs are quite rare, occurring in approximately 1% of treated patients [12]. Most reports of ocular irAEs are limited to single-digit case series and case reports [12]. Nevertheless, as use of ICI increases, ocular adverse events are becoming more relevant. Ocular toxicities may range from transient blurred vision and ocular discomfort to uveitis and optic neuropathy. Ocular toxicity may be sight-threatening and has a significant impact on a patient's quality of life. Specialized and multidisciplinary teams including ophthalmologists, oncologists, internal medicine, etc. are critical to prevent further aggravation of irAEs.

The National Cancer Institute has created Common Terminology Criteria for Adverse Events (CTCAE), which provides descriptive terminology to report grading (severity) of medication adverse events (toxicities) [11]. The CTCAE includes grading tables for the severity of ocular pathology (Table 1). These include blurred vision, cataract formation, conjunctivitis, flashing lights, floaters, dry eye, extraocular muscle paresis, retinopathy, and uveitis among others [11].

The grading system is divided into five categories: grades 1–5 [11]. Grade 1 with mild to no symptoms is discovered only by observation and requires no intervention. Grade 2 is defined as mildly limiting age-appropriate activities of daily living (ADL) with minimal, local, noninvasive intervention indicated. Visual acuity is 20/40 or better (or loss of 3 lines or fewer from baseline). Grade 3 occurs when there is a severe or medically significant adverse effect; however, it is not immediately life-threatening. Hospitalization may be indicated due to disabling or limited ability to perform ADLs. Vision is worse than 20/40 with more than 3 lines decreased from baseline but better than 20/200. For grade 4 toxicities that are life-threatening, urgent intervention is required. Visual acuity is worse than 20/200 and qualifies as blindness. Grade 5 involves death that is related to the adverse event [11].

In general, patients with mild (i.e., grade 1) toxicity can be monitored closely for the progression of adverse events. Patients who develop moderate to severe toxicity (i.e., grade 2 or above) should consider reducing the dose or withholding treatment. Grade 3 and above toxicity should prompt consideration of holding or permanently discontinuing treatment. Rapid and aggressive use of systemic corticosteroids may be required followed by a slow taper. Other treatments such as plasmapheresis, intravenous immunoglobulin, and other immunosuppressants may be used [7].

3 Immunotherapy Considerations

Adverse events are most common with the use of nivolumab compared to any other ICI [13]. The reported ocular toxicity rate of ipilimumab is 1.3% including anterior uveitis, optic neuropathy, and thyroid orbitopathy [14]. Atezolizumab carries the highest association with ocular inflammation, while ipilimumab has the greatest association with uveitis [15]. Adverse events with CTLA-4 inhibitors appear to be dose dependent, but this may not be necessarily true for PD-1 and PD-L1 inhibitor monotherapy [13]. Additionally, the combination of ipilimumab with nivolumab is associated with greater toxicity than either ICI alone. Several studies have also shown that patients who had systemic manifestations such as colitis were also more likely to have uveitis or episcleritis [14].

Table 1 Common terminology criteria for adverse events: grading/severity

Grade 1	Grade 2	Grade 3	Grade 4	Grade 5
Mild	*Moderate*	*Severe*	*Sight-threatening/ life-threatening*	*Death*
Asymptomatic or mild symptoms	Symptomatic with moderate decrease in VA	Symptomatic with marked decrease in VA	Life-threatening consequences	Death
	BCVA >20/40 or <3 lines of decreased vision from baseline	BCVA < 20/40 or >3 lines of decreased vision from baseline (up to 20/200)	BCVA <20/200	
Intervention not indicated	Medical intervention indicated	Invasive intervention indicated	Urgent intervention indicated	

VA visual acuity; *BCVA* best-corrected visual acuity

4 Pathogenesis of ICI

The pathogenesis of ICI leading to ocular toxicity is not well understood. One study proposed that CTLA-4 inhibitors impair the survival and function of T cells which yields to the formation of autoimmune inflammatory disorders [16]. Conversely, PD-1 and PD-L1 inhibitors not only affect T cell function but also produce pathological autoantibodies [16]. This may be why PD-1 inhibitors are more likely to result in ocular myasthenia [16]. Further studies need to be conducted to elucidate the mechanism of adverse events.

5 Clinical Manifestations of ICI Toxicities

5.1 Eyelids, Eyebrows, and Eyelashes

5.1.1 Blepharitis and Meibomian Gland Dysfunction (MGD)

Blepharitis is a chronic inflammatory condition of the eyelids [17]. Meibomian glands in the eyelids secrete the oily layer of the tear film. This prevents tear evaporation, and thus, plays an important role in maintaining normal lubrication of the eye. Patients may present with itching, blurry vision improved with blinking, a foreign body sensation, and dry eye symptoms. Examination may reveal crusting of the eyelids and margin inflammation with inspissated oil glands [17]. It is hypothesized that treatment with checkpoint immunotherapy may trigger a T cell-mediated autoimmune response in the eyelids leading to ocular surface disease [18]. Ipilimumab has less than 1% incidence of blepharitis [17].

Management of symptoms includes daily eyelid scrubs and the use of therapeutic medications such as antibiotics and combination steroids to reduce infection and inflammation [17, 18]. Warm compresses may also be helpful as well as omega-3 fatty acids. There have been no case reports thus far of discontinuation of ICI due to blepharitis or MGD.

5.1.2 Stevens-Johnson Syndrome/Toxic Epidermal Necrolysis (SJS/TEN)

Stevens-Johnson syndrome (SJS) and toxic epidermal necrolysis (TEN) belong to a spectrum of rare but potentially life-threatening complications affecting the skin and mucous membranes [19]. This dermatological emergency manifests as patches of the skin and mucous membrane inflammation that rapidly progress to epidermal necrosis and sloughing. SJS typically involves less than 10% of the total body surface area, while TEN accounts for greater than 30% of total body surface area. Medications are the causative factor in 80% of cases [19]. Patients treated with nivolumab have been reported to develop SJS [2, 20, 21]. Additionally, TEN was reported with both pembrolizumab and atezolizumab [22].

A high level of suspicion and close monitoring is recommended as SJS and TEN are potentially fatal [2]. The duration from onset of drug exposure to the development of eruption is variable, and there may be delay of several months or several cycles of treatment. SJS is automatically classified as grade 3 or higher toxicity on the CTAE scale, while TEN is grade 4 or higher [11]. Thus, discontinuation of ICI is necessary. Treatment is largely supportive, but medical therapy may include corticosteroid, intravenous immunoglobulin, cyclosporine, and TNF-α inhibitors [2].

5.2 Conjunctiva and Sclera

5.2.1 Conjunctivitis

Conjunctivitis is the inflammation of the transparent conjunctiva and typically presents as a pink hue over the white part of the eye [17]. This can be associated with swelling or chemosis, increased tearing, and discharge. It is generally not accompanied by eye pain or vision changes. Although conjunctivitis may be induced from any of the ICI, it can also be caused by infectious and allergic etiologies [23]. Therefore, patient history is important [17]. Conjunctivitis was reported in two cases with irritation and injection after nivolumab [24].

Most cases of conjunctivitis are self-limited [17]. Symptoms may last 4–6 weeks. If there is suspicion for bacterial infectious etiology, a short course of antibiotic ointment may be prescribed. Allergic conjunctivitis may be treated with over-the-counter antihistamines and mast cell inhibitors [17]. There have been no reported cases requiring cessation of ICI due to conjunctivitis [24]. One case was treated with topical corticosteroids [24].

5.2.2 Sclera

Scleral disease has been reported in all the ICI; however, they are rare presentations. Together scleritis and episcleritis make up 1% of adverse events with ICI [25].

5.2.3 Episcleritis

Episcleritis is the inflammation of the tissue between the conjunctiva and sclera [17]. Patients will report a sudden onset redness, irritation, and watering of the eye. There is minimal pain and vision is preserved. Examination may reveal vasodilation of the superficial episcleral vessels without swelling or thinning of the sclera. Cases of episcleritis have been reported with ipilimumab [8, 26]. Episcleritis can be managed with topical lubricants, oral nonsteroidal anti-inflammatory drugs (NSAIDs), or topical corticosteroid [17].

5.2.4 Scleritis

Scleritis involves the deeper connective tissue and appears darker and more violaceous compared to episcleritis [25]. This condition can be localized, nodular, or diffuse with vasodilation. Pain ranges from mild to out of proportion to examination findings based on the severity of disease. Rarely, necrosis may be seen in the most severe type. However, necrotizing scleritis has not been reported as an adverse event with ICI. Diagnosis of scleritis is based on location, redness, pain, and tenderness to touch. B-scan ultrasonography may help to diagnose posterior scleritis when a classic T-sign is observed due to the presence of fluid in Tenon's space [27]. Nivolumab had one case report of scleritis treated with oral corticosteroids [27]. Scleritis is generally managed with NSAIDs and topical corticosteroid [25]. Severe cases may require oral corticosteroids and cessation of the ICI if poorly controlled [27].

5.3 Cornea and Tear Film

ICI can affect the cornea leading to dry eye, corneal ulcers, and deposits. The most common adverse event is dry eye. Clinical trial reports of CTLA4 and PD-1-targeting antibodies showed that the incidence of dry eye is 1.2–24.2% [10]. Another study suggested that dry eye occurred in one in four treated patients [12]. The most common ICI associated with dry eye are ipilimumab, nivolumab, and pembrolizumab [13]. Dry eyes are often not reported in clinical trials and are often underdiagnosed even in clinical practice [12].

5.3.1 Dry Eye Syndrome

Dry eye syndrome results in burning, gritty, sandy, or foreign body sensation [25]. Some may experience increased redness, sensitivity to light, and blurred vision. Corneal defects associated with dry eyes are variable. Blurry vision often improves with blinking. Diagnosis is achieved primarily from the patient's history and symptoms. Staining with fluorescein, rose bengal, or lissamine green can reveal epithelial defects. Additionally, dry eye can be documented with rapid tear breakup time (TBUT) of <10 s (normal is >10 s) and reduced tear secretion using the Schirmer tests.

A retrospective review of the FDA Adverse Event Reporting System (FAERS) database from 2015 to 2020 demonstrated 75 reports of dry eye syndrome secondary to PD1/PD-1 inhibition [28]. Nivolumab represented 51 cases (68%) followed by pembrolizumab with 22 cases (29%). There was only one documented incidence each of dry eye with atezolizumab (1%) and durvalumab (1%) [28].

Lubrication with artificial tears is the first line of treatment as they are simple to administer and available over the counter [25]. Lid hygiene and warm compresses also play an important role in tear quality. Patients may benefit from punctal occlusion if they have reflex excess tearing caused by dry eyes. Severe cases may be improved with topical corticosteroids or ophthalmic cyclosporine [25]. Autologous serum tears have also been used with success.

5.3.2 Corneal Epithelial Defects, Keratitis, and Corneal Melts

Persistent corneal epithelial defects are often secondary to poor healing of the epithelial layer of the cornea [25]. Symptoms associated with corneal epithelial defects are similar to dry eye but more severe. Patients may experience blurred vision, burning, and eye pain. Measurement of visual acuity is critical. Nonhealing epithelial defects are at increased risk of developing infectious keratitis and corneal ulcers [25]. However, not all corneal ulcers are related to exposure. Parker et al. described a peripheral corneal ulcer secondary to nivolumab use which was resolved after discontinuation of nivolumab [23]. Corneal ulcers or infiltrates can appear as white-tan-colored lesions in the clear cornea. These conditions are sight-threatening and require immediate ophthalmologic attention [23].

Aggressive lubrication with preservative-free artificial tears or ointments is helpful. However, patients with corneal epithelial defects are often not improved on topical lubrication alone [25]. Patients generally are treated with topical antibiotics to prevent superinfection. Some cases may benefit from a bandage contact lens or temporary tarsorrhaphy although care must be taken to ensure there is no infection present [25]. Nivolumab-induced ulcerative keratitis was treated successfully with topical corticosteroids alone [29]. Another patient on atezolizumab developed autoimmune keratitis that was treated with both topical and oral corticosteroids [30].

Corneal thinning and melt are severe epithelial defects [29, 30]. They are often difficult to diagnose unless viewed through a slit lamp with a thin beam transecting the cornea. These are vision-threatening conditions that may lead to corneal perforation if left untreated. There has been one case report of corneal perforation following the use of nivolumab that did not improve with corticosteroids (both systemic and subconjunctival) [31].

5.4 Cataracts

Cataracts are opacities of the lens of the eye and are generally associated with age. Cataracts are classified as nuclear sclerotic, cortical, or posterior subcapsular based on the location in the lens where the opacification occurs. Patients will typically complain of painless, progressive vision loss. There may be symptoms of glare or halos around lights at night. Cataract formation from ICI is rare and typically found as a sequela of chronic or severe uveitis [12, 32, 33]. Posterior subcapsular cataracts are most reported in pembrolizumab, ipilimumab, and nivolumab [32, 33]. There were two cases of cataract formation with the use of nivolumab [34]. There have been no reports of cataracts with the use of atezolizumab, avelumab, or durvalumab to date. Treatment is surgical excision of the cataract and placement of an intraocular lens.

5.5 Uveitis

The uvea is composed of the iris, ciliary body, and choroid. Uveitis can be divided into four broad categories, anterior, intermediate, posterior, and panuveitis, depending on the location of the inflammation. Presentation typically occurs within 2 months after starting ICI therapy; however, there has been a case report of a patient with anterior uveitis presenting 2 years after treatment with nivolumab [12, 35]. Inflammation of the uveal tract can produce variable ophthalmic complaints depending on the location of involvement including vision loss, floaters, pain, redness, and photophobia [17]. The incidence of uveitis ranges from 0.3 to 6% [10]. Conrady et al. performed a literature review of 33 cases of uveitis secondary to ICI [36]. One-third of patients experienced anterior uveitis alone; one-third demonstrated anterior uveitis with posterior segment changes such as macular edema, retinitis, or papillitis; and one-third had panuveitis [36]. The odds ratio for uveitis ranged from 4.6 to 10.8 [12]. The risk of uveitis is greatest with the use of ipilimumab, nivolumab, pembrolizumab, and atezolizumab [13].

5.5.1 Anterior Uveitis

Anterior uveitis is characterized by white cells in the anterior chamber of the eye [17]. When it affects the iris, it is frequently referred to as iritis. When the ciliary body is also involved, it is known as iridocyclitis. Symptoms of anterior uveitis are pain, photophobia, and redness. Examination often reveals limbal flush (inflammation around the cornea and sclera). The cornea may demonstrate keratic precipitates. The key finding is white cells in the anterior chamber. The severity of anterior uveitis is determined by the number of cells seen in high-power magnification on a slit lamp. In addition, there may be a haze or flare noted which represents protein in the aqueous humor caused by disruption of the blood-aqueous barrier [17]. In severe inflammation, posterior synechiae or scarring of the iris to the lens may occur resulting in an abnormal pupil shape on attempted dilation [25].

5.5.2 Intermediate Uveitis

Leukocytes in the vitreous or inflammation of the ciliary body is referred to as intermediate uveitis [17]. Unlike anterior uveitis, intermediate uveitis is typically painless; however, vision changes such as vision loss and floaters are more prevalent [17].

5.5.3 Posterior Uveitis and Panuveitis

Posterior uveitis involves the choroid [17]. Severe choroiditis can affect the retina and optic nerve. Vision loss can be profound without pain [17]. Patients may present with floaters, photopsias, and blind spots [12]. Fluorescein angiography (FA) and indocyanine green angiography (ICG) play an important role in the diagnosis of posterior uveitis [25]. Panuveitis involves all three compartments of the eye and may present with all symptoms from eye pain to vision loss [17].

Prompt referral to an ophthalmologist is critical for the proper management of uveitis [17]. Treatment involves the initiation of topical cycloplegics and corticosteroids to prevent scarring and reduce ciliary spasms of the eye which cause pain [35]. Sometimes periocular and intraocular steroids are necessary in cases with involvement of the macula. Systemic corticosteroids are used to treat posterior or panuveitis. If systemic steroids were used, the American Society of Clinical Oncology (ASCO) recommended suspending the ICI until the patient is either off all steroids or is receiving a daily dose of 10 mg of oral prednisone or less [12]. Grade 2–4 drug toxicities may require discontinuation of ICI. In fact, most patients with uveitis in a case series (five out of seven patients) ultimately have had their treatment discontinued [12]. Patients may see a reversal of vision loss after treatment; however, a small minority may have permanent vision loss. A rechallenge can be considered in patients with mild irAE once symptoms resolve [14].

Shahzad et al. developed an algorithm based on their review of literature and international guidelines on the management of uveitis [12]. It is designed for multidisciplinary teams for use in clinical settings [12]. For patients with mild to moderate symptoms, ICI may be continued but requires a referral to ophthalmology in 1–2 weeks. For patients with moderate to severe symptoms or neurological symptoms such as diplopia, color vision, or visual field deficits, ICI should be paused, and urgent referral should be made to an ophthalmologist. Ophthalmologists can diagnose uveitis and begin management with corticosteroids and escalate therapy as needed. Additional testing such as fluorescein angiography, autofluorescence, and optical coherence tomography (OCT) may be performed. After monitoring treatment response, the ophthalmologist and oncologist can then create a multidisciplinary assessment and tailor ICI therapy [12].

Poorly controlled uveitis may lead to cataract formation, glaucoma, or choroidal neovascularization [12, 33]. Conversely, treatment of uveitis with glucocorticoids may result in elevated intraocular pressures and subsequent optic nerve damage leading to glaucoma and irreversible blindness. Thus, patients with uveitis should be followed closely [17].

5.5.4 Vogt-Koyanagi-Harada (VKH)-Like Syndrome

A recent review of 126 cases of ICI-associated uveitis found that 35% of panuveitis cases were part of Vogt-Koyanagi-Harada (VKH)-like syndrome [12]. VKH is an inflammatory disease process against melanocytes characterized by chronic diffuse granulomatous panuveitis [25, 35]. VKH is mediated by T lymphocytes similar to the mechanism of action of ICI, with presumed mechanisms to make ICI have a high incidence of VKH. CTLA-4 and PD1 and PD-L1 antibodies may disrupt the immune tolerance to melanocytes and trigger VKH [25]. VKH-like syndrome has been reported in patients receiving combination therapy ipilimumab and pembrolizumab as well as nivolumab [37, 38].

Classically, VKH presents as a bilateral panuveitis with exudative retinal detachments. Vision loss can be profound in both eyes. Associated symptoms include cutaneous changes—vitiligo, poliosis, alopecia, and neurological deficits—tinnitus, hearing loss, meningismus, and headache. Cerebrospinal fluid analysis may reveal pleocytosis. However, VKH-like syndrome may have some distinct features. For example, VKH-like syndrome did not feature pleocytosis or meningismus symptoms [39]. The diagnosis of VKH should be in the absence of prior ocular trauma or surgery and any other ocular disease based on clinical or laboratory evidence [35].

VKH has four stages with different clinical features [35, 39]. Stage I is the prodromal stage in which the patient may suffer nonspecific viral illness with nausea, vomiting, and headache for up to a week. Stage 2 presents with ophthalmic symptoms and signs of uveitis. This may lead to serous retinal detachments and subsequent vision loss. During stage 3, convalescence, choroidal depigmentation results in a sunset glow fundus. At this point, the patient generally develops vitiligo and poliosis due to an autoimmune attack on melanocytes. Stage 4 is the chronic recurrent stage in which recurrent uveitis is predominant. Patients may develop complications from uveitis as described above. Ipilimumab and nivolumab have been implicated in a presentation very similar to classic VKH [35, 40]. The time to onset after immunotherapy ranges from 2 weeks to 13 months [17].

Treatment is the same as the management of uveitis with topical and systemic corticosteroids [17]. Most cases of drug-induced VKH require stopping ICI. In one case report, treatment with ICI was continued with the use of subconjunctival steroids, and no recurrence of symptoms has occurred to date [37].

5.5.5 Uveal Effusion

Uveal effusion is a rare adverse event with the use of ICI, particularly with PD-1 and PD-LI inhibitors atezolizumab, nivolumab, or pembrolizumab [41]. Only three patients have been reported to develop large uveal effusions. These first appeared between 1 and 3 months after two infusions of ICI [41]. Two out of three patients discontinued therapy with resolution of uveal effusion after several weeks. The last patient succumbed to melanoma [41]. Similarly, Telfah described two patients on pembrolizumab who presented with vision loss bilaterally and were found to have choroidal effusions leading to exudative retinal detachments [42]. The first patient developed irAE 1 year after initiating treatment, while the second suffered vision loss more acutely within weeks. Once the ICI was stopped, the vision returned to baseline in both patients. One of the patients resumed ICI after 4 months; however, his symptoms recurred, and ICI was permanently discontinued [42].

5.6 Retina and Vitreous

ICI can produce variable toxicity to the retina. The retinal vasculature may be at risk in developing intraretinal hemorrhages, cotton wool spots, and choroidal neovascularization. Damage to the retinal pigment epithelium may lead to pigmentary retinopathy or intraretinal fluid known as macular edema. Involvement of photoreceptors may lead to flashes or night blindness.

5.6.1 Retinal Tears and Detachments

According to the retrospective review of the FAERS study from 2015 to 2020, there were 49 reported cases of retinal detachments secondary to PD-1 and PD-L1 inhibition [28]. Nivolumab had 30 associated cases (61%), while pembrolizumab had 11 reported cases (22%). Eight cases were reported with the use of atezolizumab [28]. Treatment of retinal detachments includes scleral buckle, pars plana vitrectomy, or cryotherapy.

5.6.2 Macular Edema

Cystoid macular edema is defined as multiple cyst-like fluid spaces in the central retina resulting in swelling or edema. Patients present with painless blurry vision or metamorphopsia, or the perception that straight lines appear wavy. Most cases of macular edema occur in conjunction with uveitis or optic neuropathy.

5.6.3 Choroidal Neovascularization

Only one case report has documented choroidal neovascularization with ipilimumab treatment thus far [43]. The patient presented with blurred vision 1 year after starting ICI therapy. Macular edema and choroidal neovascularization were confirmed on OCT. The patient was treated with intravitreal anti-vascular endothelial growth factor (anti-VEGF) therapy with resolution of symptoms 2 years later without discontinuation of ipilimumab [43].

5.6.4 Other

Grade 3 chorioretinitis was seen in one patient treated with ipilimumab which led to treatment discontinuation [44]. There has been one case report of a patient treated with pembrolizumab who developed a white dot syndrome known as birdshot-like chorioretinopathy 2 years after treatment [45]. Combined FA/ICG showed hypocyanescent lesions without retinal vasculitis in both eyes. The patient underwent testing for HLA-A29 which generally is positive in 95% of patients with birdshot chorioretinopathy; however, this patient was negative. The patient was treated with triamcinolone injections in both eyes with partial resolution [45]. There has been one case report of retinal vasculitis which developed after pembrolizumab treatment which improved after vitrectomy and external beam radiotherapy for vitreous metastases [46]. Another case report details the development of melanoma-associated retinopathy (MAR) with atypical chorioretinal lesions after treatment with pembrolizumab [47]. On the other hand, another study reported photoreceptor toxicity secondary to nivolumab [48].

5.7 Neuro-ophthalmology

Neuro-ophthalmic adverse events are extremely rare but visually significant. Ocular myasthenia risk was only associated with nivolumab and pembrolizumab [13]. The reported cumulative incidence of severe neurotoxicities related to ICI is estimated at less than 1% [49]. A review of ocular irAE found that neurological-related events occurred at a median of 35 days (5 weeks) after initiating ICI therapy [13, 49]. This included cases of optic neuritis and myasthenia gravis [13, 48].

5.7.1 Optic Nerve Edema and Neuropathy

Optic neuropathy may present as optic nerve edema, optic atrophy, idiopathic intracranial hypertension, or extraocular motility deficits. It has a variable presentation from asymptomatic to enlarged blind spot or constriction of visual fields. Two cases of optic neuropathy have been associated with ipilimumab [51]. The patients presented with visual disturbances such as scotomas or visual field deficits [51]. Another case report documented a patient with previously 20/20 vision who developed vision loss down to 20/200 within days after his fourth infusion of ipilimumab [52]. Examination demonstrated optic nerve edema with correlating visual field defects. OCT imaging confirmed moderate optic nerve atrophy [52]. Six months after treatment with topical steroids, the patient's vision returned to baseline; however, the visual field defects persisted [52].

5.7.2 Optic Neuritis

Optic neuritis is a rare presentation with ICI. Patients will complain of blurred vision, color vision loss, and pain with eye movements. One patient with nivolumab-induced optic neuritis complained of photopsias only [53]. Examination may reveal afferent pupillary defect if there is asymmetry of optic nerve involvement. Fundus exam may show optic nerve edema if the anterior optic nerve is involved or a normal fundus in which case may represent retrobulbar optic neuritis. MRI orbits will reveal optic nerve enhancement. Duong reported a patient who developed demyelinating disease secondary to combination ipilimumab with nivolumab therapy [49]. MRI revealed bilateral optic nerve enhancement. Cerebrospinal fluid (CSF) studies were negative for infection and neuromyelitis optica (NMO) and paraneoplastic (PNP) antibodies. The patient was treated with intravenous steroids for 5 days followed by intravenous immunoglobulin (IVIG) for 2 days and then transitioned to oral prednisone [49]. Later she relapsed and was treated with one dose of infliximab with some improvement overall in vision [49]. Another case report detailed a pediatric patient who was treated with nivolumab monotherapy and developed bilateral optic neuritis after the second infusion [54]. A large case series of 18 patients found that combination therapy created a higher short-term risk for optic neuritis, while protracted use of a single-agent ICI was associated with a delayed risk [50].

5.8 Orbital Inflammation

ICI have been reported to develop inflammation of the orbit, particularly with ipilimumab [14]. Symptoms associated with orbital inflammation are pain with eye movement, orbital congestion, proptosis, subsequent exposure keratopathy, ophthalmoplegia, diplopia, and blindness if severe. Examination should include visual acuity, pupil assessment to rule out an afferent pupillary defect, color plates to look for desaturation, extraocular motility testing in addition to slit lamp, and dilated fundus examination. Imaging with CT scan and MRI of the orbits helps elucidate extraocular muscle enlargement and involvement of muscle tendons [17].

5.8.1 Thyroid Eye Disease

Thyroid eye disease (TED) is also known as Graves' disease. It occurs when there is an abnormal expression of thyrotropin receptor antibody and T cell response. The T cell response seen in TED is similar to the mechanism of action in CTLA-4 and PD1/PD-L1 antibodies [55]. The result is inflammation of the orbit and extraocular muscles sparing the tendons [55]. Other associated symptoms include eye pain, redness, diplopia, and blurred vision from compressive ophthalmopathy [25]. Signs of TED may be eyelid retraction, and lid lag in downgaze with proptosis, and restrictive strabismus. Symptoms can present after the first dose of ICI but may be delayed even 2 years later [56]. Hertel measurements can be used to monitor for progression [57]. Enlargement of extraocular muscles and fat on imaging may lead to compressive optic neuropathy [25]. Laboratory workup for thyroid function may assist with diagnosis; however, normal test results do not necessarily exclude disease if clinical suspicion is high [56]. Treatment may range from lubrication and NSAIDs for redness and pain to corticosteroids and even decompressive surgery if vision is threatened by compressive orbitopathy [25]. Fresnel prisms can be used to control diplopia [57].

A case report described a patient who developed severe Graves' disease with proptosis and diplopia after two doses of ipilimumab [55, 58]. The patient's blood work returned elevated antithyroglobulin and thyroid-stimulating hormone receptor antibodies, while TSH, T3, and T4 were within normal limits [55, 58]. Imaging revealed diffuse enlargement of all extraocular muscles consistent with TED [55]. The patient required oral corticosteroids and orbital decompression with resolution of symptoms. Similarly, pembrolizumab has also been linked to new-onset Graves' ophthalmopathy [57]. Thyroid function studies may be unremarkable. Imaging revealed asymmetric proptosis consistent with TED. Treatment is the cessation of ICI and initiation of corticosteroid.

5.8.2 Orbital Myositis

Orbital myositis has been reported in patients treated with ICI. A patient treated with ipilimumab developed ophthalmoplegia and proptosis after the third infusion [59]. Imaging with MRI revealed diffuse EOM enlargement that involved the tendons. Typically, the tendons are spared in thyroid ophthalmopathy. Ultrasound demonstrated hypo-reflectivity of the extraocular muscles which was more consistent with myositis or orbital inflammatory syndrome [59]. Ipilimumab was discontinued and the patient required prolonged steroid taper over 5 months [59]. Another case was diagnosed with orbital inflammatory syndrome and hypophysitis, secondary to ipilimumab [60]. The patient similarly presented with ophthalmoplegia. Treatment with ICI was stopped, and the patient underwent oral corticosteroid treatment with mild residual abduction deficit remaining [60].

5.8.3 Myasthenia Gravis

Myasthenia gravis (MG) is a neuromuscular disorder of the postsynaptic neuromuscular junction that causes variable muscle weakness involving the eyes, mouth, limbs, and respiration. Nivolumab had the highest association with an OR of 22.82 followed by pembrolizumab with an OR of 20.17 [13, 15]. Ipilimumab has also been implicated in the development of MG [61]. Patients with ocular MG may present with variable ptosis and diplopia [62]. Kamo described two cases of patients taking pembrolizumab who developed autoimmune myositis resembling MG with the involvement of the levator palpebrae superioris and extraocular muscles [63]. However, MG-related antibodies were negative [63]. Diagnosis is clinical as autoantibodies to acetylcholine receptors, binding, blocking, and modulating may be negative. The patients may be managed with discontinuation of ICI and the start of steroids or intravenous immunoglobulin may be considered [15]. Additionally, patients can be treated with plasmapheresis and pyridostigmine [51].

5.8.4 Giant Cell Arteritis

Giant cell arteritis (GCA) or temporal arteritis is inflammation of the large vessels of the body. GCA has been reported more frequently for ipilimumab ($n = 10$) than for nivolumab ($n = 3$) or pembrolizumab ($n = 4$) [64]. Vision can be affected profoundly. Two patients presented with blurred vision, headache, jaw claudication, and myalgias after treatment with ipilimumab [51, 65]. Both patients were treated with high-dose systemic corticosteroids [51, 65]. The third patient presented with scalp necrosis 6 weeks after initiation of nivolumab [64]. She did not complain of any visual changes at the time. Temporal artery biopsy confirmed GCA [64].

5.9 Glaucoma

Glaucoma is a disease of the optic nerve that can lead to irreversible vision loss [66]. Characteristic features of glaucoma include cupping of the optic disc and corresponding visual field deficits due to retinal ganglion cell loss. Glaucoma is thought to arise from increased resistance to aqueous outflow which may be associated with elevated intraocular pressures [66]. The mechanism is not well understood, but studies have shown that lowering intraocular pressure is effective at preventing progression of glaucoma [66]. ICI have indirectly been linked to the development of glaucoma such as a complication of poorly controlled uveitis or from autoimmune thyroid disease [12, 33]. To date there have been no reports of direct formation of glaucoma from ICI.

5.9.1 Hypotony

Hypotony is the presence of low intraocular pressure defined as below 6 mmHg [67]. Ocular hypotony has been documented in a patient on treatment with pembrolizumab. Nguyen described sequential vision loss down to 20/200 after mild blunt trauma [67]. Examination revealed a pressure of 0 mmHg with minimal inflammation. Intraoperatively, the patient had profound ciliary body atrophy. The patient underwent multiple tests and procedures to reverse the hypotony including high-dose systemic steroids, but the response was limited [67].

6 Patient Education and Multidisciplinary Approach

Early recognition and treatment initiation is essential to the management of irAEs. Communication between ophthalmologists, primary care physicians, and oncologists can help guide diagnosis and management for patients with ocular irAE related to checkpoint immunotherapy [68]. Patient education also provides awareness and promotes discussion on what to expect during cancer treatment [69, 70]. With improved education, patients are more likely to adhere to treatment regimens and have a better overall prognosis. Oncological societies such as the American Cancer Society, cancer centers, and pharmaceutical companies are launching patient education programs to share important signs and symptoms that may herald an adverse event [69, 70]. A multidisciplinary approach will minimize the impact of ocular toxicity.

7 Conclusion

ICI has provided new hope in the treatment of advanced malignancies. Despite their success, ICI have been associated with a broad spectrum of adverse events. Although ocular side effects account for 1% of total adverse events, they are becoming more commonplace as more people undergo treatment with ICI. Recognizing ocular adverse events early is important as they can impact a patient's quality of life. Most irAEs are mild and do not require discontinuation of ICI. Treatment with corticosteroids assists with more moderate cases. Patients with severe and sight-threatening adverse events should have their immunotherapy discontinued. This may come at a cost as tumor progression can be noted after cessation of ICI. Management should involve ophthalmologists and oncologists. Risks and benefits should be addressed with patients. With improved education, patients are more likely to adhere to treatment regimens and have a better overall prognosis of advanced malignancies. In conclusion patients who present with ocular complaints should be referred to an ophthalmologist for early identification and intervention.

References

1. Pennock GK, Chow LQ. The evolving role of immune checkpoint inhibitors in cancer treatment. Oncologist. 2015;20(7):812–22. https://doi.org/10.1634/theoncologist.2014-0422. Epub 2015 Jun 11.
2. Tattersall IW, Leventhal JS. Cutaneous toxicities of immune checkpoint inhibitors: the role of the dermatologist. Yale J Biol Med. 2020;93(1):123–32.
3. Dobosz P, Dzieciątkowski T. The intriguing history of cancer immunotherapy. Front Immunol. 2019;10:2965. https://doi.org/10.3389/fimmu.2019.02965.
4. Darvin P, Toor SM, Sasidharan Nair V, Elkord E. Immune checkpoint inhibitors: recent progress and potential biomarkers. Exp Mol Med. 2018;50(12):1–11. https://doi.org/10.1038/s12276-018-0191-1.
5. Wierenga APA, Cao J, Luyten GPM, Jager MJ. Immune checkpoint inhibitors in uveal and conjunctival melanoma. Int Ophthalmol Clin. 2019;59(2):53–63. https://doi.org/10.1097/IIO.0000000000000263.
6. Immune checkpoint inhibitors and their side effects. In: Immunotherapy, American Cancer Society; 2019.
7. Postow M, et al. Toxicities associated with checkpoint inhibitor immunotherapy. UpToDate, Wolters Kluwer; 2021.
8. Attia P, Phan GQ, Maker AV, Robinson MR, Quezado MM, Yang JC, Sherry RM, Topalian SL, Kammula US, Royal RE, Restifo NP, Haworth LR, Levy C, Mavroukakis SA, Nichol G, Yellin MJ, Rosenberg SA. Autoimmunity correlates with tumor regression in patients with metastatic melanoma treated with anti-cytotoxic T-lymphocyte antigen-4. J Clin Oncol. 2005;23(25):6043–53. https://doi.org/10.1200/JCO.2005.06.205. Epub 2005 Aug 8.
9. Ito F, Ernstoff MS. Immune checkpoint inhibitors in cancer. Elsevier; 2019.
10. Abdel-Rahman O, Oweira H, Petrausch U, Helbling D, Schmidt J, Mannhart M, Mehrabi A, Schöb O, Giryes A. Immune-related ocular toxicities in solid tumor patients treated with immune checkpoint inhibitors: a systematic review. Expert Rev Anticancer Ther. 2017;17(4):387–94. https://doi.org/10.1080/14737140.2017.1296765. Epub 2017 Feb 24.
11. Common Terminology Criteria for Adverse Events (CTCAE) Version 5.0. National Institutes of Health, U.S. Department of Health and Human Services; 2017.
12. Shahzad O, Thompson N, Clare G, Welsh S, Damato E, Corrie P. Ocular adverse events associated with immune checkpoint inhibitors: a novel multidisciplinary management algorithm. Ther Adv Med Oncol. 2021;13:1758835921992989. https://doi.org/10.1177/1758835921992989.
13. Fang T, Maberley DA, Etminan M. Ocular adverse events with immune checkpoint inhibitors. J Curr Ophthalmol. 2019;31(3):319–22. https://doi.org/10.1016/j.joco.2019.05.002.
14. Papavasileiou E, Prasad S, Freitag SK, Sobrin L, Lobo AM. Ipilimumab-induced ocular and orbital inflammation—a case series and review of the literature. Ocul Immunol Inflamm. 2016;24(2):140–6. https://doi.org/10.3109/09273948.2014.1001858. Epub 2015 Mar 11.
15. Bindiganavile S, Bhat N, Lee A, Gombos S, Al-Zubidi N. Targeted cancer therapy and its ophthalmic side effects: a review. J Immunother Precis Oncol. 2021;4(1):6–15.
16. Inno A, Metro G, Bironzo P, Grimaldi AM, Grego E, Di Nunno V, Picasso V, Massari F, Gori S. Pathogenesis, clinical manifestations and management of immune checkpoint inhibitors toxicity. Tumori. 2017;103(5):405–21. https://doi.org/10.5301/tj.5000625. Epub 2017 May 10.

17. Liu C, et al. Ocular side effects of systemically administered chemotherapy. UpToDate, Wolters Kulwer; 2021.
18. Brouwer NJ, Haanen JBAG, Jager MJ. Development of ocular rosacea following combined ipilimumab and nivolumab treatment for metastatic malignant skin melanoma. Ocul Oncol Pathol. 2017;3(3):188–92. https://doi.org/10.1159/000455150. Epub 2017 Feb 2.
19. Oakley AM, Krishnamurthy K. Stevens Johnson syndrome. [Updated 2020 Nov 20]. In: StatPearls [Internet]. Treasure Island, FL: StatPearls Publishing; 2021. https://www.ncbi.nlm.nih.gov/books/NBK459323/.
20. Keerty D, Koverzhenko V, Belinc D, LaPorta K, Haynes E. Immune-mediated toxic epidermal necrolysis. Cureus. 2020;12(8):e9587. https://doi.org/10.7759/cureus.9587.
21. Haratake N, Tagawa T, Hirai F, Toyokawa G, Miyazaki R, Maehara Y. Stevens-Johnson syndrome induced by pembrolizumab in a lung cancer patient. J Thorac Oncol. 2018;13(11):1798–9. https://doi.org/10.1016/j.jtho.2018.05.031. Epub 2018 Jun 6.
22. Hsu TJ, Yeh HH, Lee CH, Liu KL. Stevens-Johnson syndrome and toxic epidermal necrolysis in a referral center in Taiwan. Int J Dermatol. 2021;60(8):964–72. https://doi.org/10.1111/ijd.15586.
23. Parker JS, Feagin W, Wang C, Heersink M, Parker JS. Corneal ulceration associated with Nivolumab use. Am J Ophthalmol Case Rep. 2019;14:26–7. https://doi.org/10.1016/j.ajoc.2019.01.013.
24. Zimmer L, Goldinger SM, Hofmann L, Loquai C, Ugurel S, Thomas I, Schmidgen MI, Gutzmer R, Utikal JS, Göppner D, Hassel JC, Meier F, Tietze JK, Forschner A, Weishaupt C, Leverkus M, Wahl R, Dietrich U, Garbe C, Kirchberger MC, Eigentler T, Berking C, Gesierich A, Krackhardt AM, Schadendorf D, Schuler G, Dummer R, Heinzerling LM. Neurological, respiratory, musculoskeletal, cardiac and ocular side-effects of anti-PD-1 therapy. Eur J Cancer. 2016;60:210–25. https://doi.org/10.1016/j.ejca.2016.02.024. Epub 2016 Apr 13.
25. Liu X, Wang Z, Zhao C, Wang H, Guo X, Zhou J, Duan L, Si X, Zhang L, Li Y, Wang M, Zhang M, Zhang L. Clinical diagnosis and treatment recommendations for ocular toxicities of targeted therapy and immune checkpoint inhibitor therapy. Thorac Cancer. 2020;11(3):810–8. https://doi.org/10.1111/1759-7714.13327. Epub 2020 Feb 4.
26. Khoja L, Atenafu EG, Ye Q, et al. Real-world efficacy, toxicity and clinical management of ipilimumab treatment in metastatic melanoma. Oncol Lett. 2016;11(2):1581–5. https://doi.org/10.3892/ol.2015.4069.
27. Gonzales JA, Shantha J, Acharya NR. Combination nivolumab- and cabiralizumab-associated acute bilateral anterior and posterior scleritis and anterior uveitis. Am J Ophthalmol Case Rep. 2018;10:117–8. https://doi.org/10.1016/j.ajoc.2018.02.005.
28. Sahu Y, Ensor J, Burns E, et al. Ocular adverse events due to PD-1 and PD-L1 checkpoint inhibitors: a retrospective review of FDA adverse events reporting system (FAERS). In: ESMO immuno-oncology virtual congress; 2020.
29. Losonczy G, Gijs M, Nuijts RMMA. Nivolumab-induced ulcerative keratitis-a case report. Cornea. 2021;40(5):656–8. https://doi.org/10.1097/ICO.0000000000002460.
30. Oh J. Autoimmune keratitis after atezolizumab treatment. N Engl J Med. 2020;383:1468. https://doi.org/10.1056/NEJMicm1910925.
31. Le Fournis S, Gohier P, Urban T, Jeanfaivre T, Hureaux J. Corneal graft rejection in a patient treated with nivolumab for primary lung cancer. Lung Cancer. 2016;102:28–9. https://doi.org/10.1016/j.lungcan.2016.10.008. Epub 2016 Oct 22.
32. Lee JC, Al-Humimat G, Kooner KS. Acute bilateral uveitis, hypotony, and cataracts associated with ipilimumab and nivolumab therapy: optical coherence tomography angiography findings. Case Rep Ophthalmol. 2020;11(3):606–11. https://doi.org/10.1159/000509629.
33. Basilious A, Lloyd JC. Posterior subcapsular cataracts and hypotony secondary to severe pembrolizumab induced uveitis: case report. Can J Ophthalmol. 2016;51(1):e4–6. https://doi.org/10.1016/j.jcjo.2015.09.008.
34. Maruyama D, Hatake K, Kinoshita T, Fukuhara N, Choi I, Taniwaki M, Ando K, Terui Y, Higuchi Y, Onishi Y, Abe Y, Kobayashi T, Shirasugi Y, Tobinai K. Multicenter phase II study of nivolumab in Japanese patients with relapsed or refractory classical Hodgkin lymphoma. Cancer Sci. 2017;108(5):1007–12. https://doi.org/10.1111/cas.13230. Epub 2017 May 19.
35. Witmer MT. Treatment of ipilimumab-induced Vogt-Koyanagi-Harada syndrome with oral dexamethasone. Ophthalmic Surg Lasers Imaging Retina. 2017;48(11):928–31. https://doi.org/10.3928/23258160-20171030-09.
36. Conrady CD, Larochelle M, Pecen P, Palestine A, Shakoor A, Singh A. Checkpoint inhibitor-induced uveitis: a case series. Graefes Arch Clin Exp Ophthalmol. 2018;256(1):187–91. https://doi.org/10.1007/s00417-017-3835-2. Epub 2017 Oct 27.
37. Yoshida S, Shiraishi K, Mito T, Sayama K. Vogt-Koyanagi-Harada-like syndrome induced by immune checkpoint inhibitors in a patient with melanoma. Clin Exp Dermatol. 2020;45(7):908–11. https://doi.org/10.1111/ced.14282. Epub 2020 Jul 5.
38. Gambichler T, Seifert C, Lehmann M, Lukas C, Scheel C, Susok L. Concurrent Vogt-Koyanagi-Harada disease and impressive response to immune checkpoint blockade in metastatic melanoma. Immunotherapy. 2020;12(7):439–44. https://doi.org/10.2217/imt-2019-0206. Epub 2020 Apr 19.
39. Kikuchi R, Kawagoe T, Hotta K. Vogt-Koyanagi-Harada disease-like uveitis following nivolumab administration treated with steroid pulse therapy: a case report. BMC Ophthalmol. 2020;20(1):252. https://doi.org/10.1186/s12886-020-01519-5.
40. Obata S, Saishin Y, Teramura K, Ohji M. Vogt-Koyanagi-Harada disease-Like Uveitis during Nivolumab (Anti-PD-1 Antibody) treatment for metastatic cutaneous malignant melanoma. Case Rep Ophthalmol. 2019;10(1):67–74. https://doi.org/10.1159/000496682.
41. Thomas M, Armenti ST, Ayres MB, Demirci H. Uveal effusion after immune checkpoint inhibitor therapy. JAMA Ophthalmol. 2018;136(5):553–6. https://doi.org/10.1001/jamaophthalmol.2018.0920.
42. Telfah M, Whittaker TJ, Doolittle C, G. Vision loss with pembrolizumab treatment: a report of two cases. J Oncol Pharm Pract. 2019;25(6):1540–6. https://doi.org/10.1177/1078155219841683. Epub 2019 Apr 18.
43. Modjtahedi BS, Maibach H, Park S. Multifocal bilateral choroidal neovascularization in a patient on ipilimumab for metastatic melanoma. Cutan Ocul Toxicol. 2013;32(4):341–3. https://doi.org/10.3109/15569527.2013.781618. Epub 2013 May 28.
44. Jacobsoone-Ulrich A, Jamme P, Alkeraye S, Dzwiniel V, Faure E, Templier C, Mortier L. Ipilimumab in anti-PD1 refractory metastatic melanoma: a report of eight cases. Melanoma Res. 2016;26(2):153–6. https://doi.org/10.1097/CMR.0000000000000221.
45. Acaba-Berrocal LA, Lucio-Alvarez JA, Mashayekhi A, Ho AC, Dunn JP, Shields CL. Birdshot-like chorioretinopathy associated with pembrolizumab treatment. JAMA Ophthalmol. 2018;136(10):1205–7. https://doi.org/10.1001/jamaophthalmol.2018.1851.
46. Manusow JS, Khoja L, Pesin N, et al. Retinal vasculitis and ocular vitreous metastasis following complete response to PD-1 inhibition in a patient with metastatic cutaneous melanoma. J Immunother Cancer. 2014;2:41.
47. Roberts P, Fishman GA, Joshi K, Jampol LM. Chorioretinal lesions in a case of melanoma-associated retinopathy treated with pembrolizumab. JAMA Ophthalmol. 2016;134(10):1184–8. https://doi.org/10.1001/jamaophthalmol.2016.2944.

48. Reddy M, Chen JJ, Kalevar A, Terribilini R, Agarwal A. Immune retinopathy associated with nivolumab administration for metastatic non-small cell lung cancer. Retin Cases Brief Rep. 2020;14(2):120–6. https://doi.org/10.1097/ICB.0000000000000675.
49. Duong SL, Barbiero FJ, Nowak RJ, Baehring JM. Neurotoxicities associated with immune checkpoint inhibitor therapy. J Neuro-Oncol. 2021;152(2):265–77. https://doi.org/10.1007/s11060-021-03695-w. Epub 2021 Jan 17.
50. Francis JH, Jaben K, Santomasso BD, Canestraro J, Abramson DH, Chapman PB, Berkenstock M, Aronow ME. Immune checkpoint inhibitor-associated optic neuritis. Ophthalmology. 2020;127(11):1585–9. https://doi.org/10.1016/j.ophtha.2020.05.003. Epub 2020 May 8.
51. Dalvin LA, Shields CL, Orloff M, Sato T, Shields JA. Checkpoint inhibitor immune therapy: systemic indications and ophthalmic side effects. Retina. 2018;38(6):1063–78. https://doi.org/10.1097/IAE.0000000000002181.
52. Yeh OL, Francis CE. Ipilimumab-associated bilateral optic neuropathy. J Neuroophthalmol. 2015;35(2):144–7. https://doi.org/10.1097/WNO.0000000000000217.
53. Ahluwalia A, Kohli AA. Photopsias in the setting of nivolumab therapy. J Neuroophthalmol. 2021;41(1):e25–6. https://doi.org/10.1097/WNO.0000000000000909.
54. Kartal Ö, Ataş E. Bilateral Optic neuritis secondary to nivolumab therapy: a case report. Medicina (Kaunas). 2018;54(5):82. doi:https://doi.org/10.3390/medicina54050082.
55. Borodic G, Hinkle DM, Cia Y. Drug-induced graves disease from CTLA-4 receptor suppression. Ophthalmic Plast Reconstr Surg. 2011;27(4):e87–8. https://doi.org/10.1097/IOP.0b013e3181ef72a1.
56. McElnea E, Ní Mhéalóid A, Moran S, Kelly R, Fulcher T. Thyroid-like ophthalmopathy in a euthyroid patient receiving Ipilimumab. Orbit. 2014;33(6):424–7. https://doi.org/10.3109/01676830.2014.949792. Epub 2014 Sep 10.
57. Park ESY, Rabinowits G, Hamnvik OR, Dagi LR. A case of Graves' ophthalmopathy associated with pembrolizumab (Keytruda) therapy. J AAPOS. 2018;22(4):310–2. https://doi.org/10.1016/j.jaapos.2018.01.006. Epub 2018 Apr 4.
58. Renouf DJ, Velazquez-Martin JP, Simpson R, Siu LL, Bedard PL. Ocular toxicity of targeted therapies. J Clin Oncol. 2012;30(26):3277–86. https://doi.org/10.1200/JCO.2011.41.5851. Epub 2012 May 29.
59. Sheldon CA, Kharlip J, Tamhankar MA. Inflammatory orbitopathy associated with ipilimumab. ophthalmic. Plast Reconstr Surg. 2017;33(3S Suppl 1):S155–8. https://doi.org/10.1097/IOP.0000000000000509.
60. Henderson AD, Thomas DA. A case report of orbital inflammatory syndrome secondary to ipilimumab. Ophthalmic Plast Reconstr Surg. 2015;31(3):e68–70. https://doi.org/10.1097/IOP.0000000000000081.
61. Johnson DB, Saranga-Perry V, Lavin PJ, et al. Myasthenia gravis induced by ipilimumab in patients with metastatic melanoma. J Clin Oncol. 2015;33(33):e122–4. https://doi.org/10.1200/JCO.2013.51.1683.
62. Onda A, Miyagawa S, Takahashi N, Gochi M, Takagi M, Nishino I, Suzuki S, Oishi C, Yaguchi H. Pembrolizumab-induced ocular myasthenia gravis with anti-titin antibody and necrotizing myopathy. Intern Med. 2019;58(11):1635–8. https://doi.org/10.2169/internalmedicine.1956-18. Epub 2019 Feb 1.
63. Kamo H, Hatano T, Kanai K, Aoki N, Kamiyama D, Yokoyama K, Takanashi M, Yamashita Y, Shimo Y, Hattori N. Pembrolizumab-related systemic myositis involving ocular and hindneck muscles resembling myasthenic gravis: a case report. BMC Neurol. 2019;19(1):184. https://doi.org/10.1186/s12883-019-1416-1.
64. Kreuter A, Koushk-Jalali B, Cusenza A, Oellig F, Tigges C. Nivolumab-associated giant cell arteritis with scalp necrosis. JAMA Dermatol. 2019;155(9):1086–7. https://doi.org/10.1001/jamadermatol.2019.1411.
65. Goldstein BL, Gedmintas L, Todd DJ. Drug-associated polymyalgia rheumatica/giant cell arteritis occurring in two patients after treatment with ipilimumab, an antagonist of ctla-4. Arthritis Rheumatol. 2014;66(3):768–9. https://doi.org/10.1002/art.38282.
66. Anderson DR, Normal Tension Glaucoma Study. Collaborative normal tension glaucoma study. Curr Opin Ophthalmol. 2003;14(2):86–90. https://doi.org/10.1097/00055735-200304000-00006.
67. Nguyen M, Islam MR, Lim SW, Sahu A, Tamjid B. Pembrolizumab induced ocular hypotony with near complete vision loss, interstitial pulmonary fibrosis and arthritis. Front Oncol. 2019;9:944. https://doi.org/10.3389/fonc.2019.00944.
68. Antoun J, Titah C, Cochereau I. Ocular and orbital side-effects of checkpoint inhibitors: a review article. Curr Opin Oncol. 2016;28(4):288–94. https://doi.org/10.1097/CCO.0000000000000296.
69. Naing A, Hajjar J, Gulley JL, Atkins MB, Ciliberto G, Meric-Bernstam F, Hwu P. Strategies for improving the management of immune-related adverse events. J Immunother Cancer. 2020;8(2):e001754. https://doi.org/10.1136/jitc-2020-001754.
70. Reynolds KL, Cohen JV, Zubiri L, Stern TA, editors. Facing immunotherapy. Boston: Octal Productions, LLC; 2020.

Part VI

Healthcare Barriers Worldwide: Meeting the Challenge

Awareness, Advocacy, and the Volunteer Sector

Sandra E. Staffieri

1 Introduction

'Retinoblastoma is a remarkable success story...This cancer was virtually uniformly fatal 200 years ago and is now uniformly curable if detected early.' [1]

With prompt diagnosis and access to treatment, retinoblastoma is the most survivable paediatric cancer, with survival rates in excess of 95% in high-income countries (HIC) [2]. In low-middle income countries (LMIC), however, survival is considerably lower due to late presentation of disease associated with systemic and metastatic spread, and incomplete or lack of access to treatment [3, 4].

In both HICs and LMICs, leukocoria remains the most common presenting sign of retinoblastoma. In HICs, strabismus is the second most common sign, whilst proptosis is more commonly seen as a presenting sign in LMICs [5].

Many factors contribute to parents, caregivers and healthcare providers overlooking leukocoria or strabismus as an early sign of disease. These signs may appear innocuous given the child is otherwise well, and in the case of unilateral disease, is unlikely to outwardly alter the child's visual behaviour. Leukocoria can be dismissed as an artefact of lighting or malfunction of a camera [6], and strabismus is often considered normal for many months or years longer than appropriate [7–10].

S. E. Staffieri (✉)
Department of Ophthalmology, Royal Children's Hospital, Parkville, VIC, Australia

Centre for Eye Research Australia, Royal Victorian Eye and Ear Hospital, East Melbourne, VIC, Australia

Ophthalmology, University of Melbourne Department of Surgery, Parkville, VIC, Australia
e-mail: sandra.staffieri@unimelb.edu.au

2 Improving Awareness of the Potential Significance of These Signs is Imperative

It is easy to understand why the two most common early signs of retinoblastoma, leukocoria and strabismus, might initially be dismissed by caregivers and healthcare providers. These signs are typically considered nonthreatening, particularly when the child is well and continues to behave normally.

2.1 Leukocoria

In the twentieth Edward Jackson Lecture 'The Story of Retinoblastoma', Dunphy recounts a letter written by Mr. Hayes in 1765 to Mr. William Hunter reporting a parent's description of retinoblastoma: 'At the age of 15 months, the parents noted a peculiar appearance in the left eye in the evening when the light was not strong' (pages 540–541) [11]. Over 250 years later, parents still describe leukocoria in much the same way—in any country and in any language. 'When she looks up at me from the bath", "When I changed his nappy in the dim light at night', 'In some of our photos, not all of them, there is a white glow, like a cat's eye' are examples from Australian parents [12] (unpublished data) but similarly reported in the literature [13, 14]. Whilst leukocoria can be dismissed for many months by parents/caregivers and healthcare providers, a timely referral to an ophthalmologist may provide a diagnosis of retinoblastoma in an otherwise well child.

2.2 Strabismus

Strabismus is often considered a normal phenomenon in newborns. Indeed, intermittent deviations of the eye, either inward or outward, are commonly seen in the early neonatal

B. V. Chawla, M. E. Aronow (eds.), *Global Perspectives in Ocular Oncology*, https://doi.org/10.1007/978-3-031-08250-4_34

period [15, 16]. As the sensorineural connections form during development of the binocular vision system, these transient deviations resolve spontaneously anywhere from 2 to 4 weeks [15] or 6 months of age [16]. Similarly, pseudostrabismus, resulting from broad epicanthic folds in infancy, is reported to persist up until 10 years of age [17]. As the broad epicanthic folds reduce with physical growth and development, so too does the appearance of strabismus. Thus, the perception that strabismus resolves over time and does not require medical attention has evolved in the community and even amongst medical professionals.

True primary strabismus can arise at any time throughout childhood, with a reported prevalence of between 1 and 6% [18–20]. When left untreated, primary strabismus can significantly impair vision or disrupt development of binocular vision [21, 22]. Moreover, the psychosocial impact of strabismus significantly affects quality of life or employment [23–25] as well as self-image and interpersonal relationships [23, 26].

Secondary strabismus can develop as a result of severe vision loss [27] or systemic disease [28], as well as intracranial [29] or intraocular pathology [30]. In some cases, there will be associated neurologic or systemic symptoms that prompt parents to seek medical attention for their child [31]. However, in the case of intraocular pathology, the only sign may be strabismus, particularly when the fellow eye remains unaffected and the child's visual behaviour is unchanged.

Most children presenting with strabismus will not have retinoblastoma. Nevertheless, clinical examination may identify significant disease warranting prompt attention. Children who present with strabismus and are diagnosed with retinoblastoma are more likely to receive treatment early enough that the eye is conserved [32]. Ellsworth's sentiment, more than half a century ago, that 'It is not a bad idea to consider that every child with strabismus has retinoblastoma until proven otherwise' [33] (page 20) remains true today.

The obvious early signs for retinoblastoma, such as leukocoria and strabismus, provide an opportunity for diagnosis at a time when prompt treatment will possibly preserve the child's vision or conserve the eye but most importantly, likely save their life. Thus, awareness of these potential signs of serious disease must be promoted amongst the broader community and healthcare providers to direct appropriate health-seeking and referral to an ophthalmologist and further improve current survival rates.

2.3 Who Should Be Targeted?

As stated by Knudson, 'If most solid tumors of childhood are indeed correctly attributable to mutations in germ and/or somatic cells…then childhood cancer cannot be prevented… the main effort against childhood cancer must be that of early diagnosis and treatment' [34] (page 516). In the case of achieving optimal outcomes for retinoblastoma, our initial focus must be on the early, or rather timely, diagnosis of disease. Addressing diagnostic delays starts with awareness of signs of disease. For all paediatric cancers, delays attributed to the patient/parent and healthcare providers contribute the most to overall diagnostic delays [35] and healthcare provider delays are longer than patient/parent delays [36].

Retinoblastoma is rare. Worldwide, it is estimated that approximately 8000 children are newly diagnosed with retinoblastoma per year, 80% of whom live in resource-poor countries [37]. Disparities in treatment access and survival between HIC and LMIC are well described in the literature [38–41]. However, in both HICs and LMICs, delayed diagnosis can be attributed to parents not recognising the signs of retinoblastoma and healthcare providers not responding appropriately to the parents' concerns [14, 42–46]. Although many studies exploring delayed diagnosis of retinoblastoma recommend improving parents' and healthcare providers' awareness of the common signs, only a few report successful implementation strategies to improve awareness [47, 48].

For centuries, there have been reports of parents noting the characteristic glow seen in intraocular retinoblastoma [49], and multiple studies recognise that highlighting the significance of leukocoria to parents [43, 50, 51] is a critical step to reducing time to diagnosis and improving outcomes. Awareness campaigns designed to improve timely diagnosis need to be culturally safe, effective, inexpensive and sustainable. In 2004, at the Annual Meeting of the American Society of Clinical Oncology, Epelman and co-workers [48] described a print media and television campaign in Brazil aimed at raising awareness of early signs of retinoblastoma. The target audience were parents and healthcare providers. Following the campaign, an increase in children presenting with the disease was noted. In 2007, Leander et al. [47] reported the outcomes of a similar campaign. A simple poster depicting leukocoria in a child (Fig. 1) was displayed in community centres throughout Honduras and healthcare providers were upskilled in recognising this ominous sign. Within 18 months of the campaign implementation, a significant positive impact on survival was observed. Children presenting with extraocular disease was reduced from 73% to 35% and survival increased from 14 to 48%.

A systematic review of early interventions to promote cancer awareness highlighted this study as an example of the positive impact that can be achieved by a simple awareness programme [52]. The three key components of this awareness strategy were that it provided (1) basic information supported by images, (2) messages to motivate parents to act and importantly (3) how to seek advice. Indeed, this framework for developing health information to effect behaviour change (Information-Motivation-Behaviour

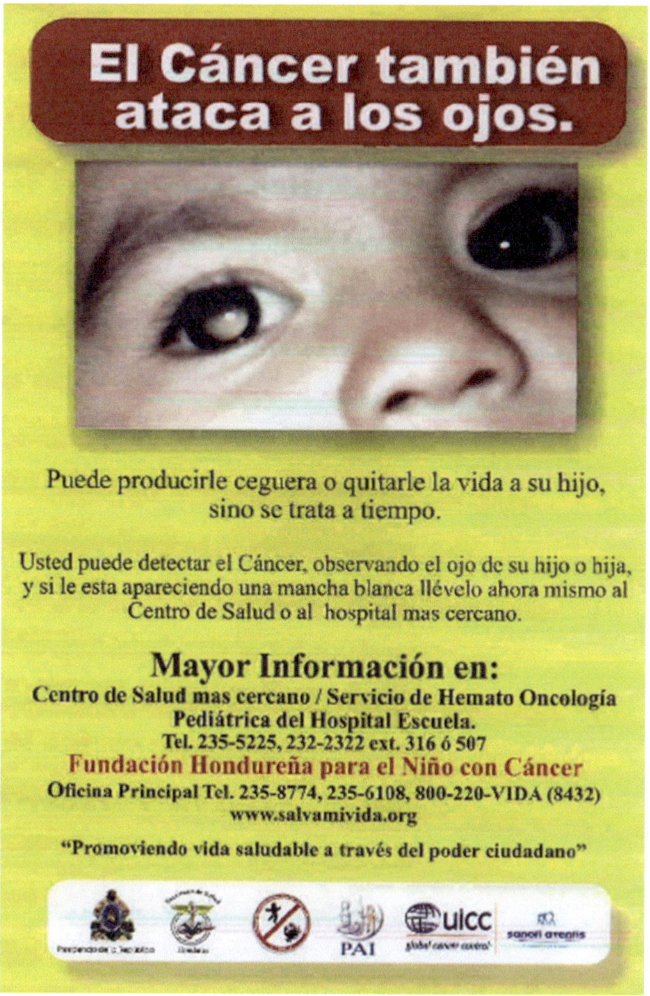

Fig. 1 Poster depicting leukocoria in a child used in Honduran awareness campaign. (With permission)

Skills Model [53], intended or not, has been effectively utilised since the early 1990s to change behaviour to improve health outcomes) [54].

It could be argued that awareness must include not only parents, but extended family members (grandparents, aunts and uncles) and childcare providers including nannies, au pairs and childcare workers in crèche and childcare centres.

2.4 Damned If You Do, Damned If You Don't

When providing any health information to consumers, the material must be presented in a way that provides parents/caregivers with useful advice that does not cause anxiety or alarm [55, 56]. With respect to leukocoria and strabismus, parents must be encouraged to remain alert and vigilant without becoming paranoid. The poster shown in Fig. 2 is an example of efforts to dampen alarm whilst still encouraging parents to act and respond to their observations. It uses language that tempers the message and minimises parental anxiety yet encourages concerned parents to seek clinical review. Furthermore, to achieve maximal uptake and engagement with health information, potential variations in health literacy of the target audience should also be considered [57].

2.5 Awareness Amongst Healthcare Providers

Educating healthcare providers has been highlighted by the work of Yousef and co-workers [58]. Their study of the ability of medical students and paediatric and ophthalmology residents in their final years of training to recognise and respond to a diagnosis of leukocoria highlighted significant gaps in knowledge relating to leukocoria as a sign of significant disease. Similarly, in Brazil 70% of overall diagnostic delay was due to delayed medical referral, emphasising the importance of raising awareness of clinicians to the early signs of retinoblastoma [59].

Healthcare providers' awareness and knowledge can be supported and extended not only during basic vocational training but also when retinoblastoma specialists present at medical conferences and professional development seminars, and through reporting in the peer-reviewed medical literature.

2.6 Retinoblastoma Awareness Campaigns: A Global Study

In 2017, retinoblastoma treatment centres, philanthropic retinoblastoma-specific organisations and non-governmental organisations (NGOs) relating to retinoblastoma around the world were invited to participate in a survey to identify the barriers and enablers of retinoblastoma awareness campaigns [9]. Respondents were represented across all continents of the world (excluding the Arctic and Antarctica). With a modest 25% participation rate, 67% of respondents reported ever having conducted an awareness campaign in their country, city or local area. Campaigns were directed towards either parents/caregivers or healthcare providers through lectures and presentations. Notably, 33% had never conducted any awareness campaign, the majority of which were from HICs.

Several barriers to conducting awareness campaigns were identified, the most common of which were lack of funding, social or cultural factors (language, health literacy) and that retinoblastoma is a rare disease.

Securing resources globally to raise awareness for a singular, rare, but important disease can be challenging. A broad strategy that aims to highlight the myriad of paediatric eye diseases that may present with leukocoria or strabismus may

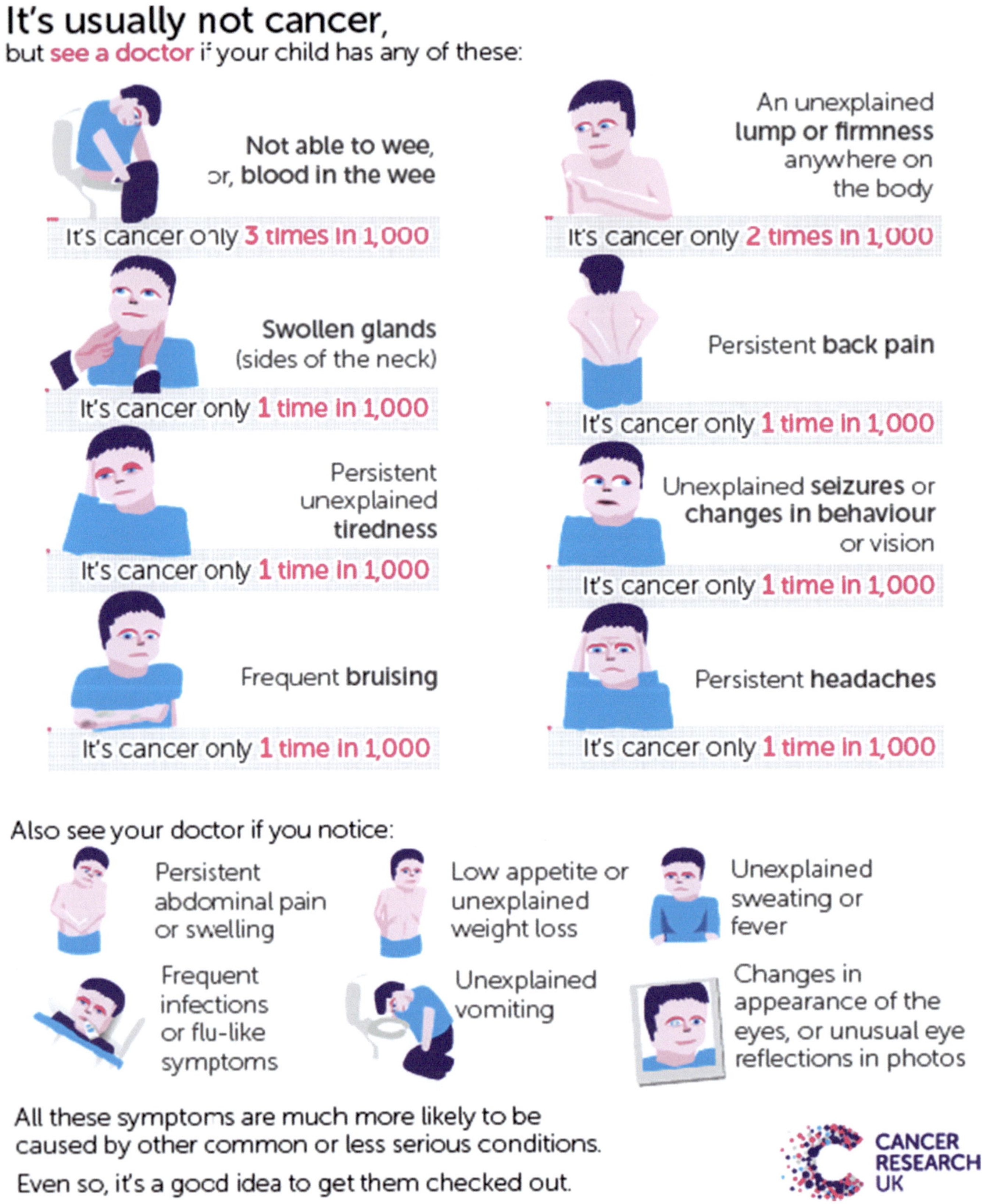

Fig. 2 Poster highlighting signs of childhood cancer

be more viable and sustainable than a campaign specifically targeted for retinoblastoma.

Social media can provide a relatively inexpensive method of delivering health messages to a wide audience that may impact health behaviour and outcomes [60, 61]. Figure 3a–d demonstrates examples of social media posts that appear regularly to promote awareness. Although social media platforms provide an opportunity for increasing the frequency of health messages, the reach is not systematic and depends on the reader seeing the post in their feed. Embedding eye health information at the time of a child's birth and providing parents with useful advice to recognise early signs of eye disease, namely, leukocoria and strabismus, ensures all parents hear the message. This initial information can then be supplemented with regular reminders through poster campaigns at community centres, social media posts (e.g. Facebook, Instagram, Twitter) or targeted television and radio campaigns.

However, even when parents are armed with information suggesting that leukocoria may be a harbinger of significant disease, the message may still be ignored. In a study exploring website search terms parents would use if they observed leukocoria in a child, and which websites these terms directed them to, parents still did not change their behavioural intention and seek health advice promptly as recommended by reputable websites [6].

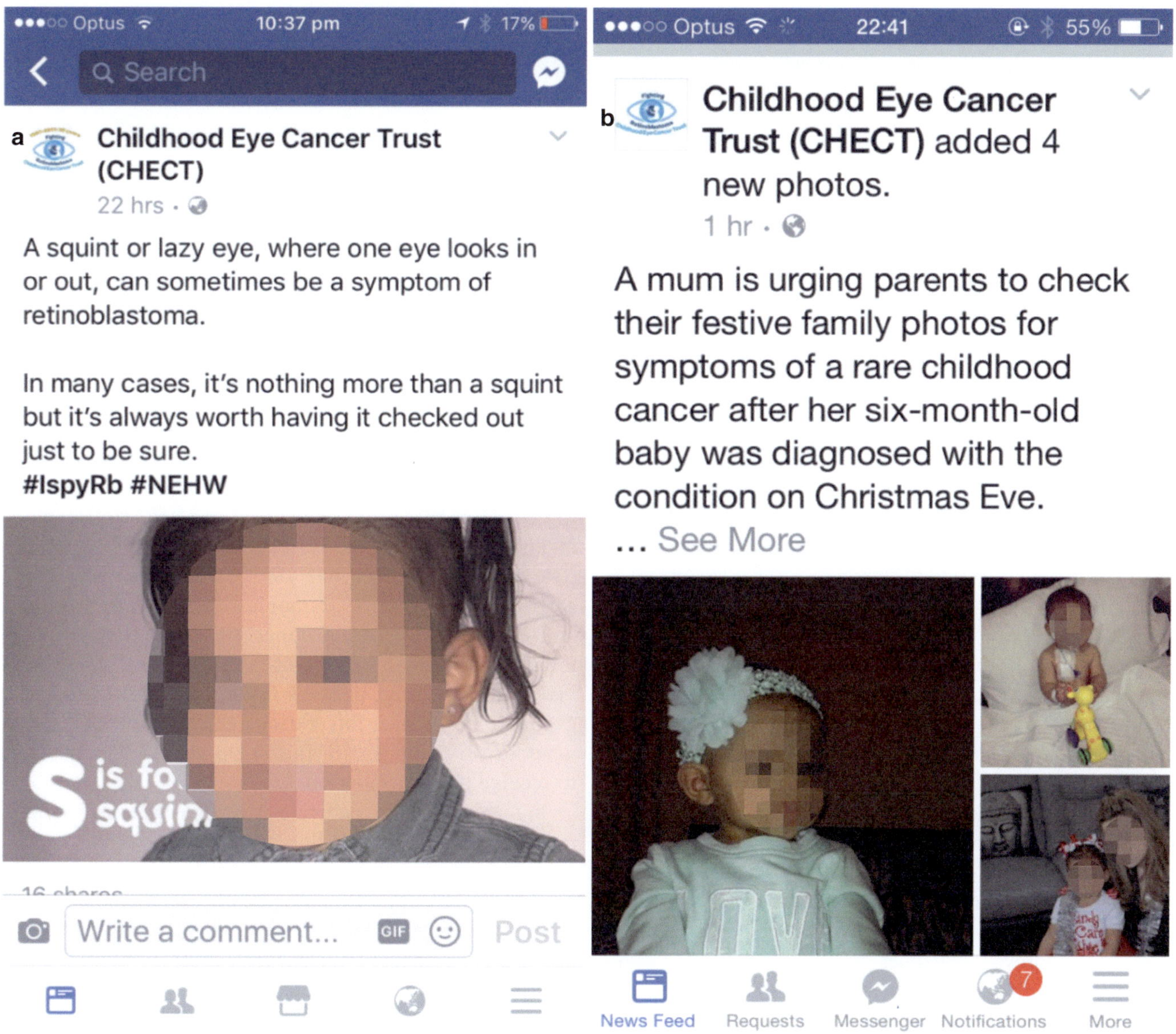

Fig. 3 (a–d) Social media posts reminding parents to check their children for signs of cancer. (Used with permission from Childhood Eye Cancer Trust)

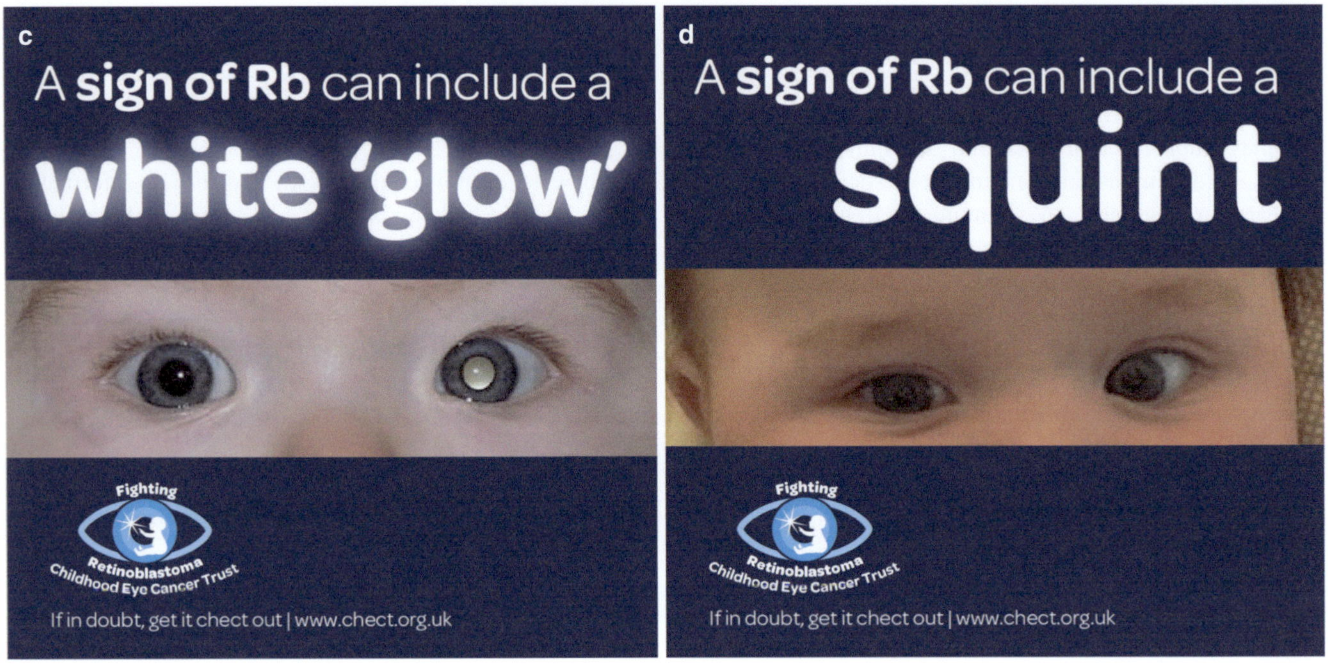

Fig. 3 (continued)

2.7 Sustainability of Awareness Programmes

Awareness strategies require sufficient financial and human resources to prepare, deliver and assess the effectiveness of any programme. In the case of retinoblastoma, 'piggybacking' onto a programme that identifies more than one ocular disease may promote investment and buy-in of stakeholders. Reporting outcomes of awareness campaigns could also drive ongoing support to deliver these health messages. The work of Leander et al. [47] regarding the campaign in Honduras and its association with improved survival outcomes is currently the only awareness campaign that is reported in sufficient detail in the peer-reviewed literature. Posner and co-workers [62] alluded to the likelihood that local awareness campaigns in the United Kingdom may have led to an increase in the number of parents attending local emergency departments with their child with strabismus/leukocoria, although the overall median parental delay during the study period increased from 2.5 to 4 weeks.

Many philanthropic, retinoblastoma-specific or non-governmental organisations continue to drive awareness campaigns in their local areas. Measuring and formally reporting improved outcomes resulting from these campaigns will further support their sustainability and promote implementation more globally.

2.8 Awareness of Survivors: Late Effects of Treatment, Risk of Second Primary Cancers and Family Planning or Surveillance of Their Children

Awareness of retinoblastoma is not solely relevant at the time of diagnosis. Affected individuals and their families should be informed of the association between harbouring germline mutations of the *RB1* gene and the development of treatment-related effects [63] and second cancers [64, 65]. Surveillance has changed the treatment landscape for survivors of retinoblastoma, and they should also receive information about individual family planning choices and screening of their offspring. Many survivors were treated decades before genetic testing was available [66], and this raises ethical questions as to whether survivors lost to follow-up should be contacted to receive new information.

In many countries, particularly LMICs, genetic testing is not widely available, and thus an inequity exists in knowledge and information that could have an impact on their long-term survival or ocular health of their offspring. Identifying strategies to ensure that all survivors know how and when to access surveillance and follow-up could be critical to their lifelong health outcomes.

3 Advocacy, Volunteering and Retinoblastoma

Initiation and promotion of awareness needs advocates—parents, survivors, organisations and clinicians—who highlight that awareness is not only necessary, but critical. Through active patient engagement, parents and survivors can participate in setting research priorities [67] and advocate for research projects or interventions as perceived by them drawing on or as a result of their lived experience [68].

3.1 Advocates Working Together

There is no greater advocate for a child than their parents, and thus it is not surprising that advocacy for retinoblastoma awareness is led or driven largely by parents and survivors individually or as part of philanthropic organisations. Parents whose child's own diagnosis might have been missed, or when a delayed diagnosis impacted the outcome, can be highly motivated to ensure that no parent experiences the same.

Medical professionals involved in treating and caring for children with retinoblastoma are familiar with the missed opportunities for more timely diagnosis and treatment options and are strong advocates for awareness. Respondents in the study on global awareness campaigns even reported self-funding campaigns and volunteering to present at professional development and training opportunities to address the observed outcomes of delayed diagnosis [9].

Finally, survivors can advocate strongly for the establishment of, or access to, screening and surveillance programmes that may optimise their health outcomes. Recognising their own risks related to their treatment in childhood or the development of second primary cancers is the first step, but accessing the care and support they need may be problematic. Healthcare providers unfamiliar with survivors' lifetime risks related to their history of retinoblastoma, because it is rare, can be a barrier to access the medical care they require.

3.2 Where Would We Be Without Volunteers?

Volunteering can have positive health benefits [69] and provide an outlet for the individual to fulfil a need to 'give back' or 'fill an unmet need'. Parent-to-parent support in the context of children with disease or disability can provide parents with the support of individuals with the same lived experience [70]. This may be provided directly through parent support groups or indirectly via social media, online forums, blogs or books publishing their lived experience. Similarly, retinoblastoma survivors supporting each other and sharing their experience and knowledge using the same mediums can be positive.

There is no shortage of NGOs, not-for-profit organisations or charitable organisations that are initiated, supported or maintained by volunteers. Parents, survivors, extended family members and clinicians alike come together and volunteer their time to drive such organisations to (1) promote awareness of the early signs of retinoblastoma to improve timely diagnosis; (2) provide information and support to parents, siblings and extended family members through diagnosis, treatment and survivorship; and (3) advocate for services and support for survivors.

Websites that include useful information describing retinoblastoma and its treatment are a valuable information resource for parents of a child newly diagnosed with retinoblastoma. Parents can also direct their extended family to these websites for information about the disease when to explain it themselves is too overwhelming.

3.3 A Final Word...

Strong advocacy to promote awareness of the early signs of retinoblastoma will support timely diagnosis and improve survival of children with retinoblastoma worldwide, as well as enhance health outcomes for survivors. This requires a team effort; parents and survivors, describing their lived experience, will continue to demonstrate the ongoing need for awareness about all facets of a retinoblastoma diagnosis—from initial diagnosis through to adulthood.

Organisations and treatment centres with more resources (human and/or financial) that share their materials with lower-resourced countries can establish cost-efficiencies and facilitate a collaborative approach to global awareness for retinoblastoma.

References

1. Grossniklaus HE. Retinoblastoma. Fifty years of progress. The LXXI Edward Jackson Memorial Lecture. Am J Ophthalmol. 2014;158(5):875–91.
2. Kaatsch P. Epidemiology of childhood cancers. Cancer Treat Rev. 2010;36:277–85.
3. Canturk S, Qaddoumi I, Khetan V, Ma Z, Furmanchuk A, Antoneli CB, et al. Survival of retinoblastoma in less-developed countries impact of socioeconomic and health-related indicators. Br J Ophthalmol. 2010;94(11):1432–6.
4. Chantada GL. Retinoblastoma: lessons and challenges from developing countries. Ellsworth Lecture 2011. Ophthalmic Genet. 2011;32(4):196–203.

5. Reddy SC, Anusya S. Clinical presentation of retinoblastoma in Malaysia: a review of 64 patients. Int J Ophthalmol. 2010;3(1):64–8.
6. Staffieri SE, Kearns LS, Sanfilippo PG, Craig JE, Mackey DA, Hewitt AW. Crowd-sourced ontology for photoleukocoria: identifying common internet search terms for a potentially important pediatric ophthalmic sign. Transl Vis Sci Technol. 2018;7(1):18.
7. Nirmalan PK, Sheeladevi S, Tamilselvi V, Victor AC, Vijayalakshmi P, Rahmathullah L. Perceptions of eye diseases and eye care needs of children among parents in rural south India: the Kariapatti Pediatric Eye Evaluation Project (KEEP). Indian J Ophthalmol. 2004;52(2):163–7.
8. Ebeigbe JA, Emedike CM. Parents' awareness and perception of children's eye diseases in Nigeria. J Optom. 2017;10(2):104–10.
9. Staffieri SE. "A glint or a squint should make you think!" Towards the earlier diagnosis of retinoblastoma. [Dissertation]. Melbourne, Victoria: University of Melbourne; 2019.
10. Donaldson L, Subramanian A, Conway ML. Eye care in young children: a parent survey exploring access and barriers. Clin Exp Optom. 2018;101(4):521–6.
11. Dunphy EB. The story of retinoblastoma. The XX Edward Jackson Memorial Lecture. Am J Ophthalmol. 1964;58:539–52.
12. Staffieri SE. Retinoblastoma: awareness, diagnosis, treatment and outcome. 2013.
13. Damasco VC, Dire DJ. A child with leukocoria. Pediatr Emerg Care. 2011;27(12):1170–4.
14. Wirix M, Parys-Vanginderdeuren R, Casteels I, Uyttebrouck A. Delayed diagnosis of retinoblastoma. Bull Soc Belge Ophtalmol. 2000;278:37–41.
15. Horwood AM. Maternal observations of ocular alignment in infants. J Pediatr Ophthalmol Strabismus. 1993;30(2):100–5.
16. Sondhi N, Archer SM, Helveston EM. Development of normal ocular alignment. J Pediatr Ophthalmol Strabismus. 1988;25(5):210–1.
17. Jacobs HB. Pseudostrabismus: an audit. Br J Ophthalmol. 1978;62(11):763–4.
18. Graham PA. Epidemiology of strabismus. Br J Ophthalmol. 1974;58(3):224–31.
19. Robaei D, Rose KA, Kifley A, Cosstick M, Ip JM, Mitchell P. Factors associated with childhood strabismus: findings from a population-based study. Ophthalmology. 2006;113(7):1146–53.
20. Friedman DS, Repka MX, Katz J, Giordano L, Ibironke J, Hawse P, et al. Prevalence of amblyopia and strabismus in white and African-American children aged 6 through 71 months: the Baltimore Pediatric Eye Disease Study. Ophthalmology. 2009;116(11):2128–34.e1-2.
21. Birch EE, Wang J. Stereoacuity outcomes following treatment of infantile and accommodative esotropia. Optom Vis Sci. 2009;86(6):647–52.
22. Birch EE. Amblyopia and binocular vision. Prog Retin Eye Res. 2013;33:67–84.
23. Menon V, Saha J, Tandon R, Mehta M, Khokhar S. Study of the psychosocial aspects of strabismus. J Pediatr Ophthalmol Strabismus. 2002;39(4):203–8.
24. Chang MY, Velez FG, Demer JL, Isenberg SJ, Coleman AL, Pineles SL. Quality of life in adults with strabismus. Am J Ophthalmol. 2015;159(3):539–44.e2.
25. Mojon-Azzi SM, Mojon DS. Strabismus and employment: the opinion of headhunters. Acta Ophthalmol. 2009;87(7):784–8.
26. Mojon-Azzi SM, Potnik W, Mojon DS. Opinions of dating agents about strabismic subjects' ability to find a partner. Br J Ophthalmol. 2008;92(6):765–9.
27. Kim IG, Park JM, Lee SJ. Factors associated with the direction of ocular deviation in sensory horizontal strabismus and unilateral organic ocular problems. Korean J Ophthalmol. 2012;26(3):199–202.
28. Hunter DG, Ellis FJ. Prevalence of systemic and ocular disease in infantile exotropia: comparison with infantile esotropia. Ophthalmology. 1999;106(10):1951–6.
29. Williams A, Hoyt CS. Acute comitant esotropia in children with brain tumors. Arch Ophthalmol. 1989;107(3):376–8.
30. Berk TA, Oner HF, Saatci OA. Underlying pathologies in secondary strabismus. Strabismus. 2000;8(2):69–75.
31. Taylor RH. Guidelines for the management of strabismus in childhood. 2012.
32. Abramson DH, Beaverson K, Sangani P, Vora RA, Lee TC, Hochberg HM, et al. Screening for retinoblastoma: presenting signs as prognosticators of patient and ocular survival. Pediatrics. 2003;112(6 Pt 1):1248–55.
33. Ellsworth RM. Hereditary and preventive aspects of retinoblastoma. Sight Sav Rev. 1969;39:17–20.
34. Knudson AG Jr. Genetics and the etiology of childhood cancer. Pediatr Res. 1976;10(5):513–7.
35. Dang-Tan T, Trottier H, Mery LS, Morrison HI, Barr RD, Greenberg ML, et al. Delays in diagnosis and treatment among children and adolescents with cancer in Canada. Pediatr Blood Cancer. 2008;51(4):468–74.
36. Dang-Tan T, Franco EL. Diagnosis delays in childhood cancer: a review. Cancer. 2007;110(4):703–13.
37. Kivela T. The epidemiological challenge of the most frequent eye cancer: retinoblastoma, an issue of birth and death. Br J Ophthalmol. 2009;93(9):1129–31.
38. Rodriguez-Galindo C, Friedrich P, Alcasabas P, Antillon F, Banavali S, Castillo L, et al. Toward the cure of all children with cancer through collaborative efforts: pediatric oncology as a global challenge. J Clin Oncol. 2015;33(27):3065–73.
39. Singh G, Daniels AB. Disparities in retinoblastoma presentation, treatment, and outcomes in developed and less-developed countries. Semin Ophthalmol. 2016;31(4):310–6.
40. Dimaras H, Dimba EA, Gallie BL. Challenging the global retinoblastoma survival disparity through a collaborative research effort. Br J Ophthalmol. 2010;94(11):1415–6.
41. Gallie BL, Zhao J, Vandezande K, White A, Chan HS. Global issues and opportunities for optimized retinoblastoma care. Pediatr Blood Cancer. 2007;49(7 Suppl):1083–90.
42. De Sutter E, Hoepping W. First symptoms in retinoblastoma. Bull Soc Belge Ophtalmol. 1983;207:45–51.
43. Haik BG, Siedlecki A, Ellsworth RM, Sturgis-Buckhout L. Documented delays in the diagnosis of retinoblastoma. Ann Ophthalmol. 1985;17(11):731–2.
44. Goddard AG, Kingston JE, Hungerford JL. Delay in diagnosis of retinoblastoma: risk factors and treatment outcome. Br J Ophthalmol. 1999;83(12):1320–3.
45. Butros LJ, Abramson DH, Dunkel IJ. Delayed diagnosis of retinoblastoma: analysis of degree, cause, and potential consequences. Pediatrics. 2002;109(3):E45.
46. Chantada G, Fandino A, Manzitti J, Urrutia L, Schvartzman E. Late diagnosis of retinoblastoma in a developing country. Arch Dis Child. 1999;80(2):171–4.
47. Leander C, Fu LC, Pena A, Howard SC, Rodriguez-Galindo C, Wilimas JA, et al. Impact of an education program on late diagnosis of retinoblastoma in Honduras. Pediatr Blood Cancer. 2007;49(6):817–9.
48. Epelman S, Epelman C, Erwenne C, Melaragno R, Teixeira LF, Adde M, et al. National campaign for early diagnosis of retinoblastoma in Brazil. J Clin Oncol. 2004;22(Suppl 14:abstract 8561).
49. Hayes R, (as communicated to Mr William Hunter S. Medical Observations and Enquiries. London: William Johnston; 1767.
50. Atchaneeyasakul LO, Wongsiwaroj C, Uiprasertkul M, Sanpakit K, Thephamongkhol K, Trinavarat A. Prognostic factors and treat-

ment outcomes of retinoblastoma in pediatric patients: a single-institution study. Jpn J Ophthalmol. 2009;53(1):35–9.
51. Chawla B, Hasan F, Azad R, et al. Clinical Presentation and survival of retinoblastoma in Indian children. Br J Ophthalmol. 2016;100:172–8.
52. Austoker J, Bankhead C, Forbes LJ, Atkins L, Martin F, Robb K, et al. Interventions to promote cancer awareness and early presentation: systematic review. Br J Cancer. 2009;101(Suppl 2):S31–9.
53. Fisher JD, Fisher WA. Changing AIDS-risk behavior. Psychol Bull. 1992;111(3):455–74.
54. Chang SJ, Choi S, Kim S-A, Song M. Intervention strategies based on information-motivation-behavioral skills model for health behavior change: a systematic review. Asian Nurs Res. 2014;8(3):172–81.
55. Abraham C. Developing evidence-based content for health promotion materials. In: Abraham C, Kools M, editors. Writing health communication—an evidence-based guide. London, UK: Sage Publications; 2012.
56. Simpson JK. Appeal to fear in health care: appropriate or inappropriate? Chiropr Man Ther. 2017;25:27.
57. Ryan L, Logsdon MC, McGill S, Stikes R, Senior B, Helinger B, et al. Evaluation of printed health education materials for use by low-education families. J Nurs Scholarsh. 2014;46(4):218–28.
58. Yousef YA, AlNawaiseh T, AlJabari R, Muhsen S, Al-Nawaiseh I. Retinoblastoma awareness among first contact physicians in Jordan. Ophthalmic Genet. 2019:1–5.
59. Mattosinho CCS, Grigorovski N, Lucena E, et al. Prediagnostic intervals in retinoblastoma: experience at an oncology center in Brazil. J Glob Oncol. 2017;3(4):323–30. https://pubmed.ncbi.nlm.nih.gov/28831440/.
60. Neiger BL, Thackeray R, Van Wagenen SA, Hanson CL, West JH, Barnes MD, et al. Use of social media in health promotion: purposes, key performance indicators, and evaluation metrics. Health Promot Pract. 2012;13(2):159–64.
61. Welch V, Petkovic J, Pardo Pardo J, Rader T, Tugwell P. Interactive social media interventions to promote health equity: an overview of reviews. Health Promot Chronic Dis Prev Can. 2016;36(4):63–75.
62. Posner M, Jaulim A, Vasalaki M, Rantell K, Sagoo MS, Reddy MA. Lag time for retinoblastoma in the UK revisited: a retrospective analysis. BMJ Open. 2017;7(7):e015625.
63. Freyer DR, Brugieres L. Adolescent and young adult oncology: transition of care. Pediatr Blood Cancer. 2008;50(5 Suppl):1116–9.
64. Fletcher O, Easton D, Anderson K, Gilham C, Jay M, Peto J. Lifetime risks of common cancers among retinoblastoma survivors. J Natl Cancer Inst. 2004;96(5):357–63.
65. Friedman DN, Chou JF, Oeffinger KC, Kleinerman RA, Ford JS, Sklar CA, et al. Chronic medical conditions in adult survivors of retinoblastoma: results of the retinoblastoma survivor study. Cancer. 2016;122(5):773–81.
66. Gregersen PA, Urbak SF, Funding M, Overgaard J, Jensen UB, Alsner J. Danish retinoblastoma patients 1943–2013—genetic testing and clinical implications. Acta Oncol. 2016;55(4):412–7.
67. Gelkopf MJ, Avramov I, Baddeliyanage R, Ristevski I, Johnson SA, Flegg K, et al. The Canadian retinoblastoma research advisory board: a framework for patient engagement. Res Involv Engagem. 2020;6:7.
68. White E, Baddeliyanage R, Shaikh F, Dimaras H. Meaningful patient engagement in research: lessons from retinoblastoma. Pediatrics. 2019;143(6):e20182166.
69. Yeung JWK, Zhang Z, Kim TY. Volunteering and health benefits in general adults: cumulative effects and forms. BMC Public Health. 2017;18(1):8.
70. Bray L, Carter B, Sanders C, Blake L, Keegan K. Parent-to-parent peer support for parents of children with a disability: a mixed method study. Patient Educ Couns. 2017;100(8):1537–43.

Overcoming Challenges in the Delivery of Care: The Thailand Story

Duangnate Rojanaporn

1 Introduction

The perspective in ocular oncology varies worldwide in terms of epidemiology, ethnicity, disease severity, socioeconomic status, treatment modalities, and treatment outcomes. These lead to challenges in the delivery of care in ocular oncology patients globally, especially in developing countries. To overcome these challenges, the understanding of ocular oncology perspectives in each country is mandatory in order to utilize available local resources, and develop strategies to maximize the treatment outcomes for the patients. The field of ocular oncology has been developed enormously over the past decades. The goal of management in ocular oncology patients in order of importance is saving patients' lives, globe, and vision. In the past, the majority of patients with malignant intraocular tumors were treated with enucleation. At present, globe preservation and even visual preservation can be achieved with recent advanced in treatment modalities. This chapter will focus on our experiences in the delivery of care of patients with intraocular tumors in Thailand, our unique challenges in the region that have been encountered and overcome.

2 Ocular Oncology in Thailand

In the past, before we established our ocular oncology service, patients with intraocular tumors were treated with local ophthalmologists in their region, which includes general ophthalmologists, retina specialists, oculoplastic surgeons, or pediatric ophthalmologists. The treatment protocol which varies between each treatment centers based on the available treatment modalities in each local treatment centers results in variable treatment outcomes. Some retinoblastoma treatment centers required pathological diagnosis of retinoblastoma before systemic chemotherapy can be given. Moreover, single patient may be diagnosed, treated, and followed up by different ophthalmologists. The available treatment modalities were enucleation, systemic chemotherapy, and external beam radiotherapy.

There are seven tertiary referral centers that provide treatment for ocular oncology patients in Thailand, four in Bangkok (capital city) and three in each part of Thailand, north, northeast, and south. Our ophthalmology department is a part of the Faculty of Medicine Ramathibodi Hospital, Mahidol University, located in Bangkok, which serves as one of the main tertiary referral centers in our country.

In 2012, we established our ocular oncology service for the first time in Thailand at Ramathibodi Hospital, aiming to be the referral center for ocular oncology patients in Thailand and South East Asia region, to deliver the standard of care, and to improve the patients' quality of life. The delivery of care for ocular oncology patients is challenging and requires a multidisciplinary team, including ocular oncologists, pediatric ophthalmologists, pediatric oncologists, medical oncologists, radiologists, neurologists, neurosurgeons, anesthesiologists, pathologists, ocularists, and other medical personnel. A good teamwork is extremely mandatory to achieve the best patients' outcomes.

Our center is currently the only center in Thailand and South East Asia region that has all the treatment modalities for ocular oncology patients including systemic chemotherapy, intra-arterial chemotherapy (IAC), subtenon chemotherapy, intravitreal chemotherapy, cryotherapy, transpupillary thermotherapy (TTT), external beam radiotherapy (EBRT), plaque brachytherapy with Ruthenium-106 (Ru-106), tumor endoresection, tumor exoresection, enucleation, and exenteration.

Intra-arterial chemotherapy (IAC) for retinoblastoma was introduced by Kaneko et al. in 2004 [1], before it was modified and popularized by Abramson et al. in 2008 [2]. We first performed IAC in our center in 2009, using melphalan, topotecan, and carboplatin. Intra-arterial chemotherapy in our center was performed by neurointerventionists using the similar technique as described by Abramson et al. [2]. With

D. Rojanaporn (✉)
Department of Ophthalmology, Faculty of Medicine, Ramathibodi Hospital, Mahidol University, Bangkok, Thailand
e-mail: duangnate.roj@mahidol.ac.th

B. V. Chawla, M. E. Aronow (eds.), *Global Perspectives in Ocular Oncology*, https://doi.org/10.1007/978-3-031-08250-4_35

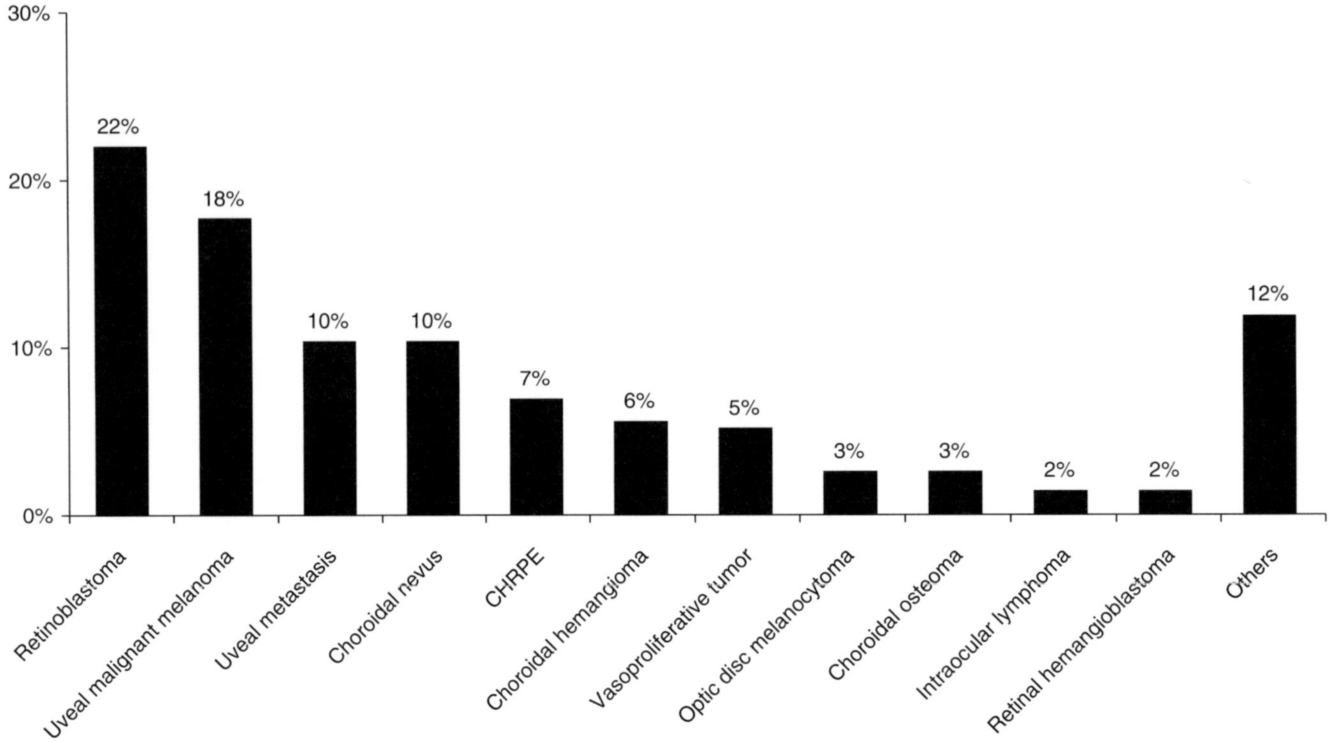

Fig. 1 Prevalence of intraocular tumor in Ramathibodi Hospital, Bangkok, Thailand, during January 2012 to January 2021

IAC, our globe survival was significantly improved, especially in patients with group D eyes [3].

Brachytherapy is the preferred treatment modality for various intraocular tumors, especially uveal melanoma. Various radioisotopes have been used worldwide for many years, with Iodine-125 and Ruthenium-106 the most commonly used isotopes. In 2013, we started brachytherapy for the first time in South East Asia. Since the number of patients in our center is not high, Ruthenium-106 is used in our center due to its long half-life. We treated various intraocular tumors with Ruthenium-106 brachytherapy including uveal melanoma, retinoblastoma, choroidal hemangioma, retinal vasoproliferative tumor, uveal metastasis, and adenoma of the retinal pigment epithelium. Dosimetry was calculated by medical physicists and radiation oncologists, who transferred each fundus drawings into a computerized treatment planning system, using the plaque simulator software (Bebig GmbH, Berlin, Germany).

3 Our Experiences

During January 2012 to January 2021, there were 613 patients with intraocular tumors in our center. The most common intraocular tumor in our center was retinoblastoma (22.2%), followed by uveal malignant melanoma (17.9%), uveal metastasis (10.4%), choroidal nevus (10.1%), congenital hypertrophy of the retinal pigment epithelium (CHRPE) (7.0%), choroidal hemangioma (5.7%), retinal vasoproliferative tumor (5.2%), optic disc melanocytoma (3.1%), choroidal osteoma (2.6%), intraocular lymphoma (2.3%), and retinal hemangioblastoma (1.5%) (Fig. 1).

4 Retinoblastoma in Thailand

Retinoblastoma is the seventh most common childhood cancer in Thailand, with the incidence of 3.1 per million population, with the 5-year overall survival probability of 73%, based on the nationwide multicenter population-based prospective study of the incidence and survival rate of childhood cancer from Thai Pediatric Oncology Group (ThaiPOG) [4]. There are seven centers that provide treatment for retinoblastoma in Thailand, four in Bangkok (capital city) and three in each part of Thailand, north, northeast, and south. The survival rate of retinoblastoma in Thailand varies among each center and region of the country. Previous report from three cancer centers in north, northeast, and south of Thailand during 1990 and 2009, which included 75 retinoblastoma patients, showed survival rates of 40%, 50%, and 75%, respectively [5]. The survival rate of retinoblastoma patients from a single institute in Bangkok, which included 90 retinoblastoma patients during 1997–2006 [6], and 144 patients during 2005–2018 [7], showed survival rates of 85%, and 90.3%, respectively [6, 7]. The overall survival rate of 81 retinoblastoma patients from our center during 2007–2018 was 93.8% [8] (Table 1).

Table 1 Patient and globe survival of retinoblastoma in Thailand

Authors (Reference)	Study period	Region	Number of patients/ eyes	Patients with Extraocular RB (%)	Eyes with advanced intraocular RB/ICRB D/ICRB E (%)	Overall survival rate	Overall globe salvage rate	Globe salvage rate in unilateral RBICRB A/B/C/D/E	Globe salvage rate in bilateral RBICRB A/B/C/D/E
Wiangnon S et al. [4]	2003–2005	Nationwide	97/NA	NA	NA	73%	NA	NA	NA
Wongmas P et al. [5]	1990–2009	North Northeast South	20/NA 31/NA 24/NA	NA	NA	40% 50% 75%	NA	NA	NA
Atchaneeyasakul L et al. [6]	1997–2006	Bangkok, single center	90/121	14.4%	72.7%/11.5%/61.2%	85%	16.2%	3.5% NA/NA/50%/0%/0%	29.6% 100%/100%/87.5%/45.5%/0%
Prajantawanich K et al. [7]	2005–2018	Bangkok, single center	144/194	2.7%	79.4%/12.9%/66.5%	90.3%	23.2%	NA	NA
Rojanaporn D et al. [8]	2007–2018	Bangkok, single center	81/124	11.1%	74.85/27%/47.8%	93.8%	51.7%	37.5% NA/100%/100%/50%/18.8%	57.8% 100%/94.4%/100%/64.7%/28.2%

All seven retinoblastoma treatment centers in Thailand have participated in the global retinoblastoma study [9]. The data from the study showed that in year 2017, there were 55 eyes of 42 patients diagnosed with retinoblastoma all over the country. Half of the patients lived in central area of the country. Only two patients from the same family had familial retinoblastoma (4.7%). Twenty-six patients were male (62%). Twenty-nine patients had unilateral retinoblastoma (69%). The mean age of diagnosis was 22.9 months (range, 0–120 months). The frequent presenting symptoms were leukocoria (66%), strabismus (7%), and proptosis (7%). According to the International Retinoblastoma Staging System (IRSS) [10], the patients were classified as IRSS stages 0, 1, 2, 3, and 4 in 33 (78.6%), 17 (40.5%), 2 (4.8%), 1 (2.4%), and 2 (4.8%) patient(s), respectively. For intraocular retinoblastoma classification, six centers used the International Classification of Retinoblastoma (ICRB) [11], and one center used the International Intraocular Retinoblastoma Classification (IIRC) [12]. According to ICRB and IIRC classification, the eyes were classified as groups A, B, C, D, and E in 1 (1.8%), 5 (9.1%), 5 (9.1%), 21 (38.2%), and 20 (36.4%) eye(s), respectively [9].

Diagnostic and treatment modalities are different among each center. Magnetic resonance imaging (MRI), computed tomography (CT), pathology, intravenous chemotherapy (IVC), and cryotherapy are available in all centers. External beam radiotherapy (EBRT) and laser treatment are available in six centers. Six centers have the ability to perform IAC, but only two centers have experiences of performing the procedure. Plaque brachytherapy is available in one center. Genetic testing is available in two centers. Primary treatment included IVC with/without other treatments (58%), enucleation (31%), and IAC (7%).

5 Retinoblastoma in our Center

Retinoblastoma is the most common intraocular tumor in our center. According to our recent study which included 124 eyes of 81 patients with retinoblastoma during 2007–2018, the most common presentation was leukocoria (76.5%), followed by strabismus (9.9%) and buphthalmos (3.7%). No sex bias was noted in our study (male 49.4%, female 41.6%). The median age at diagnosis was 8 months (range, 1–48 months). About half of patients had bilateral retinoblastoma (53.1%), which had significantly lower median age of onset (5 months) compared to unilateral retinoblastoma (46.9%, 17 months). The median lag time between symptom onset and visit to the oncology service was 6 weeks (range, 1–80 weeks). Orbital retinoblastoma, diagnosed based on clinical and radiological manifestations, was found in 9 of 81 patients (11.1%). Most patients presented with intraocular retinoblastoma (89.9%), in which the majority of them had advanced stage of disease (74.8%), as International Classification of Retinoblastoma (ICRB) groups D (27%) and E (47.8%). At the median follow-up period of 38.4 months (range, 0.2–148.2 months), the overall survival rate was 93.8%. The overall globe salvage rate for intraocular retinoblastoma was 51.7%, which was 37.5% for unilateral intraocular retinoblastoma (ICRB group B, 100%; group C, 100%; group D, 50%; and group E, 18.8%), and 57.8% for bilateral intraocular retinoblastoma (ICRB group A, 100%; group B, 94.4%; group C, 100%; group D, 64.7%; and group E, 28.2%) [8].

6 Staging of Retinoblastoma

We performed complete ophthalmic examination under anesthesia (EUA) in all patients, which included binocular indirect ophthalmoscopy (BIO) with 360° indentation, Schiotz tonometry, and ultrasonography. Fundus imaging and fluorescein angiography were performed using a wide-angle contact fundus camera (RetCam 3, Clarity Medical Systems, Inc., Pleasanton, CA). Magnetic resonance imaging (MRI) of the brain and orbits was performed in all patients to identify the presence of extraocular extension and intracranial malignancy. Intraocular tumors were classified according to the International Classification of Retinoblastoma (ICRB) [11], the International Intraocular Retinoblastoma Classification (IIRC) [12], and the American Joint Committee on Cancer (AJCC) (eighth edition) [13], while extraocular tumors were classified according to the International Retinoblastoma Staging System (IRSS) [10] and AJCC (eighth edition). Lumbar puncture and bone marrow biopsy were performed in all patients with extraocular tumors for disease staging.

7 Treatment of Retinoblastoma

Treatment strategies were planned based on the disease stage, laterality, tumor location, visual prognosis, and input from the patient's family. EUA was performed monthly during the course of treatment to evaluate treatment response.

For bilateral intraocular retinoblastoma patients, the primary treatment was intravenous systemic chemotherapy (IVC), followed by tumor consolidation with TTT, cryotherapy, or plaque brachytherapy. Secondary IAC can be performed for patients with incomplete tumor response after IVC (Fig. 2).

For unilateral intraocular retinoblastoma patients, patients in ICRB groups A and B with macula- and/or

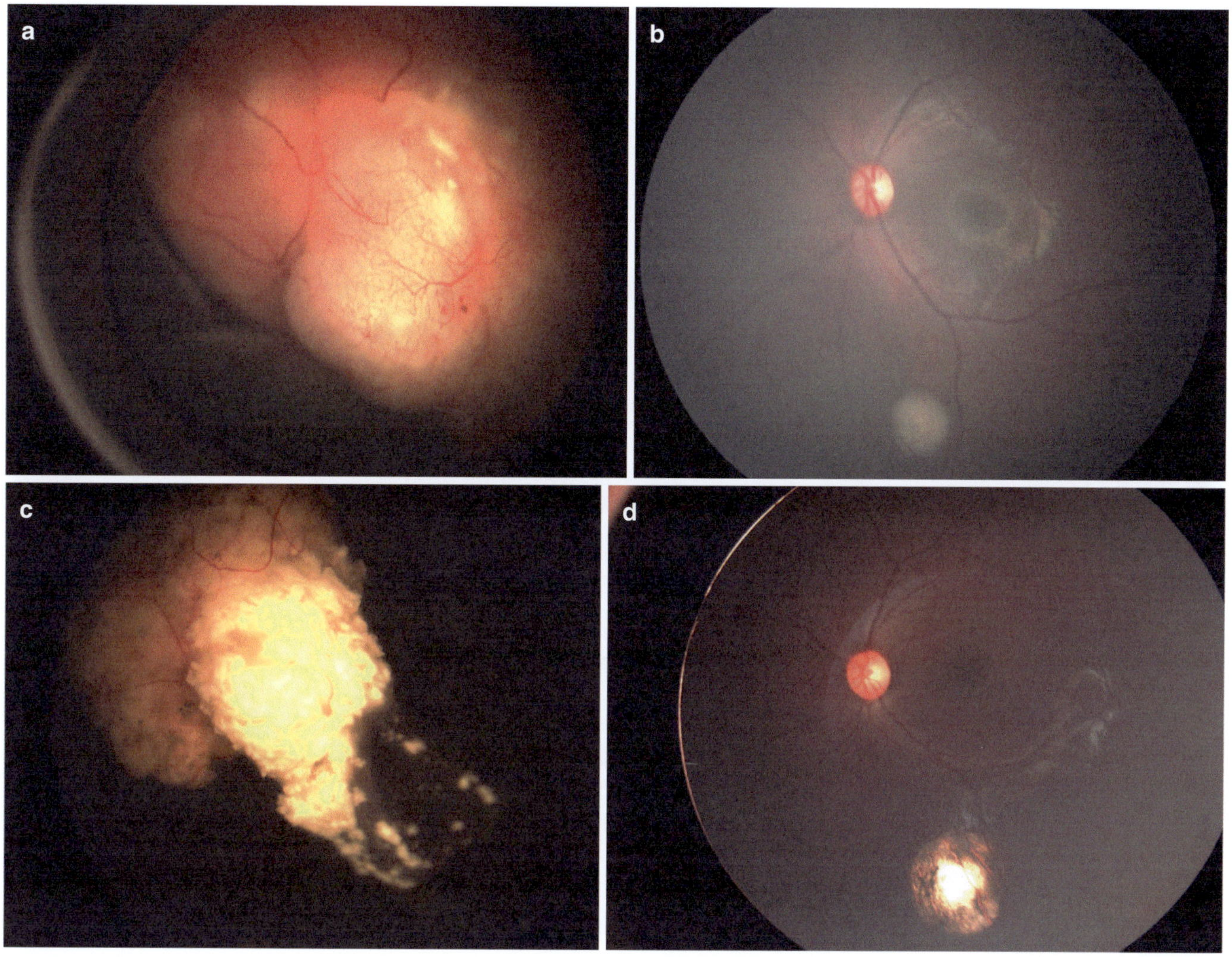

Fig. 2 (**a**) A 7-month-old girl with bilateral retinoblastoma classified as ICRB group E OD and (**b**) ICRB OS was treated with six courses of intravenous chemotherapy with vincristine, carboplatin, and etoposide, followed by tumor consolidation with transpupillary thermotherapy OS. Following the treatment, complete tumor regression was achieved in both eyes [(**c**) OD, (**d**) OS]

papilla-sparing tumors were treated locally with cryotherapy (peripheral tumor) or transpupillary thermotherapy (posterior tumor). For ICRB group B patients with macular and/or papillary involvement and patients in ICRB group C and less advanced ICRB group D were treated with IAC or IVC, based on age of patients at the time of treatment, the feasibility of catheterization during IAC, and input from patients' families (Fig. 3).

For unilateral advanced ICRB group D and ICRB group E, primary enucleation was recommended to the parents. In Thailand, like other Asian countries, the refusal of enucleation is not uncommon. Samsara is a common Buddhist belief, and enucleation is assumed to affect one's well-being in the next life, making the procedure highly stigmatized. In these cases, where parents strongly denied enucleation, IAC was offered as an alternative treatment to prevent the parents from abandoning the treatment and loss of follow-up. Enucleation was more acceptable to these parents after the failure of IAC. Additionally, in our experiences, we found that showing photos of other patients, who wear ocular prosthesis after enucleation, to the parents made them feel more comfortable to enucleation, and made the procedure more acceptable to them.

After enucleation, each enucleated eye was examined meticulously by the ocular pathologist to identify high-risk histopathological features; if present, post-enucleation adjuvant chemotherapy will be given in order to reduce the risk of systemic metastasis, as previously reported [14].

Intravitreal chemotherapy with melphalan and/or topotecan was reserved for eyes with vitreous seeds, which poorly respond to IVC and/or IAC. Safety enhancement procedures were performed to prevent extraocular extension of the tumor [8, 15, 16].

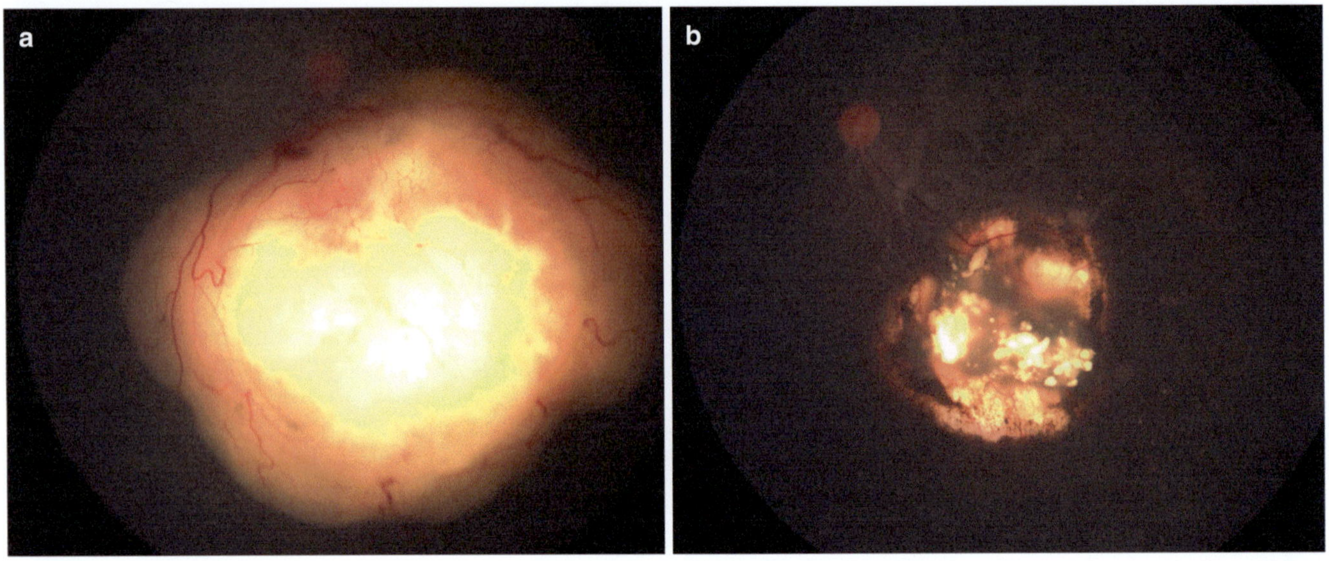

Fig. 3 (**a**) An 8-month-old boy with unilateral retinoblastoma classified as ICRB group D OS was treated with three courses of intra-arterial chemotherapy with melphalan, topotecan, and carboplatin. (**b**) Following the treatment, complete tumor regression was achieved

Table 2 Dosage of intravenous chemotherapy for intraocular and extraocular retinoblastoma

Agents/course interval	Standard dose (BW < 12 kg) for ICRB groups A, B, C, and postenucleation patients with high-risk pathological features	Intensified dose for ICRB groups D and E (BW < 12 kg)	High dose for extraocular retinoblastoma
Vincristine	1.5 mg/m^2/day on day 1 (0.05 mg/kg/day)	1.5 mg/m^2/day on day 1 (0.05 mg/kg/day)	0.025 mg/kg/day on day 1
Etoposide	150 mg/m^2/day on days 1–2 (5 mg/kg/day)	180 mg/m^2/day on days 1–2 (6 mg/kg/day)	12 mg/kg/day on days 1–2
Carboplatin	560 mg/m^2/day on day 1 (18.6 mg/kg/day)	420 mg/m^2/day on days 1–2 (14 mg/kg/day)	28 mg/kg/day on day 1
Course interval	Continue every 4 weeks for a total of six cycles	Continue every 4 weeks for a total of six cycles	Continue every 3 weeks for a total of six cycles

For orbital retinoblastoma patients, we use the combination of high-dose IVC (three to six cycles), followed by enucleation or exenteration, external beam radiation therapy (EBRT), and adjuvant chemotherapy, for a total of 12 cycles, as previously reported [17, 18].

For IVC, we use the combination of vincristine, etoposide, and carboplatin as previously described [8, 17, 19] (Table 2). For IAC, we use melphalan, topotecan, and/or carboplatin as described in our previous report [3].

8 Genetic Testing

We screened *RB1* mutations in our patients by using direct sequencing in combination with multiplex ligation-dependent probe amplification (MLPA). From our previous study of 52 retinoblastoma patients, 27 patients (52%) had unilateral retinoblastoma, and 25 patients (48%) had bilateral retinoblastoma. Germline mutation was detected in 92% of bilateral retinoblastoma patients. Interestingly, we found the high incidence of germline mutation in our unilateral retinoblastoma patients (33%) [20].

9 Three-Dimensional Organoid Model

Our group was the first to establish and characterize a three-dimensional, self-organizing organoid model derived from chemotherapy-naïve retinoblastoma tumors by harvesting tumor tissue from retinoblastoma patients who underwent primary enucleation [21]. We found that organoids had histological features, as well as gene and protein expression of the parental tissue [21]. This patient-derived organoid may enable the creation of a faithful model to be used in examining novel therapeutics for retinoblastoma in the future research [21, 22].

10 Future Challenges and Plans

A multicenter study and national system of retinoblastoma registration are required to establish a nationwide picture of retinoblastoma. Education of public and primary healthcare providers, along with the implementation of a retinoblastoma screening program, should be promoted to detect retinoblastoma at early stage. This would allow patients to gain better treatment outcomes. In addition, proper retinoblastoma management necessitates multidisciplinary cooperation, by a multidisciplinary team that should include ocular oncologists, pediatric ophthalmologists, pediatric oncologists, medical oncologists, radiologists, neurologists, neurosurgeons, anesthesiologists, pathologists, ocularists, and other medical personnel. As such specialized providers are not available in many areas of the country, comprehensive referral centers may present one solution toward better provision of retinoblastoma care in Thailand.

11 Uveal Melanoma

Uveal melanoma is the second most common intraocular tumor in our center. We retrospectively analyzed clinical characteristics and outcomes of uveal melanoma patients diagnosed in our center during January 2012 to January 2021. Of 97 uveal melanoma patients, 9 patients were excluded from the analysis due to incomplete data and follow-up. Of 88 included patients, 43 patients were male (48.9%). The mean age at diagnosis was 51.7 years (range, 15–86 years). Most patients were Asian (93%; Thai 90%, Myanmar 1%, Cambodia 2%). Six patients were Caucasian (6%).

The most common tumor location was choroid (75 patients, 85.2%), followed by ciliary body (11 patients, 12.5%) and iris (2 patients, 2.3%). The mean tumor thickness measured by ultrasonography was 9.5 millimeters (mm) (range, 2.0–18.0 mm). The tumor was classified according to COMS classification [23], as small-, medium-, and large-sized tumor in 2 (2.27%), 42 (47.72%), and 44 (50.0%) patients, respectively. According to the eighth AJCC classification [24], the tumors were classified as T1, T2A, T2B, T3A, T3B, T3C, and T4 in 14 (15.9%), 16 (18.2%), 36 (40.9%), 14 (15.9%), 4 (4.6%), 2 (2.3%), 2 (2.3%) patients, respectively. The mean logMAR visual acuity at presentation was 1.07 (range, 0.0 to no light perception).

Our available treatment modalities included transpupillary thermotherapy, ruthenium plaque brachytherapy (Ru-106), tumor endoresection, tumor exoresection, enucleation, orbital exenteration, and external beam radiotherapy. The risk and benefit of each treatment options were advised to all patients. Enucleation was the most common primary treatment (46 patients, 52.3%), followed by RU-106 plaque brachytherapy (Fig. 4) (24 patients, 27.3%), tumor endoresection with adjunctive Ru-106 brachytherapy (Fig. 5) (17 patients, 19.3%), and tumor exoresection (Fig. 6) (1 patient, 1.1%). The pathological report was analyzed in 55 patients. The most common histopathological melanoma cell type was mixed spindle and epithelioid cell type (47 patients, 87.5%), followed by epithelioid cell type (6 patients, 10.9%) and spindle B-cell type (3 patients, 5.5%).

At the mean follow-up time of 32.9 months (range, 1.3–129.5 months), the overall globe salvage rate was 46.6%. The globe salvage rate in globe-sparing therapy group was 97.6%. The mean final logMAR visual acuity by globe-sparing therapy was 1.20 (range, 0.0 to no light perception).

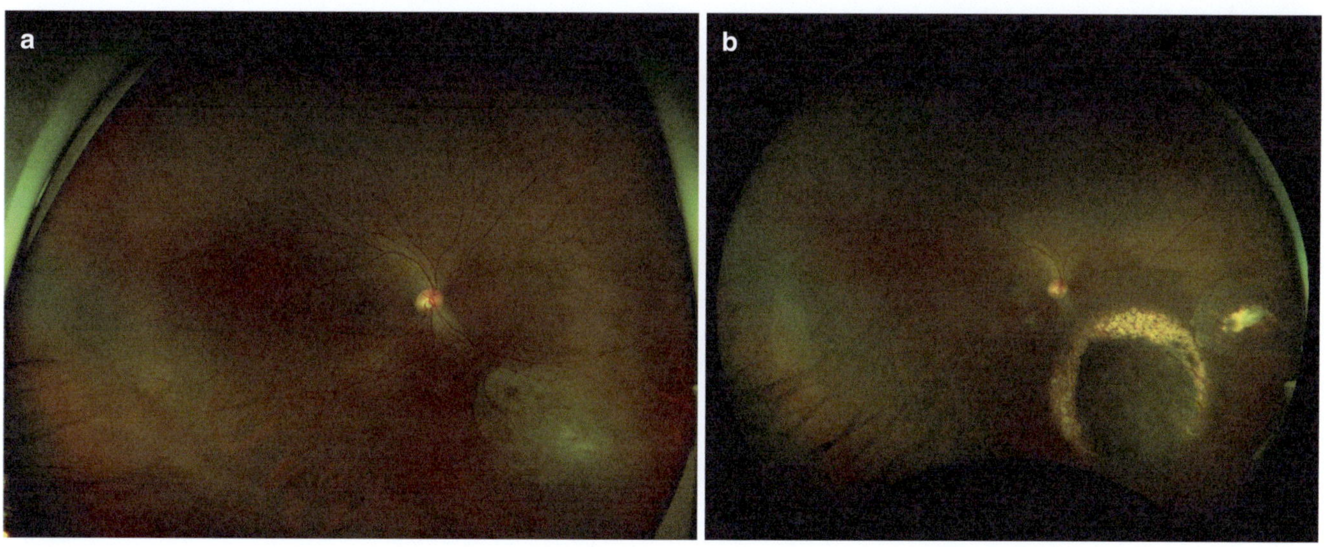

Fig. 4 (**a**) A 36-year-old male with medium-sized choroidal malignant melanoma OD was treated with ruthenium plaque brachytherapy. (**b**) Following the treatment, complete tumor regression was achieved

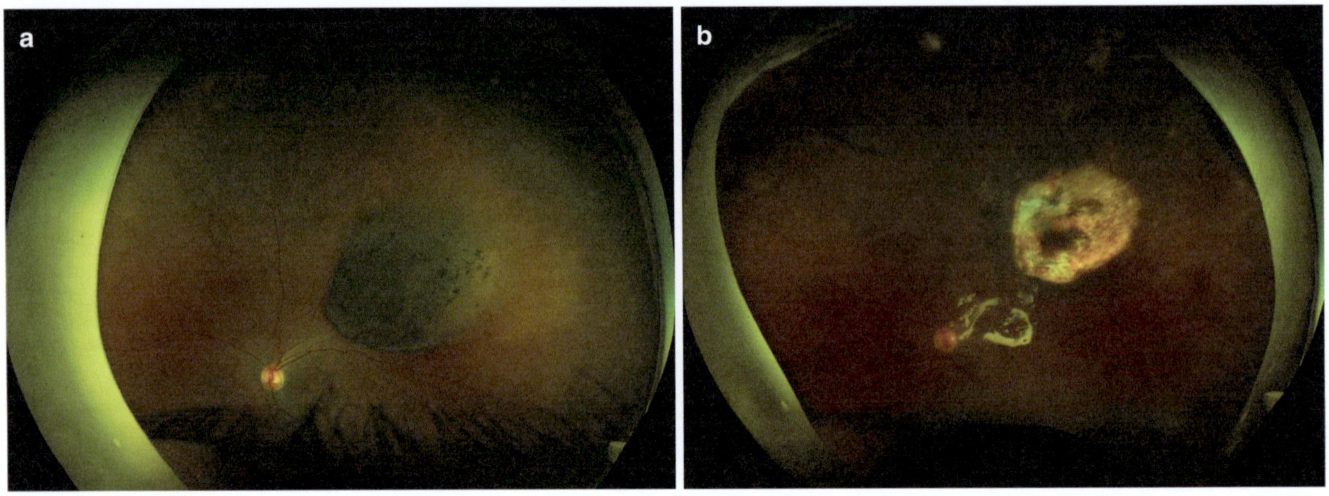

Fig. 5 (**a**) A 41-year-old female with large-sized choroidal melanoma OS was treated with tumor endoresection combined with adjunctive ruthenium plaque brachytherapy. (**b**) Following the treatment, the retina was well attached without tumor recurrence

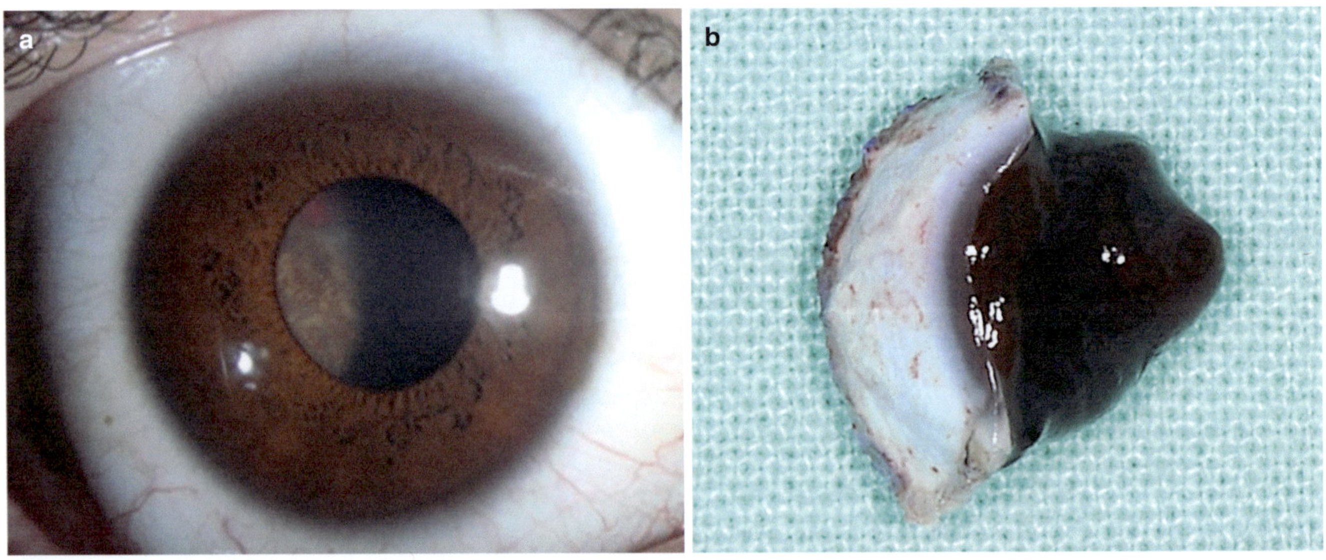

Fig. 6 (**a**) A 24-year-old male with large-sized ciliary body malignant melanoma OD. (**b**) The tumor was completely excised with tumor exoresection technique (partial lamellar sclerouvectomy)

The tumor recurrence rate in globe-sparing therapy group was 14.6%. The overall survival rate was 92%. Eight patients died from tumor metastases. One patient, who underwent tumor endoresection, died from pulmonary air embolism without the usage of air during vitrectomy [25]. Thirteen patients (14.8%) developed distant organ metastases, which were the liver (30.8%), lung (15.4%), bone (7.7%), and multiple organs (46.1%).

12 Uveal Metastases

Of 64 patients with uveal metastases in our center during January 2012 to January 2021, 56 patients had unilateral metastasis (87.5%). Forty-four patients were female (68.6%). The mean age at diagnosis was 56.0 years (range, 3–82 years). The most common site of uveal metastases was choroid (81%), followed by iris (7.8%). Two patients had iris and choroidal metastasis (3.1%), two patients had choroid and optic disc metastasis (3.1%), two patients had ciliary body and iris metastasis, and one patient (1.5%) had retinal metastasis. The most common primary cancer was lung carcinoma (45.3%), followed by breast carcinoma (28.1%), prostate carcinoma (4.6%), gastrointestinal tract carcinoma (4.6%), and renal cell carcinoma (3.1%). Other uncommon primary cancers were acute myeloid leukemia, hepatocellular carcinoma, neuroblastoma, testes carcinoma, and skin malignant melanoma. The main treatment was systemic chemotherapy, especially if the patient had other organ metastases, or active primary cancer (Fig. 7). In patients with brain and ocular

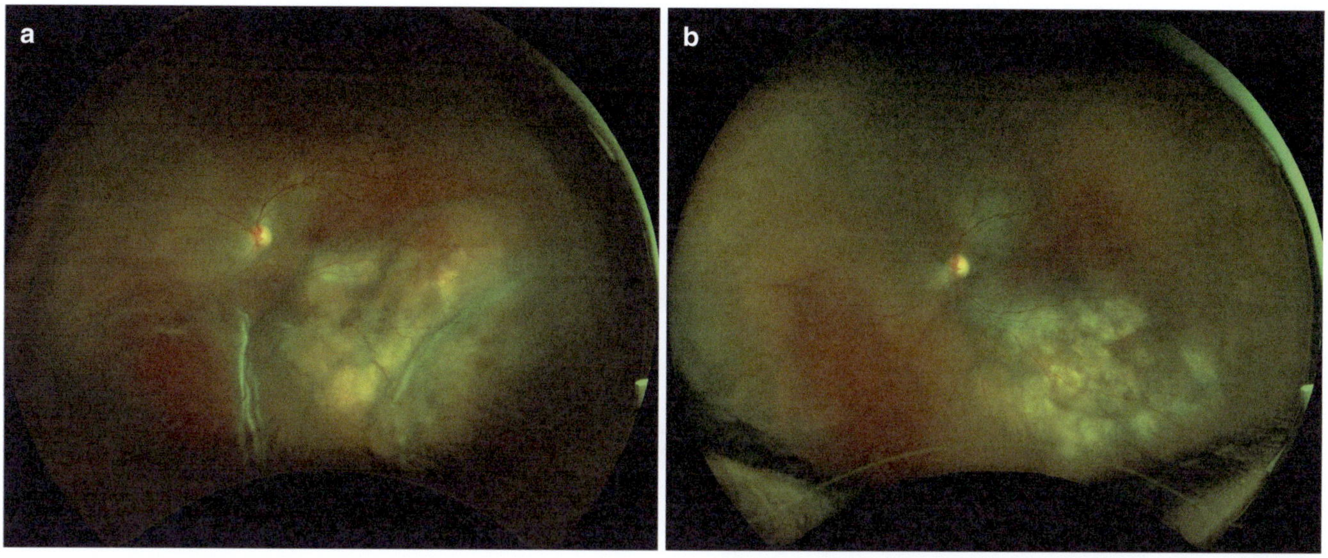

Fig. 7 (**a**) A 61-year-old female with lung carcinoma developed unilateral choroidal metastasis with extensive exudative retinal detachment OS. Systemic chemotherapy was given for other organ metastases. (**b**) The choroidal metastatic tumor was regressed and exudative retinal detachment was resolved after systemic chemotherapy

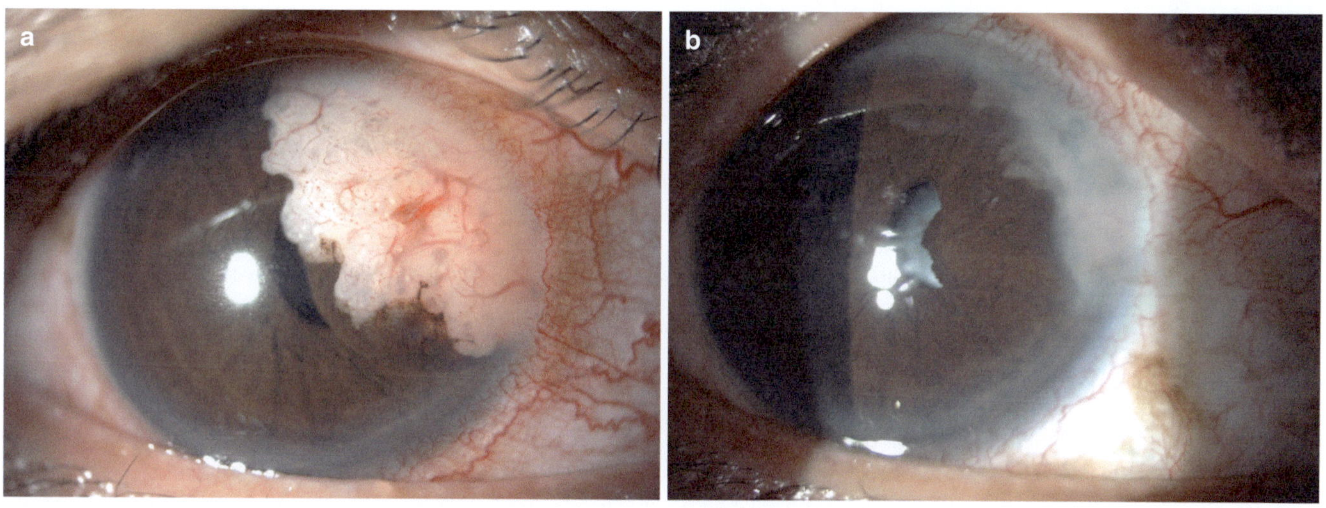

Fig. 8 (**a**) A 44-year-old-male with breast carcinoma developed unilateral iris and ciliary body metastasis OD. The metastatic iridociliary tumor did not respond to systemic chemotherapy. (**b**) Ruthenium plaque brachytherapy was applied to the metastatic iridociliary tumor, which resulted in complete tumor regression and secondary cataract

metastases, external beam radiotherapy can be delivered to the eye and brain altogether. If there were no active primary cancer, no other organ metastases, or poor treatment response following chemotherapy, local ocular treatment with photodynamic therapy, Ruthenium-106 brachytherapy, or external beam radiotherapy can be performed (Fig. 8). Enucleation was reserved for patients with painful blind eyes to improve the patient's quality of life.

13 Hemangioma

Of 35 patients diagnosed with hemangioma in our center during January 2012 to January 2021, circumscribed choroidal hemangioma (CCH) was the most common hemangioma found in the eye (77.1%), followed by diffuse choroidal hemangioma (DCH) associated with Sturge-Weber syndrome (SWS) (17.1%). One patient with SWS had optic disc

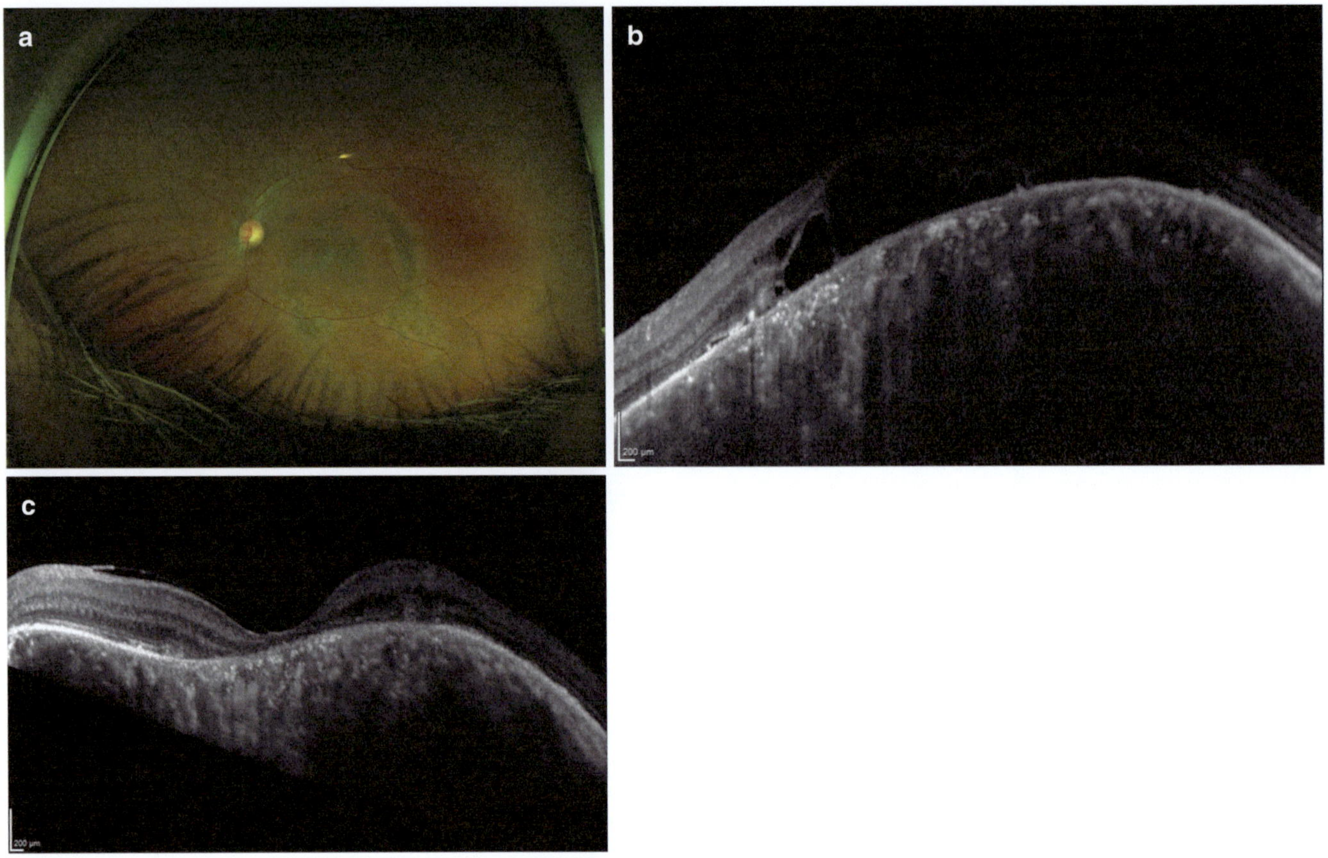

Fig. 9 (**a**) A 63-year-old male with circumscribed choroidal hemangioma in macula area OS. (**b**) Optical coherence tomography showed submacular fluid and cystoid macular edema over the tumor, (**c**) which were resolved following photodynamic therapy

hemangioma (2.9%), and one patient had iris hemangioma (2.9%). The mean age at diagnosis was 42.0 years (range, 5–73 years), with female predominance (68.6%). Observation was recommended in asymptomatic patients with inactive tumor [25]. In symptomatic patients with retinal edema or exudative retinal detachment, standard dose of photodynamic therapy (PDT) was the preferred treatment [26] (Fig. 9). Plaque brachytherapy, or low-dose external beam radiotherapy, was reserved for large tumor, or tumor with extensive retinal detachment, which is difficult to treat with PDT [26] (Fig. 10).

14 Retinal Vasoproliferative Tumor

There were 32 patients with retinal vasoproliferative tumor (VPT) in our center during January 2012 to January 2021. Nineteen patients were male (59.3%). The mean age at diagnosis was 43.3 years (range, 13–84 years). Twenty patients had primary VPT (62.5%), and 12 patients had secondary VPT (37.5%). The ocular diseases associated with secondary VPT were Coats disease (33.3%), uveitis (25.0%), retinitis pigmentosa (25%), familial exudative vitreoretinopathy (8.3%), and chronic retinal detachment (8.3%). The management of VPT is based on visual symptoms, tumor size, tumor location, and other associated vitreoretinal findings. Asymptomatic and stable VPT were carefully observed. Treatment was required in patients with active VPT, progressive exudation, detachment, vitreous hemorrhage, or remote macular changes [27]. For small active VPT, we performed cryotherapy with double freeze-thaw technique (Fig. 11). Ruthenium brachytherapy was preserved for thick active VPT (Fig. 12). Pars plana vitrectomy was performed in patients with epimacular membrane, vitreomacular traction, macular hole, vitreous hemorrhage, or tractional retinal detachment.

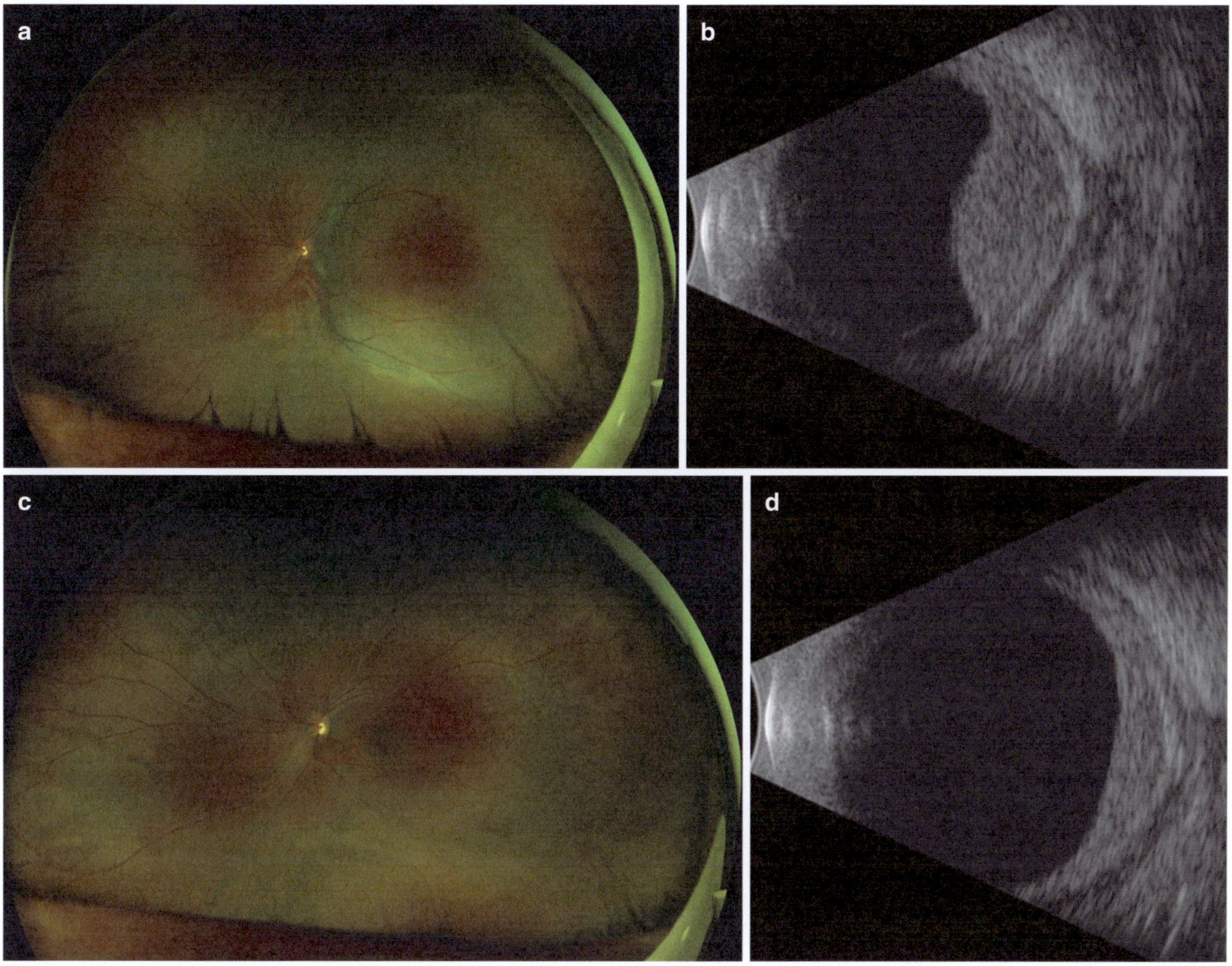

Fig. 10 (**a**) A 21-year-old male with circumscribed choroidal hemangioma and exudative retinal detachment OS (optos), (**b**) (ultrasonography). (**c**) Ruthenium plaque brachytherapy was applied to the tumor, which resulted in the resolution of exudative retinal detachment, and regression of the hemangioma (optos), (**d**) (ultrasonography)

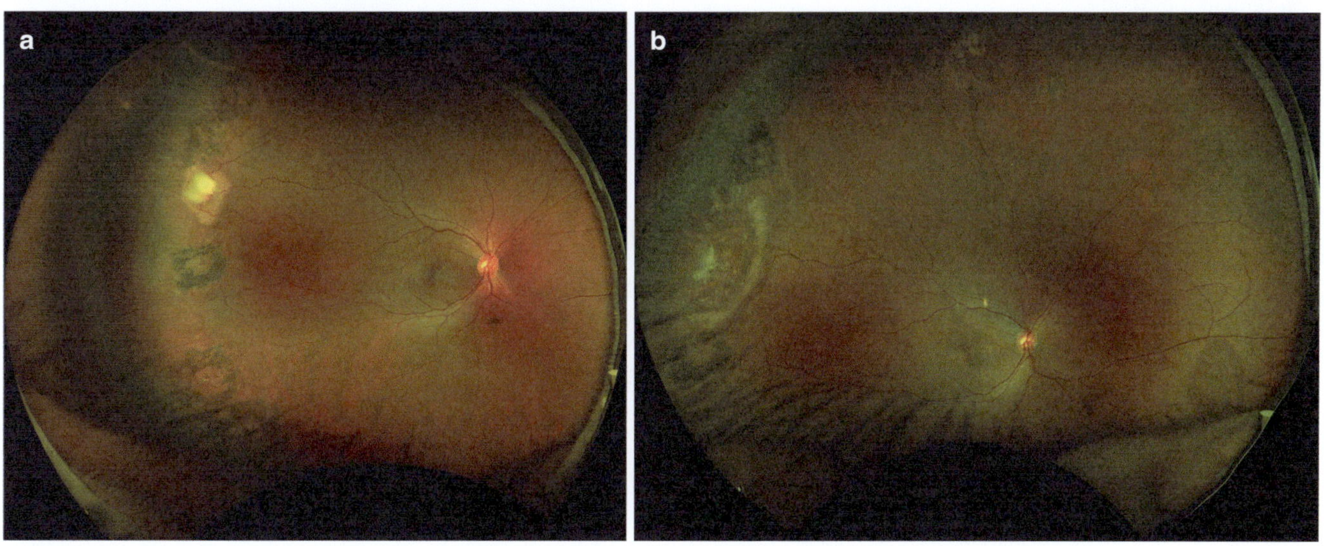

Fig. 11 (**a**) A 46-year-old female with familial exudative vitreoretinopathy developed secondary small retinal vasoproliferative tumor OD. (**b**) The tumor was regressed following a single session of cryotherapy

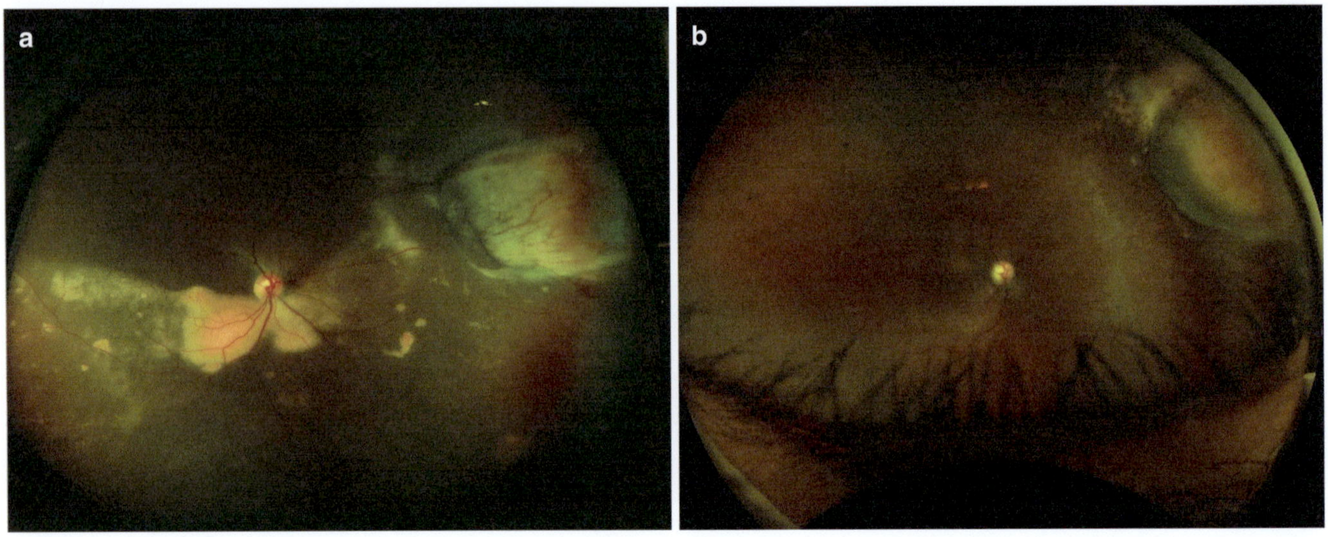

Fig. 12 (**a**) A 33-year-old male with a large-sized primary retinal vasoproliferative tumor producing extensive exudative retinal detachment, and subretinal exudates OS. (**b**) Ruthenium plaque brachytherapy was applied to the tumor, which resulted in the resolution of exudative retinal detachment, subretinal exudates, and regression of the vasoproliferative tumor

15 Conclusion

In our experiences, there were many challenges that we have encountered and overcome. First of all, Thailand is a developing country, where resources are limited in terms of medical personnel, medical equipment, and budgets. The utilization of our limited resources at its best may overcome these challenges. We formed our multidisciplinary ocular oncology team with ocular oncologists, oculoplastic surgeons, pediatric ophthalmologists, pediatric oncologists, medical oncologists, radiologists, neurologists, neurosurgeons, anesthesiologists, pathologists, ocularists, and other medical personnel. A good teamwork with constant communications is extremely mandatory to achieve the best patients' outcomes.

Ocular oncology is relatively new in Thailand. Therefore, introduction and education of ocular oncology to general ophthalmologists, retina specialists, and medical personals are mandatory. We formed our particular team of surgical nurses who have expertise in ocular oncology surgeries. Our medical personnel are familiar with the use and the maintenance of medical equipment. We have promoted our ocular oncology unit by presenting our treatment outcomes in publications and national, regional, and international meetings. We found that spending times with patients to discuss about their diagnosis, treatment options, and treatment plan allow for the patients' better understanding of the treatment necessity, which may improve the patients' compliance for the treatment and follow-up. For all Thai patients, most of medical expenses, except intra-arterial chemotherapy and brachytherapy, are covered by the government. On the other hand, the patients have to manage their own travel expenses. These are the main reasons of treatment abandonment, and the loss of follow-up. To minimize these problems, we established a special charity fund under the hospital foundation, particularly for ocular oncology patients, to cover these expenses, in order to maximize the benefits of the patients to receive the best treatment that they deserve, and for them to maintain their regular follow-up visits.

References

1. Yamane T, Kaneko A, Mohri M. The technique of ophthalmic arterial infusion therapy for patients with intraocular retinoblastoma. Int J Clin Oncol. 2004;9(2):69–73. https://doi.org/10.1007/s10147-004-0392-6.
2. Abramson DH, Dunkel IJ, Brodie SE, Kim JW, Gobin YP. A phase I/II study of direct intraarterial (ophthalmic artery) chemotherapy with melphalan for intraocular retinoblastoma initial results. Ophthalmology. 2008;115(8):1398–404, 1404.e1. https://doi.org/10.1016/j.ophtha.2007.12.014. Epub 2008 Mar 14.
3. Rojanaporn D, Chanthanaphak E, Boonyaopas R, Sujirakul T, Hongeng S, Ayudhaya SSN. Intra-arterial chemotherapy for retinoblastoma: 8-year experience from a Tertiary Referral Institute in Thailand. Asia Pac J Ophthalmol (Phila). 2019;8(3):211–7. https://doi.org/10.22608/APO.2018294. Epub 2019 Feb 4.
4. Wiangnon S, Veerakul G, Nuchprayoon I, Seksarn P, Hongeng S, Krutvecho T, Sripaiboonkij N. Childhood cancer incidence and survival 2003-2005, Thailand: study from the Thai Pediatric Oncology Group. Asian Pac J Cancer Prev. 2011;12(9):2215–20.
5. Wongmas P, Jetsrisuparb A, Komvilaisak P, Suwanrungruang K, Choeyprasert W, Sriplung H, Wiangnon S. Incidences, trends and long term outcomes of retinoblastoma in three cancer registries, Thailand. Asian Pac J Cancer Prev. 2015;16(16):6899–902. https://doi.org/10.7314/apjcp.2015.16.16.6899.
6. Atchaneeyasakul LO, Wongsiwaroj C, Uiprasertkul M, Sanpakit K, Thephamongkhol K, Trinavarat A. Prognostic factors and treatment outcomes of retinoblastoma in pediatric patients: a single-institution study. Jpn J Ophthalmol. 2009;53(1):35–9. https://doi.org/10.1007/s10384-008-0614-y. Epub 2009 Jan 30.

7. Prajantawanich K, Sanpakit K, Narkbunnam N, Vathana N, Takpradit C, Phuakpet K, Pongtanakul B, Atchaneeyasakul LO, Sinlapamongkolkul P, Buaboonnam J. Clinical outcomes and prognosis of Thai retinoblastoma patients. Pediatr Int. 2021;63(6):671–7. https://doi.org/10.1111/ped.14498. Epub 2021 May 26.
8. Rojanaporn D, Attaseth T, Dieosuthichat W, Leelawongs K, Pakakasama S, Anurathapan U, Chanthanaphak E, Singhara Na Ayudhaya S, Aroonroch R, Hongeng S. Clinical presentations and outcomes of retinoblastoma patients in relation to the advent of new multimodal treatments: a 12-year report from Single Tertiary Referral Institute in Thailand. J Ophthalmol. 2020;2020:4231841. https://doi.org/10.1155/2020/4231841.
9. Global Retinoblastoma Study Group, Fabian ID, Abdallah E, Abdullahi SU, Abdulqader RA, Adamou Boubacar S, et al. Global retinoblastoma presentation and analysis by national income level. JAMA Oncol. 2020;6(5):685–95. https://doi.org/10.1001/jamaoncol.2019.6716. Erratum in: JAMA Oncol. 2020 Nov 1;6(11):1815.
10. Chantada G, Doz F, Antoneli CB, Grundy R, Clare Stannard FF, Dunkel IJ, Grabowski E, Leal-Leal C, Rodríguez-Galindo C, Schvartzman E, Popovic MB, Kremens B, Meadows AT, Zucker JM. A proposal for an international retinoblastoma staging system. Pediatr Blood Cancer. 2006;47(6):801–5. https://doi.org/10.1002/pbc.20606.
11. Shields CL, Mashayekhi A, Au AK, Czyz C, Leahey A, Meadows AT, Shields JA. The international classification of retinoblastoma predicts chemoreduction success. Ophthalmology. 2006;113(12):2276–80. https://doi.org/10.1016/j.ophtha.2006.06.018. Epub 2006 Sep 25.
12. Linn Murphree A. Intraocular retinoblastoma: the case for a new group classification. Ophthalmol Clin N Am. 2005;18(1):41–53, viii. https://doi.org/10.1016/j.ohc.2004.11.003.
13. Mallipatna A, Gallie BL, Chévez-Barrios P, Lumbroso-Le Rouic L, Chantada GL, Doz F. Retinoblastoma. In: Amin MB, Edge SB, Greene FL, editors. AJCC cancer staging manual. 8th ed. New York: Springer; 2017. p. 819–31.
14. Honavar SG, Singh AD, Shields CL, Meadows AT, Demirci H, Cater J, Shields JA. Postenucleation adjuvant therapy in high-risk retinoblastoma. Arch Ophthalmol. 2002;120(7):923–31. https://doi.org/10.1001/archopht.120.7.923.
15. Munier FL, Soliman S, Moulin AP, Gaillard MC, Balmer A, Beck-Popovic M. Profiling safety of intravitreal injections for retinoblastoma using an anti-reflux procedure and sterilisation of the needle track. Br J Ophthalmol. 2012;96(8):1084–7. https://doi.org/10.1136/bjophthalmol-2011-301016. Epub 2012 Feb 24.
16. Francis JH, Xu XL, Gobin YP, Marr BP, Brodie SE, Abramson DH. Death by water: precautionary water submersion for intravitreal injection of retinoblastoma eyes. Open Ophthalmol J. 2014;8:7–11. https://doi.org/10.2174/1874364101408010007.
17. Honavar SG, Singh AD. Management of advanced retinoblastoma. Ophthalmol Clin N Am. 2005;18(1):65–73, viii. https://doi.org/10.1016/j.ohc.2004.09.001.
18. Chawla B, Hasan F, Seth R, Pathy S, Pattebahadur R, Sharma S, Upadhyaya A, Azad R. Multimodal therapy for stage III retinoblastoma (International Retinoblastoma Staging System): a prospective comparative study. Ophthalmology. 2016;123(9):1933–9. https://doi.org/10.1016/j.ophtha.2016.05.034. Epub 2016 Jul 21. Erratum in: Ophthalmology. 2016;123(12):2634.
19. Leahey AM. Systemic chemotherapy: a pediatric oncology perspective. In: Ramasubramanian A, Shields CL, editors. Retinoblastoma. New Delhi: Jaypee Brothers Medical Publisher; 2012. p. 81–5.
20. Rojanaporn D, Boontawon T, Chareonsirisuthigul T, Thanapanpanich O, Attaseth T, Saengwimol D, Anurathapan U, Sujirakul T, Kaewkhaw R, Hongeng S. Spectrum of germline *RB1* mutations and clinical manifestations in retinoblastoma patients from Thailand. Mol Vis. 2018;24:778–88.
21. Saengwimol D, Rojanaporn D, Chaitankar V, Chittavanich P, Aroonroch R, Boontawon T, Thammachote W, Jinawath N, Hongeng S, Kaewkhaw R. A three-dimensional organoid model recapitulates tumorigenic aspects and drug responses of advanced human retinoblastoma. Sci Rep. 2018;8(1):15664. https://doi.org/10.1038/s41598-018-34037-y.
22. Kaewkhaw R, Rojanaporn D. Retinoblastoma: etiology, modeling, and treatment. Cancers (Basel). 2020;12(8):2304. https://doi.org/10.3390/cancers12082304.
23. Design and methods of a clinical trial for a rare condition: the collaborative ocular melanoma study. COMS Report No. 3. Control Clin Trials. 1993;14(5):362–91. https://doi.org/10.1016/0197-2456(93)90052-f.
24. Kivelä T, Simpson RE, Grossniklaus HE, et al. Uveal melanoma. In: AJCC cancer staging manual. 8th ed. New York, NY: Springer; 2016. p. 805–17.
25. Rojanaporn D, Tipsuriyaporn B, Chulalaksiriboon P, Virankabutra T, Morakul S, Damato B. Fatal air embolism after choroidal melanoma endoresection without air infusion. Ocular Oncology and Pathology. 2021;7(5):321–5.
26. Shields CL, Dalvin LA, Lim LS, Chang M, Udyaver S, Mazloumi M, Vichitvejpaisal P, Su GL, Florakis E, Mashayekhi A, Shields JA. Circumscribed choroidal hemangioma: visual outcome in the pre-photodynamic therapy era versus photodynamic therapy era in 458 cases. Ophthalmol Retina. 2020;4(1):100–10. https://doi.org/10.1016/j.oret.2019.08.004. Epub 2019 Aug 22.
27. Shields CL, Kaliki S, Al-Dahmash S, Rojanaporn D, Shukla SY, Reilly B, Shields JA. Retinal vasoproliferative tumors: comparative clinical features of primary vs secondary tumors in 334 cases. JAMA Ophthalmol. 2013;131(3):328–34. https://doi.org/10.1001/2013.jamaophthalmol.524.

Building a Retinoblastoma Service in China

Junyang Zhao and Honggai Yan

Retinoblastoma (RB) is the most common malignant tumor arising from the retina in children. It endangers the vision and life of patients. The worldwide incidence of RB is 1:15,000–1:120,000 live birth [1]. If left untreated, the mortality rate is 100% [2]. Timely and effective treatment can save life and preserve vision.

The survival of children with RB like other cancers is markedly dependent on early diagnosis after detection of symptoms such as leukocoria, strabismus, red eye, lacrimation, and photophobia. In China, for many years, patients from remote areas faced late diagnosis and misdiagnosis. There was high rate of extraocular disease at initial presentation leading to poor outcome. For those patients, more than 95% patients underwent upfront enucleation. The mortality was 30–50% and less than 5% patients had eye preservation.

China is the third largest by geography and is the most populated country in the world. China has a vast territory with more than 9.6 million square kilometers and includes 32 provinces. It is 5200 km from east to west and 5500 km from north to south. China's territory spans more than 60° longitude from east to west, across five time zones. The population is more than 1.4 billion and more than ten million newborn babies per year. There are about 1100 new cases of retinoblastoma each year [3]. Because of the large geographic area, Chinese patients with RB are scattered, and it is difficult to establish a unified treatment. Suboptimal care yields poor outcome; therefore, establishing a standard of care is key to improving survival.

There were many barriers to optimizing RB care in China. First, there was a lack of standard protocol in peripheral hospitals. Physicians in peripheral hospitals have few exposures to RB, therefore lack the experience in making the correct diagnosis or treatment. Second, long travel time and distance to tertiary centers was another barrier for patients living in remote areas. Beijing is the capital of China with the largest hospitals and most advanced equipment and physicians specialized in RB. But the commute to major cities like Beijing can be long for families in other parts of China (Fig. 1). For example, the distance from Urumqi to Beijing is 2417 km, patients would require 3 h and 40 min by plane. Due to financial considerations, plane is not the primary choice of transportation for most Chinese families. Trains or buses are more frequently used, which means longer commute time to treatment centers in Beijing. Third, low follow-up rate due to financial challenges leads to high prevalence of late-stage presentation and low eye salvage rate. Based on our survey, the loss of income for parents due to travel accounted for 38.63% of the financial burden. The cost of food, transportation, and accommodation accounted for 28.71% of the burden. Each visit to Beijing takes up 5–7 days. One follow-up involves flying to Beijing, receiving clinic testing, booking an operating room, examination under anesthesia, and then flying back home [4]. The burden of care constitutes a major reason for poor outcome in patients from remote areas.

Collaboration with local hospitals is necessary in China. Our goal is to establish centers of excellence closer to the patients' family to decrease the burden of travel. This will save time for the patients by 1–2 days for each visit. The shorter commute time decreases loss of income and reduces the nonmedical costs. From 2007 to now, we have built more than 30 collaboration centers across China that cover more than 95% areas and populations of China (Fig. 2). This network ensures patients living in a big city or remote areas can receive the same high-quality care in a timely manner. For each new center in the network, we send retinoblastoma experts to train local physicians on RB diagnosis and treatment and establish standardized protocol (Fig. 3). Experts from Beijing also routinely visit local centers for guidance

J. Zhao (✉)
Department of Pediatric Oncology Center, Beijing Children's Hospital, Capital Medical University, National Center for Children's Health, Beijing, China

H. Yan
Department of Ophthalmology, Beijing Children's Hospital, Capital Medical University, National Center for Children's Health, Beijing, China

B. V. Chawla, M. E. Aronow (eds.), *Global Perspectives in Ocular Oncology*, https://doi.org/10.1007/978-3-031-08250-4_36

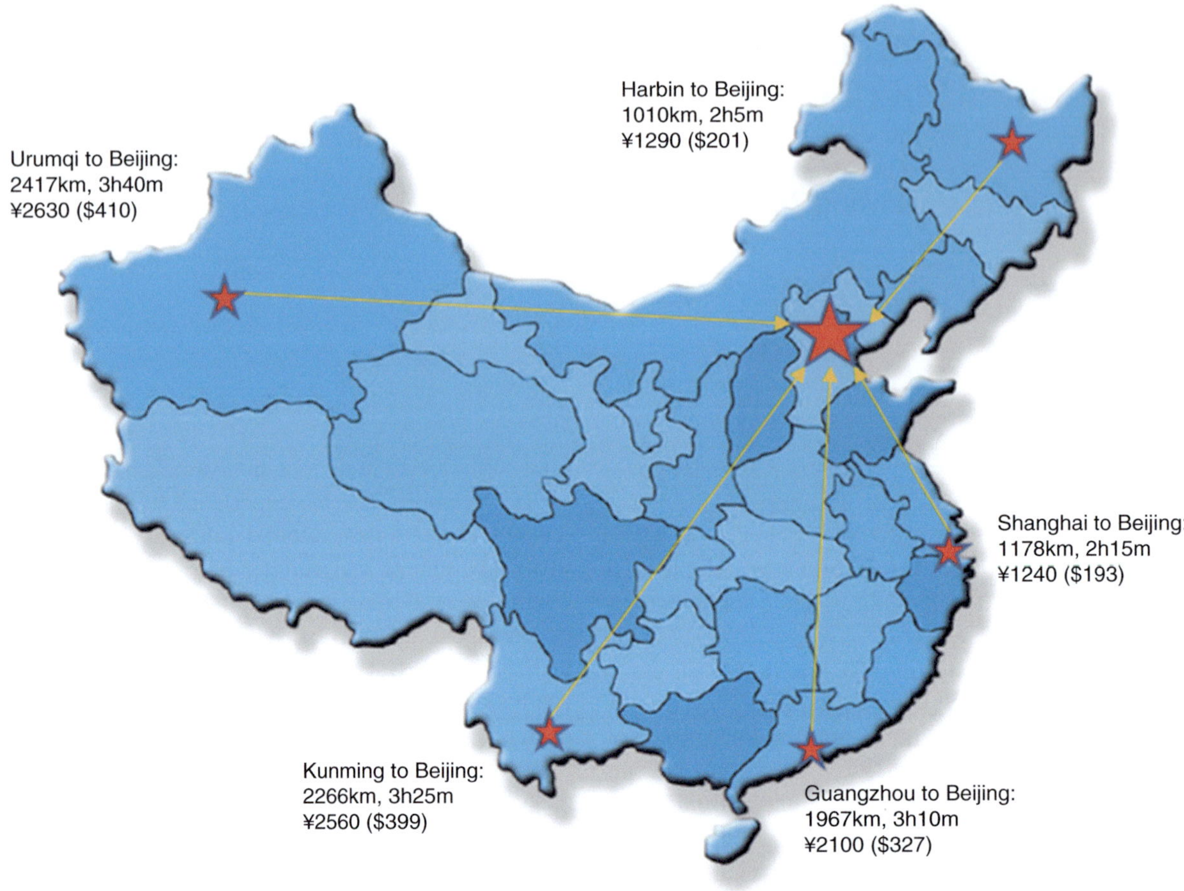

Fig. 1 The distance between Beijing and some cities

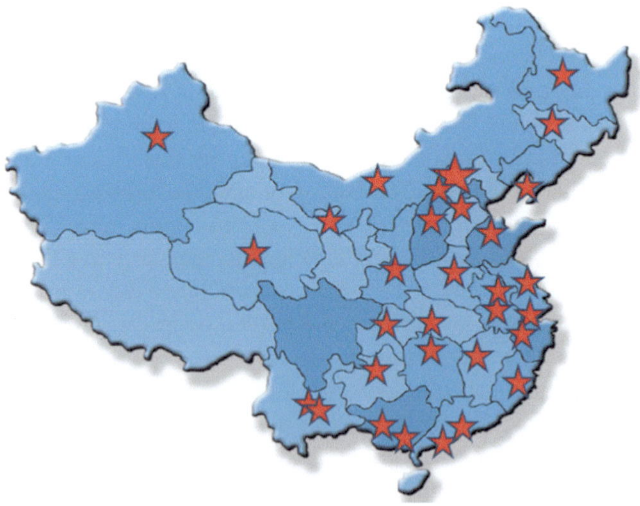

Fig. 2 The collaboration centers in China

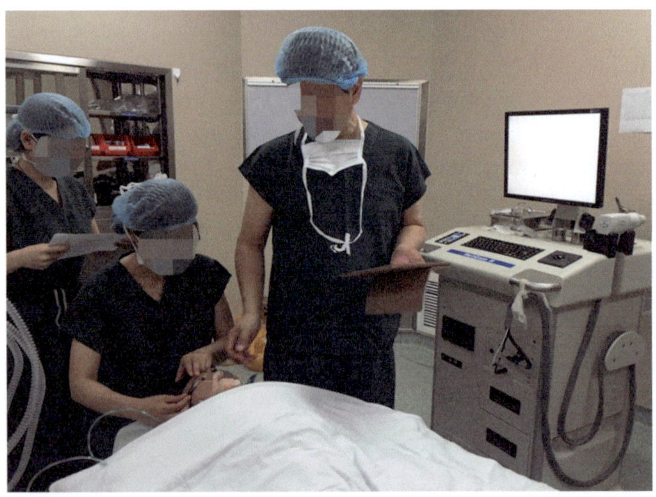

Fig. 3 Doctor Junyang Zhao was training physicians in local hospitals

(Fig. 4). All patients will be enrolled in different groups on WeChat based on geography. The experts' schedule to peripheral centers is available on the virtual bulletin board. Patients make appointment for examination via the contact person in the local center. The RB specialist will travel to the local hospital for treatments and training on the pre-scheduled date. We offer on-site training to local physicians and offer suggestions for improvement and standardization. In addi-

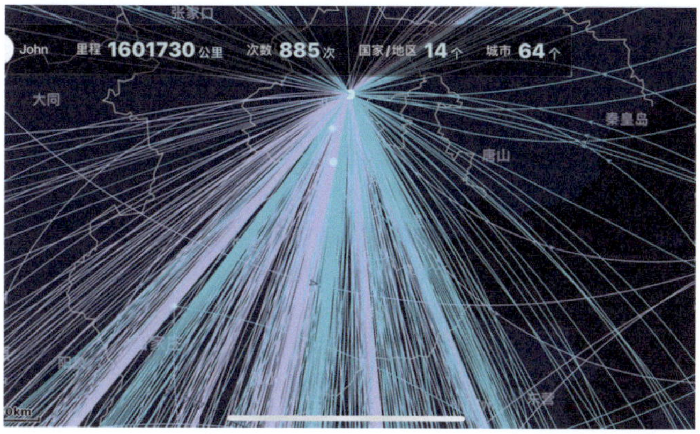

Fig. 4 One of the experts' flight from Beijing to other cities in the past 10 years

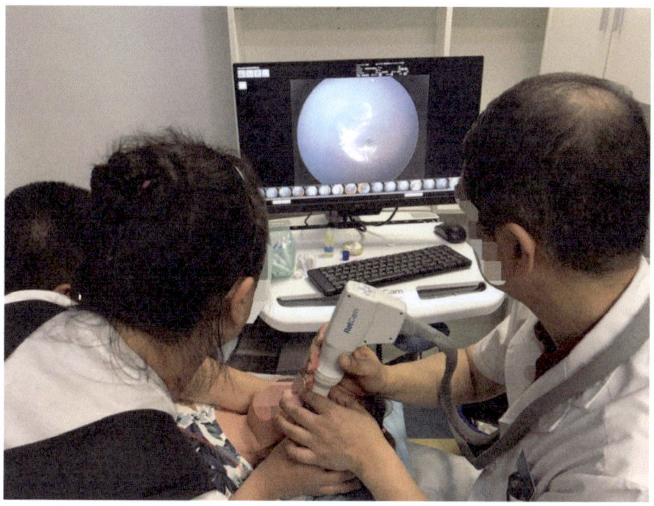

Fig. 5 Topical anesthesia fundus examination by RetCam

tion, for patients with stable disease following chemotherapy, we offer fundus examination under topical anesthesia in clinic to reduce the wait time for patients. For topical anesthesia examination, the caregiver applies dilation drops to the child's eyes 30 min prior to examination and applies topical anesthesia eyes upon entering the examination room. During exam, the caregiver holds the child down on the bed (not necessary for older children). The ophthalmologist retracts the eyes and examines the fundus (Fig. 5).

A uniform protocol across centers is important to ensure a good outcome. The same criteria and same medical care are delivered to all children irrespective of their location. Local training includes staging of the tumor, treatment, and follow-up. The staging classification standards include IIRC, cTNM, and pathology staging: seventh pTNM (AJCC Cancer Staging Manual). Treatment protocols include surgeries (enucleation, pars plana vitrectomy), focal therapies (cryotherapy, laser, transpupillary thermotherapy), chemotherapies (intravenous, intra-arterial, intravitreal), and radiotherapies (plaque brachytherapy, external beam technique).

Since the implementation of multicenter network, the number of treated RB patients is 1257 cases. 1160 (92.3%) patients were under follow-up. 97 (7.7%) patients were lost to follow-up. Confirmed dead patients were 99 (7.9%) cases. Including those lost to follow-up, potential deceased patients were 99–196 cases (7.9–15.6%). The mortality, loss of follow-up, and enucleation rates were significantly lower than those before the establishment of the multicenter model. Eye salvage, survival, and follow-up rate were significantly improved. It also reduced financial burden to the patient's family and the healthcare system. Through treatment and observation of a large number of Chinese RB patients, we implemented a novel treatment method, offering tumor endoresection to patients with intravitreal tumor implantation which improved the eyeball preservation rate [5].

Our aim is to establish a Chinese guideline of RB to better serve the RB patients in China. The guideline advocates for all patients with RB, including monocular retinoblastoma, to receive genetic testing to guide treatment and follow-up. Eye examination should be performed in every newborn baby to ensure early detection, diagnosis, and treatment of retinoblastoma in China.

References

1. Fabian ID, Onadim Z, Karaa E, Duncan C, Chowdhury T, Scheimberg I, Ohnuma SI, Reddy MA, Sagoo MS. The management of retinoblastoma. Oncogene. 2018;37(12):1551–60.
2. Jin L, Zhang W, Pan H, Li T, Liu B, Zhao J, Wang B. Retrospective investigation of retinoblastoma in Chinese patients. Oncotarget. 2017;8(65):108492–7.
3. Zhao J, Li S, Shi J, Wang N. Clinical presentation and group classification of newly diagnosed intraocular retinoblastoma in China. Br J Ophthalmol. 2011;95(10):1372–5.
4. Zhou Y, Cai S, Jin M, Jiang C, Xu N, Duan C, Peng X, Zhao J, Ma X. Economic burden for retinoblastoma patients in China. J Med Econ. 2020;23(12):1553–7.
5. Zhao J, Li Q, Wu S, Jin L, Ma X, Jin M, Wang Y, Gallie B. Pars plana vitrectomy and endoresection of refractory intraocular retinoblastoma. Ophthalmology. 2018;125(2):320–2.

Retinoblastoma, the African Context

Vera Adobea Essuman, Vera M. Beyuo,
and Helen Dimaras

1 Introduction: Retinoblastoma Worldwide

Retinoblastoma a rare retina cancer, with a worldwide incidence of 1 in 15,000–20,000 live births, is the commonest intraocular childhood cancer in the world [1, 2]. The incidence (per live births) is constant; however, differences exist due to variations in birth rates per population [1, 2]. Approximately 8000–9000 new cases of retinoblastoma are diagnosed annually around the world [1–3] with over 80% of these cases being found in Asia and Africa due to higher birth rates [3]. The incidence also varies inversely with the level of socio-economic development [4] with more than 90% of children with retinoblastoma living in low- and middle-income countries (LMICs). Ninety percent of cases presenting with metastatic disease and virtually all cases that abandon therapy are found in these LMICs [5]. While survival rates in developed countries such as the United States and Canada are nearly 100%, they are much lower in developing nations [6, 7]. Survival rates range from 80 to 89% in more developed Latin American countries to as low as 20–46% in certain African countries [6–12]. As a result of lower survival rates, there are an estimated 3000–4000 deaths annually due to retinoblastoma [5]. There is no sex predilection in the incidence of retinoblastoma globally [1, 2, 13–15].

V. A. Essuman (✉)
Ophthalmology Unit, Department of Surgery, University of Ghana Medical School, College of Health Sciences, University of Ghana, Accra, Greater Accra, Ghana
e-mail: vaessuman@ug.edu.gh

V. M. Beyuo
Eye Department, Korle Bu Teaching Hospital, Accra, Greater Accra, Ghana

H. Dimaras
Ophthalmology & Vision Sciences, The Hospital for Sick Children and University of Toronto, Toronto, ON, Canada
e-mail: helen.dimaras@sickkids.ca

Retinoblastoma is uniformly fatal if not detected early and appropriate treatment applied [1]. However, with early detection and treatment, survival is assured, sometimes with preservation of vision [1]. The progressive improvement in survival in developed countries over the century has been attributed to improvement in enucleation surgery and radiation, and more recently, to the advent of chemotherapy [16].

2 Retinoblastoma in Africa

2.1 The Burden

Africa shares the burden of retinoblastoma, where it is found to be the most common and important life-threatening ocular neoplasm [1, 2, 8, 17]. Unlike in Europe, North America, Australia and Asia where retinoblastomas account for 2–4% of total neoplasms in children, African populations have higher proportions, with retinoblastoma reported to account for 10–15% of childhood cancers [18] and 2% of childhood deaths from malignancies in autopsy studies in some countries in sub-Saharan Africa (SSA) [19]. The incidence of retinoblastoma is not distributed equally around the world. It varies with the level of socio-economic development, higher in low settings such as Africa, Mexico, Brazil and Asia. The average age-adjusted incidence rate of retinoblastoma in the United States and Europe is 2–5/106 children. However, it appears to be higher (6–10/106 children) in Africa, India and among children of Native American descent in the North American continent [20]. This difference is suggested in rare studies, but there are limitations to its interpretation. A recent global survey on retinoblastoma suggests that the incidence in LMICs may be hard to calculate due to incomplete data, where completeness of data decreased going from high-income countries (HICs), upper-middle-income countries, lower-middle-income countries to lower-income countries [21].

B. V. Chawla, M. E. Aronow (eds.), *Global Perspectives in Ocular Oncology*, https://doi.org/10.1007/978-3-031-08250-4_37

It is unknown if environmental or biological factors could influence the incidence of retinoblastoma. Few studies have suggested that in industrialized countries, an increased incidence of retinoblastoma was associated with poverty and low levels of maternal education [22, 23]. Despite more than 90% of affected patients living in resource-poor countries, there are few studies on disease characteristics in these populations [11].

2.2 Clinical Presentation, Risk Factors for Late Disease Presentation and Poor Patient Outcome

Recent work done globally on retinoblastoma has reemphasized the association of low national economic levels with late disease presentation, Africa being part of countries with poor disease stage at presentation [21, 24].

In Africa, over 70% of children present with unilateral retinoblastoma, a proportion relatively higher than that observed in developed countries [25, 26]. The apparent high prevalence of unilateral disease in African population compared to developed countries could be due to lapses in making diagnosis in the second eye of a bilateral disease leading to misclassification. These include challenges in performing examination under anaesthesia, lack of equipment such as indirect ophthalmoscopes and complementary lenses to examine the peripheral retina as well as some patients who may be lost to follow-up before the diagnosis can be made [9].

The median age at diagnosis in several sub-Saharan African countries has been found to be relatively high (30–36 months) compared to that reported for developed countries like the United States which is 18 months [25–31] (Table 1). In Canada, the mean age at diagnosis is 27 months (SD 18) for unilateral retinoblastoma and bilateral cases present earlier: 15 months for bilateral disease in Canada (Gallie BL, unpublished) and 25 months (16·8) for bilateral disease in Kenya [30]. Bilateral disease largely signifies heritable or germline type of retinoblastoma [1] with implication on management and transmission. A delay of more than 6 months from the first clinical sign to diagnosis is associated with 70% mortality in developing countries [30]. It is therefore important to report age at diagnosis separately for unilateral and bilateral cases. As indicated earlier, in SSA, there could be overestimation of the prevalence of unilateral retinoblastoma with under-representation of bilateral cases due to challenges with diagnosis.

The commonest presentation of retinoblastoma is leukocoria as occurs worldwide (Fig. 1) [8, 28, 31]. However, in SSA, this tends to be associated with signs of severe intraocular disease characterized by hyphaema, pseudohypopyon, buphthalmia and glaucoma, among others (Fig. 2) [8, 26, 29] as well as late disease stage both clinically and histopathologically characterized by orbital and optic nerve extensions (Fig. 3) [8, 24, 28, 31, 32].

Various factors have been found to be contributory to late disease presentation in Africa. These factors include lack of knowledge or awareness of the disease and its outcome as well as failure to recognize danger signs [33, 34], preference to seek alternate medicine in the form of spiritual and/or herbal treatment first, difficulty in accessing referral centres and financial constraints [25–27, 35].

Unfortunately, higher mean age at presentation is associated with more advanced disease and poorer prognosis [1, 8, 26, 27, 30, 32]. Higher occurrence of poorly differentiated tumours and presence of other histopathological high-risk features (HHRF) for metastasis are also associated with poor prognosis [36, 37]. Additional factors identified as risk factors for presentation with advanced disease include lower national income level, African residence and older age [24, 33].

Table 1 Age and laterality at presentation of retinoblastoma in sub-Saharan Africa

Author	Country	% Unilateral	Median age at presentation	Median age at presentation unilateral	Median age at presentation bilateral
Lukamba et al. [25]	Cote d'Ivoire, DR Congo	84%	NA	36 months	24 months
Essuman et al. [28]	Ghana	82.6%	36 months	NA	NA
Fousseyni Traoré et al. [29]	Mali	57% (early stage RB)	36 months	NA	12 months
Lukasa et al. [9]	DR Congo	77.5%	NA	32 months	28 months
Nwosu et al. [26]	Nigeria	77.4%	28 months	NA	NA
Nyamori et al. [30]	Kenya	NA	NA	36 months	25 months
Kruger et al. [25]	South Africa	78% (1993–2000) 67% (2001–2008)	32 months (1993–2000) 26 months (2001–2008)	35 months	NA

NA not available

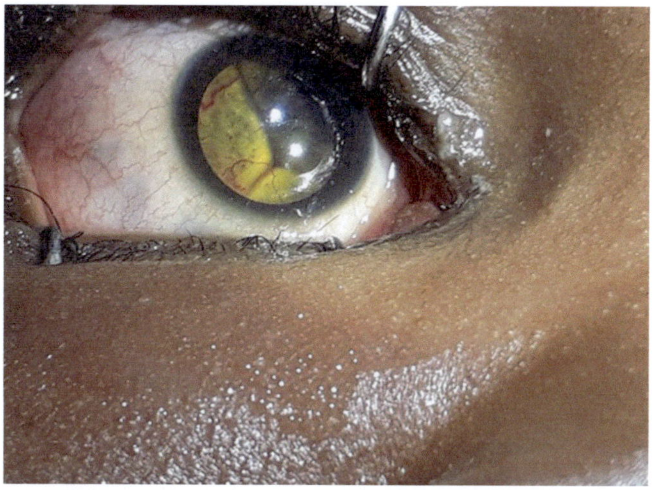

Fig. 1 The right eye of a 2-year-old child showing leukocoria

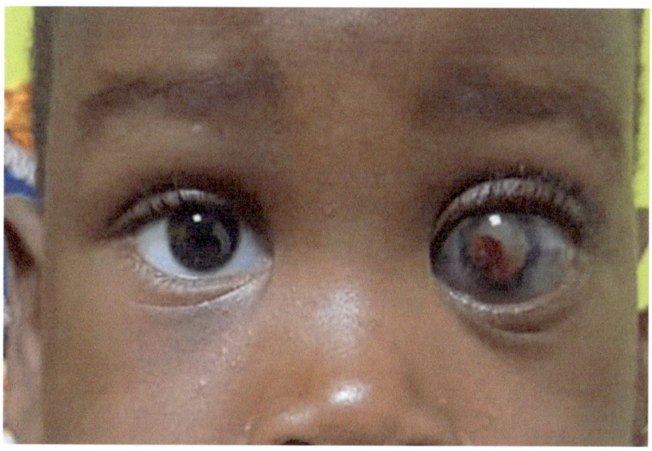

Fig. 2 Photo of 18 months old with left retinoblastoma showing buphthalmos, megalocornea, hyphaema and leukocoria

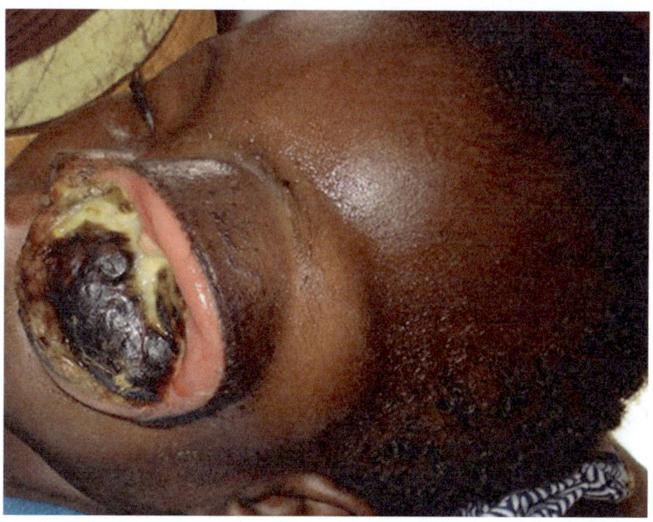

Fig. 3 A 3-year-old with left orbital retinoblastoma showing proptosis with a fungating mass

Abandonment and refusal of treatment are recognized factors associated with late disease presentation and poor patient outcomes in SSA [10, 26, 35, 38].

3 Retinoblastoma Treatment in Africa

Generally, there has been a lot of progress in the treatment of retinoblastoma in the past century worldwide. With the first enucleation done in the late 1800s in the United States [39], other forms of treatment came on the scene with progressive improvement in technique and outcome: chemotherapy in 1953 by Carl Kupfer [40], photocoagulation with the xenon arc in 1959 [41] and introduction of cryotherapy in the 1960s by Harvey Lincoff et al. for retinoblastoma [42].

Currently, new forms of treatment including chemotherapy (systemic, periocular, intravitreal, intra-arterial, chemoplaques), brachytherapy, etc. have been added over the decades. These strides have been realized in the developed countries which, together with early detection tools and measures, have improved on survival from about 30% in 1930s to almost 100% in recent times [6].

Unfortunately, in the African setting, not much has changed over the past decades. There has been very slow progress in these treatment advancements, hence not keeping up with the pace seen in developed countries. A recent international, multicentre, registry-based analysis of RB management revealed that lower national income levels (as seen in Africa) were associated with significantly higher rates of metastasis-related mortality, local treatment failure and lower globe salvage [24].

Enucleation, and occasionally exenteration, has been the first line of treatment, sometimes with systemic chemotherapy and external beam radiation, because of advanced disease. The introduction of systemic chemotherapy in the 1990s and 2000s on the African scene has helped with the treatment of advanced disease but to a limited extent due to other factors contributing to the occurrence of advanced disease. Kodinliye, in the 1960s, advocated for the provision of cobalt-60 external beam radiation facilities, but the ocular morbidity and mortality attributable to RB did not decline despite its availability in the West African region [43, 44].

Currently, a number of retinoblastoma treatment centres have resources for diagnosis, systemic chemotherapy, surgery (enucleation), radiotherapy (external beam radiation) and focal treatment (laser and cryotherapy) [45]. Brachytherapy is available only in Cape Town, South Africa; high-dose chemotherapy with autologous stem cell transplant is available in Egypt; and intra-arterial chemotherapy, IAC, is available in University of Alexandria Main Hospital, Egypt [45], and recently in Ghana [46] and Kenya [12 March 2021, Personal Communication with Dr. Kahaki Kimani]. These relatively newer treatment modalities in the African setting, i.e. brachytherapy, IAC and stem cell transplants, may be limited in use due to the high cost associated with their use as well as the late stage of disease presentation. These may be reserved for treatment of second eyes in patients with bilateral disease with moderate stage disease with good visual potential.

4 Cost of Treatment of Retinoblastoma

The cost of treatment continues to be a limiting factor to access of care with the sequelae of poor outcome in survival [25–27]. Countries with National Health Insurance Schemes (NHIS) provide some relief to affected patients, but this is not adequate, since in some countries such as Ghana, the NHIS does not cover the cost of diagnostic imaging, chemotherapy and in some settings, even enucleation. The cost of treatment then becomes an important determinant of advanced disease presentation and poor patient outcome.

5 National Retinoblastoma Strategies and Twinning Programme

National retinoblastoma strategies have been shown to be effective in developing agreed-upon evidence-based clinical guidelines, training medical personnel, attracting resources for healthcare delivery improvements and raising public awareness of early signs of disease. The multipronged strategy can result in early detection of the disease and improved patient management, allowing gains in survival and reduction in morbidity, in both developed and developing countries [47–49]. A collaboration between the University of Nairobi/Kenyatta National Hospital (Kenya) and the Hospital for Sick Children/University of Toronto (Canada) led to the establishment of the Kenyan National Retinoblastoma Strategy (KNRbS), the first of its kind in Africa. This strategy has seen improvement in early detection and the medical care of children with retinoblastoma, better stage of disease at presentation with improvement in patient survival [48]. Ethiopia [started in 2017] and Ghana [started 2018] are in the process of establishing national retinoblastoma strategies in collaboration with Emory University, Atlanta [for Ethiopia], and University of Toronto [for Ghana]. These strategies are taking inspirations from the KNRbS and hopefully should impact positively on patient outcomes in these countries.

Twinning programmes are collaborations aimed at capacity building at a single institution in a developing country, usually through support from a partnering institution in a developed country. Such collaborations have been documented between well-established centres in the Northern Hemisphere and paediatric oncology centres in Africa, e.g. Korle Bu Teaching Hospital (KBTH) and St Jude Hospital in the United States on one hand and World Child Cancer Twinning Programme between the Royal Hospital for Sick Children, Edinburgh and KBTH. These programmes have led to improvement in childhood cancer management generally with retinoblastoma benefitting from the systemic chemotherapy and pathology services.

6 Research on Retinoblastoma in Africa

A look at published literature reveals that whereas retinoblastoma research in developed countries consists of many studies covering the basic sciences, molecular genetics or evaluation of therapeutic interventions to salvage eyes and vision, studies in Africa are mainly clinical observational studies. There is paucity of cohort studies or clinical trials on retinoblastoma in Africa [1, 37]. The rare African studies utilizing basic science or clinical trial methods were usually completed in collaboration with colleagues from well-resourced countries, who provided funding and technical expertise. This may signal lack of capacity or funding for such studies on the part of researchers in Africa [50, 51]. While international collaboration is helpful to get such studies off the ground in the short term, in the long term, reliance on international partners may inadvertently stifle African-led science and innovation. For Africa to see significant improvement in patient outcomes from retinoblastoma, investment in research capacity building is necessary to improve the breadth, scope and quality of African scholarship in retinoblastoma.

7 The Way Forward

Early Detection: Ensuring that parents recognize and seek prompt attention for the early signs of retinoblastoma is imperative to improving outcomes for retinoblastoma everywhere, including Africa. Efforts to increasing public awareness, as well as ensuring timely, evidence-based treatment, are available and accessible to all, which would dramatically improve retinoblastoma outcomes in Africa. In Honduras, where a retinoblastoma public education programme was employed, there was significant improvement in numbers presenting with late disease: a reduction from 73% of 59 diagnosed cases to 35% of 23 diagnosed cases of extraocular disease during the first eight previous years (July 1995–June 2003) and the post-campaign period (June 2003–January 2005), respectively [52].

Partnerships for Capacity Building: Establishment of national strategies which focus on early detection, improved medical care, psychosocial support and funding for care will be needed going forward. Twinning programmes between African centres and well-established centres in the developed countries aiming at capacity building for medical care and collaborative research will be needed; the latter focussed on clinical trials for therapeutic interventions for advanced disease, basic science and genetic studies as well as quality of life studies to improve on patient outcomes.

Funding: International partnerships could help navigate funding barriers faced by African partners. However, efforts to look at how retinoblastoma is covered by national health insurance schemes could go a long way to ensure sustainability of retinoblastoma care.

Research and Learning Health Systems: This should aim to improve on technical expertise in medical care, capacity building for research and exchange of knowledge to provide answers for retinoblastoma challenges [53] in the African context, including unique sociocultural influencers and barriers to retinoblastoma care and optimal outcomes. Given the high retinoblastoma mortality in Africa, efforts should be directed to identify the actual magnitude of the problem through robust research which is crucial to improve the quality of the provided healthcare services [54]. Health service research could provide insight into access, utilization and quality of service in LMICs [55].

National Retinoblastoma Control Registries: Development of up-to-date retinoblastoma control registries is also one of the key steps to meet the challenge of the detrimental outcome of retinoblastoma [2]. These registries could provide a realistic estimation of the magnitude of the problem and help better allocation of the available resources [53]. Global development partners could provide the expertise and fund needed to develop these data registries and health surveys and train a new generation of national scientists to achieve the goal of providing optimum care to cancer patients [54].

8 Conclusion

Africa has seen some improvement in the management of retinoblastoma but still has the challenge of late disease presentation with poor patient outcome due to problems with access to care, affordability and lack of resources for care, among others. African leadership for retinoblastoma and local expertise has grown, access to novel therapies has improved and with tailored global support and collaboration where deemed necessary, there is great potential to improve retinoblastoma survival in Africa.

References

1. Dimaras H, Corson TW, Cobrinik D, et al. Retinoblastoma. Nat Rev Dis Primers. 2015;1:15021.
2. Kivela T. The epidemiological challenge of the most frequent eye cancer: retinoblastoma, an issue of birth and death. Br J Ophthalmol. 2009;93:1129–31.
3. Fabian ID, Rosser E, Sagoo MS. Epidemiological and genetic considerations in retinoblastoma. Community Eye Heal J. 2018;31(101):29–30.
4. Magrath I, Steliarova Foucher E, Epelman S, Ribeiro RC, Harif M, Li CK, et al. Paediatric cancer in low-income and middle-income countries. Lancet Oncol. 2013;14(3):e104–16.
5. Chantada GL, Qaddoumi I, Canturk S, et al. Strategies to manage retinoblastoma in developing countries. Pediatr Blood Cancer. 2011;56:341–8.
6. Houston SK, Murray TG, Wolfe SQ, Fernandes CE. Current update on retinoblastoma. Int Ophthalmol Clin. 2011;51:77–91.
7. Dimaras H, White A, Gallie B. The Kenyan National Retinoblastoma Strategy: building local capacity in the diagnosis and management of pediatric eye cancer in Kenya. Ophthalmol Rounds. 2008;6:1–6.
8. Kaimbo WK, Mvitu MM, Missotten L. Presenting signs of retinoblastoma in Congolese patients. Bull Soc Belge Ophtalmol. 2002;283:37–41.
9. Kazadi Lukusa A, Aloni MN, Kadima-Tshimanga B, Mvitu-Muaka M, Gini Ehungu JL, Ngiyulu R, Ekulu Mfutu P, Budiongo Nzazi A. Retinoblastoma in the Democratic Republic of Congo: 20-year review from a tertiary hospital in Kinshasa. J Cancer Epidemiol. 2012;2012:920468.
10. Bekibele CO, Ayede AI, Asaolu OO, Brown BJ. Retinoblastoma: the challenges of management in Ibadan, Nigeria. J Pediatr Hematol Oncol. 2009;31:552–5.
11. Canturk S, Qaddoumi I, Khetan V, Ma Z, Furmanchuk A, Antoneli CB, Sultan I, Kebudi R, Sharma T, Rodríguez-Galindo C, Abramson DH, Chantada GL. Survival of retinoblastoma in less-developed countries impact of socioeconomic and health-related indicators. Br J Ophthalmol. 2010;94:1432–6.
12. Schefler AC, Abramson DH. Retinoblastoma: what is new in 2007–2008. Curr Opin Ophthalmol. 2008;19:526–34.
13. Pendergrass TW, Davis S. Incidence of retinoblastoma in the United States. Arch Ophthalmol. 1980;98:1204–10.
14. Moll AC, Kuik DJ, Bouter LM, et al. Incidence and survival of retinoblastoma in The Netherlands: a register based study 1862-1995. Br J Ophthalmol. 1997;81:559–62.
15. MacCarthy A, Birch JM, Draper GJ, et al. Retinoblastoma in Great Britain 1963-2002. Br J Ophthalmol. 2009;93:33–7.
16. Shields CL, Meadows AT, Leahey AM, Shields JA. Continuing challenges in the management of retinoblastoma with chemotherapy. Retina. 2004;24(6):849–62.
17. Shields CL, Shields JA. Basic understanding of current classification and management of retinoblastoma. Curr Opin Ophthalmol. 2006;17:228–34.
18. Yeole BB, Advani S. Retinoblastoma: an epidemiological appraisal with reference to a population in Mumbai, India. Asian Pac J Cancer Prev. 2002;3:17–21.
19. Gyasi R, Tettey Y. Childhood deaths from malignant neoplasms in Accra. Ghana Med J. 2007;41(2):78–81.
20. Stiller C, Parkin D. Geographic and ethnic variations in the incidence of childhood cancer. Br Med Bull. 1996;52:682–703.
21. Global Retinoblastoma Study Group, Fabian ID, Abdallah E, Abdullahi SU, Abdulqader RA, Adamou Boubacar S, Ademola-Popoola DS, et al. Global retinoblastoma presentation and analysis by national income level. JAMA Oncol. 2020;6(5):685–95. https://doi.org/10.1001/jamaoncol.2019.6716.
22. de Camargo B, de Oliveira Ferreira J, de Souza Reis R, Ferman S, de Oliveira Santos M, Pombo-de-Oliveira M. Socioeconomic status and the incidence of non-central nervous system childhood embryonic tumours in Brazil. BMC Cancer. 2011;11:160.
23. Fajardo-Gutierrez A, Juarez-Ocana S, Gonzalez-Miranda G, et al. Incidence of cancer in children residing in ten jurisdictions of the Mexican Republic: importance of the Cancer registry (a population-based study). BMC Cancer. 2007;7:68.

24. Tomar AS, Finger PT, Gallie B, Kivelä TT, Mallipatna A, Zhang C, Zhao J, Wilson MW, Brenna RC, Burges M, Kim J, Khetan V, Ganesan S, Yarovoy A, Yarovaya V, Kotova E, Yousef YA, Nummi K, Ushakova TL, Yugay OV, Polyakov VG, Ramirez-Ortiz MA, Esparza-Aguiar E, Chantada G, Schaiquevich P, Fandino A, Yam JC, Lau WW, Lam CP, Sharwood P, Moorthy S, Long QB, Essuman VA, Renner LA, Semenova E, Català J, Correa-Llano G, Carreras E, for the American Joint Committee on Cancer Ophthalmic Oncology Task Force. Global retinoblastoma treatment outcomes: association with national income level. Ophthalmology. 2020;128(5):740–53. https://doi.org/10.1016/j.ophtha.2020.09.032.
25. Lukamba RM, Yao JA, Kabesha TA, Budiongo AN, Monga BB, Mwembo AT, Bey P, Chenge GB, Desjardins L, Luboya ON, Doz F, Stefan CD. Retinoblastoma in Sub-Saharan Africa: case studies of the Republic of Côte d'Ivoire and the Democratic Republic of the Congo. J Glob Oncol. 2018;4:1–8.
26. Nwosu SN, Okpala N, Nnubia C, Akudinobi C. Retinoblastoma in Onitsha, Nigeria. Niger J Ophthalmol. 2019;27(1):8.
27. Kruger M, Reynders D, Omar F, Schoeman J, Wedi O, Harvey J. Retinoblastoma outcome at a single institution in South Africa. South African Med J. 2014;104(12):859–63.
28. Essuman V, Ntim-Amponsah C, Akafo S, Renner L, Edusei L. Presentation of retinoblastoma at a paediatric eye clinic in Ghana. Ghana Med J. 2010;44(1):10–5.
29. Traoré F, Sylla F, Togo B, Kamaté B, Diabaté K, Diakité AA, et al. Treatment of retinoblastoma in Sub-Saharan Africa: experience of the paediatric oncology unit at Gabriel Toure Teaching Hospital and the Institute of African Tropical Ophthalmology, Bamako. Mali Pediatr Blood Cancer. 2018;65(8):1–7.
30. Nyamori JM, Kimani K, Njuguna MW, Dimaras H. The incidence and distribution of retinoblastoma in Kenya. Br J Ophthalmol. 2012;96(1):141–3. http://bjo.bmj.com/content/96/1/141
31. Klauss V, Chana HS. Ocular tumors in Africa. Soc Sci Med. 1983;17:1743–50.
32. Akang EE, Ajaiyeoba IA, Campbell OB, Olurin IO, Aghadiuno PU. Retinoblastomas in Ibadan Nigeria: II—Clinicopathologic features. West Afr J Med. 2000;19(1):6–11.
33. Fabian ID, Stacey AW, Foster A, et al. Travel burden and clinical presentation of retinoblastoma: analysis of 1024 patients from 43 African countries and 518 patients from 40 European countries. Br J Ophthalmol. 2021;105(10):1435–43. https://doi.org/10.1136/bjophthalmol-2020-316613.
34. Essuman VA, Braimah IZ, Ndanu TA, Ntim-Amponsah CT. Presentation of children with advanced retinoblastoma for treatment in Ghana—the Caretakers' perspective. West Afr J Med. 2018;35(1):9–14.
35. Essuman VA, Braimah IZ, Essuman A, Abaidoo B, Ndanu TA, Ntim-Amponsah CT. Challenges in the management of retinoblastoma at peripheral eye clinics in Ghana. Postgrad Med J Ghana. 2019;8(1):54–61.
36. Mukhtar AU, Kagame K. Pathological study of retinoblastoma in. Mbarara, Uganda. Cent Afr J Med. 2000;46:13–6.
37. Owoeye JF, Afolayan EA, Ademola-Popoola DS. Retinoblastoma—a clinico-pathological study in Ilorin, Nigeria. Afr J Health Sci. 2006;13:117–23.
38. Boubacar T, Fatou S, Fousseyni T, Mariam S, Fatoumata DT, Toumani S, Abdoul-Aziz D, Marouf KM. A 30-month prospective study on the treatment of retinoblastoma in the Gabriel Toure Teaching Hospital, Bamako, Mali. Br J Ophthalmol. 2010;94(4):467–9. https://doi.org/10.1136/bjo.2009.159699. Epub 2009 Oct 12.
39. Abramson DH. Retinoblastoma in the 20th century: past success and future challenges the Weisenfeld lecture. Invest Ophthalmol Vis Sci. 2005;46(8):2683–91.
40. Kupfer C. Retinoblastoma treated with intravenous nitrogen mustard. Am J Ophthalmol. 1953;36:1721–172.
41. Meyer-Schwickerath G. Lichtkoagulation. Graefes. Arch Ophthalmol. 1954;156(2–34):10.
42. Lincoff H, McLean J, Long R. The cryosurgical treatment of intraocular tumors. Am J Ophthalmol. 1967;63:389–99.
43. Kodilinye HC. Retinoblastoma in Nigeria: problems of treatment. Am J Ophthalmol. 1967;63:469–81.
44. Ademola-Popoola DS, Opocher E, Reddy MA. Contemporary management of retinoblastoma in the context of a low-resource country. Niger Postgrad Med J. 2019;26:69–79.
45. One Retinoblastoma World Map. www.1rbw.org.
46. https://www.graphic.com.gh/news/general-news/intra-arterial-chemotherapy-used-to-treat-eye-cancer-in-children.html. Accessed April 2020.
47. Canadian Retinoblastoma Society. National Retinoblastoma Strategy Canadian guidelines for Care: Stratégie thérapeutique du rétinoblastome guide clinique canadien. Can J Ophthalmol. 2009;44(Suppl 2):S1–88. https://doi.org/10.3129/i09-194.
48. Hill JA, Kimani K, White A, Barasa F, Livingstone M, Gallie BL, Dimaras H, Daisy's Eye Cancer Fund & The Kenyan National Retinoblastoma Strategy Group. Achieving optimal cancer outcomes in East Africa through multidisciplinary partnership: a case study of the Kenyan National Retinoblastoma Strategy group. Glob Health. 2016;12(1):23. https://doi.org/10.1186/s12992-016-0160-1.
49. Kenyan National Retinoblastoma Strategy Group. Retinoblastoma best practice guidelines. 2014.
50. Alfaar AS, Nour R, Bakry MS, et al. A change roadmap towards research paradigm in low-resource countries: retinoblastoma model in Egypt. Int Ophthalmol. 2017;37(1):111–8. https://doi.org/10.1007/s10792-016-0233-4.
51. Elahi A. Challenges of data collection in developing countries—the Pakistani experience as a way forward. Stat J IAOS. 2008;25(1–2):11–7.
52. Leander C, Fu LC, Peña A, Howard SC, Rodriguez-Galindo C, Wilimas JA, Ribeiro RC, Haik B. Impact of an education program on late diagnosis of retinoblastoma in Honduras. Pediatr Blood Cancer. 2007;49(6):817–9.
53. Chantada GL. Retinoblastoma: lessons and challenges from developing countries. Ellsworth Lecture 2011. Ophthalmic Genet. 2011;32(4):196–203. https://doi.org/10.3109/13816810.2011.592173.
54. Kruk ME, Gage AD, Arsenault C, et al. High-quality health systems in the Sustainable Development Goals era: time for a revolution. Lancet Glob Health. 2018;6(11):e1196–252. https://doi.org/10.1016/S2214-109X(18)30386-3.
55. Hanna TP, Kangolle AC. Cancer control in developing countries: using health data and health services research to measure and improve access, quality and efficiency. BMC Int Health Hum Rights. 2010;10:24. https://doi.org/10.1186/1472-698X-10-24.

The Brazilian Experience: The Retinoblastoma Awareness Campaign

Sidnei Epelman

1 Introduction

Childhood cancer often receives little attention in the less developed societies because other problems, such as infection, poor hygiene, and malnutrition, are given higher priority. As these problems are gradually controlled, pediatric cancer becomes an important cause of mortality, and many less developed countries have started programs to address this problem. Pediatric cancer in low-income countries has unique problems that influence the care and outcome of children with the disease.

Retinoblastoma is a rare, unique, and most common cancer that forms in the eyes of children, often before they are born. It is a complicated disease triggered by genetic mutations in one or more cells in the retina. Usually, it affects 1 in 14.000 live births to 1 in 34.000, with around 400 children newly diagnosed each year in Brazil [1, 2]. Interestingly, it is an uncommon cancer in the high-income countries accounting for only 3% of all childhood cancer; in opposite, it is one of the more common malignancies in countries with limited resources [3]. Population-based reports show a higher incidence in some countries like Brazil, which can be as high as three to seven times that of Western Europe [2]. Investigations studying causes of increased prevalence in certain populations include the presence of human papillomavirus in the tumor since HPV infection is more prevalent in the developing countries. But that was not well demonstrated and is probably not seen in particular in nonfamilial cases [2].

It was estimated to be responsible for 17% of all neonatal cancers [4]. Approximately 20–30% of patients have bilateral disease, with the presence of germline mutations of the RB1 gene [1]. It may occur sporadically or may be genetic. The genetic form of retinoblastoma can be diagnosed in 40% of cases, but the majority of these are new germline mutations than true hereditary cases. Among the nonhereditary cases, comprising of 60% of the patients, 90% are unilateral or unifocal. It is important to emphasize that patients with bilateral disease tend to present at a younger age than those with unilateral disease with better visual potential in the eye with the smaller tumor size [4].

According to literature data, the most common reason that concerned the family was the presence of leukocoria, often observed on flash photographs.

2 Early Diagnosis

Most cancers present at an advanced stage in developing countries when cure is improbable even with best treatments. A major element in improved survival rates in many cancers in the United States and Europe has been shown to be the much earlier stage of disease at diagnosis brought about by public education and in some cases screening for premalignant lesions or early cancer.

In most countries with limited resources, primary healthcare workers are rarely provided with sufficient education about the early signs of cancer or where to refer suspected cases. This could readily be remedied by short training courses (ideally, coupled to continuing education programs), brochures, or posters and establishing links between those who deliver primary health care and referral centers [5].

Early detection refers to the diagnosis of a cancer at a point in its evolution when it remains localized and small in size and has a high chance of being cured, often by a simple surgical approach. The two approaches to early detection are education and screening. The term "downstaging," although meaning different things to different people, refers to improving the stage distribution of diagnosed cases (i.e., increasing the proportion of early stage cancers) by any of a variety of means. One is to raise awareness about the early signs and

S. Epelman (✉)
Pediatric Oncology Department, Santa Marcelina Hospital, São Paulo, Brazil

TUCCA - Associação para Crianças e Adolescentes com Câncer, Santa Marcelina Hospital, São Paulo, Brazil
e-mail: epelman@inctrbrasil.org

B. V. Chawla, M. E. Aronow (eds.), *Global Perspectives in Ocular Oncology*, https://doi.org/10.1007/978-3-031-08250-4_38

symptoms of cancer in the population at risk as well as among primary care doctors, nurses, and paramedical personnel [6].

Early detection, of course, can only be successful when linked to effective treatment. It is unethical to initiate an early detection program in the absence of adequate treatment facilities.

The methodology of early detection as follows:

1. Develop a strategic plan at the national level.
2. Educate the primary care health professionals.
3. Education of target populations:
   (a) Education by first-line clinician and health staff through community outreach program
   (b) Education through media campaign
      - Expected result: groups at risk aware of early signs and symptoms and empowered to take care of their health
4. Improve patient navigation of the health system, with more rapid diagnosis and treatment.

Early diagnosis of cancer is also a mandatory goal in oncology; it affords the opportunity of treatment with curative intent while disease burden is still in earliest stages. Nowadays, early detection and immediate referral of patients with retinoblastoma increases the possibility of saving lives and eyes with useful vision. The consequences are improvement of prognosis and cure attained with minimal late effects.

Access to quality health care has become an increasingly important public health concern. Of importance are the factors that influence the delays to propose an adequate strategy to solve those issues. Unfortunately, physician delays were longer than those related to parents' or patients' recognition of underlying disease. Therefore, an awareness campaign for early diagnosis of retinoblastoma is very important and useful [6, 7].

High cure rates require access to medical care, referral to a treatment center, and completion of the therapy necessary. Cure rates in low-income countries are in general at least 20–30% lower than those in high-income countries. In 50% of the cases worldwide, there were extraocular signs and symptoms, which were associated with poorer survival rate (0–50% vs. 95%), a reality that is possible to change.

Four stages of diagnosis and treatment were reported as the time between development of symptoms, initial health-care contact, referral to the treating oncologist, and initiation of treatment. They are not solved only with a campaign alone and other strategies should be incorporated to treat the patients as soon as possible [7].

Literature shows that access to care is a multifactorial problem encountered by those with cancer in low- and middle-income countries. Causes such as poverty, illiteracy, lack of investment in public health, discontinuation of treatment, long distances from major centers, and very few comprehensive cancer centers all contribute to delays in diagnosis and treatment. In addition, even for those who reach adequate medical centers, the disease may be too advanced resulting in an overall worse prognosis or no clinical condition to deliver the appropriate cancer care [7, 8].

Lack of cancer registries in many countries or registries that only cover or represent some areas often do not reflect the true incidence of diseases such as retinoblastoma, particularly for those living in rural or remote areas [7]. Also, as a consequence, the analysis of any intervention is very difficult to achieve reliable results [9].

It is also important to emphasize that unfortunately screening, a strategy to identify disease in an asymptomatic population, was still not well demonstrated to show the efficacy of a retinoblastoma screening program. There is also no test capable of detecting disease in the preclinical phase. Currently, the red reflex test is the main screening tool used by primary care physicians for the detection of retinoblastoma. The proper performance of the red reflex test is mandatory in many countries and can detect cases of retinoblastoma [10]. Leukocoria is the most common initial sign of retinoblastoma and is first apparent when the tumor is still contained within the eye. It reflects light and remains intraocular and curable for 3–6 months after the first sign of leukocoria. It is first noticed by parents when the pupils of the child's eyes dilate naturally in dim light, with a beam of light shining over the parents' shoulder. In a UK study, 25% of children with leukocoria waited more than 4 weeks for primary care referral to an ophthalmologist. Flash photography can enable early detection of leukocoria. Anecdotal evidence suggests that parents who notice this photoleukocoria now commonly search the Internet and promptly seek medical attention [11].

3 Campaign for Early Diagnosis and Educational Actions

Awareness campaigns to educate the public on the signs and symptoms of retinoblastoma are likely to increase the rates of early diagnosis and a higher chance of cure and better vision potential for affected eyes. In low-income countries where advanced disease is seen in the majority of cases of retinoblastoma, such awareness campaign becomes more relevant. Increased awareness, improved patient education, and easy and quick referral for ocular complaints suggestive of leukocoria may lead to more children with access to eye-sparing treatment modalities. Therefore, to increase the number of saving eyes, it is mandatory to decrease the delay in diagnosis, a reality already documented in most developing countries [11, 12].

Parents, rather than health-care professionals, are usually the first to notice the initial ocular signs of an ocular tumor. The initial presenting sign in the majority of cases was detected by a family member or even a friend. Therefore, the most effective instrument to increase early detection is focusing education to laypeople since the time frame for observation is much greater for parents. Educating people on the signs and symptoms could also empower parents to influence a hesitant professional to refer to a specialist, a picture that occurs not rarely. Public education about leukocoria and retinoblastoma is crucial since it is an easy sign for laypeople but does not correlate with very early stage. Primary care physicians play a major role in the detection of retinoblastoma.

Another central information to analyze is the causes of delay in diagnosis. It can be divided into poor health services, lack of awareness, and socioeconomic difficulties. A study questionnaire was developed by the International Network for Cancer and Treatment Research (www.inctr.org), an organization dedicated to cancer control in developing countries, to understand problems faced by parents of children with retinoblastoma prior to treatment in many countries with limited resources and the importance of identifying factors contributing to late diagnosis. The relevant conclusion was that there are regional differences related to the child's extent of disease at diagnosis. Families from rural areas or who were of lower socioeconomic status had children with more advanced disease at diagnosis as well as illiterate fathers [2]. Improving public awareness through culturally relevant campaigns should be developed particularly in countries where such initiatives don't exist and resources for treatment are scarce, including professional education for health-care professionals including ophthalmologists.

There is a very limited information looking at causes of delays in diagnosis and the presenting features in countries with limited resources and their correlation with stage and survival. All information may be useful for planning early diagnosis strategies. A paper attempted to look at causes of late diagnosis and found that the role of primary health-care professionals was crucial in this regard as described in the INCTR questionnaire. It was still surprising that 25% or more ophthalmologists missed the diagnosis. Even in the United States, more patients were initially detected by the family or a friend than by pediatricians or ophthalmologists. Most children whose retinoblastoma is diagnosed initially present with leukocoria detected by a parent, despite routine pediatric screening for leukocoria via the red reflex test. Therefore, the campaigns are important in all countries and not limited to low-income countries.

A relevant paper demonstrated the importance of retinoblastoma public awareness campaign in a high-income country such as the United Kingdom. Parents are attending emergency units more compared with the 1990s [11]. More eyes are being salvaged despite a similar number of children requiring adjuvant chemotherapy. High-risk Rb and Group E eyes do not correlate with increased lag time in the United Kingdom where the majority of patients presented within 6 months of signs. Similar findings have been found in virtually all pediatric cancers. Other determinants such as tumor biology may be more relevant. Even in Canada where the presentation of retinoblastoma occurs earlier than in developing countries, awareness campaigns are recommended by the government, which is an attempt to reduce the number of advanced Rb cases, and lead to even earlier detection, resulting in better visual outcome.

Other countries like Mexico developed a large public education campaign with posters in public places, schools, and health-care centers [2]. There also was demonstrated the need of a development of a national protocol and continuous educational program. In Honduras, an awareness campaign was also initiated to promote early detection. The information was disseminated to parents during annual vaccination campaigns in government health clinics. The number of patients presenting with extraocular disease decreased from 75% to 35% in 8 years [13]. The nationwide awareness campaign led by the Kenyan National Retinoblastoma Strategy group is educating the public and health-care workers about implications of leukocoria [14]. Effectiveness of campaigns will be validated when their incidence of early and late stages of disease at presentation is measured.

In Brazil, a national campaign for early diagnosis of retinoblastoma was initiated in 2002. At that time, a public service announcement highlighting leukocoria (cat's eye reflex) as a symptom of cancer was broadcast on several television stations throughout the country and offered a toll-free telephone number for more information. The video was translated to ten different languages and is still available free of charge. This first video is called attention to leukocoria on a flash photograph, observed as white reflection in the eye, instead of the usual red eye reflex. Many parents and relatives now notice the white reflex in family photographs and then seek medical attention. That initial campaign also included educational material provided to the population, primary health-care workers, and ophthalmologists and pediatricians as posters and flyers. We had the information of many cases diagnosed through the campaign, but the real number of those who benefited from the strategy is not available since the information or registry is not mandatory. Besides the diagnosis of retinoblastoma, other vision-threatening conditions that can lead to blindness are also detected through as congenital cataract, congenital glaucoma, Coats' disease, toxocariasis, and retinopathy of prematurity—for which prompt medical attention is needed. Therefore, it can be considered a campaign to fight blindness in the childhood and not only retinoblastoma. Other initiatives were developed throughout the periods, and new videos (tucca@tucca.org.br) and materials for the Internet, brochures, flyers, social media, television, radio, newspapers,

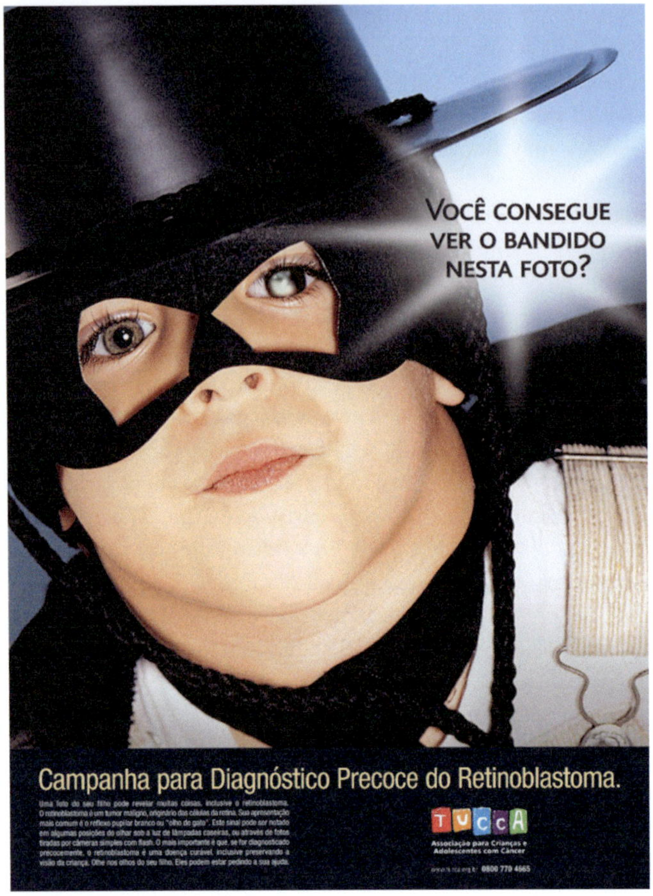
Você consegue ver o bandido nesta foto?
Campanha para Diagnóstico Precoce do Retinoblastoma.
Uma foto do seu filho pode revelar muitas coisas, inclusive o retinoblastoma. O retinoblastoma é um tumor maligno, originário das células da retina. Sua apresentação mais comum é o reflexo pupilar branco ou "olho de gato". Este sinal pode ser notado em algumas posições do olhar sob a luz de lâmpadas caseiras, ou através de fotos tiradas por câmeras simples com flash. O mais importante é que, se for diagnosticado precocemente, o retinoblastoma é uma doença curável, inclusive preservando a visão da criança. Olhe nos olhos do seu filho. Eles podem estar pedindo a sua ajuda.
TUCCA
Associação para Crianças e Adolescentes com Câncer
0800 770 4665

Fig. 1 RB campaign poster

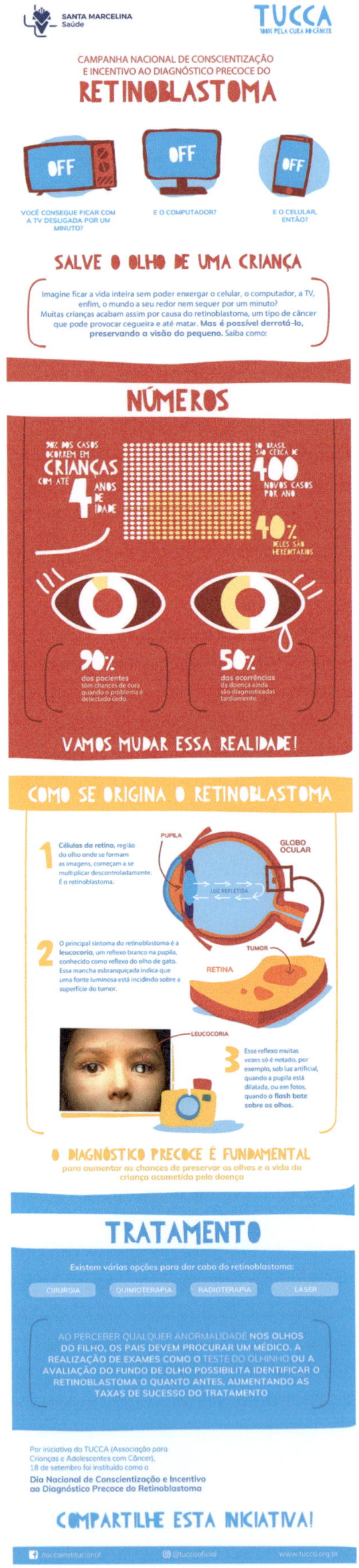

Fig. 2 National Retinoblastoma Awareness Day infographic

and mobile apps were used to deliver the main messages (Figs. 1, 2, 3, and 4) [9]. In 2012, a decree was signed by the president of the country when September 18 became the awareness day for the early diagnosis of retinoblastoma. Every year since that year, an agenda is organized with many actions to call attention to the day and the campaign. The symbol of Brazil, Corcovado in Rio de Janeiro, turns off the lights for certain period of time to show that darkness can be a consequence of late diagnosis in a child with retinoblastoma. Other monuments in many different cities also turn off the lights as part of the chain developed that particular day to call attention as well.

Actually, many parents use the Internet to research a white pupil, and arrive at their first physician visit with a great deal of good information on leukocoria and its common causes. That is an important instrument at our campaign. We developed a reliable site to ensure the information on retinoblastoma is current and accurate but also using keywords like white pupil or cat's eye reflex.

The results in a retrospective cohort including 262 patients with retinoblastoma treated between 2001 and 2018 from our pediatric oncology department at Santa Marcelina Hospital in Sao Paulo showed the following results that also demonstrated the importance of awareness campaign for such disease in low-middle income country. Extraocular dis-

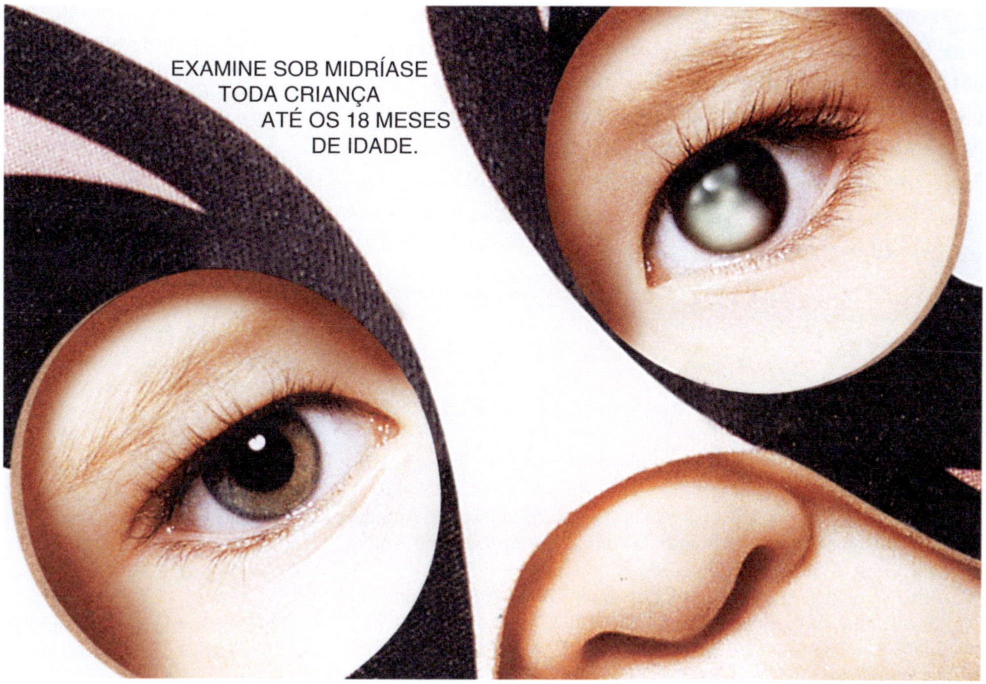
EXAMINE SOB MIDRÍASE
TODA CRIANÇA
ATÉ OS 18 MESES
DE IDADE.

Fig. 3 RB campaign information pamphlet for pediatricians

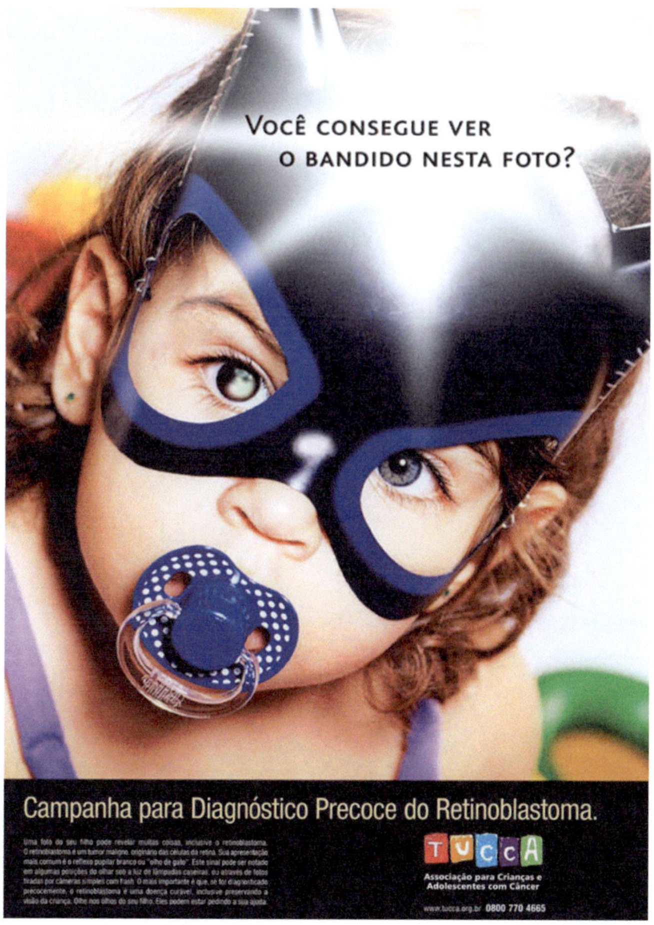
VOCÊ CONSEGUE VER
O BANDIDO NESTA FOTO?
Campanha para Diagnóstico Precoce do Retinoblastoma.
TUCCA
Associação para Crianças e Adolescentes com Câncer
www.tucca.org.br 0800 770 4665

Fig. 4 RB campaign poster

ease was significantly associated with older age at diagnosis ($p < 0.001$), non-white race ($p < 0.001$), family history of cancer ($p < 0.001$), and lag time greater than 2.5 months ($p < 0.001$). In the multivariate analysis, only age (>36 months, OR = 6.51, 95% CI), race (non-white, OR = 2.61, 95% CI), and lag time (>2.5 months, OR = 2.40, 95% CI 1.01–5.74) remained associated with extraocular disease. After 2012, we could observe a significant decrease in the number of patients with extraocular disease (2013–2018 = 9.7% × 2001–2012 = 20.6%) and also a reduction in the number of patients submitted to enucleation (2013–2018 = 38.9% × 2001–2012 = 69.1%). Although not statistically significant, a larger proportion of patients coming from North, Northeast, and Midwest regions was registered after the establishment of the Retinoblastoma Comprehensive Treatment Center in 2012 (2013–2018 = 46% × 2001–2012 = 31.9%). We have not observed a significant change in lag time over time ($p = 0.918$) [15].

4 Conclusion

In Brazil an increased awareness of retinoblastoma has contributed to more timely recognition of the disease, referral for specialized care, diagnosis, and treatment initiation at a comprehensive cancer center. This in turn holds the possibility of less advanced stage disease and lower disease- and treatment-related mortality.

Awareness campaigns to educate the public on the signs and symptoms of leukocoria have increased the rates of early detection of retinoblastoma, and the likelihood of parents taking their child to a specialist sooner. Awareness campaigns in developing countries, where the majority of Rb cases present as advanced disease, have met with some success. With those interventions, more children are cured, many with useful vision.

References

1. Ortiz MV, Dunkel IJ. Retinoblastoma. J Child Neurol. 2016;31(2):227–36.
2. Epelman S. Preserving vision in retinoblastoma through early detection and intervention. Curr Oncol Rep. 2012;14(2):213–9.
3. Galindo CR, Wilson MW, Chantada G, Fu L, Qaddoumi I, Antoneli C, Leal-Leal C, et al. Retinoblastoma: one world, one vision. Pediatrics. 2008;122(3):e763–70.
4. Toli A, Perente A, Labiris G. Evaluation of the red reflex: an overview for the pediatrician. World J Methodol. 2021;11(5):263–77.
5. Dang-Tan T, Franco EL. Diagnosis delays in childhood cancer: a review. Cancer. 2007;110(4):703–13.
6. Dang-Tan, Trottier H, Mery LS, Morrinson HI, Barr RD, et al. Delays in diagnosis and treatment among children and adolescents with cancer in Canada. Pediatr Blood Cancer. 2008;51:468–74.
7. Magrath I, Steliarova-Foucher E, Epelman S, Ribeiro RC, Harif M, Li CK, et al. Paediatric cancer in low-income and middle-income countries. Lancet Oncol. 2013;14(3):e104–16.
8. Tuong B, Green AD, Friedrich P, Ribeiro KB, Galindo CR. Ethnic, racial and socioeconomic disparities in retinoblastoma. JAMA Pediatr. 2015;169(12):1096–104.
9. Epelman S, Epelman C, Erwenne C, Melaragno R, Teixeira L, Adde M, et al. National Campaign for early diagnosis of retinoblastoma in Brazil. Proc ASCO. 2005;22:8561.
10. Vempuluru VS, Kaliki S. Screening of Retinoblastoma: a systematic review of current strategies. Asia Pac J Ophthalmol. 2021;10:192–9.
11. Posner M, Jaulim A, Vasalaki M, Rantell K, Sagoo MS, et al. Lag time for retinoblastoma in the UK revisited: a retrospective analysis. BMJ Open. 2017;7:e015625.
12. Bey P, Traore F, Sylla F, Chenge G, Ilunga J, et al. Retinoblastoma: an exemplary tumor in young children that can be cured in low-income countries. Cancer Control. 2014:111–4.
13. Leander C, Fu LC, Pena A, Howard SC, Rodriguez-Galindo C, Wilimas JA, et al. Impact of an education program on late diagnosis of retinoblastoma in Honduras. Pediatr Blood Cancer. 2007;49(6):817–9.
14. Gallie B. Canadian guidelines for retinoblastoma care. Can J Ophthalmol. 2009;44(6):639–42.
15. Epelman S. Facing the challenge: the successful establishment of a comprehensive retinoblastoma center in a country with limited resources. Personal communication; 2022.

Part VII

Reflections

Creating a Science Project: Advice from Personal Experience

Martine J. Jager

1 Introduction

There may be several reasons why you would like to create a science project. As a student, it may be an obligatory part of school/college, or you may perhaps want to work on your skills and increase your chances of a future residency or PhD position. As an academic employee, you may be expected to "engage in research." The best reason, in my opinion, would be more intrinsic: *you want to answer a scientific question*. Dr. Peter G. Watson became the major force in scleritis care after he had seen a scleritis case on the first day of his residency and his supervisor asked him what one should do to cure the patient. He wanted to know. For me, simple curiosity is the basis of my research. What is the reason we see what we see? If we understand what happens, we can do something about it. What makes the patient ill?

Research can be done at various levels, and the most exciting is a project where you accidentally get a Eureka moment. These are rare in one's career. I have known people who waited for this their whole life to start a project… It is better to plan projects to answer a question, and always keep an open eye for surprises. My PhD supervisor, Professor Jon van Rood, called such moments "serendipity"; he had an open eye for unusual situations and became one of the discoverers of the HLA (human leukocyte antigen) system [1].

At scientific conferences, people often ask me: "how do I start with research?" If there is already a question, one should look for practical solutions. Most often, this is not the case, and we start with exploring possibilities. The answer to a clinician is simple: collect data on the cases you see. Anything unusual may trigger your interest, and a proper review of data may lead to a published paper: you can describe one special case or a series of cases, or you may use your data as a starting point for a translational research or experimental project or for prospective treatment studies. I will use papers I am familiar with as examples and demonstrate what knowledge we achieved through the different approaches.

M. J. Jager (✉)
Department of Ophthalmology, Leiden University Medical Center (LUMC), Leiden, The Netherlands
e-mail: m.j.jager@lumc.nl

2 A Case

When you have a patient in front of you with a problem that you do not fully understand, it is worthwhile to check the literature. Finding a similar story may guide you to the right diagnosis and then to proper treatment. The value of case reports is that they are often specific and carry educational value. It is not so easy to publish a case, however, as journals often consider case reports of minor importance compared to larger series. There are specific journals that do publish case reports. A case should have a beginning (the problem) and an end: the outcome (for better or worse), and an educational message.

An example of an educational case is, for instance, "Development of ocular rosacea following combined ipilimumab and nivolumab treatment for metastatic malignant skin melanoma" [2]. When the reported patient was referred to Leiden, information on the side effects (immune-related adverse effects = irAEs) of the new treatment with immune checkpoint inhibitors was only just emerging. We were consulted regarding a 68-year-old gentleman who was undergoing treatment with anti-CTLA4 and anti-PD-1 monoclonal antibodies for metastases of a cutaneous melanoma. He had developed red eyelids and inflamed conjunctivae, with gritty eyes. When examined, it appeared as a severe bilateral case of rosacea, with dry eyes. We concluded that this had to be inflammatory, not infectious, and not caused by the melanoma itself; the patient was treated with corticosteroid drops, a steroidal/antimicrobial ointment for the eyelids, and eyelid scrubbing. This treatment resolved the inflammation. It showed us that immune checkpoint inhibitors would stimulate not only the patient's immune response against tumor antigens but also against the patient's own tissues. One may also conclude that rosacea as well as dry eyes is most likely

B. V. Chawla, M. E. Aronow (eds.), *Global Perspectives in Ocular Oncology*, https://doi.org/10.1007/978-3-031-08250-4_39

the effect of a local immune response against yet unknown antigens (reviewed by Hori et al. [3]).

3 A Diagnostic Series

Sometimes, a few cases present with a similar appearance and an association is made with a shared factor such as a specific drug. Drs. Van Dijk and Boon [4] were actively studying patients with central serous retinopathy when some patients with an atypical serous maculopathy were referred to the LUMC in Leiden. They had been treated for metastatic cutaneous melanoma with a MEK (mitogen-activated protein kinase kinase) inhibitor, pimasertib. This led to a collaborative prospective observational study between the clinics of Leiden and Rotterdam in The Netherlands [5]. Using optical coherence tomography, all eight cases in the study were found to have some degree of serous subretinal fluid and a preserved visual acuity. The paper gave a fine description of a newly-observed side effect. One patient developed symptoms, but this patient had a bilateral vein occlusion, which had previously been described as a complication of MEK inhibitors [6, 7].

Clinical observations are essential: not only when describing new side effects or a new disease entity, but also to describe a new technique. When you do something new, set up a system where you can evaluate your new approach. You can learn from your data: what goes wrong and what goes right, and others may learn from your good and bad results. This is true for drugs, but also for procedures (implantation of a new type of intraocular lens, modifying a corneal transplantation approach), as well as for imaging.

An example of a report on a new technique is, for instance, the analysis of retinal vessel oxygenation using retinal oximetry: vessel oximetry determines the level of oxygen in arteries and veins of the retina and can provide information about the difference between the incoming arteries and outgoing retinal veins. Dr. Brouwer ("Retinal oximetry is altered in eyes with choroidal melanoma but not in eyes with choroidal nevi," [8]) analyzed whether the presence of a choroidal nevus or melanoma influenced the level of oxygen in the retinal blood vessels. A total of 45 patients with a choroidal melanoma and 42 patients with a nevus were analyzed, and while arterial saturation was the same, oxygen saturation in veins of eyes with a choroidal melanoma was slightly lower than in the contralateral eye and compared to nevus-containing eyes. Brouwer's hypothesis for this finding is that the increased metabolism of the tumor consumes oxygen, and that the whole eye may show some level of inflammation, leading to a higher total oxygen consumption.

A clinical study like this one was possible by the availability of a new imaging device in combination with a specific patient population. It requires a lot of logistical preparation. Approval needs to be obtained from a (institutional) medical ethics committee, and patients need to provide informed consent. Clinicians seeing the reported patients need to be aware of the study to refer them for possible inclusion. Over time, however, this can lead to a beautiful dataset and a fine paper, providing new information.

4 Retrospective and Prospective Data Collection

When your clinic sees a lot of specific patients, you may wish to create a database describing all cases. My first analysis was based on the notebook of my cornea teacher, professor Dr. C.L. Dake, who had written down every cornea transplantation he ever performed. I went through the charts of all his patients and evaluated the patients' visual acuity [9]. I learned from this that the visual prognosis that clinicians often predicted was not achieved by most of the patients, which led me to be cautious when advising patients regarding their chances of visual rehabilitation through a full-thickness corneal transplant. It also led to my enthusiasm when I saw the first patient who had undergone a partial-thickness transplant (a posterior lamellar keratoplasty) by Dr. Gerrit Melles in Rotterdam (the Netherlands), as visual recovery was much faster and better than what I had observed with the standard full-thickness procedure [10–12].

In oncology, many of the well-known clinicians have developed extensive registries. Drs. Carol and Jerry Shields have published very many papers based on patients seen in their specialized clinic at the Wills Eye Hospital in Philadelphia (USA), but their analyses were made possible because of their well-planned and structured method for data collection. They use their database for descriptions of diseases, translational studies (e.g., genetics vs tumor characteristics), and prognostication [13–17]. Dr. Bertil Damato has similarly been able to develop the Liverpool Uveal Melanoma Prognosticator Online (LUMPO), an online prognostication tool which combines patient age, tumor size, and genetic information [18]. Dr. Tero Kivela has been able to collect data from different centers for the creation of categories for the American Joint Committee on Cancer (AJCC) TNM staging for prognostication (seventh edition) [19–21]. The availability of the AJCC categories allows comparison between studies with a different patient mix from multiple centers.

One of the essential parts of creating prognostication tools is having good information on patient survival. Especially in Northern Europe, national registries regarding patient death certificates are available, and information can be obtained for research purposes; this leads to only sporadic cases with loss of follow-up. In Leiden (The Netherlands), records of eyes that were enucleated for uveal melanoma have systematically been collected since 1972. In 1984, I started to work with eye pathologist Dr. Didi de Wolff-Rouendaal and we collected data on all eyes enucleated for uveal melanoma in Leiden. We could retrospectively add her reports since 1972, and with her successors, Dr. Sjoerd van Duinen and Dr. Robert Verdijk, collected data from over 1200 uveal melanoma patients. Using patient follow-up information from the Dutch national registry, we were able to analyze five decades of enucleations for UM ([22]: "Five decades of enucleations for uveal melanoma in one center; more tumors with high risk factors, no improvement in survival over time"). As only a minority of patients in the Netherlands undergo an enucleation and the majority of uveal melanoma are treated with ruthenium plaques or proton beam irradiation, analyses were performed on size categories, as defined by the AJCC, so that one could see that we were dealing consistently with large tumors. We observed no changes in survival of patients with stage III tumors over these five decades, indicating the urgent need for new treatments.

Retrospective studies provide a great opportunity for students to work on. Often these can be performed quite independently, can be well scheduled, and result in a scientific answer that is worth publishing. These are important aspects compared to either very clinical or more fundamental work. It should be noted however that while case series may result in interesting observations, other studies are needed to truly answer questions on the fundamental understanding of disease or development (and testing) of new treatments.

5 Translational Studies

When one has a fine pathology or genetics department, translational studies are within reach. These are usually collaborative studies (between clinical and supporting departments), and the interest of all parties has to be kept in mind. Being generous with co-authorships—while acknowledging the IJCC authorship policies—is one way of showing your appreciation to your collaborators. For myself, my first experience in oncology came from an invitation from the pathology department. I was interested in studying HLA expression in cornea tissues that became available from patients after a corneal transplantation. A pathologist, Dr. Dirk Ruiter, was studying HLA expression in cutaneous melanoma and had the appropriate monoclonal antibodies that I needed for my study. As I worked in the Ophthalmology Department, he asked me to help him and select a series of uveal melanoma for a new study, and to help him with the evaluation of the tissue staining. As a resident in ophthalmology, I had diagnosed my very first uveal melanoma patient, and was keen on helping out. A medical student, Dr. Jeroen van der Pol, was anxious to help. We had a great time trying to get everything to work, as Dr. Ruiter had a fabulous technician. When we found out that doing immunohistochemistry on paraffin sections was not always possible, a collection of frozen material was started in Leiden with great support from Dr. de Wolff-Rouendaal. One needs a fine laboratory to collect such material, and the Department of Ophthalmology had its own lab facilities. As mentioned above, Dr. de Wolff-Rouendaal provided standardized data on uveal melanoma pathology. This pathology database, together with a biobank, excellent immunohistochemistry, and later genetic analyses, led to many translational studies.

One of the very first papers was clinically one of the most important: Dr. van der Pol et al. [23] published—"Heterogeneous expression of melanoma-associated antigens in uveal melanomas." This was as far as we know the very first paper showing expression of pigment-related genes in uveal melanoma. One of the most often and most highly expressed genes was gp100, which is the target of a specific treatment for uveal melanoma metastases. The bispecific antibody known as tebentafusp is directed against a combination of CD3 and gp100 [24] and applied in clinical studies to stop metastases from growing [25].

Several of our translational studies involved the already mentioned HLA antigens, and in the 1980s, it was generally assumed that tumor cells could escape from immunomonitoring and killing through loss of their HLA antigens. When I first saw the outcome of our HLA staining and the survival results, I had difficulty believing them. So, always be ready for a surprise! In uveal melanoma, we noticed the opposite of what was generally accepted: tumors with a high HLA Class I expression were the ones that gave rise to metastases [26]! My second Eureka moment. Tumors with the lowest expression were the ones that did not kill the patient. When the editor of the journal *Human Immunology*, Professor J.J. van Rood, heard about this, he asked me to write a paper about it. This led to the review: "HLA expression in uveal melanoma: there is no rule without some exception" [27]. (My first Eureka moment was during my PhD when I accidentally discovered a new polymorphic antigen system on human peripheral blood monocytes [28, 29]).

Translational studies may try to answer a specific question or can be an inventory, for instance, a summary of genetic aberrations, or a series of cases where you do a test on tumor tissue, ocular fluid, or blood. For translational studies, one often needs laboratory facilities or collaboration with a lab, for instance, for genetic testing. We benefitted in many studies from an extensive microarray analysis on 64 primary uveal melanomas as ordered by Dr. P.A. van der Velden, which provided information on the expression of thousands of genes [30]. Together with excellent histopathologic information on tumor size and cell type, as well as patient follow-up data, the value of genes for prognostication or the relation with blood vessel density could be determined.

Over the years, we kept asking the question: which factors determine malignancy in uveal melanoma? This research led to several discoveries in uveal melanoma, which, however, often led to the next question:

- A high HLA Class I expression is associated with high numbers of infiltrating T cells [31].
- UM cells protect themselves from complement-mediated lysis by expressing complement inhibitors [32].
- A high HLA expression is associated with the development of metastases [33].
- Metastases have a higher HLA Class I expression than the primary tumor [26].
- Individual HLA Class I alleles may be downregulated, while others are highly expressed [34].
- Normal distribution of genetic HLA Class I and II polymorphisms in UM patients [35].
- Vascular endothelial growth factor-A is produced by the tumor and the retina in eyes with UM [36].
- UM contain numerous tolerizing dendritic cells [37].
- Epigenetics play a role in HLA Class II expression in UM [38].
- The inflammatory phenotype is associated with loss of one chromosome 3 [39].
- The majority of macrophages are pro-angiogenic M2 macrophages [40].
- Loss of one chromosome 3 is associated with the presence of regulatory T cells [41].
- Hypoxia induces monocyte migration in UM [42].
- High-risk UM can be divided in group IIa and IIb, with different gene expression patterns [30].
- HLA expression is upregulated in UM by infiltrating leukocytes [43].
- Loss of BAP1 guides the development of an inflammatory environment [44].
- PRAME is expressed on UM metastases, making it a potential target for immunotherapy [45].
- Nevi already carry *GNAQ* and *GNA11* mutations, previously thought to be characteristic of UM [46].
- Aqueous humor biomarkers help to identify three groups of UM [47].
- Ischemia is genetically determined and related to loss of one chromosome 3/BAP1 loss [48].
- Tumor angiogenesis is related to a tumor's genetic evolution [49].
- Loss of BAP1 is associated with upregulation of the NFkB pathway and an increased HLA Class I expression [50].

We have learned a lot from these translational studies, which results in a model: loss of one chromosome 3, together with a pathogenic mutation in the BAP1 gene, leads to tumor ischemia. The subsequent production of cytokines attracts leukocytes, which stimulate the expression of a wide range of interferon-regulated proteins (including HLA), leading to an inflammatory phenotype. The presence of ischemia and M2 macrophages stimulates blood vessel formation. Cells from such tumors find their way into the bloodstream and settle in the liver. This story will develop further, as we do not know what causes cells to specifically settle in the liver. How do different mutations in UM such as those in those in the BAP1 and SF3B1 gene give rise to metastases [51, 52]? What makes cells stay dormant in the liver? Why do inhibitors of active pathways not stop liver metastases from growing? Why do monoclonal checkpoint inhibitors not work when many checkpoints are being expressed? How does the immune privilege of the ocular environment influence tumor cell behavior?

While translational research may lead to more insight in tumor behavior, it can also provide ocular oncologists with better parameters to predict patient prognosis. Our studies did that at different levels:

- Gene expression profiling can provide markers for prognostication [53].
- Chromosome 3 loss corresponds to BAP1 immunohistochemistry [54].
- ddPCR can be used to identify extra copies of 8q, which are relevant to prognosis [55].
- PRAME is an independent prognostic marker of low-risk UM [56].
- The combination of tumor size and chromosome categorization provides better prognostication than any test alone [57].

The study by Dr. Zuidervaart et al. [53] was an analysis of mRNA expression patterns in (uveal) melanoma cell lines, which helped to identify two groups of cell lines. Differentiating markers were tested on primary tumors and identified a low and a high risk of developing metastases. The high-risk phenotype was characterized by high levels of angiogenic factors. The data were presented at a fabulous meeting in Leiden in 2002 and provided Dr. J.W. Harbour with a Eureka moment: he had the idea to test the gene expression profile of primary tumors instead of using a few individual markers; this led to the development of the gene expression Class I/Class II testing [58], and the development of a commercial test.

The group of Dr. Jens Kiilgaard in Denmark first showed that combining size and genetic data may provide better accuracy of prognostication [59]. Working in a collaboration between the LUMC and the University of Copenhagen, Dr. Dogrusöz extended the prior findings of Drs. Bagger and Kiilgaard using larger numbers and published a study on using tumor size as well as chromosome data for prognostication [57]. A large tumor size and loss of chromosome 3 carry a higher risk of metastases when they occur together.

6 Functional Studies

All these data suggest many functional relationships exist, but those have to be proven through functional studies. For these, one needs a laboratory with technical and animal facilities, depending on what one wants to study. Dr. Bruce Ksander in Boston (USA) and Dr. Tim Murray (Miami, USA) have provided the world with a series of UM cell lines, which have been the workhorses for in vitro and murine functional studies. Their collaboration provided cell lines Mel202 and Mel270 and two cell lines from metastases of the same patient (OMM2.3 and OMM2.5), Mel285 and Mel290 [60, 61]. As cell lines may accidentally be exchanged in the lab or between labs, it is always essential to write in a paper from which lab cell lines were obtained, and it is appropriate to refer to the original paper where the creation of the cell line was described and how it can be identified [62]. Recognizing the hard work of the maker is the least one can do when using somebody else's creation. Creating a new cell line is hard work. In our lab, Dr. De Waard-Siebinga tried to follow Dr. Ksander's example to create new cell lines, for which goal she cultured 22 fresh primary UM. Out of these came cell line 92.1 [63]. This cell line has since been used extensively for testing drugs. Around the same time, Dr. Gré Luyten developed cell lines in Rotterdam. One of these (OMM1) came from a metastasis and is therefore popular in drug screening studies [64]. Most research projects use cell lines obtained from others. We received Dr. Ksander's cell lines in the early 1990s, and have, with his permission, distributed our own and his cell lines to people worldwide, with the help of departmental funds that paid for a technician to keep growing cells and to send them all around the world. Although many people take cell lines for granted, and do not even mention their origin in their paper, this effort has helped to determine the effect of many different drugs on human UM cell lines. Over 25 years later, it became possible to trace the previously mentioned cell lines back to their original tumors and report on their mutational status through a collaboration between Leiden, the Bascom Palmer Eye Institute (Miami), and the Schepens Eye Research Institute (Boston) [65].

The Curie Institute in Paris, France, developed a new technique to obtain cell lines: placing tumor tissue in the skin of immunodeficient mice has resulted in a series of new cell lines, which display a variety of genetic backgrounds. Several of these lack BAP1 expression and several originate from metastases, offering a wide range of useful testing materials [66]. Dr. Sergio Roman-Roman and Dr. Didier Decaudin from the Curie Institute, Paris, France, have been so kind to generously provide them to other centers worldwide.

7 In Vivo Experiments

When working with animals, a lot of expertise is needed, and collaborations are essential. In the field of ocular tumor immunology, we had the luck to have a lot of experts in Leiden, such as Dr. Kees Melief, Dr. Martin Kast, Dr. René Toes, Dr. Rienk Offringa, Dr. Thorbald van Hall, and Dr. Ferry Ossendorp.

Mouse models can be used to determine the effectiveness of potential therapies. Dr. Schurmans [67] was the first to set up a murine ocular tumor model in Leiden, thanks to the support of Dr. Jerry Niederkorn from Dallas, Texas, USA.

Sutmuller et al. [68] subsequently tested the potential to kill intraocular tumors with cytotoxic T cells: would the melanoma antigen gp100 be a good target for therapy with cytotoxic T cells? He placed cells of human UM cell line OMM-1 in the eye of HLA-A2 transgenic mice. Adoptive transfer of cytotoxic T cells directed against human HLA-A2/gp100-expressing tumor cells was able to effectively remove the tumors from the eye. For experiments like this, one needs an exquisite lab with excellent mouse facilities. Data such as these indicated the effectiveness of immune responses against gp100, and helped to develop tebentafusp: the already mentioned combination of a soluble T cell receptor and an anti-CD3 single chain variable fragment [24]. Tebentafusp is now in clinical trials for the treatment of UM metastases.

Other studies involve macrophages. As I did my PhD study with monocytes, the function of monocytes/macrophages has always intrigued me. De Waard-Siebinga had noticed many macrophages in primary UM [31]. We wondered what their function might be. Previously, cornea studies had shown that depletion of macrophages through clodronate-filled liposome injections would block immune rejection of corneal transplants [69]. Thanks to the presence of very smart and dexterous PhD students who would later become excellent eye surgeons, we were able to analyze the effect of macrophage depletion using two different mouse models.

We first used a model based on tumor cells transformed by the early region 1 of human adenovirus type 5 (Ad5E1) [70]. Prior experiments had shown that these tumor cells grow in a mouse eye, but after a few weeks, the mouse develops an immune response, which leads to spontaneous resolution of the intraocular tumor. This tumor killing depends on CD4 T cells [71]. We wondered whether macrophages played any role in the elimination of these tumors. Indeed, depletion of macrophages led to progressive tumor growth and inhibited tumor eradication. They were essential for tumor antigen presentation to the immune system. In the mouse, tumor antigens could be found in the regional lymph nodes.

We later used another model with B16F10 cells placed in the anterior chamber of C57Bl/6 mice to study the role of macrophages in young and old mice. During aging, the polarity of the macrophages changes from the type that is needed to fight infections to a pro-angiogenic type. When macrophages were depleted from the eye in an old mouse at the time of tumor implantation, tumors would no longer grow [72]. We think that they were needed for blood vessel development. Shortly after, we discovered that most macrophages in human high-risk UM are typical pro-angiogenic macrophages [40]. Overall, our data show that loss of one chromosome 3 and a mutation in BAP1 gene lead to a tumor with ischemia, attracting macrophages that produce all kinds of cytokines [73]. The production of cytokines such as VEGF stimulate vessel development, providing UM cells with a route to escape from the eye. The acquired knowledge about the changing role of macrophages during aging helps to understand other diseases as well, such as age-related macular degeneration and severe pulmonary COVID-19 [74].

8 Prospective Studies

A prospective study is very useful to compare different therapeutic approaches but it needs careful planning and hard work. In our institution, we learned a valuable lesson when we started our first prospective study. We developed a trial to treat radiation retinopathy that followed radiation of an eye with a UM. We compared the therapeutic effect of the VEGF inhibitor ranibizumab versus an intravitreal corticosteroid, triamcinolone acetonide. The current new inhibitors of angiopoietin may be similarly investigated. While we were including patients for this study, we happened to get audited (i.e., the monitoring process to assess adherence to laws and regulations, as required under Dutch law); during the preparation for this audit, we found an inadequate patient consent form, which is a real no-no. We showed it to the auditors prior to the audit, and the hospital closed the study. Our honesty in confessing the error prior to the audit prevented any punitive actions, but also stopped the trial and our attempt to improve the care for radiation retinopathy. Obviously, this was a great setback; however, something good did come out of it: the process resulted in the creation of a specialized departmental trial bureau.

9 Setting Up Collaborations

Many of our papers have been written with collaborators from other departments, often in other countries. Politics (at the institutional level or between institutes) may interfere with potential collaborations, however, as sometimes the leadership prefers certain connections and dissuades others. For ages, Leiden and Rotterdam (two cities about a half-hour drive by car) did not collaborate as Professor Oosterhuis and Professor Manschot held opposing views on radiation therapy: one considered a radioactive plaque the best option for small-to-medium tumors, while the other argued that removing the eye was needed to prevent systemic spreading of tumor cells from these melanomas [75, 76]. It took years to overcome this divide: building connections needs trust. When you promise to do something, really try to do it. Do not expect that collaboration is a one-way street. Once you have asked somebody to work with you, next time they may need your help, and you are expected to give it. That is how relationships are built. Helping other people is one of the best ways to go forward.

At meetings, get to know people. Go to meetings that may not necessarily be in your specialization. I learned very much from attending the meetings of The Netherlands Society of Immunology, and then trying to translate new findings to my own field. I recently learned that my great friend Dr. Junko Hori in Japan did the same [77]. Both of us worked with the great eye immunologist Dr. Wayne Streilein. It is good to realize that people from other research fields may have helpful know-how. And listen to your patients! For example, a lady singer told me about a presumed side effect of a drug she was taking, and I had never heard of it. She was a particularly good observer and described that her eyes became grittier on stage (with all the lights) when she was taking a diuretic. When I looked in the literature, a paper from the 1970s indeed described a similar side effect. Patients may also come up with questions that you had not yet thought about. Working with patient organizations may (again) be an effective way to learn more about the effects of a disease or a treatment.

Collaborations with other centers provide an excellent opportunity for students to work on projects abroad. Over the years, many students that I supervised have worked in other institutions, and some international collaborations have resulted in fruitful projects for decades. There is a major benefit in these projects, as the receiving institutions obtain a motivated extra help-force for projects, and the students learn from a scientific experience as well as from the personal experience by working abroad.

10 Collaborative Studies

In Europe, ocular oncologists and researchers come together in the European Ophthalmic Oncology Group, which meets twice a year. People can invite others to join in collaborations. European studies developed by the European Ophthalmic Oncology Group are, for instance, the following: a study spearheaded by Dr. Al-Jamal on analyzing choroidal and ciliary body melanoma in children [78], Dr. Jouhi's "Small fatal choroidal melanoma study" [79], and

Dr. Cunha Rola's study on a "multicenter external validation study of the Liverpool Uveal Melanoma Prognosticator online" [80].

The different TNM-AJCC studies used follow-up data from several European groups ("Staging of ciliary body and choroidal melanomas based on anatomic extent: a collaborative study by the European Ophthalmic Oncology Group," [81]), as did the worldwide study of Dr. B. Gallie, who analyzed the relation between the risk of developing metastases following a local recurrence in UM [82]. The studies spearheaded by Dr. J.W. Harbour are focused on oncologists in the USA (Collaborative Ocular Oncology Report, [83]) and bring together many data from many clinics.

One of the papers that came out of a very extensive translational European/American collaboration was The Cancer Genome Atlas (TCGA) Uveal Melanoma study, which reported on the analysis of 80 UM using different testing platforms (mutations, chromosome numbers, mRNA, miRNA, lncRNA, epigenetic modifications, survival) [84]. The tumors came from several different labs (mainly from Europe), while the testing labs were based in the USA. A group of scientists from many backgrounds evaluated these results and wrote the paper. The original data were made available to any researcher worldwide under the Beau Biden Cancer Moonshot program initiated by then Vice President Joe Biden. We simplified the identification of the four identified groups by proposing a new categorization (Categories A, B C, and D), based on chromosome 3 and 8q status, which was further developed and evaluated by Dr. Carol Shields [85, 86]. The four categories work well for prognostication on a genetic basis. Combining genetics with tumor size leads to even better prognostication [87]. Chromosome 3 and 8q aberrations have been noticed to have a greater impact on survival in patients with a light iris versus a dark iris color [88].

In Europe, financial stimulus packages have been provided to stimulate collaborative research. I strongly believe that collaboration between people with different experiences and knowledge is essential for providing new knowledge. All participants should contribute and all should gain from it, and the patients will gain the most. Thanks to the networks that we had developed over the years, we were able to get two Horizon 2020 grants, one for corneal regenerative medicine (Horizon 2020 grant Arrest Blindness) and one for developing a treatment for UM (Horizon 2020 grant UM Cure). Centers in France, the UK, Poland, Italy, The Netherlands, and Portugal collaborated to provide materials; test drugs in vitro, in zebrafish, and in murine xenograft models; and develop more insight in the genetics and immunology of UM. During the application as well as the research meetings, patients heavily participated, and specific patient-oriented meetings were held in several countries to share information.

11 Visibility

When data are not published, they do not exist. It is essential to show the world what you have done so that others can learn from it and use the knowledge you gained for asking better questions and developing new knowledge. This is also true for negative results, as you may help others find a better way. Hopefully, journals will accept such so-called "negative" results, when you have performed a study to answer a question but you did not find something new. Publishing such results may stimulate others to plan a project differently. Speak about your work at conferences and use the modern social networks to spread information. I learned this from the example of the outstanding work of the Champalimaud Institute, Lisbon, Portugal, partner in the Horizon 2020 project UM Cure. By building a website and keeping information up to date by placing interviews with researchers on their website, they continuously informed researchers and patients about the progress of UM Cure. Small meetings help to build collaborations, and by inviting patients as well, you really find out what patients want.

12 Education: *Nature Reviews* Uveal Melanoma

It is important to transfer knowledge and a superb way is by writing reviews. This provides the writer with a good overview of the scientific area, and the reader with a fast way to learn about a new topic. For starting scientists, writing a review is an especially useful exercise to get into a field. And even for more-experienced scientists, it can be a great experience. I very much enjoyed working on an extensive review of the clinical and basic knowledge about UM: *Nature Reviews* Uveal Melanoma [89]. It was fabulous to see how effective the leaders in the field are when working on a paper. Furthermore, working with a *Nature Reviews* journal gave me more insight in the level of support that a high-ranking journal provides; collaborating with a group of experienced and superb authors was for me a great and very enjoyable experience. The result was an up-to-date overview of the clinical, pathologic, and genetic background of UM. Papers like this can benefit clinicians, researchers, and patients around the world, and it was with disappointment that I learned that *Nature* does not (yet) provides open-access publishing, limiting access to the paper, that all of us wrote without getting paid. This touches upon the earning models of publishers and journals, which is a much-debated topic and provided an educational moment for me.

13 Outreach

When one has a good overview of a scientific field, it may be useful to call attention to urgent medical needs, and try to influence decision-makers. Those who deal with giving out grants often do not distinguish between cutaneous and uveal melanoma. Rodrigues and other partners of the UM Cure 2020 project wrote a position paper to call attention to the discrepancies between uveal and other melanomas [90]. Genetically, UM are characterized by specific mutations that differ from those in cutaneous melanoma. Immune checkpoint inhibitors are rarely effective in UM, and the presence of immune cells in the primary tumor is associated with a bad prognosis, not with protection. Knowledge of these discrepancies is important, as it urges specific funding for UM. As UM is a rare disease, obtaining funds for research is challenging. Publishing about these issues may help to call attention to this disease. Working together with patient groups will help as well.

14 Conclusion

When one wishes to engage in research, many options are available ranging from single case reports to larger clinical or translational projects. For most ophthalmologists, writing a single paper in one's lifetime is a major achievement. Once published, however, one may start to enjoy it and look for further options. This review shows the opportunities which I encountered, and this may perhaps give you ideas for projects of your own. Apart from the mere scientific view, however, I am very happy for the great collaborations that I experienced in the past years, and am grateful that it led to great (personal) friendships. I hope your research does the same for you.

Acknowledgments Many thanks to I. de Waard-Siebinga, D-J. R Blom, W.R.O. Goslings, J. Slooff-Kool, F. van Klink, L.R.H.M. Schurmans, M.H.M. Hurks, J.A.W. Blok, W. Zuidervaart, G.S.O.A. Missotten, Z.F.H.M. Boonman, S. Keijser, M. Polak, L.V. Ly, M. El Filali, J.J.J. Bosch, W. Maat, I. Bronkhorst, J.S. Parker, J. Cao, K. van Dijk, M. Dogrusöz, T.H. van Essen, T.H.K. Vu, D. Spinozzi, R.S. Birbal, Z. Souri, L. Baydoun, A. Miron, I. Vasuliauskaite, R. Singh, K. Glinkina, M.J. de Lange, G. Gezgin, A.P.A. Wierenga, N.J. Brouwer, C. Chau, R.J. Nell, M.C. Gelmi, S. Ma, R.V. Huis in't Veld, K.C. de Sousa Pontes, T. Jehs, L.E. Houtzagers, C. van Weeghel, C.D.M. Roelofsen, N. Meijer, A.M.W. ten Voorde, all students, P.A. van der Velden, M. Versluis, G.P.M. Luyten, M. Marinkovic, J. Bleeker, and my other colleagues in the Department of Ophthalmology of the LUMC and around the world.

References

1. Jager MJ, Brand A, Claas FHJ. Jon van Rood: the pioneer and his personal view on the early developments of HLA and immunogenetics. Transpl Immunol. 2019;52:1–26. https://doi.org/10.1016/j.trim.2018.12.006.
2. Brouwer NJ, Haanen JBAG, Jager MJ. Development of ocular rosacea following combined ipilimumab and nivolumab treatment for metastatic malignant skin melanoma. Ocul Oncol Pathol. 2017;3:188–92.
3. Hori J, Kunishige T, Nakano Y. Immune checkpoints contribute corneal immune privilege: implications for dry eye associated with checkpoint inhibitors. Int J Mol Sci. 2020;21911:3962. https://doi.org/10.3390/ijms21113962.
4. Van Dijk EHC, Boon CJF. The differential diagnosis of central serous chorioretinopathy and other diseases associated with subretinal fluid in the macula. Progress Ret Eye Res. 2021;84(Pt 3b):100955. https://doi.org/10.1016/j.preteyeres.2021.100955.
5. Van Dijk EHC, Kruit WHJ, Jager MJ, Luyten GPM, Vingerling JR, Boon CJF. Pimasertib-associated ophthalmological adverse events. Acta Ophthalmol. 2018;96(7):712–8. https://doi.org/10.1111/aos.13677.
6. LoRusso PM, Krishnamurthi SS, Rinehart JJ, et al. Phase I pharmacokinetic and pharmacodynamic study of the oral MAPK/ERK kinase inhibitor PD-0325901 in patients with advanced cancers. Clin Cancer Res. 2010;16:1924–37.
7. Leijen S, Middleton MR, Tresca P, et al. Blockade of the MEK/ERK signalling cascade by AS703026, a novel selective MEK1/2 inhibitor, induces pleiotropic anti-myeloma activity in vitro and in vivo. Clin Cancer Res. 2012;18:4794–805.
8. Brouwer NJ, Marinkovic M, Bleeker JC, El Filali M, Stefansson E, Luyten GPM, Jager MJ. Retinal oximetry is altered in eyes with choroidal melanoma but not in eyes with choroidal nevi. Retina. 2020;40(11):2207–15.
9. Jager MJ, Hermans LJA, Kok JHC. Visual results after corneal transplantation. Doc Ophthalmol. 1989;72:265–72.
10. Melles GR, Eggink FA, Lander F, Pels E, Rietveld FJ, Beekhuis WH, Binder PS. A surgical technique for posterior lamellar keratoplasty. Cornea. 1998;17(6):618–26.
11. Melles GR, Lander F, van Dooren BT, Pels A, Beekhuis WH. Preliminary clinical results of posterior lamellar keratoplasty through a sclerocorneal pocket incision. Ophthalmology. 2000;107(10):1850–6.
12. Melles GRJ, Ong TS, Ververs B, van der Wees J. Descemet membrane endothelial keratoplasty (DMEK). Cornea. 2006;25(8):987–90.
13. Shields CL, Furuta M, Thangappan A, Nagori S, Mashayekhi A, Lally DR, et al. Metastasis of uveal melanoma millimeter-by-millimeter in 8033 consecutive eyes. Arch Ophthalmol Chic Ill. 2009;127:989–98. https://doi.org/10.1001/archophthalmol.2009.208.
14. Shields CL, Kancherla S, Patel J, Vijayvargiya P, Suriano MM, Kolbus E, et al. Clinical survey of 3680 iris tumors based on patient age at presentation. Ophthalmology. 2012a;119(2):407–14. https://doi.org/10.1016/j.ophttha.2011.07.059.
15. Shields CL, Kaliki S, Furuta M, Mashayekhi A, Shields JA. Clinical spectrum and prognosis of uveal melanoma based on age at presentation in 8,033 cases. Retina. 2012b;32(7):1363–72. https://doi.org/10.1097/IAE.0b013e31824d09a8.
16. Shields CL, Say EAT, Hasanreisoglu M, Saktanasate J, Lawson BM, Landy JE, et al. Cytogenetic abnormalities in Uveal Melanoma Based on tumor features and size in 1059 patients. Ophthalmology. 2017;124:609–18. https://doi.org/10.1016/j.ophtha.2016.12.026.
17. Shields CL, Sioufi K, Srinivasan A, Di Nicola M, Masoomiam B, Barna LE, et al. Visual outcome and millimeter incremental risk of metastasis in 1780 patients with small choroidal melanoma managed

by plaque radiotherapy. JAMA Ophthalmol. 2018;136(12):1325–33. https://doi.org/10.1001/jamaophthalmol.2018.3881.
18. Damato B, Duke C, Coupland SE, Hiscott P, Smith PA, Campbell I, et al. Cytogenetics of uveal melanoma: a 7-year clinical experience. Ophthalmology. 2007;114:1925–31.
19. Kujala E, Damato B, Coupland SE, Desjardins L, Bechrakis NE, Grange J-D, Kivelä T. Staging of ciliary body and choroidal melanomas based on anatomic extent. J Clin Oncol. 2013a;31(22):2825–31.
20. Kivela T, Simpson ER, Grossniklaus HE, Jager MJ, Singh AD, Caminal JM, Pavlick AC, Kajula E, Coupland SE, Finger PT. Uveal Melanoma. American Joint Committee on Cancer 2017. In: Amin MB, et al., editors. AJCC cancer staging manual. 8th ed; 2017. p. 805–67. https://doi.org/10.1007/978-3-319-40618-3_67.
21. AJCC Ophthalmic Oncology Task Force. International validation of the American Joint Committee on Cancer's 7th edition classification of uveal melanoma. JAMA Ophthalmol. 2015;133(4):376–83. https://doi.org/10.1001/jamaophthalmol.2014.5395.
22. Roelofsen CDM, Wierenga APA, Van Duinen S, Verdijk RM, Bleeker J, Marinkovic M, Luyten GPM, Jager MJ. Five decades of enucleations for Uveal Melanoma in one center; more tumors with high risk factors, no improvement in survival over time. Ocul Oncol Pathol. 2021;7(2):133–41. https://doi.org/10.1159/000509918.
23. van der Pol JP, Jager MJ, de Wolff-Rouendaal D, Ringens PJ, Vennegoor C, Ruiter DJ. Heterogeneous expression of melanoma-associated antigens in uveal melanomas. Current Eye Res. 1987;6:757–65.
24. Damato BE, Dukes J, Goodall H, Carvajal RD. Tebentafusp: T cell redirection for the treatment of metastatic uveal melanoma. Cancers. 2019;11:971.
25. Nathan P, Hassel JC, Rutkowski P, Baurain J-F, Butler MO, Schlaak M, et al. Overall survival benefit with tebentafusp in metastatic uveal melanoma. N Engl J Med. 2021;385(13):1196–206. https://doi.org/10.1056/NEJMoa2103485.
26. Blom DJR, Luyten GPM, Mooy CM, Kerkvliet S, Zwinderman AH, Jager MJ. Human Leukocyte Antigen Class I expression: marker of poor prognosis in uveal melanoma. Invest Ophthalmol Vis Sci. 1997a;38:1865–72.
27. Jager MJ, Hurks HMH, Levitskaya J, Kiessling R. HLA expression in uveal melanoma: there is no rule without some exception. Hum Immunol. 2002;63:444–51.
28. Jager MJ, Claas FH, D'Amaro J, Baldwin WM, van Rood JJ. Two alloantigens on human monocytes; a diallelic system? Hum Immunol. 1987;19(3):215–24. https://doi.org/10.1016/0198-8859(87)90116-9.
29. Jager MJ, Claas FH, Schot JD, gratama JW, de Lange G, van Rood JJ. Genetics of two human monocyte antigens. Hum Immunol. 1988;22(3):163–70. https://doi.org/10.1016/0198-8859(88)90025-0.
30. De Lange MJ, Van Pelt SI, Versluis M, Jordanova ES, Kroes WGM, Ruivenkamp C, et al. Heterogeneity revealed by integrated genomic analysis uncovers a molecular switch in malignant uveal melanoma. Oncotarget. 2015;6(35):37824–35. https://doi.org/10.18632/oncotarget.5637.
31. De Waard-Siebinga I, Hilders CGJM, Hansen BE, van Delft JL, Jager MJ. HLA expression and tumor-infiltrating immune cells in uveal melanoma. Graefes Arch Clin Exp Ophthalmol. 1996;234:34–42.
32. Goslings WRO, Blom DJR, De Waard-Siebinga I, Van Beelen E, Luyten GPM, Claas FHJ, et al. Membrane-bound regulators of complement in uveal melanoma. CD46, CD55, and CD59 in uveal melanoma. Invest Ophthalmol Vis Sci. 1996;37:1884–91.
33. Blom DJR, Schurmans LRHM, De Waard-Siebinga I, De Wolff-Rouendaal D, Jager MJ. A comparative analysis of HLA expression in a primary uveal melanoma, its cell line and four of its metastases. Br J Ophthalmol. 1997b;81:989–93.
34. Hurks HMH, Metzelaar-Blok JAW, Mulder A, Claas FHJ, Jager MJ. High frequency of allele-specific down-regulation of HLA Class I expression in uveal melanoma cell lines. Int J Cancer. 2000;85:697–702.
35. Metzelaar-Blok JAW, Hurks HMH, Naipal A, De Lange P, Keunen JEE, Claas FHJ, Doxiadis IIN, Jager MJ. Normal HLA class I, -II, and MICA gene distribution in uveal melanoma. Mol Vis. 2005;21(11):1166–72.
36. Missotten GSOA, Notting IC, Schlingemann RO, Zijlmans HJ, Lau C, Eilers PH, Keunen JE, Jager MJ. Vascular endothelial growth factor-A in eyes with uveal melanoma. Arch Ophthalmol. 2006;124:1428–34.
37. Polak M, Borthwick NJ, Johnson P, Hungerford JL, Higgins B, Di Palma S, Jager MJ, Cree IA. Presence and phenotype of dendritic cells in uveal melanoma. Br J Ophthalmol. 2007;91:971–6.
38. Holling TM, Van Eggermond MCJA, Jager MJ, van den Elsen PJ. Epigenetic silencing of MHC2TA transcription in cancer. Biochem Pharmacol. 2006;72:1570–6.
39. Maat W, Ly LV, Jordanova ES, de Wolff-Rouendaal D, Schalij-Delfos NE, Jager MJ. Monosomy of chromosome 3 and an inflammatory phenotype occur together in uveal melanoma. Invest Ophthalmol Vis Sci. 2008;49:505–10.
40. Bronkhorst IHG, Ly LV, Jordanova ES, Vrolijk H, Versluis M, Luyten GPM, Jager MJ. Detection of M2 macrophages in uveal melanoma and relation to survival. Invest Ophthalmol Vis Sci. 2011;52:643–50.
41. Bronkhorst IHG, Vu THK, Jordanova ES, Luyten GPM, van der Burg SJ, Jager MJ. Different subsets of tumor-infiltrating lymphocytes correlate with macrophage influx and monosomy 3 in uveal melanoma. Invest Ophthalmol Vis Sci. 2012;53:5370–8.
42. Bronkhorst IHG, Jehs TML, Dijkgraaf EM, Luyten GPM, van der Velden PA, van der Burg SH, Jager MJ. Effect of hypoxic stress on migration and characteristics of monocytes in uveal melanoma. JAMA Ophthalmol. 2014;132(5):614–21.
43. Van Essen TH, van Pelt SI, Bronkhorst IHG, Versluis M, Nemati F, Luyten GPM, van Hall T, van den Elsen PJ, van der Velden PA, Decaudin D, Jager MJ. Upregulation of HLA expression in Uveal melanoma by infiltrating leukocytes. PLOS One. 2016;11(10):e0164292. https://doi.org/10.1371/journal.pone.0164292.
44. Gezgin G, Dogrusöz M, van Essen TH, Kroes WGM, Luyten GPM, van der Velden PA, et al. Genetic evolution of uveal melanoma guides the development of an inflammatory microenvironment. Cancer Immunol Immunother. 2017a;66(7):903–12. https://doi.org/10.1007/s00262-017-1991-1.
45. Gezgin G, Luk SJ, Cao J, Dogrusöz M, van der Steen DM, Hagedoorn RS, et al. PRAME as a potential target for immunotherapy in uveal melanoma metastases. JAMA Ophthalmol. 2017b;135(6):541–9. https://doi.org/10.1001/jamaophthalmol.2017.0729.
46. Vader MJC, Madigan MC, Versluis M, Suleiman HM, Gezgin G, Gruis NA, et al. GNAQ and GNA11 mutations and downstream YAP activation in choroidal nevi. Br J Cancer. 2017;117(6):884–7. https://doi.org/10.1038/bjc.2017.259.
47. Wierenga APA, Gezgin G, van Beelen E, Eijkmans M, Versluis M, Verdijk RM. Soluble HLA in the aqueous humour in uveal melanoma is associated with unfavourable tumour characteristics. Cancers. 2019;11(8):1202. https://doi.org/10.3390/cancers11081202.
48. Brouwer NJ, Wierenga APA, Gezgin G, Marinkovic M, Luyten GPM, Kroes WGM, et al. Ischemia is related to tumour genetics in uveal melanoma. Cancers. 2019a;11:1004. https://doi.org/10.3390/cancers11071004.
49. Brouwer NJ, Gezgin G, Wierenga APA, Bronkhorst IHG, Marinkovic M, Luyten GPM, et al. Tumour angiogenesis in Uveal Melanoma is related to genetic evolution. Cancers. 2019b;11:979. https://doi.org/10.3390/cancers11070979.

50. Souri Z, Wierenga APA, van Weeghel C, van der Velden PA, Kroes WGM, Luyten GPM, et al. Loss of BAP1 is associated with upregulation of the NFkB pathway and increased HLA Class I expression in uveal melanoma. Cancers. 2019;11:1102. https://doi.org/10.3390/cancers11081102.
51. Harbour JW, Onken MD, Roberson ED, Duan S, Cao L, Worley LA, Council ML, Matalall KA, Helms C, Bowcock AM. Frequent mutation in metastasizing uveal melanomas. Science. 2010;330(6009):1410–3. https://doi.org/10.1126/science.1194472.
52. Yavuzyigitoglu S, Koopmans AE, Verdijk RM, et al. Uveal melanomas with SF3B1 mutations: a distinct subclass associated with late-onset metastases. Ophthalmology. 2016;123(5):1118–28. https://doi.org/10.1016/j.ophtha.2016.01.023.
53. Zuidervaart W, Van der Velden PA, Hurks HMH, Van Nieuwpoort FA, Out-Luiting CJ, Singh AD, Frants RR, Jager MJ, Gruis NA. Gene expression profiling identifies tumour markers potentially playing a role in uveal melanoma development. Br J Cancer. 2003;89:1914–9.
54. Van Essen TH, van Pelt SI, Versluis M, Bronkhorst IHG, van Duinen SG, Marinkovic M, et al. Prognostic parameters in uveal melanoma and their association with BAP1 expression. Br J Ophthalmol. 2014,98(12):1738–43. https://doi.org/10.1136/bjophthalmol-2014-305047.
55. Versluis M, de Lange MJ, van Pelt SI, Ruivenkamp CAL, Kroes WGM, Cao J, et al. Digital PCR validates 8q dosage as prognostic tool in uveal melanoma. PLOS One. 2015;10(3):e0116371. https://doi.org/10.1371/journal.pone/0116371.
56. Field MG, Decatur CL, Kurtenbach S, Gezgin G, Van der Velden PA, Jager MJ, et al. PRAME as an independent biomarker for metastasis in low-risk uveal melanoma. Clin Cancer Res. 2016;22(5):1234–42. https://doi.org/10.1158/1078-0432.CCR-15-2071.
57. Dogrusöz M, Bagger M, van Duinen SG, Kroes WG, Ruivenkamp CAL, Böhringer S, et al. The prognostic value of AJCC staging in uveal melanoma is enhanced by adding chromosome 3 and 8q status. Invest Ophthalmol Vis Sci. 2017;58:833–42.58. https://doi.org/10.1167/iovs.16-20212.
58. Onken MD, Worley LA, Ehlers JP, Harbour JW. Gene expression profiling in uveal melanoma reveals two molecular classes and predicts metastatic death. Cancer Res. 2004;64(20):7205–9. https://doi.org/10.1158/0008-5472.CAN-04-1750.
59. Bagger M, et al. The prognostic effect of American Joint Committee on Cancer staging and genetic status in patients with choroidal and ciliary body melanoma. Invest Ophthalmol Vis Sci. 2014;56:438–44.
60. Ksander BR, Rubsamen PE, Oslen KR, Cousins SW, Streilein JW. Studies of tumor-infiltrating lymphocytes from a choroidal melanoma. Invest Ophthalmol Vis Sci. 1991;32:3198–208.
61. Chen PW, Murray TG, Uno T, Salgaller ML, Reddy R, Ksander BR. Expression of MAGE genes in ocular melanoma during progression from primary to metastatic disease. Clin Exp Metastasis. 1997;15:509–18.
62. Folberg R, Kadkol SS, Frenkel S, Valyi-Nagy K, Jager MJ, Pe'er J, Maniotis AJ. Authenticating cell lines in ophthalmic research laboratories. Inves Ophthalmol Vis Sci. 2008;49(11):4697–701. https://doi.org/10.1167/iovs.08-2324.
63. De Waard-Siebinga I, Blom D-JR, Griffioen M, Schrier PI, Hoogendoorn E, Beverstock G, Danen EHJ, Jager MJ. Establishment and characterization of an uveal melanoma cell line. Int J Cancer. 1995;62:155–61.
64. Luyten GP, Naus NC, Mooy CM, Hagemeijer A, Kan-Mitchell J, Van Drunen E, Vuzevski V, de Jong PT, Luider TM. Establishment and characterization of primary and metastatic uveal melanoma cell Lines. Int J Cancer. 1996;66:380–7.
65. Jager MJ, Magner JA, Ksander BR, Dubovy SR. Uveal melanoma cell lines: where do they come from? An American Ophthalmological Society Thesis. Trans Am Ophthalmol Soc. 2016;114:T5.
66. Amirouchene-Angelozzi N, Nemati F, Gentien D, Nicolas A, Dumont A, Carita G, Camonis J, Desjardins L, Cassoux N, Piperno-Neumann S, Mariani P, Sastre X, Decaudin D, Roman-Roman S. Establishment of novel cell lines recapitulating the genetic landscape of uveal melanoma and preclinical validation of mTOR as a therapeutic target. Mol Oncol. 2014;8(8):1508–20. https://doi.org/10.1016/j.molonc.2014.06.004.
67. Schurmans LRHM, De Boer AT, Diehl L, Van der Voort EIH, Kast WM, Melief CJM, Toes REM, Jager MJ. Successful immunotherapy of an intraocular tumor in mice. Cancer Res. 1999;59:5250–4.
68. Sutmuller RPM, Schurmans LRHM, Van Duivenvoorde LM, Tine JA, Van der Voort EIH, Toes REM, Melief CJM, Jager MJ, Offringa R. Adoptive T cell immunotherapy of human uveal melanoma targeting gp100. J Immunol. 2000;165:7308–15.
69. Slegers TP, Broersma L, van Rooijen N, Hooymans JM, van Rij G, van der Gaag R. Macrophages play a role in the early phase of corneal allograft rejection in rats. Transplantation. 2004;77(11):1641–6. https://doi.org/10.1097/01.tp.0000129410.89410.f2.
70. Boonman ZFHM, Wang S, van Rooijen N, Melief CJM, Toes REM, Jager MJ. Macrophages are vital in spontaneous intraocular tumor eradication. Invest Ophthalmol Vis Sci. 2006;47:2959–65.
71. Wang S, Boonman ZF, Li HC, He Y, Jager MJ, Toes RE, Niederkorn JY. Role of TRAIL and IFN-gamma in CD4+ T cell-dependent tumor rejection in the anterior chamber of the eye. J Immunol. 2003;171(6):2789–96. https://doi.org/10.4049/jimmunol.171.6.2789.
72. Ly LV, Baghat A, Versluis M, Jordanova ES, Luyten GPM, van Rooijen N, van Hall T, van der Velden PA, Jager MJ. In aged mice, outgrowth of intraocular melanoma depends on proangiogenic M2 type macrophages. J Immunol. 2010;185:3481–8.
73. de Lange MJ, Nell RJ, Lalai RN, Versluis M, Jordanova ES, Luyten GPM, Jager MJ, van der Burg SH, Zoutman WH, van Hall T, van der Velden PA. Digital PCR-based T-cell quantification-assisted deconvolution of the microenvironment reveals that activated macrophages drive tumor inflammation in uveal melanoma. Mol Cancer Res. 2018;16(12):1902–11. https://doi.org/10.1158/1541-7786.
74. Jager MJ, Seddon JM. Eye diseases direct interest to complement pathway and macrophages as regulators of inflammation in COVID-19. Asia Pacific J Ophthalmol. 2020;10(2):114–29. https://doi.org/10.1097/APO.0000000000000346.
75. Manschot WA, van Strik R. Is irradiation a justifiable treatment of choroidal melanoma? Analysis of published results. Br J Ophthalmol. 1987;71(5):348–55. https://doi.org/10.1136/bjo.71.5.348.
76. Oosterhuis JA, Lommmatsch PK, Wessing A. Is radiation a justifiable treatment of choroidal melanoma? Br J Ophthalmol. 1988;72(4):317–20. https://doi.org/10.1136/bjo.72.4.317.
77. Hori J, Yamaguchi T, Keino H, Hamrah P, Maruyama K. Prog Retin Eye Res. 2019;72:100758. https://doi.org/10.1016/j.preteyeres.2019.04.002.
78. Al-Jamal R, Cassoux N, Desjardins L, Damato B, Konstantinidis L, Coupland S, et al. The pediatric choroidal and ciliary body melanoma study. A survey by the European Ophthalmic Oncology Group. Ophthalmology. 2016;123:898–907. https://doi.org/10.1016/j.ophtha.2015.12.024.
79. Jouhi S, Jager MJ, De Geus SJR, Desjardins L, Eide N, Grange J-D, et al. The small fatal choroidal melanoma study. A Collaborative Survey by the European Ophthalmic Oncology Group. Am J Ophthalmol. 2019;202:100–8. Pii: Sooo2-9394(19)30062-5. https://doi.org/10.1016/j.ajo.2019.01.031.
80. Cunha Rola AMB, Taktak AFG, Eleuteri A, Kalirai H, Heimann H, Hussain R, et al. Multicenter external validation of the Liverpool uveal melanoma prognosticator online: an OOG collaborative study. Cancers. 2020;12(2):477. https://doi.org/10.3390/cancers12020477.

81. Kujala E, Damato B, Coupland SE, Desjardins L, Bechrakis NE, Grange J-D, Kivela T. Staging of ciliary body and choroidal melanomas based on anatomic extent: a collaborative study by the European Ophthalmic Oncology Group. J Clin Oncol. 2013b;31(22):2825–231. https://doi.org/10.1200/JCO.2012.45.2771.
82. Gallie BL, Simpson ER, Saakyan S, Amiryan A, Valskiy V, Finger PT, et al. (The Ophthalmic Oncology Task Force.) Local recurrence significantly increases the risk of metastatic uveal melanoma. Ophthalmology. 2016;123(1):86–91. https://doi.org/10.1016/j/ophtha.2015.09.014.
83. Onken MD, Worley LA, Char DH, et al. Collaborative Ocular Oncology Report number 1: prospective validation of a multigene prognostic assay in uveal melanoma. Ophthalmology. 2012;119(8):1596–603. https://doi.org/10.1016/j.ophtha.2021.02.017.
84. Robertson AG, Shih J, Yau C, Gibb EA, Mungall KL, Hess JM, et al., Uzunangelov V, et al. Integrative analysis identifies four molecular and clinical subsets in uveal melanoma. Cancer Cell. 2017;32(2):204–220.e15. https://doi.org/10.1016/j.ccell.2017.07.003.
85. Jager MJ, Brouwer NJ, Esmaeli B. The Cancer genome Atlas project: an integrated view of uveal melanoma. Ophthalmology. 2018;125(8):1139–42. https://doi.org/10.1016/j.ophth.2018.03.011.
86. Vichitvejpaisal P, Dalvin LA, Mazloumi M, Ewens KG, Ganguly A, Shields CL. Genetic analysis of uveal melanoma in 658 patients using the cancer genome atlas classification of uveal melanoma as A, B, C, and D. Ophthalmology. 2019;126(10):1445–53. https://doi.org/10.1016/j.ophtha.2019.04.027.
87. Gelmi MC, Bas Z, Malkani K, Ganguly A, Shields CL, Jager MJ. Adding the cancer genome atlas chromosome classes to american joint committee on cancer system offers more precise prognostication in uveal melanoma. Ophthalmology. 2022 Apr;129(4):431–7. https://doi.org/10.1016/j.ophtha.2021.11.018.
88. Wierenga APA, Brouwer NJ, Gelmi MC, Verdijk RM, Stern MH, Bas Z, Malkani K, van Duinen SG, Ganguly A, Kroes WGM, Marinkovic M, Luyten GPM, Shields CL, Jager MJ. Chromosome 3 and 8q aberrations in uveal melanoma show greater impact on survival in patients with light iris versus dark iris color. Ophthalmology. 2022 Apr;129(4):421–30. https://doi.org/10.1016/j.ophtha.2021.11.011.
89. Jager MJ, Shields CL, Cebulla CM, Abdel-Rahman M, Grossniklaus H, Stern M-H, et al. Uveal melanoma. Nat Rev Dis Primers. 2020;6(1):24. https://doi.org/10.1038/s41572-020-0158-0.
90. Rodrigues M, de Koning L, Coupland SE, Jochemsen AG, Marais R, Stern M-H, et al. So close, yet so far: discrepancies between uveal and other melanomas. A position paper from UM Cure 2020. Cancers. 2019;11:1032. https://doi.org/10.3390/cancers11071032.

Ocular Oncology Practice During the COVID-19 Pandemic

Victor M. Villegas and Timothy G. Murray

1 Introduction

Practicing ocular oncology during the COVID-19 pandemic has been an ongoing challenge [1–3]. The constant changes in local, national, and international incidence rates of SARS-CoV-2 have created shifting healthcare policies in our communities, hospitals, and outpatient facilities [4]. Incorporating new technologies such as telemedicine, automated check-in/checkout, and virtual waiting rooms has optimized our abilities to care for our patients without sacrificing quality and safety [5]. The leading ocular oncology practices seamlessly adapt to the patients' needs in order to deliver the best possible service [6]. The following chapter will provide clinical care strategies during the COVID-19 pandemic to help ocular oncologists achieve effective utilization of available resources during this or other pandemics and ensure the safety of patients and healthcare workers.

2 Clinic Evaluations

There is international consensus that all patients with malignant tumors should continue to undergo a complete ophthalmological examination, relevant testing, possible biopsy, and corresponding definitive therapy [1–3, 7]. Therefore, most ocular oncologists continue to work regardless of the ongoing pandemic. However, altering the ocular oncology practice to accommodate for new and follow-up patients at times when many patients may have limited or delayed access to medical care can create new challenges [1–3, 8, 9].

Understanding the individual characteristics of your practice will maximize the efforts to adapt to this new reality [10, 11]. Established practices may acclimatize differently than new ones. Surgically driven physicians may also employ different strategies to evaluate patients safely and in a timely fashion as compared to medical practices.

Similar to pre-COVID-19, one of the most critical aspects that defines utilization of resources of any practice is clinical volume. Small (25 patients/day), medium (50 patients/day), and large (75 patients/day) volume practices have different staffing, imaging, and clinical support requirements. It is important to continually reassess clinical volume (new evaluations vs. follow-up vs. procedures) and resource allocation as the clinic volumes change during the COVID-19 pandemic.

3 Screening and Triage

To avoid a significant bottleneck at the front desk and unnecessary COVID-19 exposure, a shift toward online or by phone appointments and registration should be undertaken [1, 2]. New and follow-up patients should undergo telephone triage to ensure that the face-to-face evaluation is appropriate, to ensure that the patient is not at high risk of COVID-19 infection, or has had contact with any known or suspected COVID-19 patient. Specific questions regarding fever, shortness of breath, cough, and malaise during the last 14 days should be performed. Many patients exposed to COVID-19 or suspected to have the disease may have their appointment delayed. However, patients with intractable eye pain, visual loss, photophobia, or malignancy may need to be evaluated in a pre-designated area with complete personal protective equipment (PPE) prior to referral to for COVID-19 treatment [7]. If the patient is asymptomatic or has mild disease, in-

V. M. Villegas
Department of Ophthalmology, University of Puerto Rico, San Juan, PR, USA

Bascom Palmer Eye Institute, University of Miami Miller School of Medicine, Miami, FL, USA

Department of Surgery, Ponce Health Sciences University, Ponce, PR, USA
e-mail: v.villegas@villegasmd.com

T. G. Murray (✉)
Miami Ocular Oncology and Retina (MOOR), Miami, FL, USA
e-mail: tmurray@murraymd.com

B. V. Chawla, M. E. Aronow (eds.), *Global Perspectives in Ocular Oncology*, https://doi.org/10.1007/978-3-031-08250-4_40

person evaluation may be performed after resolution of disease or negative testing is documented. We recommend a second level of triage for all new patients prior to in-person encounters.

Onsite triage may be performed with temperature screening and COVID-19 questionnaires. Any patient with a positive screening test should be isolated and disposition by the physician should promptly performed.

4 Check-In and Checkout

Front desk holdup due to patients arriving at unscheduled times and/or rapid turnover of follow-up patients should be avoided [1, 2]. Small practices may prefer having patients call the reception to check in as soon as they are in the parking lot or outside the building. Medium or larger practices may consider an online automated receptionist. Once the patient's physical presence is needed, communication can be performed via the designated platform to have them then walk into the clinic.

Checkout may also be adapted to minimize physical proximity with the front desk staff. In general cash payments should be avoided during the COVID-19 pandemic. Copays and deductibles can be performed electronically without the patient being physically at the front desk. Follow-up times may also be communicated by phone, email, or online platforms.

5 Waiting Rooms

A packed waiting room may be a terrifying experience for immunocompromised patients undergoing chemotherapy during the COVID-19 pandemic [4]. The classic waiting room setup with rows of chairs stacked next to each other may not be practical during these times. Signage to limit certain chairs in the waiting room may be a reasonable strategy to employ social distancing measures inside the office. However, the most powerful tool to minimize the time patient's wait inside medical offices and potential exposure to infection is to have a virtual waiting room. Having patients wait in their car may be the best strategy to decompress the clinical space. A critical component of an efficient virtual waiting room is to know how much time it takes for patients to get to your physical office once the staff contacts them. The existing waiting room in your practice may be repurposed using social distancing for patients that are awaiting dilation, have particular mobility problems, or are next in line for physical evaluation. Training the staff to properly manage the virtual waiting room may take some time. However, once in place, this process may allow some practices to grow beyond their pre-COVID-19 volumes. Large volume practices may consider investing in a coordinator that focuses on keeping the virtual waiting room in synchrony.

6 Electronic Medical Record

A number of ophthalmology-focused EMRs are available in the market and may help optimize your ocular oncology practice during the pandemic. The most advanced EMRs provide up-to-date government and insurance compliance with seamless optimization of billing. Recent updates in many EMRs have integrated particular features including specific screening questions regarding COVID-19. Prepopulating of the EMR by prior to physical check-in may also be a vital step to minimize encounter time and exposure risk [5]. This may be particularly important to new patients to the practice. Having the staff inquire and electronically upload any radiologic imaging, biopsy results, genetic tests, and previous medical records may also help eliminate handoffs at the front desk. Overall, try to individualize and tailor the EMR to each patient in order to fill the needs of each individual as much as possible. At this time, specifics regarding missed or delayed therapies, medical appointment, and diagnostic studies due to the COVID-19 pandemic should be documented.

7 Multimodal Imaging

Ocular oncologists perform a significant number of imaging studies as compared to other ophthalmologists. Spectral-domain optical coherence tomography (sdOCT), photography, ultrasonography, and angiography are among the most common tests performed. Some practices may consider limiting how many patients undergo advanced testing at peak times during the pandemic; however, to individualize care, it is important to reassess some patients regularly. Consider tailoring your imaging utilization depending on prevalence of COVID-19 in your community.

To decrease the total office physical encounter time, assess if an imaging bottleneck is present for the utilization of imaging [6]. Consider hiring a dedicated ophthalmic photographer or echographer to speed the process and minimize clinic COVID-19 exposure. Practices that have not upgraded to sdOCT angiography should consider it. This could potentially decrease the time allotted to contrast-based angiography and in some situations may provide the dual benefits of standard macular sdOCT and fluorescein angiography. However, considerations regarding computer hardware demands and the extra time associated with performing sdOCT angiography should also be undertaken.

8 Intravitreal and Laser Therapy

Ocular oncologists may treat a wide range of diseases, ranging from radiation retinopathy to vitreoretinal lymphoma, with a myriad of intraocular therapeutic agents [12]. Intravitreal therapy, the most common form of injectable therapy performed in our clinics, may be performed in the physician evaluation room or may be performed in a separate room. Small volume practices with limited space may benefit from performing intravitreal injections in the evaluation room. However, large volume practices will decrease the bottleneck effects of intravitreal injections by using one or more rooms exclusively for intravitreal injections. This also allows for dedicated nurses that monitor and educate the patient before, during, and after intravitreal injections.

Although select patients with stable visual acuity and without new complains may undergo intravitreal therapy without extensive testing or dilation to improve efficiency and minimize exposure risk during the COVID-19 pandemic, the ability to individualize therapy and extend between treatment is reduced with this strategy. Therefore, the physician should weight the risk of additional testing in the office vs. the potential to extend therapy. Switching patients to longer-acting intravitreal agents may provide additional safety.

We have continued to perform photodynamic therapy (PDT) and transpupillary thermotherapy (TTT) at comparable rates as compared to pre-pandemic levels. However, due to the close contact nature of these procedures, we routinely request COVID-19 testing similar to surgical patients. Topical povidone-iodine is effective against coronaviruses and should be used for surgical prep.

9 Clinic Flow and Patient Focus

F [13] However, several unaccountable factors can interfere with ideal flow such as late or too early arriving patients, emergencies, and equipment and staffing availability. The best way to decrease inefficiency in the clinic is to allow regular meetings for staff input. Due to the increasing number details associated with organizing a safe clinic during the COVID-19 pandemic, all the members of the clinical team should help identify the weaknesses associated with reaching synchrony, minimize COVID-19 exposure, and help generate solutions. This may become particularly important as prevalence of COVID-19 evolves, staff availability changes, or new technology is introduced into the practice.

Focus the practice on the process the patient has to encounter during a visit. During the COVID-19 pandemic, immunocompromised patients should be identified and quickly moved through imaging and clinical evaluations. Having the patient feel safe and understand the clinical scenario easily will provide vital reassurance of your expertise. Emboldened and well-educated patients will unquestionably be invested in compliance and optimal clinical outcomes.

10 Universal Precautions

Every person in your clinic, patients and staff, should be considered to be at risk of COVID-19 [1–3]. Protection of healthcare workers is of paramount importance, and universal PPE consisting of surgical mask should be worn by all staff. No attendants should be allowed in the clinical area, except in the case of children and senior citizens where only one attendant should be allowed during consultation. All patients should have surgical mask or a do-it-yourself (DIY) face mask (but not a valved respirator mask). If available, eye protection should also be used by the clinician. Slit-lamp shields and not speaking during slit-lamp biomicroscopic examinations are appropriate. The optimal level of PPE and standard guidelines may continue to change depending on the prevalence of SARS-CoV-2 in the community and availability of PPE resources [14].

11 High Risk of SARS-CoV-2 Patients

Encourage all symptomatic or high-risk patients (i.e., high risk of infection through exposure or travel) for SARS-CoV-2 to stay home, and follow the standard medical recommendations by the Centers for Disease Control and Prevention (CDC) [14]. In the event that a high-risk patient enters the clinic, immediately perform isolation of the patient and undertake further assessment by the physician to determine appropriate management.

Evaluate patients known to have SARS-CoV-2 or deemed to be high risk in a controlled hospital setting with PPE for the mouth, nose, and eyes. All high-risk patients should wear a surgical mask at all times to minimize aerosolization of the virus. Clinical staff should use an N-95 mask, gown, gloves, and eye protection (face shield or goggles) to evaluate and perform procedures in patients considered high risk. The examination room should be thoroughly cleaned after the encounter.

12 Operation Room Safety Protocols

We routinely perform SARS-CoV-2 polymerase chain reaction testing to all patients 24–28 h prior to any interaction at the operating room. This minimizes exposure to some patients. However, this may be difficult if testing is scarce. Despite preoperative testing, it is important to utilize appropriate PPE (N-95 masks) resources available to ensure the safety of everybody inside the operating room [15]. The highest risk procedures include intubation, extubation, manual ventilation, open suctioning of the respiratory tract, high flow nasal oxygen, administration of humified oxygen, surgeries involving high-speed drilling, and mucosal exposure. Overall, local anesthesia with monitored anesthesia care is preferred over general anesthesia. In cases were general anesthesia is performed, an interval of 20–30 min between cases is recommended for aerosol clearance. Diathermy cauterization should be minimized due to risks for aerosolization [16, 17]. Instead, bipolar cautery on low settings is preferred. High vacuum and high flow devices should be utilized when available to minimize aerosols, including under the drapes during monitored anesthesia care.

Endoscopic surgery, high-speed drilling, and sinus exposure should be avoided. In cases were these procedures need to be undertaken, full PPE including face shields should be implemented.

13 Radiation Oncology Guidelines

The specifics regarding radiation oncology guidelines during the COVID-19 pandemic have been previously described [18, 19]. Most external beam radiotherapy is fractioned and treatment is extended over 4–6 weeks. Due to the COVID-19 pandemic, a shift toward hypofractionated external beam radiation protocols is underway to minimize COVID-19 exposure in immunocompromised patients. Most currently, brachytherapy protocols remain unchanged.

14 Disease-Specific Recommendations

1. Uveal Melanoma

   Uveal melanoma continues to represent a diagnostic and therapeutic challenge in spite of being the most common primary intraocular malignant tumor in adults (Fig. 1) [20]. The mechanisms and risk factors leading to primary uveal melanoma continue to be poorly elucidated [21]. The incidence of uveal malignant melanoma has been reported to be as high as 1 case per 200,000 per year. During the last 20 years, there has been widespread use of brachytherapy for the treatment of uveal melanoma; however, significant morbidity and mortality is still associated with this disease [22].

   Despite the pandemic, we continue to evaluate initial patients with uveal melanoma as soon as possible because most patients have significant anxiety regarding the diagnosis. However, we perform a chart review prior to evaluation in order to determine if the patient truly warrants and expedited appointment. During the initial evaluation, we perform a complete ophthalmological exam including sdOCT, ultrasonography (A/B scan), and fluorescein and indocyanine green angiography. Currently, management options and indication of brachytherapy versus enucleation remain unchanged [23, 24]. We continue to perform brachytherapy with retrobulbar block and monitored anesthesia care. Screening for metastatic disease continues to be performed based on gene expression profile with patients with high-risk tumors undergoing lifelong yearly abdominal magnetic resonance imaging with and without intravenous gadolinium.

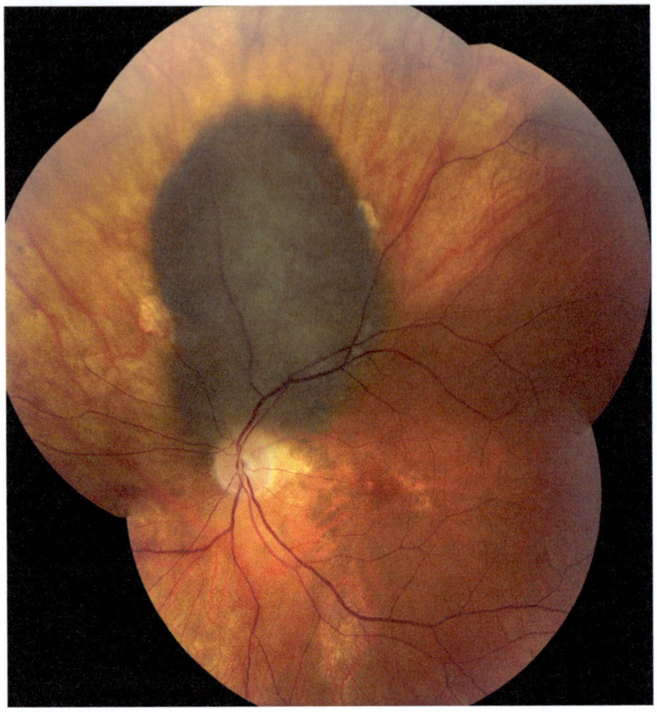

Fig. 1 Color fundus montage photography of a juxtapapillary medium choroidal melanoma

   Follow-up of patients after primary therapy remains every 3–4 months to monitor for the development of radiation retinopathy. Once radiation retinopathy is detected, intravitreal therapy with anti-VEGF agents is guided by sdOCT and performed every 4–6 weeks [25]. We have shifted to using intravitreal triamcinolone acetonide more frequently to allow a longer interval between treatments (8–12 weeks). However, monotherapy with intravitreal corticosteroids is limited by intraocular pressure increase. Once an increase in intraocular pressure is documented, we start patients with topical glaucoma therapy and return to anti-VEGF agent monotherapy until intraocular pressure is less than 20 mmHg [26].

2. High-Risk Choroidal Nevi and Small Choroidal Melanoma

   Small choroidal melanoma (less than 2.5 mm in thickness) continues to represent a diagnostic and therapeutic challenge [27]. Definitive treatment of small choroidal melanoma continues to be controversial because of the similarities with atypical choroidal nevi. Under normal circumstances, we typically observe high-risk lesions every 3–4 months. If growth is documented, we perform a two-pronged approach: fine needle aspiration biopsy and concomitant thermotherapy [28]. However, because of the ongoing pandemic, we are being more conservative with follow-up of high-risk nevi and may follow-up select lesions every 6 months.
3. Retinoblastoma

   Retinoblastoma (RB) continues to be the most common primary intraocular malignancy of childhood (Fig. 2). However, enucleation continues to be the international gold standard of management [29]. During the last 20 years, globe-salvaging therapies with chemoreduction and focal consolidation have significantly improved the morbidity associated with RB therapy [30]. Still, some developing countries with limited access to medical care continue to struggle with the high morbidity and mortality associated with the natural course of the disease. During the pandemic, RB continues to be a diagnostic and therapeutic priority for ocular oncologists.

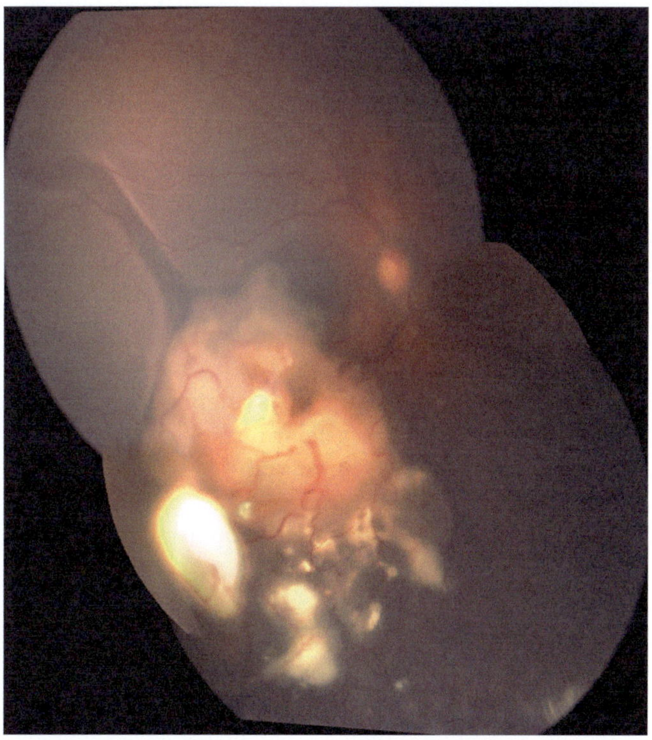

Fig. 2 Color fundus montage photography of exophytic Group D retinoblastoma with diffuse subretinal seeding

Due to the aggressive and malignant nature, early diagnosis is of critical importance because small tumors have the best prognosis. We evaluate all children with leukocoria or suspected to have an intraocular mass within the first week under anesthesia.

Management of RB tumors remains mostly unchanged as compared to pre-pandemic times and requires a multidisciplinary approach that may include an ocular oncologist, pediatric oncologist, pediatric ophthalmologist, pediatrician, interventional radiologist, and ocular pathologist. Individualized treatment, considering factors such as the International Classification (IC) of RB, laterality, location of tumors, age of patient, family history, and prior treatment must be considered [1–3]. Although RB treatment is aimed at child survival, globe salvage and preservation of vision are important secondary goals. Early diagnosis remains the most crucial step in decreasing morbidity and mortality.

We continue to evaluate all children with active RB monthly under anesthesia. We routinely perform general inhalational anesthesia to avoid the risks associated with intubation and intravenous line placement [31]. Because of the risk of aerosols during this procedure, we perform SARS-CoV-2 polymerase chain reaction testing to all patients 48 h prior to examination to screen for any potential exposure [32]. Overall, over 95% of our procedures are performed without intravenous access placement, and mean procedural time is 20–30 min. We perform complete ophthalmologic exams including fundus photography, ultrasonography, laser therapy, intravitreal chemotherapy, and/or replacement of ocular prosthesis.

Our primary therapy consists of a three-drug intra-arterial chemotherapy (IAC) treatment (carboplatin, melphalan, and topotecan) in unilateral or bilateral cases. In the three-drug therapy, infusion dose ranges are 2.5–7.5 mg for melphalan, 0.3–0.6 mg for topotecan, and 25–50 mg for carboplatin. Especial attention to melphalan dosing in bilateral tandem infusions should be placed as to not exceed the myelosuppressive systemic dose (melphalan 0.5 mg/kg) [33]. In small infants, especially less than 10 kg, this may limit melphalan to only one eye per monthly IAC.

Sequential intravenous chemotherapy followed by intra-arterial chemotherapy (bridge chemotherapy) for young infants with retinoblastoma may be considered in cases where cannulation of the ophthalmic artery is not possible. We routinely use the classic three-drug intravenous treatment (carboplatin, vincristine, and etoposide) for these cases. However, significant bone marrow suppression, ototoxicity, nephrotoxicity, and risk of induction of secondary cancers have been reported with higher cumulative doses. Controversy continues to be present regarding the role of systemic chemotherapy in the prevention of trilateral RB. The combination of systemic and/or intra-arterial chemotherapy with focal ablative treatments has been shown to have better globe salvage rates than chemotherapy alone in both early and advanced RB.

Laser consolidation therapy is performed during monthly evaluation under anesthesia. Small tumors (<1.5 DD in base diameter) may only require transpupillary thermotherapy. However, most RB patients need combination therapy that includes either IAC or intravenous chemotherapy. Transpupillary thermotherapy is performed with a diode laser (810 nm) on continuous mode with a 1.2-mm spot size. Power ranges from 400 to 1500 mW with a total duration of treatment from 180 to 320 s. We perform confluent laser over the tumor with overlapping areas. While performing treatment, we move to a new area over the surface of the tumor once we detect a subtle change in color or contraction of retinal/tumoral tissue.

Screening for extraocular disease with neuroimaging continues to be performed. We routinely order brain and orbits magnetic resonance imaging with and without intravenous gadolinium during the first week after diagnosis. We repeat neuroimaging yearly; however, in advanced cases, we may consider magnetic resonance imaging two to three times per year.

4. Uveal Metastasis

The most common malignant intraocular tumors in adults continue to be uveal metastasis (Fig. 3). During the pandemic, we continue to evaluate patients suspected to have uveal metastasis promptly because early treatment helps palliate the visual burden. Oftentimes, many of these patients are afraid to lose their vision during the last months of life. However, promptly starting intravitreal therapy with anti-VEGF agents or corticosteroids may help reduce the exudative components while the systemic treatments take effect. In advanced cases, radiation (external beam radiation or brachytherapy) may help decrease the intraocular tumor burden. When metastatic disease is present, we routinely obtain a brain and orbits magnetic resonance imaging with and without intravenous gadolinium prior to the initial evaluation. In some advanced cases, concomitant orbital and brain radiation may be considered.

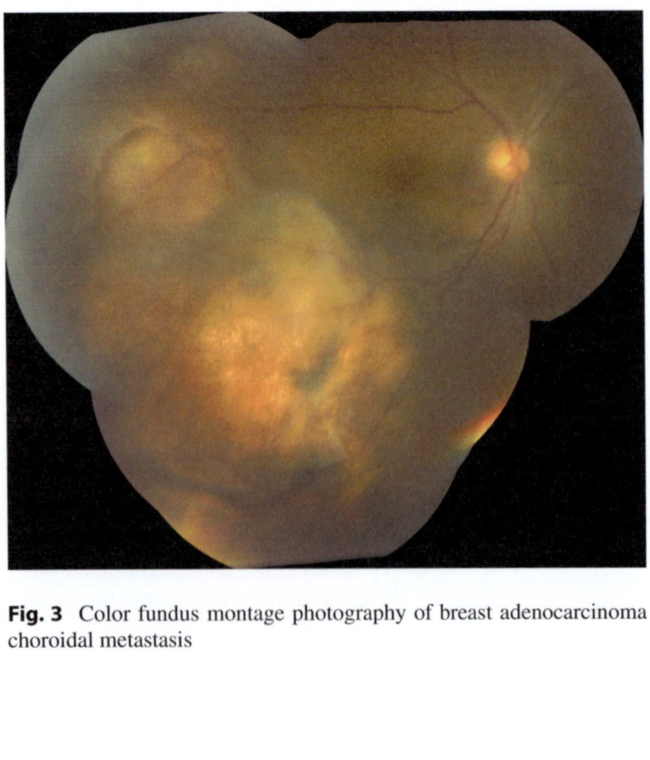

Fig. 3 Color fundus montage photography of breast adenocarcinoma choroidal metastasis

5. Vitreoretinal Lymphoma

Primary vitreoretinal lymphoma (PVRL), also known as primary central nervous system lymphoma, is a subgroup of lymphoma that may involve the brain, eyes, and meninges [34]. Most commonly, it is a high-grade B-cell lymphoma that oftentimes gets diagnosed by the ophthalmologist first. The highly lethal neoplastic process is most prevalent among older immunocompromised individuals. Intraocular presentation may precede central nervous system involvement by years. All patients referred for suspected PVRL continue to be evaluated within 1 week due to the highly aggressive nature of this neoplastic process. During the pandemic, we routinely order a brain and orbits magnetic resonance imaging with and without intravenous gadolinium prior to initial evaluation.

Diagnosis is typically performed with a vitreous sample. However, patients with evidence of brain or leptomeningeal lymphoma involvement may undergo diagnostic lumbar puncture [1, 2, 34]. Once diagnosis is confirmed, a treatment plan can be implemented. Patients without any central nervous system disease may undergo targeted ocular therapies with constant screening for signs of central nervous system progression. Controversy continues regarding systemic treatment in patients who only have evidence of intraocular disease.

Primary treatment depends on the stage of the disease. Patients with central nervous system involvement may receive high-dose methotrexate in combination with other agents [1, 2] Rituximab, a chimeric monoclonal antibody against the protein CD20, may also be used as primary systemic therapy. Historically, intraocular disease has been treated with external beam radiotherapy (either palliative or definitive). To avoid the late complications of radiation, most ocular oncologists have shifted to intravitreal therapies (methotrexate or rituximab) for PVRL. However, during the pandemic, we have started to more frequently convert patients to external beam radiotherapy to avoid repetitive long-term treatments in immunocompromised patients and minimize unnecessary COVID-19 exposure.

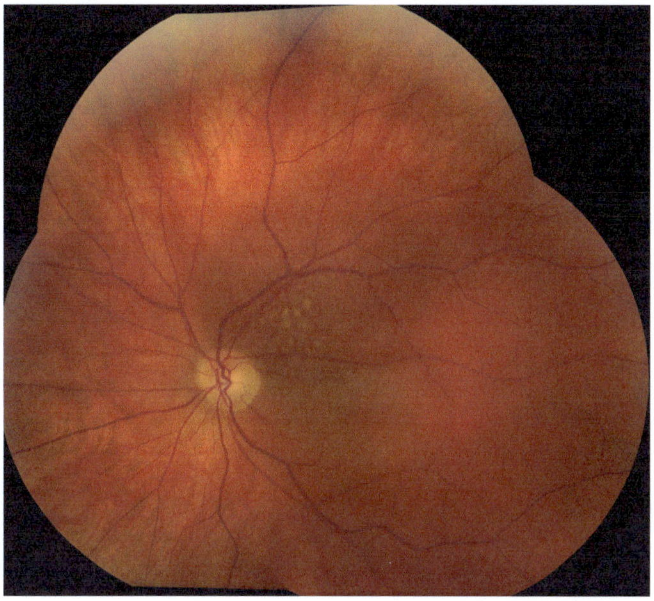

Fig. 4 Color fundus montage photography of macular circumscribed choroidal hemangioma

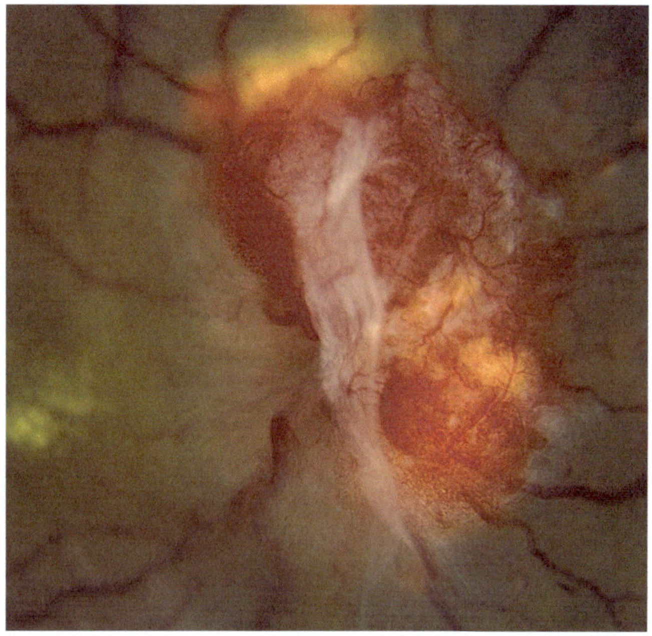

Fig. 5 Color fundus photography of exophytic epipapillary capillary hemangioblastoma in association with von Hippel-Lindau

6. Benign Intraocular Tumors

Hemangiomas of the retina or choroid are the most common benign intraocular tumors (Figs. 4 and 5). Despite their benign nature, significant visual decline may be present due to retinal detachments and intraretinal exudation [1–3, 7] During the pandemic, we may delay the evaluation of peripheral retinal or choroidal hemangiomas that are not visually threatening. However, lesions that are affecting the macula are evaluated within 2 weeks of consultation to avoid further deterioration of vision. Recent evidence suggests that some hemangiomas may respond to intravitreal therapy with anti-VEGF agents [35]. However, some posterior pole lesions may benefit from photodynamic therapy. In peripheral lesions, transpupillary thermotherapy and/or laser photocoagulation may be appropriate. In patients with serous detachments with or without tractional components, we strongly consider pars plana vitrectomy with endolaser therapy. Patients with large (>10 DD in base diameter), diffuse, or multifocal lesions may also be treated with low-dose radiation (external beam radiotherapy or brachytherapy).

Patients with benign intraocular tumors suspected of having systemic disease are particularly important during the COVID-19 pandemic since delay in care may lead to long-term sequela. In particular, patients suspected of having Gardner syndrome (Fig. 6), neurofibromatosis, von Hippel-Lindau (VHL) syndrome, tuberous sclerosis, Wyburn-Mason syndrome, and Sturge-Weber syndrome may need evaluation within 2–3 weeks of referral for diagnostic or therapeutic considerations [36, 37]. Neuroimaging should be available at the time of initial evaluation to minimize any delay in diagnosis and avoid any unnecessary close follow-up. Patients for whom the diagnosis is unclear and a malignant neoplasm is still being considered should be evaluated promptly.

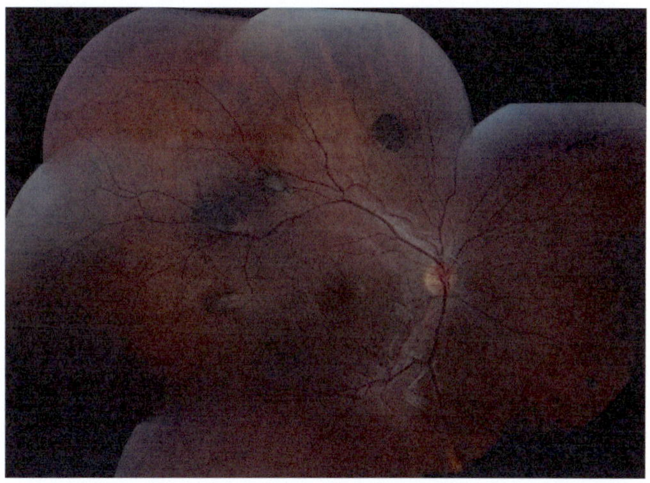

Fig. 6 Color fundus montage photography of multifocal congenital hypertrophy of the retinal pigment epithelium in association with Gardner syndrome

Telemedicine consultation is a reasonable alternative for benign lesions that may be co-managed with a colleague in the community during the COVID-19 pandemic [1–3, 7]. The availability of multimodal imaging (sdOCT, ultrasonography (A/B scan), angiography, photography, neuroimaging) is paramount to minimize any misdiagnosis. We recommend scheduling patients for in-person evaluation at a later date even after successful telemedicine consultation.

7. Conjunctival Tumors

During the pandemic, we have shifted to observation for suspected benign conjunctival lesions. When appropriate, we start topical chemotherapy for ocular surface squamous neoplasia and delay surgical excision [38, 39]. Patients with conjunctival melanoma continue to be managed urgently with wide-margins (>3 mm) surgical excision and cryotherapy. We follow-up select patients with telemedicine consultation during the first 3 months after surgical excision or after starting topical chemotherapy.

8. Eyelid Tumors

Similar to other malignant tumors, eyelid carcinomas, especially sebaceous gland carcinoma, malignant melanoma, and Merkel cell carcinoma, require urgent care. Telemedicine consultation is a reasonable alternative for initial evaluation and triage. Delay in diagnosis and treatment may lead to difficulties in excision at a later date or increase in mortality [40]. Primary management with surgical excision and pathologic analysis should be performed promptly. When indicated, chemotherapy and radiation should not be delayed.

9. Orbital Tumors

During the pandemic, malignant orbital tumors continue to be evaluated urgently due to their aggressive behavior that may progress to optic nerve compromise and death. The most common malignant orbital tumors include rhabdomyosarcoma, primary neuroectodermal tumors (PNET), sarcoma, and optic nerve glioma, lacrimal gland adenoid cystic carcinoma, adenocarcinoma, orbital metastasis, lymphoma, and other high-grade malignancy [1–3, 7]. Similarly to uveal metastasis, orbital metastasis also requires immediate attention for palliative or diagnostic purposes. When diagnosis is unclear, orbital biopsy should not be delayed and primary treatment started following the pre-pandemic standard treatment. Orbital imaging should be available at the time of initial evaluation to minimize any delay in diagnosis and avoid any unnecessary close follow-up [41].

15 Conclusion

During these unprecedented times, providing excellence in medical care requires a patient-centered systematic approach that prioritizes safety and efficiency. Understanding the details in your ocular oncology practice and anticipating the problems as the practice evolves, especially as the COVID-19 pandemic begins to resolve, is an ongoing but important challenge in maintaining outstanding care. Medical care should not be delayed or deferred in patients with malignant ocular tumors during the COVID-19 pandemic; however, implementing safety measures for patients and healthcare workers is crucial to successfully continue to practice ocular oncology. The best medical practices constantly reassess the changing pandemic risks and address them in a team-oriented approach without losing track of their passion for medicine and patient care.

Acknowledgement None of the authors have any financial interest in the material discussed in this chapter.

References

1. Manjandavida FP, Honavar SG, Kim U, et al. Ocular oncology practice guidelines during COVID-19 pandemic—an expert consensus. Indian J Ophthalmol. 2020;68(7):1281–91. https://doi.org/10.4103/ijo.IJO_1669_20.
2. Skalet AH, Allen RC, Shields CL, Wilson MW, Mruthyunjaya P, Gombos DS. Considerations for the management and triage of ocular oncology cases during the COVID-19 pandemic. Ocul Oncol Pathol. 2020;6:219–22.
3. Mazzini C, Pieretti G, Vicini G, Nicolosi C, Giattini D, Calamita R, Santoro N, Giansanti F. Ocular oncology service during the COVID-19 outbreak in Florence (Italy): practical considerations for the management of patients. Eur J Ophthalmol. 2021;31(2):NP4–7.
4. Lim LW, Yip LW, Tay HW, Ang XL, Lee LK, Chin CF, Yong V. Sustainable practice of ophthalmology during COVID-19: challenges and solutions. Graefes Arch Clin Exp Ophthalmol. 2020;258(7):1427–36.
5. Saleem SM, Pasquale LR, Sidoti PA, Tsai JC. Virtual Ophthalmology: telemedicine in a COVID-19 era. Am J Ophthalmol. 2020;216:237–42.
6. Villegas VM, Murray TG. Adapting the retina practice during the SARS-CoV-2 pandemic. Ophthalmol Manage. 2020;24:e1–8.
7. Stuart A. COVID-19 pandemic: ocular tumor triage and care. EyeNet. 2020;23(5). https://www.aao.org/eyenet/article/covid-19-pandemic-ocular-tumor-triage-and-care?april-2020.
8. Emanuel EJ, Persad G, Upshur R, Thome B, Parker M, Glickman A, et al. Fair allocation of scarce medical resources in the time of COVID-19. N Engl J Med. 2020;382(21):2049–55.
9. American College of Surgeons. COVID-19 guidelines for triage of cancer surgery patients. vol. 24. Facs.org; 2020. https://www.facs.org/covid-19/clinical-guidance/elective-case/cancer-surgery.
10. Wong TY, Bandello F. Academic ophthalmology during and after the COVID-19 Pandemic. Ophthalmology. 2020;127(8):e51–2.
11. Chen RWS, Abazari A, Dhar S, Fredrick DR, Friedman IB, Dagi Glass LR, Khouri AS, Kim ET, Laudi J, Park S, Reddy HS, Rosenberg JB, Sandler SF, Shrivastava A, Sun G, Winokur J. Living with COVID-19: a perspective from New York area ophthalmology residency program directors at the epicenter of the pandemic. Ophthalmology. 2020;127(8):e47–8.
12. Villegas VM, Murray TG. Personalized medicine and retinoblastoma treatment. Retina Specialist. 2019;5:14–6.
13. Han D, Suneja A. Make your clinics flow with synchrony: a practical and innovative guide for physicians, managers, and staff. Quality Press; 2016.
14. Mungmungpuntipantip R, Wiwanitkit V. Ocular manifestation, eye protection, and COVID-19. Graefes Arch Clin Exp Ophthalmol. 2020;258(6):1339.

15. Leung EH, Flynn HW Jr, Gayer S, Yeh S, Berrocal AM, Olmos de Koo LC, Chen RWS, Albini TA, Foroozan R. Clinical and perioperative management in ophthalmology during the COVID-19 pandemic. Int Ophthalmol Clin. 2020;60(3):141–58.
16. Patel AM, Fernandez-Miranda J, Hwang PH, Nayak JV, Dodd R, Sajjadi H. Precautions for endoscopic transnasal skull base surgery during the COVID-19 pandemic. Neurosurgery. 2020. https://www.entnet.org/sites/default/files/uploads/covid-19_endosb_lettertoeditor_neurosurgery_update3.23.20.pdf.
17. America Academy of Otolaryngology-Head and Neck Surgery. Academy supports CMS, offers specific nasal policy. Vol. 26. ENTnet.org; 2020. https://www.entnet.org/content/academy-supports-cms-offers-specific-nasal-policy.
18. Nagar H, Formenti SC. Cancer and COVID-19—potentially deleterious effects of delaying radiotherapy. Nat Rev Clin Oncol. 2020;17:332–4.
19. Filippi AR, Russi E, Magrini SM, Corvo R. Letter from Italy: first practical indications for radiation therapy departments during COVID-19 outbreak. Int J Radiat Oncol Biol Phys. 2020;107(3):597–9. https://doi.org/10.1016/j.ijrobp.2020.03.007.
20. Williams BK Jr, Di Nicola M, Lucio-Alvarez JA, Lally DR, Shields CL. Choroidal melanoma simulating adenoma of the retinal pigment epithelium arising at the site of congenital hypertrophy of the retinal pigment epithelium. Ocul Oncol Pathol. 2020;6(1):39–43.
21. Walter SD, Chao DL, Feuer W, Schiffman J, Char DH, Harbour JW. Prognostic implications of tumor diameter in association with gene expression profile for uveal melanoma. JAMA Ophthalmol. 2016;134(7):734–40. https://doi.org/10.1001/jamaophthalmol.2016.0913.
22. Jampol LM, Moy CS, Murray TG, Reynolds SM, Albert DM, Schachat AP, Diddie KR, Engstrom RE Jr, Finger PT, Hovland KR, Joffe L, Olsen KR, Wells CG, COMS Follow-up of Plaqued Eyes Working Group. The COMS randomized trial of iodine 125 brachytherapy for choroidal melanoma: IV. Local treatment failure and enucleation in the first 5 years after brachytherapy. COMS Report No. 19. Ophthalmology. 2020;127(4S):S148–57.
23. Williams BK Jr, Di Nicola M. Ocular oncology-primary and metastatic malignancies. Med Clin North Am. 2021;105(3):531–50.
24. Boldt HC, Murray TG, Binkley EM. Studies evaluating visual outcomes after brachytherapy in uveal melanoma-strengths and limitations of current investigations. JAMA Ophthalmol. 2020;138(2):146–7.
25. Murray TG, Latiff A, Villegas VM, Gold AS. Aflibercept for radiation maculopathy study: a prospective, randomized clinical study. Ophthalmol Retina. 2019;3(7):561–6.
26. Villegas VM, Gold AS, Wildner A, Latiff A, Murray TG. Intravitreal triamcinolone acetonide: a "real world" analysis of visual acuity, pressure and outcomes. Int J Ophthalmol. 2016;9(5):789–91.
27. Sobrin L, Schiffman JC, Markoe AM, Murray TG. Outcomes of iodine 125 plaque radiotherapy after initial observation of suspected small choroidal melanomas: a pilot study. Ophthalmology. 2005;112(10):1777–83.
28. Murray TG, Villegas VM, Bach A, Gold AS. Five-year follow-up of microincisional vitrectomy surgery, endolaser tumor ablation, and gene-expression profiling in small uveal melanoma. J Vitreoretin Dis. 2020.
29. Villegas VM, Hess DJ, Wildner A, Gold AS, Murray TG. Retinoblastoma. Curr Opin Ophthalmol. 2013;24(6):581–8.
30. Scelfo C, Francis JH, Khetan V, Jenkins T, Marr B, Abramson DH, Shields CL, Pe'er J, Munier F, Berry J, Harbour JW, Yarovoy A, Lucena E, Murray TG, Bhagia P, Paysse E, Tuncer S, Chantada GL, Moll AC, Ushakova T, Plager DA, Ziyovuddin I, Leal CA, Materin MA, Ji XD, Cursino JW, Polania R, Kiratli H, All-Ericsson C, Kebudi R, Honavar SG, Vishnevskia-Dai V, Epelman S, Daniels AB, Ling JD, Traore F, Ramirez-Ortiz MA. An international survey of classification and treatment choices for group D retinoblastoma. Int J Ophthalmol. 2017;10(6):961–7.
31. Vigoda MM, Latiff A, Murray TG, Tutiven JL, Berrocal AM, Gayer S. Can children undergoing ophthalmologic examinations under anesthesia be safely anesthetized without using an IV line? Clin Ophthalmol. 2011;5:503–8.
32. Ashkenazy N, Orihuela G, Rodriguez LI, Negron CI, Harbour JW, Berrocal AM. Use of a modified plastic viewing system for safer general anesthesia care in pediatric ophthalmic surgery during the COVID-19 pandemic. Ophthalmic Surg Lasers Imaging Retina. 2020;51(11):651–2.
33. Sweid A, Hammoud B, Weinberg JH, Texakalidis P, Xu V, Shivashankar K, Baldassari MP, Das S, Ramesh S, Tjoumakaris S, Shields CL, Ancona-Lezama D, Lim LS, Dalvin LA, Jabbour P. Intra-arterial chemotherapy for retinoblastoma in infants 10 kg: 74 treated eyes with 222 IAC sessions. AJNR Am J Neuroradiol. 2020;41(7):1286–92.
34. Grommes C, Rubenstein JL, DeAngelis LM, Ferreri AJM, Batchelor TT. Comprehensive approach to diagnosis and treatment of newly diagnosed primary CNS lymphoma. Neuro-Oncology. 2019;21:296–305.
35. Russell JF, Villegas VM, Schwartz SG, Weng CY, Davis JL, Flynn HW Jr, Harbour JW. Multimodal imaging in the diagnosis of exophytic juxtapapillary retinal capillary hemangioblastoma. Am J Ophthalmol. 2021;225:128–36.
36. Villegas VM, Schwartz SG, Flynn HW Jr, Capó H, Berrocal AM, Murray TG, Harbour JW. Distinguishing torpedo maculopathy from similar lesions of the posterior segment. Ophthalmic Surg Lasers Imaging Retina. 2014;45(3):222–6.
37. Bach A, Gold AS, Villegas VM, Wildner AC, Ehlies FJ, Murray TG. Spontaneous exudative retinal detachment in a patient with Sturge-Weber, vol. 1. Eye Vis; 2014. p. 7.
38. Al Bayyat G, Arreaza-Kaufman D, Venkateswaran N, Galor A, Karp CL. Update on pharmacotherapy for ocular surface squamous neoplasia. Eye Vis (Lond). 2019;6:24.
39. Karp CL, Mercado C, Venkateswaran N, Ruggeri M, Galor A, Garcia A, Sivaraman KR, Fernandez MP, Bermudez A, Dubovy SR. Use of high-resolution optical coherence tomography in the surgical management of ocular surface squamous neoplasia: a pilot study. Am J Ophthalmol. 2019;206:17–31.
40. Owen JL, Kibbi N, Worley B, Kelm RC, Wang JV, Barker CA, Behshad R, Bichakjian CK, Bolotin D, Bordeaux JS, Bradshaw SH, Cartee TV, Chandra S, Cho NL, Choi JN, Council ML, Demirci H, Eisen DB, Esmaeli B, Golda N, Huang CC, Ibrahim SF, Jiang SB, Kim J, Kuzel TM, Lai SY, Lawrence N, Lee EH, Leitenberger JJ, Maher IA, Mann MW, Minkis K, Mittal BB, Nehal KS, Neuhaus IM, Ozog DM, Petersen B, Rotemberg V, Samant S, Samie FH, Servaes S, Shields CL, Shin TM, Sobanko JF, Somani AK, Stebbins WG, Thomas JR, Thomas VD, Tse DT, Waldman AH, Wong MK, Xu YG, Yu SS, Zeitouni NC, Ramsay T, Reynolds KA, Poon E, Alam M. Sebaceous carcinoma: evidence-based clinical practice guidelines. Lancet Oncol. 2019;20(12):e699–714.
41. de la Vega G, Villegas VM, Velazquez J, Barrios M, Murray TG, Samy Elhammady M, Sidani C. Intraorbital granular cell tumor ophthalmologic and radiologic findings. Neuroradiol J. 2015;28(2):140–4.

Pearls from a Mentor and Legend in Ophthalmic Pathology and Oncology

Anna M. Stagner

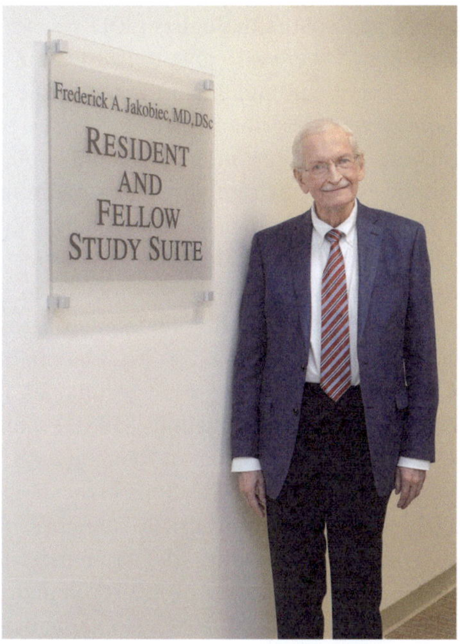

Frederick A. Jakobiec, M.D., D.Sc.

1 Introduction

Known to some by the three-letter code printed on the glass slides he reviewed as "FAJ," and to others as "Dr. J," or just "Fred," Dr. Frederick A. Jakobiec left countless trainees, mentees, and colleagues with lessons on an academically productive, but also a happy and fulfilling, career in medicine. Combining expertise in clinical ophthalmology, anatomic and ophthalmic pathology, and ocular oncology, Dr. Jakobiec became a uniquely niche expert and instilled a passion for learning in his students and colleagues. The following are four poignant lessons, among the many that are a part of his legacy.

A. M. Stagner (✉)
Department of Ophthalmology, Massachusetts Eye and Ear;
Department of Pathology, Massachusetts General Hospital,
Boston, MA, USA
e-mail: ASTAGNER@mgh.harvard.edu

2 Study the Work of Others with Different Perspectives, Apply and Modify such Knowledge to One's Own Area of Investigation, and Share with New Audiences

Dr. Jakobiec mastered the concept of the merging and swapping of knowledge between fields that traditionally have little overlap in clinical practice or readership. Bridging the worlds of diagnostic surgical pathology, ophthalmic pathology, ophthalmology, and ocular oncology, he chose to publish most of his work in the ophthalmologic literature. Even if the topic of discussion was heavy in surgical pathology concepts, he selected ophthalmology journals for manuscript submission and always included relevant clinical pearls and photographs. He taught that the pathologist should involve all of the surgeons whose patients' histopathology was being described in the authorship of a scientific publication (and vice versa). Clinical ophthalmology colleagues were exposed to, and many gained an appreciation for, pathology, through detailed descriptions and illustrations of dermatopathology, hematopathology, and soft tissue pathology in his writings on such topics as they applied to the eye and ocular adnexa. Other surgical pathologists could be quoted as saying that "he did not sign out a case without also publishing it"; meaning, he either had new insight into the entity or a new perspective from a clinician's point of view. In many cases, he simply wanted to share an amusing case with fellow ophthalmologists.

Two examples of the application of concepts studied and/or originally described in anatomic and dermatopathology to ophthalmic pathology are sebaceous neoplasia and conjunctival melanocytic proliferations. In addition to sharing such

B. V. Chawla, M. E. Aronow (eds.), *Global Perspectives in Ocular Oncology*, https://doi.org/10.1007/978-3-031-08250-4_41

entities with the ophthalmic and ocular oncology community, modifications were needed in the diagnostic and treatment algorithms of such entities in the unique environment of the eye and ocular adnexa.

Dr. Jakobiec reported a case of eyelid sebaceous carcinoma (SC) in a patient with visceral malignancies, and then described unusual periocular sebaceous tumors in patients with Muir-Torre syndrome, before and after the syndrome had an official name [1, 2]. Crossing back over into the clinical realm, based on an understanding of the unique growth pattern of sebaceous carcinoma especially within the conjunctival epithelium, a paper was published on treatment of intraepithelial spread of SC with cryotherapy to avoid exenteration, as well as the occurrence of SC in all four eyelids after radiotherapy to the face [3, 4]. Decades later, he revisited the topic of SC and applied the concepts of immunohistochemistry (IHC) previously described in the diagnosis of skin SC. Periocular SC, a basaloid tumor, could be distinguished from basal cell carcinoma or squamous cell carcinoma with clear cell features with the aid of IHC stains for androgen receptor and adipophilin [5, 6]. The identification of subtle, single cell pagetoid spread was also aided with the use of nuclear stains for androgen receptor and p16 [6]. Dr. Jakobiec also described several unusual architectural patterns of SC including a papillary growth pattern and the Borst-Jadassohn phenomenon [7, 8]. Varied and unique patterns of growth of not only carcinoma but a range of benign sebaceous tumors including sebaceoma and those tumors uniquely seen in Muir-Torre syndrome (many also with a papillary or villous architecture) were also reported in detail [9–13]. Using modern polymerase chain reaction (PCR)-based techniques later in his career, Dr. Jakobiec showed the absence of human papillomavirus (HPV) infection in SC, despite blocklike nuclear and cytoplasmic staining for p16 (a surrogate marker for high-risk HPV in other tumors and anatomic sites). Finally, again straddling between histopathology and clinical treatment in the area of immune checkpoint inhibition, a paper was published showing high expression of programmed death ligand 1 (PD-L1) in SC, a tumor without current therapeutic alternatives for locally aggressive or metastatic disease [14, 15].

The study of conjunctival melanocytic neoplasia, including nevi, melanoma, and premalignant melanocytic proliferations is another example of sharing, expanding upon, and comparing and contrasting principles of dermatopathology with ophthalmic pathology and ocular oncology, from both diagnostic and treatment perspectives. Spanning nearly 40 years, Dr. Jakobiec studied the treatment [16], the ultrastructure [17], and the immunophenotypes of conjunctival melanoma and its precursors [18]. Principles of banality in nevi were compared and contrasted with cutaneous melanocytic nevi, including the description of variant benign nevi that also occur on the ocular surface. For example, he described the common phenomenon of a robust inflammatory infiltrate in adolescent conjunctival nevi, often a concerning feature in cutaneous melanocytic proliferations. In contrast, the applicability of HMB-45 gradient staining (as is seen in benign cutaneous nevi) is a phenomenon that appears congruent in benign conjunctival nevi [18, 19]. Using the principles of head and neck lentigo maligna-type melanoma and its precursors in conceptualizing conjunctival melanocytic proliferations, Dr. Jakobiec introduced one of several new terminological classifications of "primary acquired melanosis" to the ophthalmic community. This editorial aimed to describe precursor atypical lentiginous and nested junctional conjunctival melanocytic proliferations in a manner that more accurately portrayed the histopathology of such lesions. This was also an attempt at allowing for better communication between ophthalmic and dermatopathologists, dermatologists, and ophthalmologists [20].

Ophthalmologists were also able to learn about the clinical details of benign and malignant tumors of the orbit that were previously well-described in the soft tissue pathology literature. These tumors are more commonly found in the deep soft tissues of the extremities or retroperitoneum, but also occur in the orbit: examples illustrated by Dr. Jakobiec in the ophthalmic literature in the 1970s–1980s include leiomyoma/leiomyosarcoma, fibrous histiocytoma, fibrosarcoma, hemangiopericytoma (the previous term for solitary fibrous tumor), and liposarcoma [21–26]. Later in his career, using IHC and molecular diagnostic techniques including fluorescence in situ hybridization (FISH)- and next-generation sequencing (NGS)-based fusion assays, he summarized concepts of gene translocations in the diagnosis and prognosis of, particularly, soft tissue sarcomas, including liposarcoma, synovial sarcoma, rhabdomyosarcoma, and biphenotypic sinonasal sarcoma [27–30]. Although certainly not the first to describe any of these entities, he was able to summarize the unique clinical features that may characterize such tumors in the orbit, as well as the pertinent histopathology and necessary molecular genetic tests needed for diagnosis, for ophthalmologists.

3 Physicians and Scientists Should Study What They Love, Even if It Does Not Fit the Mold, and…

3.1 …Even If One Takes an Unconventional Path or Studies an Unusual Combination of Fields

In the course of any student's formal or informal education, they will meet a teacher who exhibits palpable excitement for a chosen field. Regardless of the topic and the student's prior interest in such a field, the student becomes equally enthralled with the subject matter. The same phenomenon happens among medical students and physician trainees. A passionate, compassionate physician can inspire a trainee to enter a field of medicine they had not previously entertained, in an attempt to feel the same way about their career choice as their excited mentor. Dr. Jakobiec did this for his mentees in the field of ophthalmic pathology. He also derived an enthusiasm for an unconventional career path from his mentors, particularly the pathologist Dr. Lorenz Zimmerman at the Armed Forces Institute of Pathology, the "father" of ophthalmic pathology. A History of Science major at Harvard College, Dr. Jakobiec showed one could combine a love of the arts (particularly history and writing) with that of science; and within science, one could combine a love for anatomic pathology and ophthalmology.

A constant detailed observer (a characteristic of both great ophthalmologists and pathologists), he assumed his role as an eloquent describer of the diseases of the eye and ocular adnexa, both clinically and under the microscope. The pursuit of two residencies was unusual at the time, and is even more unusual now, but he supported continuing formal and informal education in whichever field(s) one found interest.

3.2 ...Even If It Is Not a Popular, Lucrative or Field-Changing Topic

In eye pathology sign-out one morning, a visiting pathology resident, when asked how to characterize an epithelial cyst answered, "It does not matter; it is a benign cyst." Dr. Jakobiec could not have disagreed more. The self-described "king of cysts," he loved postulating which structure each cystic cavity was derived from in order to have its distinct epithelial lining or contents. Because this truly interested him, and even if he felt the topic was not necessarily of interest to cancer biologists, he published over 40 articles describing the unique histopathologic, histochemical, and immunohistochemical features of conjunctival, orbital, eyelid skin, and lacrimal derived cysts. Each case or collection of cases was used to illustrate basic principles of ocular embryology, anatomy, and pathology.

An example of an aesthetically pleasing cyst histopathologically that was ultimately found to be clinically relevant was a cyst he descriptively termed "intratarsal keratinous cyst" [31]. Mimicking a chalazion (on examination) or an epidermoid cyst (histologically), the distinct eosinophilic cuticular lining signified derivation from the sebaceous/Meibomian gland duct. These intratarsal cysts are treated with complete excision to avoid recurrence, unlike most cysts derived from the pilosebaceous apparatus.

He particularly enjoyed postulating on the origin of cysts lined by types of epithelia not normally found at a particular anatomic site (a complex intratarsal cyst with a mixed ciliated, respiratory type, and squamous epithelial lining [32] or a conjunctival implantation cyst in orbicularis muscle) [33], or those of anatomic sites that less commonly form cysts, such as the lacrimal drainage system [34, 35]. Dr. Jakobiec also believed that eccrine glands were not usually present at the eyelid margin or in the pretarsal eyelid skin and that hidrocystomas (cysts encountered almost daily in ophthalmic pathology) were nearly all apocrine in nature. He convincingly supported his theory in an elaborately illustrated study of apocrine hidrocystomas, beginning with a review of the normal pilosebaceous-apocrine unit for ophthalmologists [36, 37].

His publications, especially later in life, started with single cases he found interesting, even if they were not necessarily rare or had been described before at other anatomic sites. Starting from nearly shrieking with excitement about the case during sign-out, he would write pages, with exceptional vocabulary, musing on the histogenesis of the entity, the differential diagnosis, and describing morphologic clues to the anatomic site. Even nonneoplastic histopathologic phenomena that one may regularly encounter in pathology practice could be turned into literary treatises. Examples include retrocorneal fibrous membranes [38], clear cell metaplasia of eccrine ducts, or the pathology of explanted buccal or cartilaginous grafts used in oculoplastic repairs [39].

4 Be a Lifelong Learner

Dr. Jakobiec was a lover of libraries and via a large financial gift, ensured that one of the remaining physical libraries within the Harvard hospital system would stand the test of time in the electronic era. Writing in cursive, he would sprawl out across the large wooden tables of the Mass Eye and Ear library with old textbooks and bound copies of journal articles open to original references. He would manually organize these written works on notecards. Dr. Jakobiec would read at least tens of journal articles a week and was constantly purchasing and making notes in textbooks and making sure he had the newest additions of each.

His interest in pathology, prior to ophthalmology residency, started with studying electron microscopy, before IHC or molecular diagnostics were a part of diagnostic pathology, or were even on the horizon as research tools. Early in the emerging days of IHC, work on ocular adnexal lymphomas and lymphoid hyperplasias in collaboration with a hematopathologist outlined the basic principles of ocular adnexal lymphoid disorders now well-known among both ophthalmologists and pathologists. Specifically, that ocular adnexal lymphomas are low-grade, small B cell lymphomas, and that reactive lymphoid hyperplasia is also common [40, 41].

Dr. Jakobiec greatly valued learning from his students. He would call individuals in the evenings to discuss, for example, how to work up a carcinoma of unknown primary or when to utilize molecular genetic tests as diagnostic tools. He would also summarize his new knowledge and translate complex molecular pathology topics into simple tables and lists in the ophthalmic literature for ophthalmologists and ophthalmic pathologists to use as references. Some of his final papers showed the utility of new, specific immunostains or molecular genetic tests as they pertained to ophthalmic pathology.

One tumor, the rare primitive intraocular neoplasm, medulloepithelioma, is a prime example of the application of new knowledge over an entire career from ultrastructural analysis to molecular genetics [42]. Collaborating with neuropathologists across the globe as well as younger trainees, Dr. Jakobiec and collaborators compared and contrasted the immunoreactivity and mutational landscape of intraocular and central nervous system (CNS) medulloepitheliomas, the latter now considered a member of the category of embryonal tumors with multilayered rosettes [43–46]. Although both show immunohistochemical positivity for LIN28A, the intraocular tumors do not show amplification of the C19MC miRNA locus that characterizes CNS medulloepitheliomas. These cytogenetic and epigenetic findings may explain why intraocular medulloepithelioma is usually cured by enucleation, while CNS "medulloepithelioma" is often fatal.

5 Choose Collaborators and Mentees Wisely and Champion Them

In finance, Dr. Jakobiec saved and invested wisely. Not particularly valuing the accumulation of property or cars and without heirs, he wanted to ensure that eye pathology, not traditionally a lucrative field, would continue to be supported at the institutions at which he taught and trained. He also hoped ophthalmology residents would have the teaching resources they needed and that faculty could be supported in the pursuit of their varied interests. In the same way, he was cautious but smart and intuitive in choosing who to work with and advocate for, having mentored many future leaders in ophthalmology early in their careers.

He felt that one should treat colleagues as friends and described that as an ophthalmology department chair, he would invite valued faculty members out to dinner and drinks to discipline behavior or offer suggestions for improvement, rather than scheduling formal in-office meetings. Cleaning out his desk following his death revealed handwritten drafts of letters in support of numerous colleagues' promotions, many of them unsolicited. He taught his mentees that as they progressed in their own careers, they should keep an eye out for students who impressed and inspired. It was these trainees for whom a faculty member should spend time promoting, doing anything possible to support the student's goals and career objectives.

Sharing meals with numerous colleagues at Legal Sea Foods in Boston, he amassed a wide group of physician friends throughout the country, many of whom he would call nightly to discuss interesting cases, ask for or give advice to, tell jokes, or discuss politics and gossip. He seemed to extract excellence and achievement from those he chose to promote, leaving late evening voicemails about ideas for further research or pushing the completion of pending projects, right up until the evening of his death. May all physicians feel the way he did about learning, "I feel like a mosquito in a nudist colony; I don't know where to begin!"

References

1. Jakobiec FA. Sebaceous adenoma of the eyelid and visceral malignancy. Am J Ophthalmol. 1974;78:952–60.
2. Jakobiec FA, Zimmerman LE, La Piana F, Hornblass A, Breffeilh R, Lackey JK, et al. Unusual eyelid tumors with sebaceous differentiation in the Muir-Torre syndrome: rapid clinical regrowth and frank squamous transformation after biopsy. Ophthalmology. 1998;95:1543–8.
3. Lisman RD, Jakobiec FA, Small P. Sebaceous carcinoma of the eyelids: the role of the adjunctive cryotherapy in the management of the conjunctival pagetoid spread. Ophthalmology. 1989;96:1021–6.
4. Rumelt S, Hogan NR, Rubin PA, Jakobiec FA. Four-eyelid sebaceous cell carcinoma following irradiation. Arch Ophthalmol. 1998;116(12):1670–2.
5. Jakobiec FA, Mendoza PR. Eyelid sebaceous carcinoma: clinicopathologic and multiparametric immunohistochemical analysis that includes adipophilin. Am J Ophthalmol. 2014;157:186–208.
6. Jakobiec FA, Werdich X. Androgen receptor identification in the diagnosis of eyelid sebaceous carcinomas. Am J Ophthalmol. 2014;157:687–96.
7. Jakobiec FA, Stagner AM, Nowak MA, Rubin PA. Presumed primary papillary sebaceous carcinoma of the palpebral conjunctiva. JAMA Ophthalmol. 2015;133:612–4.
8. Stagner AM, Jakobiec FA. Demonstration of a Borst-Jadassohn-like phenomenon in sebaceous carcinoma of the eyelid. Ophthalmic. Plast Reconstr Surg. 2017;33(3S Suppl 1):S63–6.
9. Yonekawa Y, Jakobiec FA, Zakka FR, Fay A. Sebaceoma of the eyelid. Ophthalmology. 2012;119(12):2645.e1–4.
10. Jakobiec FA, Cortes Barrantes P, Lefebvre DR, Milman T. Intraductal sebaceous papilloma of a meibomian gland: a new entity possibly associated with the MSH6 subtype of the Muir-Torre syndrome. Surv Ophthalmol. 2020;65(2):227–38.
11. Jakobiec FA, Cortes Barrantes P, Milman T, Lee NG, Fay A. Ocular adnexal adenomatoid sebaceous gland hyperplasia: a clinical and immunopathologic analysis in relation to the Muir-Torre syndrome. Ophthalmic Plast Reconstr Surg. 2020;36(1):e6–e12.
12. Jakobiec FA, Cortes Barrantes P, Milman T. Villous sebaceous adenoma arising from the caruncular surface squamous epithelium. Ocul Oncol Pathol. 2020;6(4):280–6.
13. Jakobiec FA, Cortes Barrantes P, Milman T, Yoon M. Sebaceoma of a Meibomian gland of the upper eyelid. Ocul Oncol Pathol. 2020;6(4):297–304.
14. Stagner AM, Afrogheh AH, Jakobiec FA, Iacob CE, Grossniklaus HE, et al. p16 expression is not a surrogate marker for high-risk Human papillomavirus infection in periocular sebaceous carcinoma. Am J Ophthalmol. 2016;170:168–75.
15. Wolkow N, Jakobiec FA, Afrogheh AH, Pai SI, Faquin WC. High expression of programmed death ligand 1 and programmed

death ligand 2 in ophthalmic sebaceous carcinoma: the case for a clinical trial of checkpoint inhibitors. Am J Ophthalmol. 2020;220:128–39.
16. Jakobiec FA, Rini FJ, Fraunfelder FT, Brownstein S. Cryotherapy for conjunctival primary acquired melanosis and malignant melanoma. Experience with 62 cases. Ophthalmology. 1988;95:1058–70.
17. Jakobiec FA. The ultrastructure of conjunctival melanocytic tumors. Trans Am Ophthalmol Soc. 1984;82:599–752.
18. Jakobiec FA, Bhat P, Colby KA. Immunohistochemical studies of conjunctival nevi and melanomas. Arch Ophthalmol. 2010;128:174–83.
19. Folberg R, Jakobiec FA, Bernardino VB, Iwamoto T. Benign conjunctival melanocytic lesions. Clinicopathologic features. Ophthalmology. 1989;96:436–61.
20. Jakobiec FA. Conjunctival primary acquired melanosis: is it time for a new terminology? Am J Ophthalmol. 2016;162:3–19.
21. Jakobiec FA, Jones IS, Tannenbaum M. Leiomyoma. An unusual tumour of the orbit. Br J Ophthalmol. 1973;57(11):825–31.
22. Jakobiec FA, Howard GM, Jones IS, Tannenbaum M. Fibrous histiocytomas of the orbit. Am J Ophthalmol. 1974;77(3):333–45.
23. Jakobiec FA, Tannenbaum M. The ultrastructure of orbital fibrosarcoma. Am J Ophthalmol. 1974;77(6):899–917.
24. Jakobiec FA, Howard GM, Jones IS, Wolff M. Hemangiopericytoma of the orbit. Am J Ophthalmol. 1974;78(5):816–34.
25. Jakobiec FA, Howard GM, Rosen M, Wolff M. Leiomyoma and leiomyosarcoma of the orbit. Am J Ophthalmol. 1975;80(6):1028–42.
26. Jakobiec FA, Rini F, Char D, Orcutt J, Rootman J, Baylis H, Flanagan J. Primary liposarcoma of the orbit. Problems in the diagnosis and management of five cases. Ophthalmology. 1989;96(2):180–91.
27. Jakobiec FA, Nguyen J, Bhat P, Fay A. MDM2-positive atypical lipomatous neoplasm/well-differentiated liposarcoma versus spindle cell lipoma of the orbit. Ophthalmic Plast Reconstr Surg. 2010;26(6):413–5.
28. Stagner AM, Jakobiec FA, Fay A. Primary orbital synovial sarcoma: a clinicopathologic review with a differential diagnosis and discussion of molecular genetics. Surv Ophthalmol. 2017;62(2):227–36.
29. Cortes Barrantes P, Jakobiec FA, Dryja TP. A review of the role of cytogenetics in the diagnosis of orbital rhabdomyosarcoma. Semin Ophthalmol. 2019;34(4):243–51.
30. Hanbazazh M, Jakobiec FA, Curtin HD, Lefebvre DR. Orbital involvement by biphenotypic sinonasal sarcoma with a literature review. Ophthalmic Plast Reconstr Surg. 2021;37(4):305–11.
31. Jakobiec FA, Mehta M, Iwamoto M, Hatton HP, Thakker M, Fay A. Intratarsal keratinous cysts of the Meibomian gland: distinctive clinicopathologic and immunohistochemical features in 6 cases. Am J Ophthalmol. 2010;149:82–94.
32. Jakobiec FA, Cortes Barrantes P, Ma L, Lee NG. Complex intratarsal cyst with a mixed ciliated respiratory-type and squamous epithelial lining. Ocul Oncol Pathol. 2020;6(3):151–8.
33. Jakobiec FA, Hanbazazh M, Barrantes PC, Yoon MK. Conjunctival implantation cyst in the orbicularis oculi muscle: review of a possible origin from displaced stem cells with a differential diagnosis. Ophthalmic Plast Reconstr Surg. 2021;37(1):1–11.
34. Jakobiec FA, Stagner AM, Yoon MK. Canalicular cyst. Ocul Oncol Pathol. 2015;1(4):274–7.
35. Jakobiec FA, Zakka FR, Perry LP. The cytologic composition of dacryops: an immunohistochemical investigation of 15 lesions compared to the normal lacrimal gland. Am J Ophthalmol. 2013;155(2):380–96.e1.
36. Jakobiec FA, Zakka FR. A reappraisal of eyelid eccrine and apocrine hidrocystomas: microanatomic and immunohistochemical studies of 40 lesions. Am J Ophthalmol. 2011;151:358–74.
37. Jakobiec FA, Qureshi S, Zakka FR, Tu Y, Lee NG. Eyelid eccrine cyst: an exceptional lesion among dominant apocrine cysts. Ophthalmic Plast Reconstr Surg. 2017;33(5):e128–31.
38. Jakobiec FA, Bhat P. Retrocorneal membranes: a comparative immunohistochemical analysis of keratocytic, endothelial and epithelial origins. Am J Ophthalmol. 2010;150:230–42.
39. Jakobiec FA, Stagner AM, Lee NG. Clear-cell (reticulated) transformation of eyelid eccrine sweat glands. Ophthalmic Plast Reconstr Surg. 2017;33(3):e69–72.
40. Knowles DM 2nd, Jakobiec FA. Ocular adnexal lymphoid neoplasms: clinical, histopathologic, electron microscopic, and immunologic characteristics. Hum Pathol. 1982;13:148–62.
41. Knowles DM, Jakobiec FA, McNally L, Burke JS. Lymphoid hyperplasia and malignant lymphoma occurring in the ocular adnexa (orbit, conjunctiva, and eyelids): a prospective multiparametric analysis of 108 cases during 1977 to 1987. Hum Pathol. 1990;21:959–73.
42. Jakobiec FA, Howard GM, Ellsworth RM, Rosen M. Electron microscopic diagnosis of medulloepithelioma. Am J Ophthalmol. 1975;79:321–9.
43. Jakobiec FA, Trief D, Rashid A, Rose MF, Minckler D, Vanderveen D, et al. New insights into the development of infantile intraocular medulloepithelioma. Am J Ophthalmol. 2014;158:1275–96.
44. Jakobiec FA, Rose MF, Trief D, Stagner AM, Kim I, Gragoudas ES. Immunohistochemical investigations of adult intraocular medulloepitheliomas. Clin Exp Ophthalmol. 2015;43:379–85.
45. Jakobiec FA, Kool M, Stagner AM, Pfister SM, Eagle RC, Proia AD, et al. Intraocular medulloepitheliomas and embryonal tumors with multilayered rosettes of the brain: comparative roles of LIN28A and C19MC. Am J Ophthalmol. 2015;159:1065–74.
46. Korshunov A, Jakobiec FA, Eberhart CG, Hovestadt V, Capper D, Jones DTW, et al. Comparative integrated molecular analysis of intraocular medulloepitheliomas and central nervous system embryonal tumors with multilayered rosettes confirms that they are distinct nosologic entities. Neuropathology. 2015;35:538–44.

Index

B. V. Chawla, M. E. Aronow (eds.), Global Perspectives in Ocular Oncology, https://doi.org/10.1007/978-3-031-08250-4

MIX
Papier aus verantwortungsvollen Quellen
Paper from responsible sources
FSC® C105338

If you have any concerns about our products,
you can contact us on
ProductSafety@springernature.com

In case Publisher is established outside the EU,
the EU authorized representative is:
Springer Nature Customer Service Center GmbH
Europaplatz 3, 69115 Heidelberg, Germany

Printed by Libri Plureos GmbH
in Hamburg, Germany